Peter Barnes

Atlas of
PULMONARY MEDICINE
Fourth Edition

Editor

James D. Crapo, MD

Professor of Medicine
National Jewish Medical and Research Center
Director, Clinical Science PhD Program
University of Colorado Denver
Denver, Colorado
With 59 Contributors

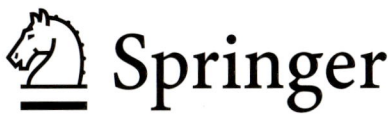

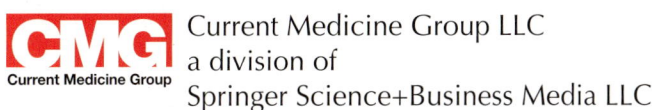

Current Medicine Group LLC
a division of
Springer Science+Business Media LLC

CURRENT MEDICINE GROUP LLC
A DIVISION OF SPRINGER SCIENCE+BUSINESS MEDIA LLC
400 MARKET STREET, SUITE 700 • PHILADELPHIA, PA 19106

Senior Developmental Editor	Elizabeth Rexon
Editorial Assistant	Bridget Jordan, Juleen Deaner
Cover Design	Wendy Vetter
Design and Layout	Dan Britt and Julia Cappiello
Illustrators	Daniel Britt, Kim Broadbent, Maureen Looney, and Wendy Wetter
Creative Director	Wendy Vetter
Production Coordinator	Carolyn Naylor
Indexer	Holly Lukens

The photographs on the cover from top to bottom, left to right are Figure 2-22 page 22; Figure 2-26A page 23; Figure 3-8A page 32; Figure 2-21 page 21; Figure 1-4 page 3 from edition 3, Courtesy of Webb Saring Institute, Denver, CO; and Figure 20-9A page 274. The photographs on the back from top to bottom are Figure 5-7B page 73 from edition 3, and Figure 2-26B page 23.

Library of Congress Cataloging-in-Publication Data

Atlas of pulmonary medicine / editor, James D. Crapo. -- 4th ed.
    p. ; cm.
 Includes bibliographical references and index.
 ISBN 978-1-57340-297-2 (alk. paper)
 1. Respiratory intensive care--Atlases. 2. Respiratory organs--Diseases--Atlases. I. Bone, Roger C. II. Crapo, James D. III. Title: Atlas of pulmonary medicine. IV. Title: Pulmonary medicine.
 [DNLM: 1. Lung Diseases--Atlases. WF 17 B7125 2008]

RC735.R48B66 2008
616.2--dc22

2008009160

ISBN 978-1-57340-297-2

Although every effort has been made to ensure that drug doses and other information are presented accurately in this publication, the ultimate responsibility rests with the prescribing physician. Neither the publishers nor the authors can be held responsible for errors or for any consequences arising from the use of information contained herein. Products mentioned in this publication should be used in accordance with the prescribing information prepared by the manufacturers. No claims or endorsements are made for any drug or compound at present under clinical investigation.

© 2008 By Current Medicine Group LLC a division of Springer Science+Business Media LLC. No part of this publication may be reproduced, stored in a retrieval system, or transmitted in any form by any means electronic, mechanical, photocopying, recording, or otherwise without prior consent of the publisher.

For more information, please call 1 (800) 427-1796 or (215) 574-2266 or email us at inquiry@phl.cursci.com

www.currentmedicinegroup.com

10 9 8 7 6 5 4 3 2 1

Printed in China by Hong Kong Graphics and Printing LTD.

This book was printed on acid-free paper.

All rights reserved. This work may not be translated or copied in whole or in part without the written permission of the publisher (Springer Science+Business Media, LLC, 233 Spring Street, New York, NY 10013, USA), except for brief excerpts in connection with reviews or scholarly analysis. Use in connection with any form of information storage and retrieval, electronic adaptation, computer software, or by similar or dissimilar methodology now known or hereafter developed is forbidden. The use in this publication of trade names, trademarks, service marks, and similar terms, even if they are not identified as such, is not to be taken as an expression of opinion as to whether or not they are subject to proprietary rights.

springeronline.com

PREFACE

The fourth edition of the *Atlas of Pulmonary Medicine* has been extensively revised and updated to keep abreast of progress in this field. The goal in creating this fourth edition has been to present the central elements of each major class of pulmonary disease in a form that is easily assimilated by the busy clinician and/or student of chest disease. The focus is on images, tables, and algorithms that clearly convey the critical elements of the pathogenesis, diagnosis, and treatment of the major lung diseases that are encountered in a general medical practice.

Each chapter has been thoroughly reviewed and revised to reflect the rapid evolution of knowledge in pulmonary medicine. For the first time the atlas is being presented in full color, and the images will be available on CD-ROM, therefore viewable in multiple formats and available for lectures and teaching.

James D. Crapo, MD

CONTRIBUTORS

Danielle Antin-Ozerkis, MD
Assistant Professor of Medicine,
 Pulmonary, and Critical Care Medicine
Department of Internal Medicine
Yale University School of Medicine
New Haven, Connecticut

Antonio Anzueto, MD
Professor of Medicine
Department of Pulmonary and
 Critical Care Medicine
University of Texas Health
 Sciences Center
Section Chief, Pulmonary Critical Care
Department of Medicine
South Texas Veterans Health
 Care System
San Antonio, Texas

David Ashkin, MD
Medical Executive Director
AG Holley State Tuberculosis Hospital
Co-Principal Investigator
Southeast National Tuberculosis Center
Lantana, Florida
State Tuberculosis Health Officer
Florida Department of Health
Tallahassee, Florida
Affiliate Assistant Professor
University of South Florida
 College of Medicine
Tampa, Florida
Adjunct Assistant Professor
University of Florida College
 of Medicine
Gainesville, Florida
Visiting Assistant Professor
Division of Pulmonary and Critical
 Care Medicine
University of Miami School of Medicine
Miami, Florida

**Peter J. Barnes,
 DM, DSc, FMedSci, FRS**
Professor and Head of Respiratory
 Medicine
National Heart and Lung Institute
Imperial College
London, United Kingdom

Seth Mark Berney, MD
Professor of Medicine
Chief
Division of Rheumatology
Director
Center of Excellence for Arthritis
 and Rheumatology
Department of Medicine
Louisiana State University
Shreveport, Louisiana

Richard C. Boucher, MD
Kenan Professor of Medicine
Director
Cystic Fibrosis/Pulmonary Research
 and Treatment Center
University of North Carolina at
 Chapel Hill
Chapel Hill, North Carolina

Robert W. Bradsher, MD
Ebert Professor of Medicine
Department of Internal Medicine
Director
Division of Infectious Diseases
University of Arkansas for
 Medical Sciences
Central Arkansas Veterans
 Healthcare System
Little Rock, Arkansas

G. Douglas Campbell Jr, MD
Professor
Department of Medicine
Division of Pulmonary and Critical
 Care Medicine
Louisiana State University Health
 Sciences Center
Shreveport, Louisiana

Michelle Cao, DO
Clinical Fellow, Stanford University
 Sleep Medicine Program
Stanford University Sleep
 Disorders Clinic
Stanford University Medical Center
Stanford, California

Raymond D. Coakley, MD
Assistant Professor of Medicine
Cystic Fibrosis Research and
 Treatment Center
University of North Carolina
Chapel Hill, North Carolina

Thomas V. Colby, MD
Geraldine C. Zeiler Professor of
 Cytopathology
Department of Pathology
Mayo Clinic
Scottsdale, Arizona

Harold R. Collard, MD
Assistant Professor
Department of Medicine
University of California San Francisco
San Francisco, California

Peter Doelken, MD
Associate Professor of Medicine
Division of Pulmonary and Critical
 Care Medicine
Medical University of South Carolina
Charleston, South Carolina

Raed A. Dweik, MD
Department of Pulmonary, Allergy, and
 Critical Care Medicine
Cleveland Clinic
Cleveland, Ohio

Georgie A. Eapen, MD
Assistant Professor
Department of Pulmonary Medicine
The University of Texas MD Anderson
 Cancer Center
Houston, Texas

Gary R. Epler, MD
Clinical Associate Professor
Department of Pulmonary and Critical
 Care Medicine
Harvard Medical School
Boston, Massachusetts

M. Yesim Ersoy, MD
Postdoctoral Fellow
Department of Pulmonary Medicine
University of Texas MD Anderson
 Cancer Center
Houston, Texas

Carol Farver, MD
Department of Anatomic Pathology
 and Pathobiology
Department of Pulmonary, Allergy, and
 Critical Care Medicine
Cleveland Clinic
Cleveland, Ohio

Matthew Fei, MD
Clinical Fellow, Division of Pulmonary
 and Critical Care Medicine
Department of Medicine
University of California
San Francisco, California

Stanley B. Fiel, MD
Professor of Medicine
University of Medicine and Dentistry
New Jersey School of Medicine
Newark, New Jersey
The deNeufville Professor and
 Regional Chair
Department of Medicine
Morristown Memorial Hospital
Morristown, New Jersey

Adam L. Friedlander, MD
Fellow
Division of Pulmonary Sciences and
 Critical Care Medicine
University of Colorado at Denver and
 Health Sciences Center
National Jewish Medical and
 Research Center
Department of Medicine
Denver, Colorado

Samuel Z. Goldhaber, MD
Professor of Medicine
Department of Cardiology
Harvard Medical School
Director
Venous Thromboembolism
 Research Group
Director
Anticoagulation Clinic
Cardiovascular Division
Brigham and Women's Hospital
Boston, Massachusetts

Michael B. Gotway, MD
Scottsdale Medical Imaging
Scottsdale, Arizona
Clinical Associate Professor
Diagnostic Radiology and
 Pulmonary/Critical Care Medicine
Department of Radiology
University of California
San Francisco, California

James F. Gruden, MD
Associate Professor of Radiology
Mayo Clinic College of Medicine
Director
Cardiothoracic Imaging
Mayo Clinic
Scottsdale, Arizona

**Christian Guilleminault,
 MD, BiolD**
Professor
Department of Psychiatry,
 Behavioral Sciences, and Neurology
Stanford University Medical School
Stanford, California

Maureen Heldmann, MD
Associate Professor
Chief-Division of Body Imaging
Department of Radiology
Louisiana State University
 Health Sciences Center School of
 Medicine in Shreveport
Shreveport, Louisiana

Laurence Huang, MD
Professor of Medicine
Department of Medicine
University of California San Francisco
Chief, HIV/AIDS Chest Clinic
Attending Physician
Department of Medicine
Division of Pulmonary and Critical
 Care Medicine
HIV/AIDS Division
San Francisco General Hospital
San Francisco, California

John T. Huggins, MD
Division of Pulmonary, Critical Care,
 Allergy, and Sleep Medicine
Medical University of South Carolina
Charleston, South Carolina

Nelly Huynh, PhD
Postdoctoral Fellow
Stanford Sleep Disorders Clinic
Stanford School of Medicine
Palo Alto, California

James R. Jett, MD
Professor of Medicine
Department of Pulmonary Medicine
Mayo College of Medicine
Rochester, Minnesota

Carlos A. Jimenez, MD
Associate Professor
Department of Pulmonary Medicine
The University of Texas MD Anderson
 Cancer Center
Houston, Texas

Joanne Julien, MD
Adjunct Assistant Professor
Division of Pulmonary, Critical Care,
 and Sleep Medicine
University of Florida
Deputy Health Officer for Tuberculosis
Bureau of Tuberculosis and
 Refugee Health
Florida Department of Heath
Medical Consultant
Southeastern National
 Tuberculosis Center
Gainesville, Florida

Talmadge E. King Jr, MD
Julius R. Krevans Distinguished
 Professorship in Internal Medicine
Chair, Department of Medicine
University of California, San Francisco
San Francisco, California

Nils Kucher, MD
Department of Cardiology
Cardiovascular Center
University Hospital
Zurich, Switzerland

Jasleen Kukreja, MD, MPH
Department of Surgery
University of California Medical School
San Francisco, California

Elif Kupeli, MD
Staff
Department of Respiratory Medicine
Private Mesa Hospital
Ankara, Turkey

Michael Lauzardo, MD, MSc
Assistant Professor
Department of Medicine
University of Florida
Deputy Health Officer for Tuberculosis
Florida Department of Health
Bureau of Tuberculosis and
 Refugee Health
Gainesville, Florida

Joseph P. Lynch III, MD
Professor of Clinical Medicine
Division of Pulmonary, Critical Care
 Medicine, and Clinical Immunology
David Geffen School of Medicine
 and UCLA
UCLA Medical Center
Los Angeles, California

Peter Mazzone, MD, MPH
Department of Pulmonary, Allergy, and
 Critical Care Medicine
Cleveland Clinic
Cleveland, Ohio

**Atul C. Mehta,
 MD, FCCP, FACP**
Department of Pulmonary, Allergy, and
 Critical Care Medicine
Cleveland Clinic Foundation
Cleveland, Ohio

Anupama Menon, MD, MPH
Assistant Professor of Medicine
Division of Infectious Diseases
University of Arkansas for
 Medical Sciences
Little Rock, Arkansas

Rodolfo C. Morice, MD
Professor
Department of Pulmonary Medicine
The University of Texas MD Anderson
 Cancer Center
Houston, Texas

Aneil Mujoomdar, MD
Clinical Fellow in Thoracic Oncology
Division of Thoracic Surgery
Brigham and Women's Hospital
Boston, Massachusetts

Jeffrey L. Myers, MD
A. James French Professor and Director
Division of Anatomic Pathology
University of Michigan
Ann Arbor, Michigan

Peter B. O'Donovan, MD, BCh
Staff Radiologist
Cleveland Clinic Foundation
Cleveland, Ohio

Otis B. Rickman, DO
Assistant Professor of Medicine
Consultant
Department of Pulmonary and
 Critical Care
Mayo Clinic College of Medicine
Rochester, Minnesota

Mark J. Rumbak, MD
Professor of Medicine
Department of Pulmonary/Critical
 Care Medicine
University of South Florida College
 of Medicine
Tampa, Florida

Hina Sahi, MD
Clinical Associate
Department of Pulmonary, Allergy, and
 Critical Care Medicine
Cleveland Clinic
Cleveland, Ohio

Steven A. Sahn, MD
Professor
Department of Medicine
Director, Division of Pulmonary, Critical
 Care, Allergy, and Sleep Medicine
Medical University of South Carolina
Charleston, South Carolina

Daniel V. Schidlow, MD
Professor and Chair
Department of Pediatrics
MCP Hahnemann University
Physician-in-Chief
St. Christopher's Hospital for Children
Philadelphia, Pennsylvania

Marvin I. Schwarz, MD
James C. Campbell Professor of
 Pulmonary Medicine
University of Colorado Health
 Sciences Center
Denver, Colorado

Cyrus Shariat, MD
Interstitial Lung Disease Program
San Francisco General Hospital
Department of Medicine
University of California San Francisco
San Francisco, California

Jaspal Singh, MD
Department of Medicine
Duke University Medical Center
Durham, North Carolina

David J. Sugarbaker, MD
Richard E. Wilson Professor of
 Surgical Oncology
Department of Surgery
Harvard Medical School
Chief
Division of Thoracic Surgery
Brigham and Women's Hospital
Boston, Massachusetts

E. Rand Sutherland, MD, MPH
Associate Professor
Department of Medicine
National Jewish Medical and
 Research Center
University of Colorado at Denver and
 Health Sciences Center
Denver, Colorado

Lynn T. Tanoue, MD
Professor of Medicine
Section of Pulmonary and Critical
 Care Medicine
Department of Internal Medicine
Yale University School of Medicine
New Haven, Connecticut

Victor F. Tapson, MD
Professor of Medicine
Department of Medicine
Duke University School of Medicine
Durham, North Carolina

Nicole Elizabeth Vignes, MD
Resident Physician
Department of Internal Medicine
Vanderbilt University
Nashville, Tennessee

Sally E. Wenzel, MD
Professor
Department of Medicine
University of Pittsburgh
Pittsburgh, Pennsylvania

CONTENTS

Chapter 1
Asthma 1
E. Rand Sutherland

Chapter 2
Severe Asthma 15
Adam L. Friedlander and Sally E. Wenzel

Chapter 3
Chronic Obstructive Pulmonary Disease 27
Peter J. Barnes

Chapter 4
Cystic Fibrosis 45
Raymond D. Coakley, Richard C. Boucher, Stanley B. Fiel, and Daniel V. Schidlow

Chapter 5
Bronchiolar Disorders 69
Thomas V. Colby, Gary R. Epler, and James F. Gruden

Chapter 6
Sleep Disordered Breathing 85
Michelle Cao, Nelly Huynh, and Christian Guilleminault

Chapter 7
Lower Respiratory Tract Infections:
Acute Exacerbation of Chronic Bronchitis 99
Antonio Anzueto and G. Douglas Campbell Jr

Chapter 8
Nosocomial Infections Including Pneumonia 117
Mark J. Rumbak

Chapter 9
Tuberculosis and Nontuberculous Mycobacterial Infections 125
Michael Lauzardo, Joanne Julien, and David Ashkin

Chapter 10
HIV/AIDS and Immunocompromised Hosts 137
Laurence Huang, Matthew Fei, and Michael B. Gotway

Chapter 11
Fungal Infection 147
Anupama Menon and Robert W. Bradsher

Chapter 12
Sarcoidosis 161
Danielle Antin-Ozerkis and Lynn T. Tanoue

Chapter 13
Interstitial Lung Disease.. *179*
Joseph P. Lynch III and Jeffrey L. Myers

Chapter 14
Connective Tissue Disease *193*
Maureen Heldmann, Nicole Elizabeth Vignes, and Seth Mark Berney

Chapter 15
Pulmonary Vasculitis *207*
Talmadge E. King Jr and Cyrus Shariat

Chapter 16
Hypersensitivity Pneumonitis *215*
Harold R. Collard and Marvin I. Schwarz

Chapter 17
Venous Thromboembolism *223*
Nils Kucher and Samuel Z. Goldhaber

Chapter 18
Idiopathic Pulmonary Arterial Hypertension *235*
Victor F. Tapson and Jaspal Singh

Chapter 19
Lung Cancer *249*
Otis B. Rickman and James R. Jett

Chapter 20
Pulmonary Neoplasms Other Than Lung Cancer............................... *269*
Peter Mazzone, Carol Farver, Peter B. O'Donovan, and Raed A. Dweik

Chapter 21
Solitary Pulmonary Nodule *279*
Hina Sahi, Elif Kupeli, and Atul C. Mehta

Chapter 22
Primary Pleural and Chest Wall Tumors *291*
Aneil Mujoomdar, Jasleen Kukreja, and David J. Sugarbaker

Chapter 23
Mediastinal Masses *301*
M. Yesim Ersoy, Carlos A. Jimenez, and Rodolfo C. Morice

Chapter 24
Metastases to the Lungs.. *311*
Carlos A. Jimenez, Georgie A. Eapen, and Rodolfo C. Morice

Chapter 25
Pleural Disease *319*
Steven A. Sahn, John T. Huggins, and Peter Doelken

Index.. *331*

ASTHMA

E. Rand Sutherland

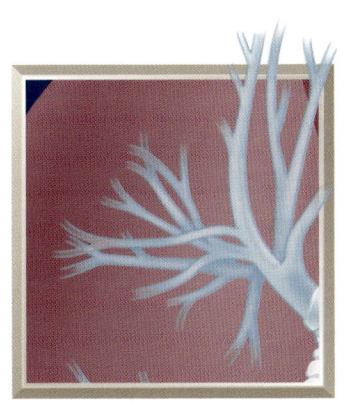
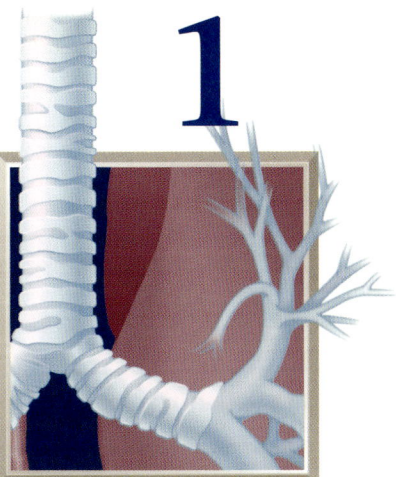
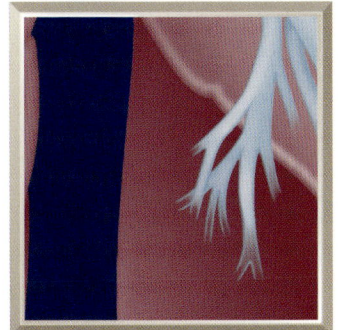

Asthma is a syndrome of airway inflammation, airway hyperresponsiveness, and bronchodilator-responsive airflow limitation that manifests itself clinically as episodic symptoms, including cough, dyspnea, and chest tightness [1]. Asthma is prevalent, affecting approximately 7% of adults and 9% of children in the United States [2], with differential impact across age groups and on ethnic and racial minorities [3]. Given its prevalence, asthma is a significant public health problem, with substantial associated morbidity, mortality, and health care resource utilization [4].

The airway inflammation that is the basis for asthma is orchestrated by numerous cells and mediators [5], with resulting architectural changes in the airway, including alteration of the airway epithelial barrier, hyperplasia of goblet cells leading to mucus hypersecretion, thickening of the basement membrane, increase in submucosal blood vessels, and an increased and hypercontractile airway smooth muscle mass [6,7]. These changes in airway structure lead to many of the clinical manifestations of asthma by causing functional abnormalities of the airway such as bronchoconstriction, hyperresponsiveness, and mucus plugging, all of which lead to airflow limitation. This alteration of airway structure and function can be detected by means of spirometry, in which there is characteristic reduction in expiratory airflows, which typically improves following administration of short-acting β_2-agonist bronchodilators. Spirometry can be augmented with full pulmonary function testing and bronchoprovocation testing as needed to confirm or further refine the diagnosis of asthma.

In 2007, the National Asthma Education and Prevention Program issued updated guidelines for the diagnosis and management of asthma [1]. This document reinforces the concepts of current impairment and future risk as important components of both asthma severity and asthma control. Assessment of asthma severity at the time of initial presentation is used to determine appropriate pharmacotherapy, which can then be adjusted in intensity guided by the degree of asthma control that is obtained after initiation of therapy. This chapter will review aspects of the public health impact of asthma, review current paradigms with regard to our understanding of asthma pathogenesis, and provide up-to-date recommendations with regard to the evaluation and management of asthma.

EPIDEMIOLOGY AND PUBLIC HEALTH IMPACT

Public Health Impact of Asthma

Morbidity
US adults with asthma	15.7 million (7.2% of US adults)
US children with asthma	6.5 million (8.9% of US children)

Mortality
Annual deaths attributable to asthma	3,780 (1.3 per 100,000 US population)

Resource Utilization
Annual office-based physician visits attributable to asthma	13.6 million
Annual emergency department visits attributable to asthma	1.8 million

Figure 1-1. Public health impact of asthma. In 2005, 7.2% of US adults and 8.9% of US children were diagnosed with asthma [2], resulting in significant utilization of outpatient and acute care resources [8, 9]. In 2004, approximately 4000 deaths were attributable to asthma [10], although the rate of asthma death in the United States declined each year between 2000 and 2004 (the most recent year for which published data are available). Much of the resource utilization in asthma is attributable to unscheduled clinician visits related to asthma exacerbations, and approximately 12 million people report at least one exacerbation per year, with children more likely than adults (5.6% vs 3.6%), women more likely than men (4.8% vs 3.5%), and male children more likely than male adults (6.5% vs 2.3%) to report at least one exacerbation per year [11].

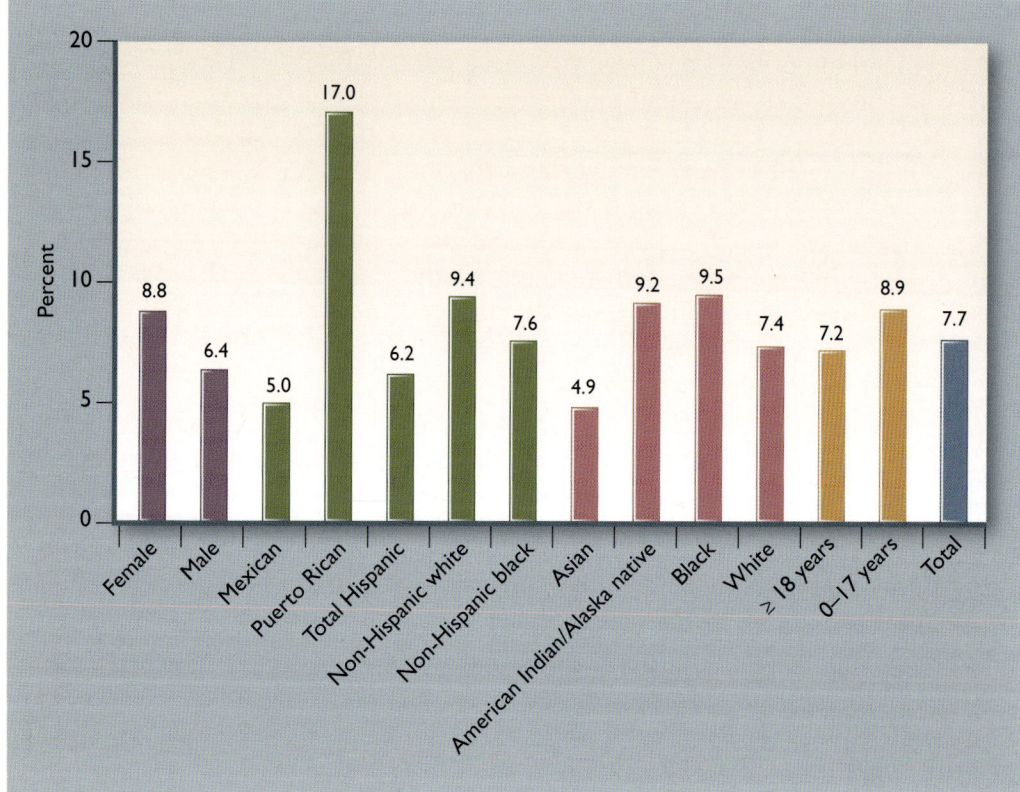

Figure 1-2. 2005 US current asthma prevalence data demonstrating total asthma prevalence (*blue bar*) as well as differential asthma prevalence by sex (*purple bars*), racial or ethnic background (*green and pink bars*), and age group (pediatric vs adult, *orange bars*) [3]. Data are age-adjusted to 2000 US standard population. These and other data [11,12] form the basis of the observation that, in the United States, low-income populations, minorities, and children living in primarily urban environments experience disproportionate asthma morbidity. The effects of asthma on children and adolescents are significant: asthma is the third-ranking cause of hospitalization among children younger than 15 years of age, accounting for 14 million days of missed school per annum and estimated annual related costs of $3.2 billion per year.

| Atlas of Pulmonary Medicine |

Economic Impact of Asthma in the United States		
	Costs (in millions of dollars)	
Direct medical expenditures	1994	1998
Hospital care		
Hospital inpatient care	1799.9	2054.6
Emergency department care	478.6	546.3
Hospital outpatient care	633	722.6
Physician's services		
Physician inpatient care	96.7	110.9
Physician office visits	647.4	742.7
Prescriptions	2452	3188.1
All direct expenditures	6107.6	7365.3
Indirect costs		
School days lost	956.7	1107.3
Loss of work		
Outside employment		
Men	365.8	415
Women	974.8	1128.2
Housekeeping	727.2	841.7
Mortality	1616.2	1813.9
All indirect costs	4640.6	5306
All costs	10748.3	12671.3

Figure 1-3. Economic impact of asthma in the United States [4]. In 1998, asthma accounted for an estimated $12.7 billion of expenditures, approximately 58% of which were direct medical expenditures related to the care of the disease, with prescription medications being the single largest cost component. Urgent care and emergency department visits and hospitalizations are key components of the direct costs of asthma, and both these costs and medication-related costs appear to be greater in patients with more severe disease. Indirect costs account for approximately 42% of total expenditures, with significant costs associated with missed school, lost employment opportunities, and mortality.

PATHOPHYSIOLOGY AND AIRWAY INFLAMMATION

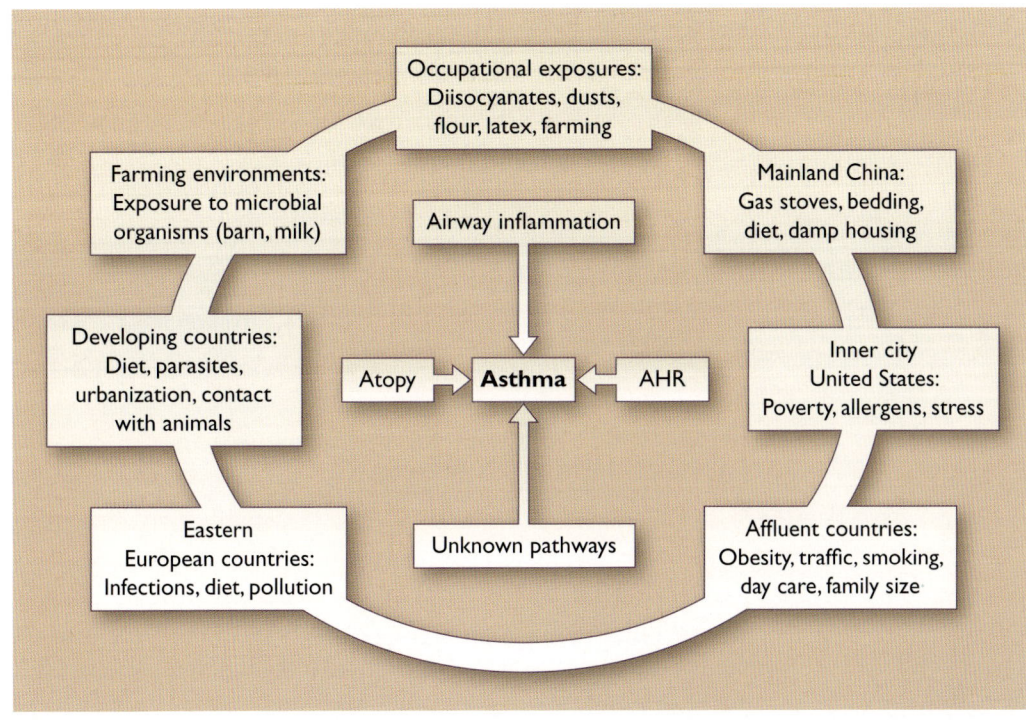

Figure 1-4. Host-environment interactions in the development of asthma. The interactions of host factors—such as atopy, airway inflammation, airway hyperresponsiveness (AHR), and genetics—with environmental factors are critical to the development of asthma. Environmental exposures, which vary in nature worldwide, interact with host pathways, and numerous genes involved in the regulation of these pathways are likely to contribute to the expression of asthma. Important environmental determinants of asthma include tobacco smoke, air pollution (such as ozone and particulate matter), allergens such as house dust mite and pet dander, infections (particularly viral), and the development of obesity [13].

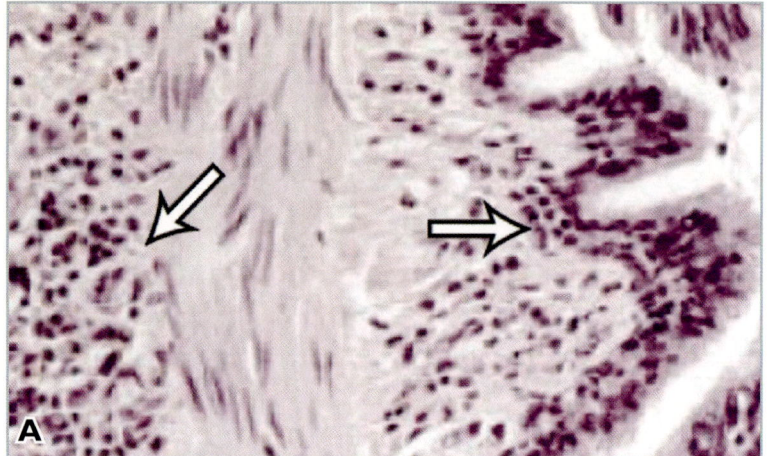
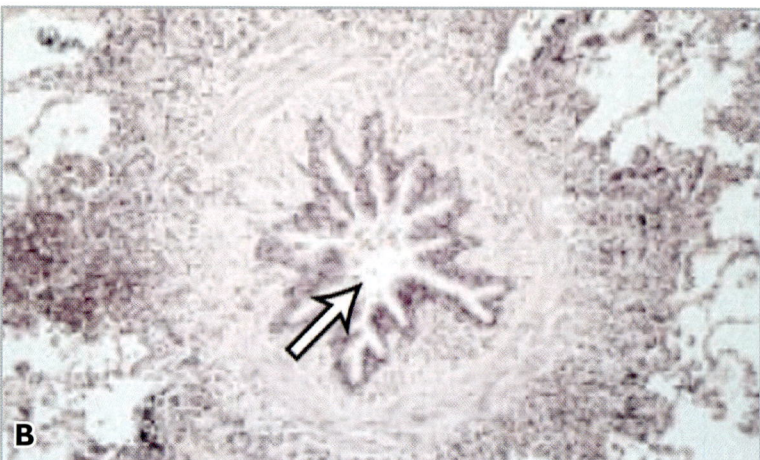

Figure 1-5. Architectural changes in airway structure that result from chronic airway inflammation. Airway inflammation in asthma involves multiple inflammatory cells, including eosinophils, CD4+ T lymphocytes, and mast cells, with eosinophilic infiltration (*arrows*) a cardinal feature of the inflammatory process (**A**). This inflammatory cell infiltrate is associated with characteristic alterations in airway wall architecture, including increased smooth muscle mass, mucous gland hypertrophy, and vascular congestion and neogenesis. These changes, along with luminal changes including plugging with mucus and inflammatory exudate, contribute to the development of airflow limitation by narrowing the airway lumen (*arrow*) (**B**), increasing airway resistance. In more severe asthma, prominent neutrophil infiltration also occurs [14]. (*From* Saetta and Turato [7]; with permission.)

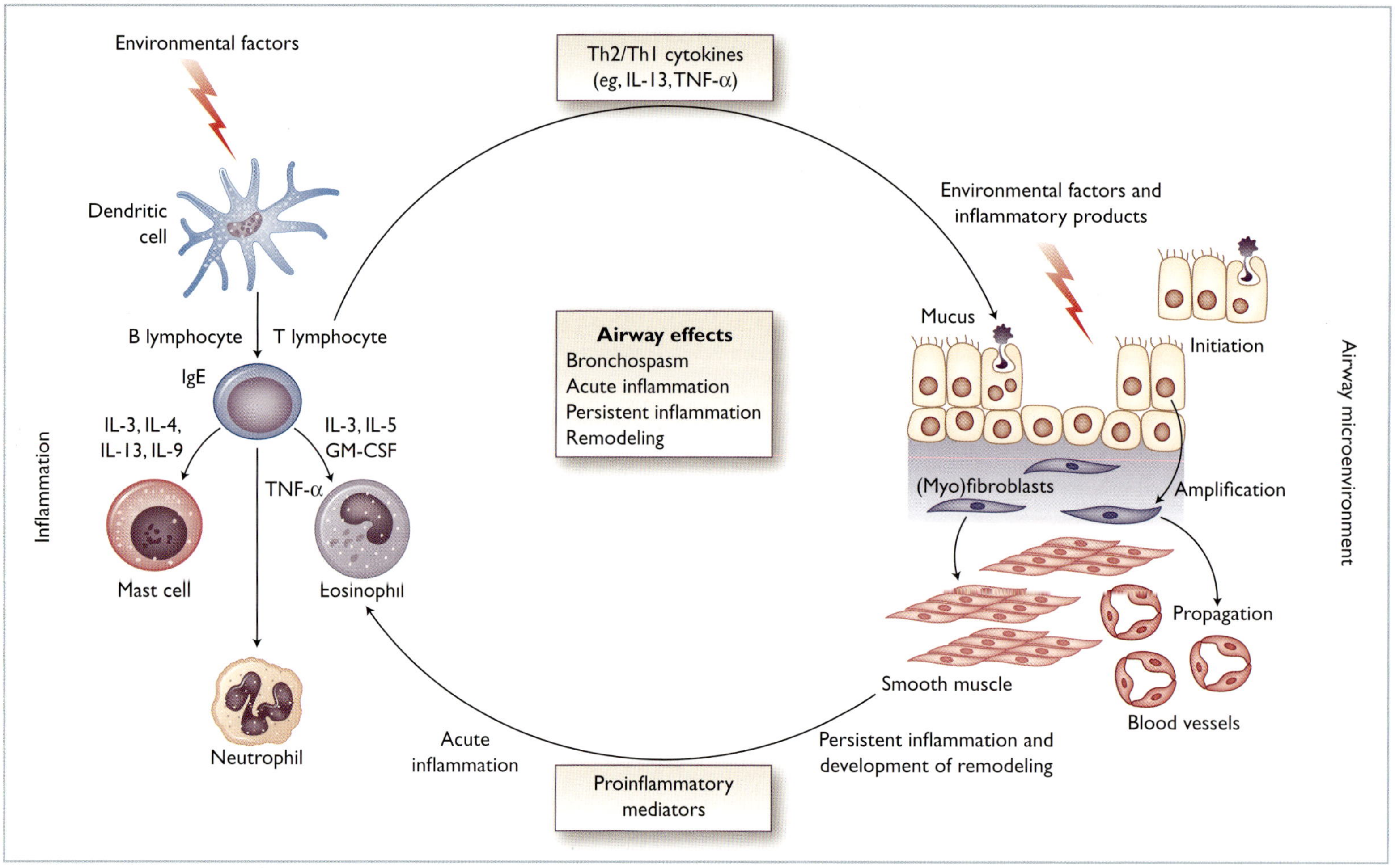

Figure 1-6. Mechanisms of airway inflammation in asthma. Airway inflammation in asthma is a complex process, orchestrated by a large number of cells and mediators [5]. Antigen-presenting dendritic cells interact with allergens encountered at the airway surface and then migrate into regional lymph nodes to interact with lymphocytes. A predisposition toward the Th2 cytokine profile plays an important role in regulating the eosinophilic inflammation characteristic of asthma. The inflammatory milieu in asthma has direct effects on airway structure and function, ultimately leading to epithelial disruption, mucus hypersecretion, airway smooth muscle proliferation activation and contraction, and an increase in the number of blood vessels. These alterations are associated with the production of proinflammatory mediators, which further propagate airway inflammation, ultimately leading to functional alterations in the airway with regard to features such as airway hyperresponsiveness, acute and chronic inflammation, and remodeling. GM-CSF—granulocyte-macrophage colony-stimulating factor; IL—interleukin; TNF—tumor necrosis factor. (*Adapted from* Holgate and Polosa [5].)

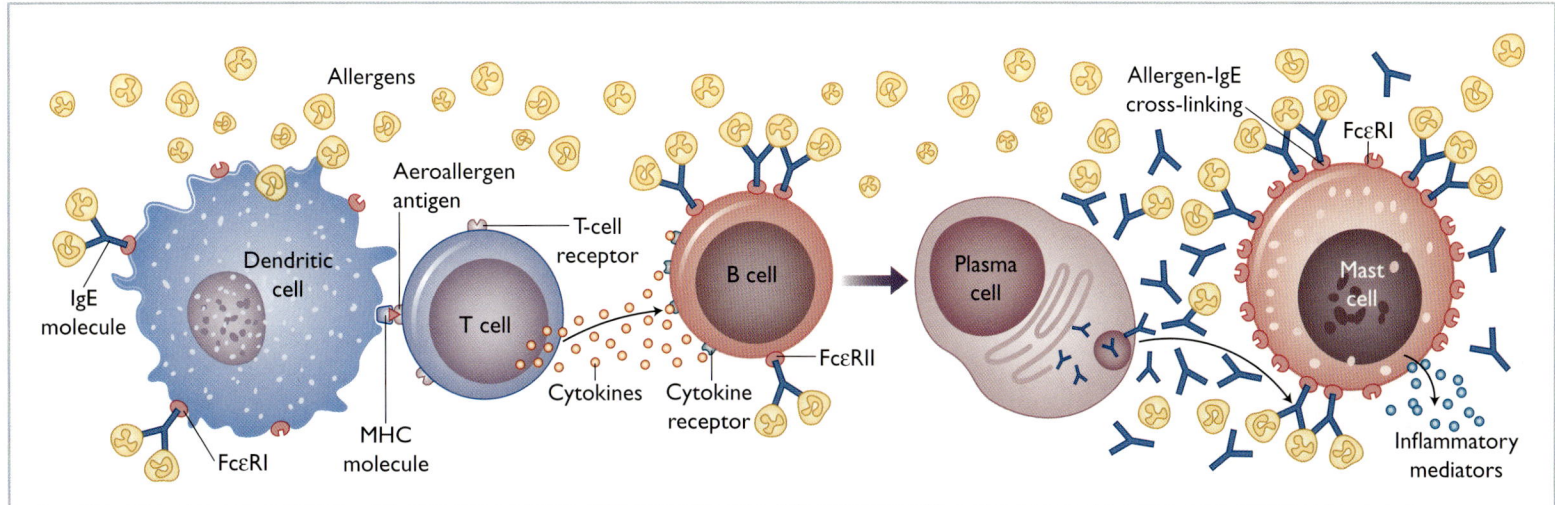

Figure 1-7. Inflammatory cell interactions in the development of allergic asthma [15]. IgE plays a critical role in the development of asthma in a significant proportion of patients [16]. In the initial phase of sensitization to an allergen, inhaled aeroallergens are presented via major histocompatibility complex (MHC) molecules to antigen-specific T cells by antigen-presenting dendritic cells in the airways. In some individuals, this interaction leads to a process by which T cells produce cytokines that ultimately lead to the development of IgE-producing plasma cells.

IgE binds to high-affinity receptors (FcεR1) found on the surface of mast cells and basophils. With subsequent exposure to the allergen to which the patient is sensitized, there is cross-linking of IgE present on the cell surface of mast cells and basophils, leading to degranulation of these cells and release of inflammatory mediators such as histamine, leukotrienes, and other chemokines/cytokines. These mediators can then facilitate acute bronchospasm, leading to associated signs and symptoms of asthma. (Adapted from Strunk and Bloomberg [17].)

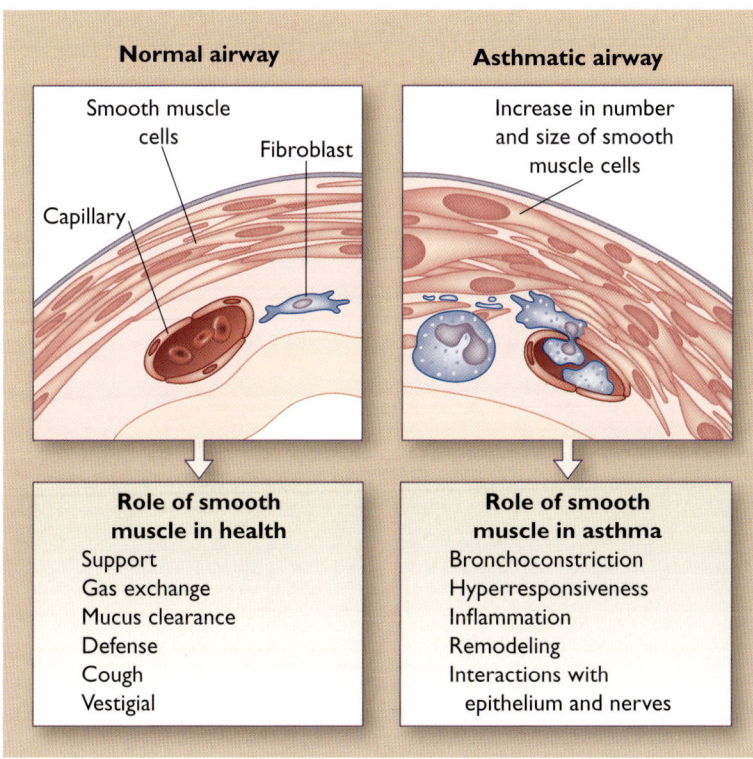

Figure 1-8. The importance of airway smooth muscle in asthma [18]. Although the exact role of airway smooth muscle in both healthy individuals (*left*) and patients with asthma (*right*) remains uncertain, it has been proposed that in the normal airway, smooth muscle provides structural support and facilitates host defense mechanisms such as mucus clearance and cough. In asthma, airway smooth muscle plays an important role in airway hyperresponsiveness by mediating acute bronchoconstriction. Furthermore, emerging data suggest that airway smooth muscle plays an important role in the pathogenesis of airway inflammation and remodeling, possibly through interactions with inflammatory cells and airway epithelium. In the asthmatic airway, there is an increase in both the number and size of airway smooth muscle cells. This increase is associated with an enhancement of their function, ultimately leading to bronchoconstriction. Controller therapies for asthma may in part exert their beneficial effects through effects on airway smooth muscle cells. (Adapted from Solway and Irvin [18].)

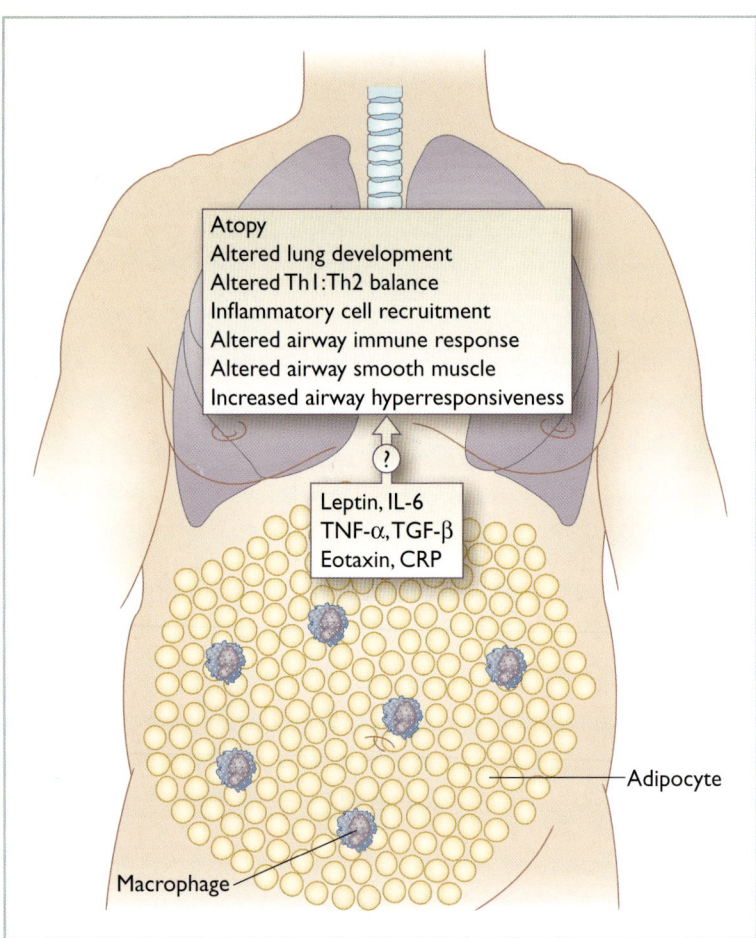

Figure 1-9. Proposed effects of obesity on the airway in asthma [19]. In obese patients, visceral adiposity is correlated with increases in circulating levels of proinflammatory cytokines, and there is evidence that adipose tissue mediates the systemic inflammation in part by recruitment of macrophages via chemokines and in part via elaboration of cytokines and chemokines such as leptin, interleukin-6 (IL-6), tumor necrosis factor-α (TNF-α), transforming growth factor-β (TGF-β), and eotaxin. Although the precise relationship between obesity and asthma remains to be determined, this systemic inflammatory environment has been postulated to have a number of effects on the lung, including the development of atopy, altered lung development, altered Th1:Th2 cytokine balance, altered airway immune response, and altered airway smooth muscle and function. These mechanisms might explain the increased risk of asthma that has been reported to occur in obese individuals [20]. CRP—C-reactive protein. (*Adapted from* Beuther *et al*. [19].)

DIAGNOSTIC TESTING IN ASTHMA

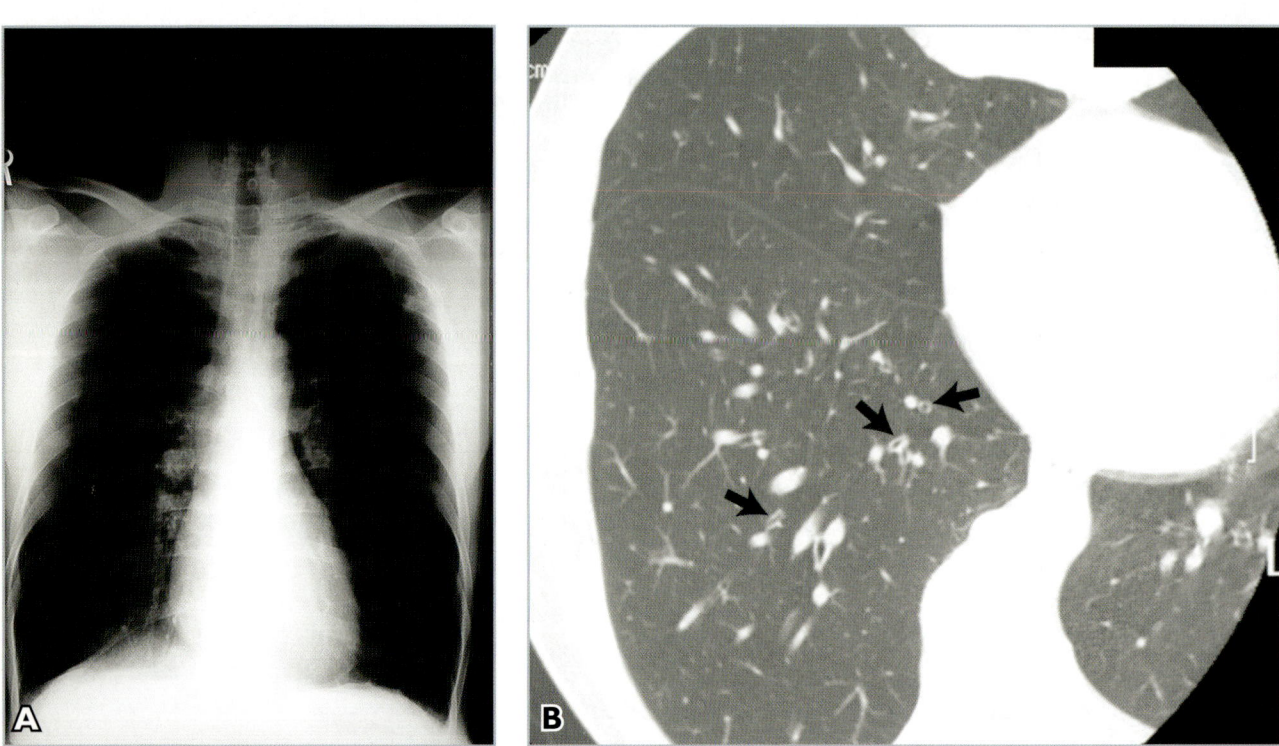

Figure 1-10. Radiographic abnormalities in asthma. **A**, Posteroanterior chest radiograph demonstrating hyperinflation, with increased lucency of the lung fields and flattening of the hemidiaphragms bilaterally [21]. **B**, High-resolution CT image demonstrating evidence of airway wall thickening due to airway inflammation (*arrows*). (**B**, *courtesy of* David Lynch, MD, National Jewish Medical and Research Center.)

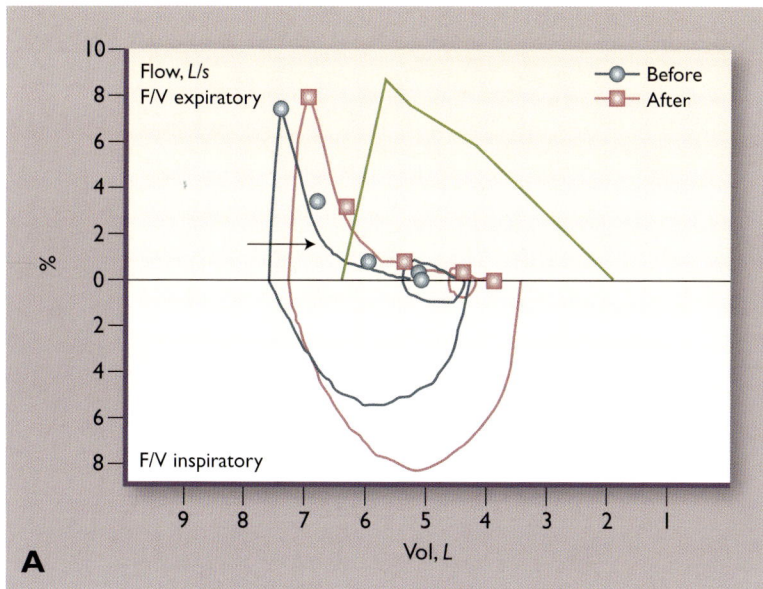

Figure 1-11. Characteristic spirometric abnormalities observed in a 65-year-old man with asthma. **A,** Spirometry, which is a critical tool for diagnosing, staging, and monitoring asthma [1], typically demonstrates evidence of expiratory airflow limitation, with concavity of the terminal expiratory portion of the flow-volume loop (*arrow*), and it can demonstrate improvement in lung function in comparing the appearance of the flow-volume loop before (*blue*) and after (*red*) albuterol. **B,** Airflow limitation manifests itself as absolute reductions in airflow compared with predicted normal airflows in both the forced expiratory volume in one second (FEV_1) and the forced vital capacity (FVC). Typically the FEV_1 is reduced out of proportion to the FVC, resulting in a reduced FEV_1/FVC ratio. In asthma, airflow limitation is typically "reversible," with improvements of 12% or more and 200 mL or more in the FEV_1 and/or FVC after administration of an inhaled short-acting β_2-agonist bronchodilator such as albuterol [22]. It is important to note that the FEV_1/FVC ratio is evaluated as an absolute value rather than as a percentage of predicted normal.

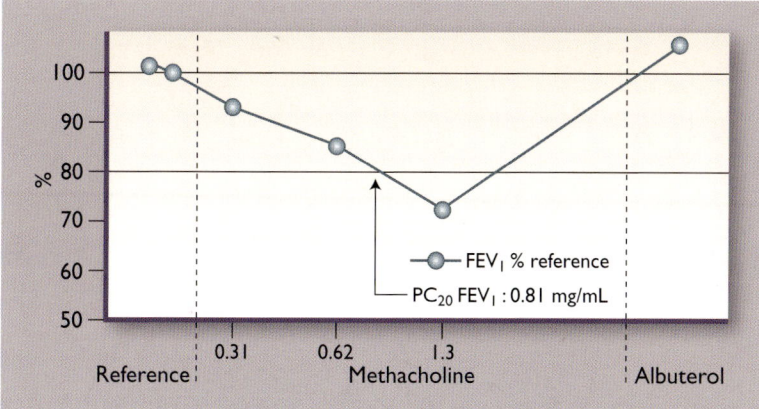

Figure 1-12. Airway hyperresponsiveness testing in asthma. To supplement findings on spirometry, additional physiologic testing can be utilized to evaluate the impact of airway inflammation on bronchoconstriction and lung volumes. In patients with asthma, inhalational challenge with a bronchoconstrictor agent such as methacholine [23] will result in a decline of 20% or more in forced expiratory volume in 1 second (FEV_1) at comparatively low concentrations of the provocative agent (eg, < 8 mg/mL of methacholine), a response not observed in healthy patients. Quantitation of the degree of airway hyperresponsiveness is obtained by means of the PC_{20} FEV_1, the concentration of methacholine that induces a 20% decline in the FEV_1 (*arrow*). Methacholine-induced bronchoconstriction typically responds quickly to albuterol.

CLINICAL MANIFESTATIONS OF ASTHMA

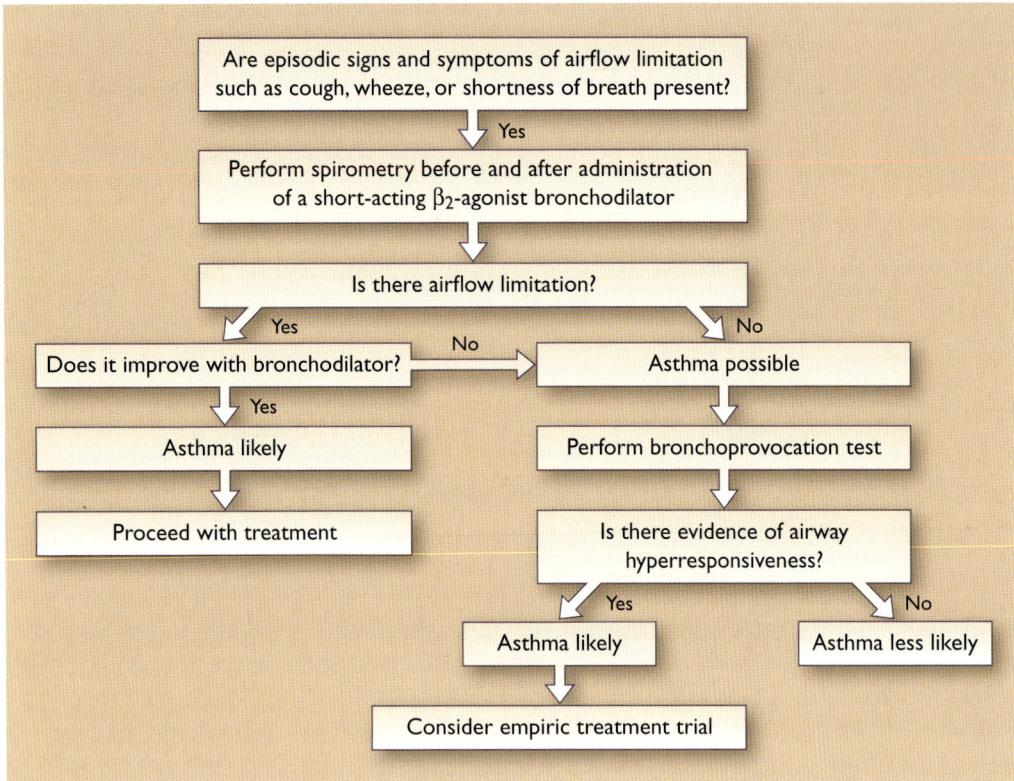

Figure 1-13. Algorithm for the diagnosis of asthma. The diagnosis of asthma should be considered in any patient with characteristic episodic signs and symptoms of airflow limitation, including cough, wheeze, or shortness of breath. In these individuals, a combination of clinical data and objective data obtained from spirometry can be used to enhance diagnostic certainty. For patients with characteristic symptoms, spirometry should be performed both before and after administration of a short-acting β_2-agonist bronchodilator such as albuterol. In patients with expiratory airflow limitation in whom the forced expiratory volume in 1 second or forced vital capacity improve by at least 12% and 200 mL, the diagnosis of asthma is likely, and it is appropriate to proceed with the initiation of asthma pharmacotherapy after assessment of severity. A subset of patients with asthma will either have normal lung function or will have lung function that does not improve after administration of a short-acting β_2-agonist. For these patients the diagnosis of asthma remains a possibility, and additional evaluation with diagnostic testing, including bronchoprovocation testing such as methacholine challenge, is appropriate. In patients who demonstrate characteristic symptoms and have either normal lung function or airflow limitation that is not responsive to bronchodilators, the presence of airway hyperresponsiveness increases the likelihood of asthma, and for these patients an empiric trial of asthma therapy to evaluate clinical response is appropriate. Asthma is less likely to be the cause of symptoms in patients who demonstrate neither bronchodilator-responsive airflow limitation nor airway hyperresponsiveness.

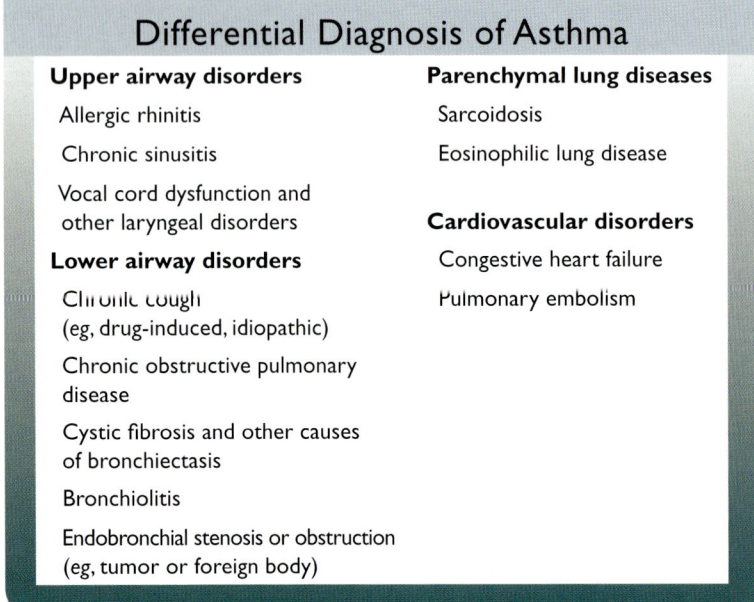

Figure 1-14. Differential diagnosis of asthma. The differential diagnosis of asthma in adults is broad, and it includes upper and lower airway disorders as well as parenchymal lung disease and cardiovascular disease.

Assessment of Asthma Severity in Adults

Components of Severity		Classification of Asthma Severity, >12 years of age			
		Intermittent	Persistent Mild	Persistent Moderate	Persistent Severe
Impairment	Symptoms	≤ 2 days/week	> 2 days/week but not daily	Daily	Throughout the day
	Nighttime awakenings	≤ 2 times/month	3–4/month	> 1 time/week but not nightly	Often 7 times/week
	Short-acting β_2-agonist use for symptom control	≤ 2 days/week	> 2 days/week but not daily, and not more than 1 time on any day	Daily	Several times per day
	Interference with normal activity	None	Minor limitation	Some limitation	Extremely limited
	Lung function	Normal FEV_1 between exacerbations			
		FEV_1 > 80% predicted	FEV_1 ≥ 80% predicted	FEV_1 > 60% but < 80% predicted	FEV_1 < 60% predicted
		FEV_1/FVC normal*	FEV_1/FVC normal*	FEV_1/FVC reduced 5%	FEV_1/FVC reduced 5%
Risk	Exacerbations requiring oral systemic corticosteroids	0–1/year	> 2/year	> 2/year	> 2/year
		Consider severity and interval since last exacerbation			
		Frequency and severity may fluctuate over time for patients in any severity category			
		Relative annual risk of exacerbations may be related to FEV_1.			

*Normal FEV_1/FVC: 8–19 years of age = 85%, 20–39 years of age = 80%, 40–59 years of age = 75%, 60–80 years of age = 70%.

Figure 1-15. Assessment of asthma severity in adults. Asthma severity is a reflection of the intrinsic intensity of the disease, and the initial assessment of asthma severity is made at the time of initial presentation, ideally before treatment with long-term controller therapies has been initiated. Guidelines from the National Asthma Education and Prevention Program [1] suggest that assessment of severity should be made on the basis of current spirometric data as well as the patient's recall of symptoms from the previous 2 to 4 weeks. Severity classification is based on evaluation of two domains: current impairment and future risk. Components of current impairment include daytime and nighttime symptoms, need for rescue bronchodilator for relief of symptoms, ability to perform normal daily activities (eg, work or school days missed), and lung function measured by spirometry. The risk of future adverse events (primarily exacerbations) due to asthma should be assessed as well and requires a careful medical history and clinical judgment, taking into account both the frequency and intensity of exacerbations. Predictors that have been reported to be associated with an increased risk of exacerbations include degree of airflow limitation, the need for two or more emergency department visits or hospitalizations for asthma in the preceding year, current smoking, and poor compliance with inhaled corticosteroid therapy [1,24,25]. FEV_1—forced expiratory volume in 1 second; FVC—forced vital capacity. (*Adapted from* Expert Panel Report 3 [1].)

Assessment of Asthma Control in Adults

Components of Control		Classification of Asthma Control		
		Well Controlled	**Not Well Controlled**	**Very Poorly Controlled**
Impairment	Symptoms	≤ 2 days/week	> 2 days/week	Throughout the day
	Nighttime awakenings	≤ 2/month	1–3 times/week	> 4 times/week
	Interference with normal activity	None	Some limitation	Extremely limited
	Short-acting β_2-agonist use for symptom control	≤ 2 days/week	> 2 days/week	Several times per day
	FEV_1 or peak flow	> 80% predicted/personal best	60%–80% predicted/personal best	< 60% predicted/personal best
	Validated questionnaires			
	ATAQ	0	1–2	3.4
	ACQ	≤ 0.75	≥1.5	N/A
	ACT	≥ 20	16–19	≤15
Risk	Exacerbations requiring oral systemic corticosteroids	0–1/year	≥ 2/year	
		Consider severity and interval since last exacerbation		
	Progressive loss of lung function	Evaluation requires long-term follow-up care		
	Treatment-related adverse effects	May vary in intensity		

ACQ—Asthma Control Questionnaire; ACT—Asthma Control Test; ATAQ—Asthma Therapy Assessment Questionnaire.

Figure 1-16. Assessment of asthma control in adults. The primary goal of long-term therapy for patients with asthma is control of the disease, and periodic assessment and ongoing monitoring are utilized to determine whether control of asthma has been achieved [1]. Like severity, evaluation of asthma control is based on domains of impairment and risk and is assessed by the degree to which elements related to these domains are minimized by treatment. Control is typically assessed at the time of follow-up after initial evaluation and can be used to make decisions about whether to maintain or adjust therapy at current levels. The goals of asthma control are to reduce impairment by 1) preventing chronic symptoms, 2) reducing the need for rescue bronchodilators, 3) maintaining normal or near normal lung function, 4) maintaining normal activity levels, and 5) meeting patient's expectations of care. Additionally, improving asthma control involves reducing risk by 1) preventing recurring exacerbations of asthma, 2) minimizing the need for unscheduled clinician visits, 3) preventing progressing decline in lung function, and 4) optimizing therapy with minimal adverse effects [1]. ACQ—Asthma Control Questionnaire; ACT—Asthma Control Test; ATAQ—Asthma Therapy Assessment Questionnaire; FEV_1—forced expiratory volume in 1 second; N/A—not available. (*Adapted from* Expert Panel Report 3 [1].)

Asthma Control Test

1. In the past 4 weeks, how much of the time did your ASTHMA keep you from getting as much done at work, school or at home?

All of the time	Most of the time	Some of the time	A little of the time	None of the time
○	○	○	○	○
1	2	3	4	5

2. During the past 4 weeks, how often have you had shortness of breath?

More than once a day	Once a day	Three to six times a week	Once or twice a week	Not at all
○	○	○	○	○
1	2	3	4	5

3. During the past 4 weeks, how often did your asthma symptoms (wheezing, coughing, shortness of breath, chest tightness or pain) wake you up at night or earlier than usual in the morning?

Four or more nights a week	Two to three nights a week	Once a week	Once or twice	Not at all
○	○	○	○	○
1	2	3	4	5

4. During the past 4 weeks, how often have you used your rescue inhaler or nebulizer medication (such as albuterol)?

Three or more times per day	One or two times per day	Two or three times per week	Once a week or less	Not at all
○	○	○	○	○
1	2	3	4	5

5. How would you rate your asthma control during the past 4 weeks?

Not controlled at all	Poorly controlled	Somewhat controlled	Well controlled	Completely controlled
○	○	○	○	○
1	2	3	4	5

Figure 1-17. Validated instrument for the assessment of asthma control. The Asthma Control Test (ACT) [26] is a self-administered tool in which patients rate the current status of their asthma with regard to symptoms, the use of rescue medications, and the overall impact of the disease on everyday functioning. This validated tool, one of several available instruments to obtain clinical data with which to assess asthma control, is used to supplement objective measures of lung function. An ACT score of 20 or higher is considered an indication of "well-controlled" asthma, with a score of 16 through 19 reflecting "not well-controlled" asthma and a score of 15 or lower reflecting "poorly controlled" asthma. (*Adapted from* Nathan et al. [26].)

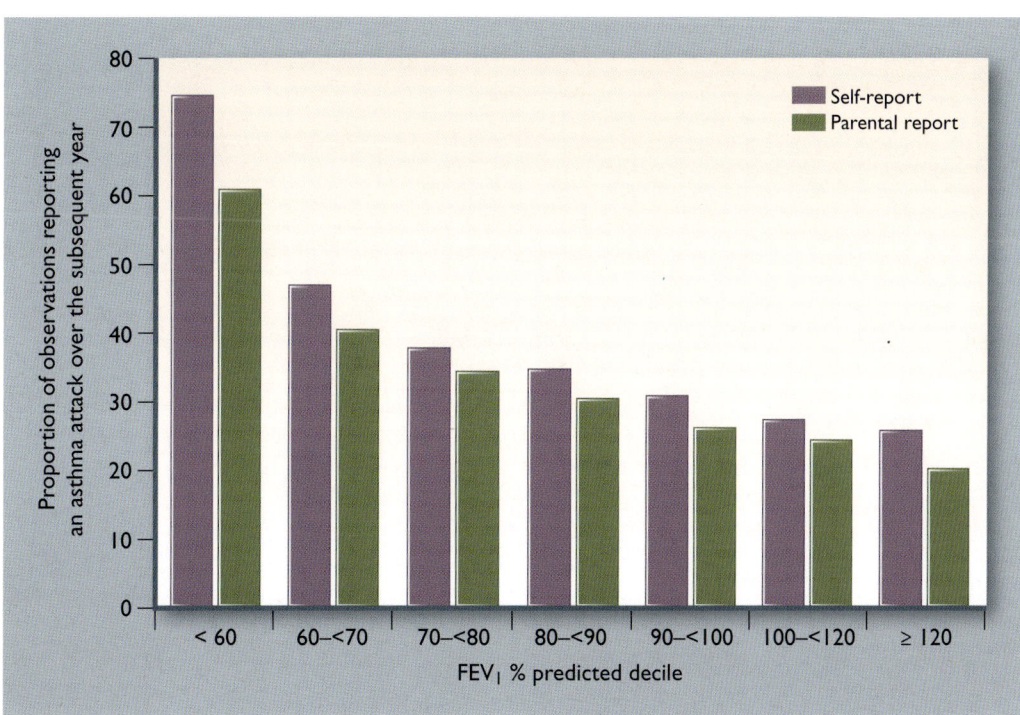

Figure 1-18. The relationship between spirometry and subsequent risk of asthma exacerbation in children. Data from a retrospective cohort study of approximately 3600 children with asthma indicate a progressive reduction in the percentage of individuals experiencing an asthma exacerbation as lung function (as measured by decile of forced expiratory volume in 1 second [FEV_1] percent predicted) increases. Prior asthma exacerbation was also found to be an important risk factor for future exacerbations, as was smoking [25]. (*Adapted from* Fuhlbrigge et al. [25].)

| Asthma |

TREATMENT OF ASTHMA

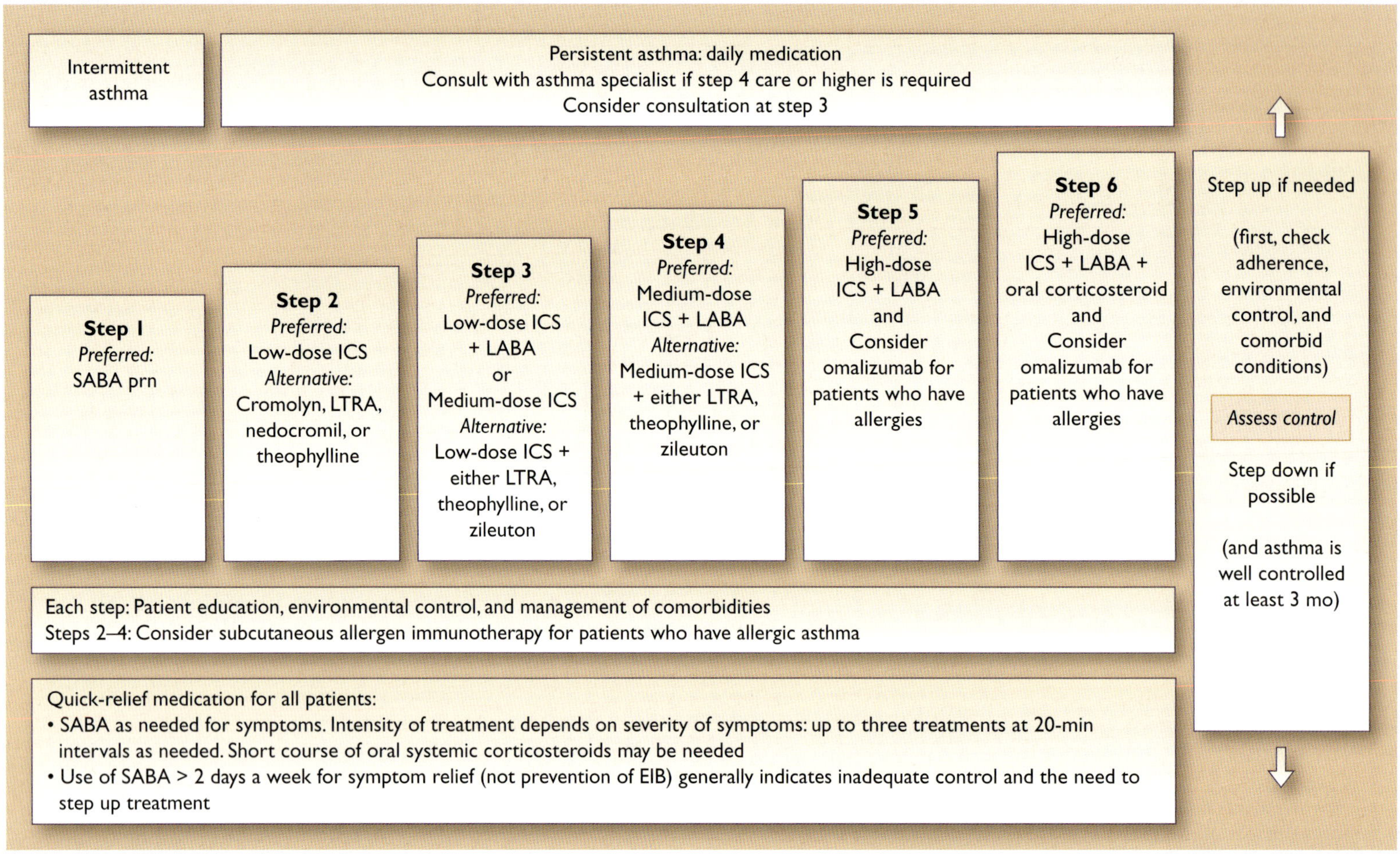

Intermittent asthma
Persistent asthma: daily medication
Consult with asthma specialist if step 4 care or higher is required
Consider consultation at step 3
Step 1
Preferred:
SABA prn
Step 2
Preferred:
Low-dose ICS
Alternative:
Cromolyn, LTRA, nedocromil, or theophylline
Step 3
Preferred:
Low-dose ICS + LABA
or
Medium-dose ICS
Alternative:
Low-dose ICS + either LTRA, theophylline, or zileuton
Step 4
Preferred:
Medium-dose ICS + LABA
Alternative:
Medium-dose ICS + either LTRA, theophylline, or zileuton
Step 5
Preferred:
High-dose ICS + LABA
and
Consider omalizumab for patients who have allergies
Step 6
Preferred:
High-dose ICS + LABA + oral corticosteroid
and
Consider omalizumab for patients who have allergies
Step up if needed
(first, check adherence, environmental control, and comorbid conditions)
Assess control
Step down if possible
(and asthma is well controlled at least 3 mo)
Each step: Patient education, environmental control, and management of comorbidities
Steps 2–4: Consider subcutaneous allergen immunotherapy for patients who have allergic asthma
Quick-relief medication for all patients:
• SABA as needed for symptoms. Intensity of treatment depends on severity of symptoms: up to three treatments at 20-min intervals as needed. Short course of oral systemic corticosteroids may be needed
• Use of SABA > 2 days a week for symptom relief (not prevention of EIB) generally indicates inadequate control and the need to step up treatment

Figure 1-19. Stepwise approach to the treatment of asthma in adults and adolescents 12 years of age or older. Although initial treatment decisions in asthma are ideally based on an assessment of asthma severity (*see* Fig. 1-20), the long-term goal of asthma therapy is to achieve control. A stepwise approach to therapy is recommended by the National Asthma Education Prevention Program to gain and maintain asthma control with regard to both impairment and risk. Intermittent asthma can be treated with as-needed (PRN) short-acting β_2-agonist (SABA) bronchodilators (reliever therapy), but once persistent asthma has been diagnosed, one or more anti-inflammatory (controller) agents such as a leukotriene modifier, inhaled corticosteroid (ICS), or ICS/long-acting β-agonist (LABA) combination are recommended to optimize asthma control. In addition to pharmacotherapy, patient education, environmental control, and management of comorbid illness are important adjunctive measures. EIB—exercise-induced bronchospasm. LTRA—leukotriene receptor antagonist. (*Adapted from* Expert Panel Report 3 [1].)

Use lowest level of treatment required to maintain control
Classification of asthma severity
Intermittent
Persistent
Mild
Moderate
Severe
Step 1
Step 2
Step 3 or 4
Step 5 or 6

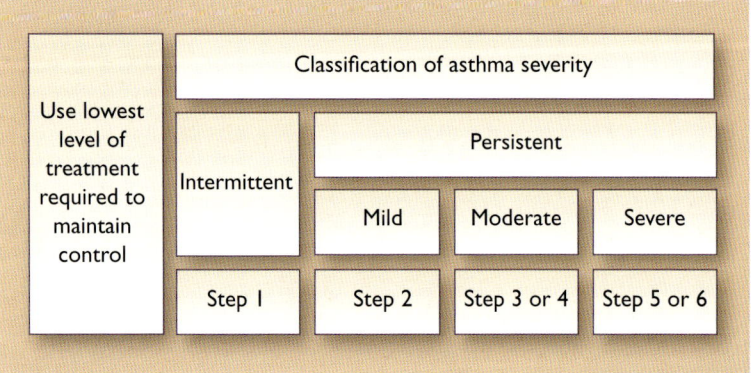

Figure 1-20. Initiating therapy based on assessment of asthma severity (*see also* Fig. 1-15) [1]. Asthma severity is assessed at the time of initial presentation, ideally before pharmacotherapy has been initiated. A treatment step appropriate to the level of asthma severity is selected as a starting point, with maintenance, upward titration, or downward titration of therapy at subsequent visits then determined by the degree of asthma control that has been achieved.

Management of Asthma During Pregnancy

- Monitoring of asthma control during prenatal visits is recommended
- Because of its favorable safety profile, albuterol is the recommended short-acting β_2-agonist
- Inhaled corticosteroids are the preferred controller agent, with budesonide the preferred agent based on a number of studies
- Intranasal corticosteroids are preferred over leukotriene modifiers or antihistamines for the management of allergic rhinitis

Figure 1-21. Management of asthma in pregnancy [27]. The health and well-being of both the mother and the baby are best served by maintaining optimal control of asthma during pregnancy. Maternal asthma has been shown to increase the risk of perinatal mortality, preeclampsia, preterm birth, and low-birth-weight infants. Moreover, suboptimally controlled asthma is associated with increased risks, whereas better-controlled asthma is associated with decreased risks. The guiding principle of asthma pharmacotherapy in pregnancy is that it is safer for pregnant women who have asthma to be treated with asthma medications during pregnancy than to have asthma symptoms and exacerbations. The National Asthma Education Prevention Program has concluded that, in pregnancy, albuterol is the preferred short-acting β-agonist and that inhaled corticosteroids are the preferred long-term controller medication. (*Adapted from* [27].)

Classification of Severity of Asthma Exacerbations

	Mild	Moderate	Severe	Life Threatening
Symptoms and signs	Dyspnea only with activity	Dyspnea interferes with usual activity	Dyspnea at rest; interferes with conversation	Too dyspneic to speak
Initial PEF (or FEV$_1$)	PEF > 70% predicted or personal best	PEF 40%–69% predicted or personal best	PEF < 40% predicted or personal best	PEF < 25% predicted or personal best
Clinical course	Usually cared for at home	Usually requires office or ED visit	Usually requires ED visit and likely hospitalization	Requires ED/hospitalization; possible ICU
	Prompt relief with inhaled SABA	Relief from frequent inhaled SABA	Partial relief from frequent inhaled SABA	Minimal or no relief from frequent inhaled SABA
	Possible short course of oral systemic corticosteroids	Oral systemic corticosteroids	Oral systemic corticosteroids	Intravenous corticosteroids
			Adjunctive therapies are helpful	Adjunctive therapies are helpful

Figure 1-22. Classification of severity of asthma exacerbations [1]. Recognizing the severity of an asthma exacerbation is critical to appropriate triage and therapeutic decision making. A written asthma action plan is useful in helping patients recognize early indicators of an impending exacerbation, such as increased symptoms and decreased lung function. ED—emergency department; FEV$_1$—forced expiratory volume in 1 s; ICU, intensive care unit; PEF—peak expiratory flow; SABA—short-acting β_2-agonist. (*Adapted from* [1].)

Risk Factors for Death from Asthma

Asthma History
- Previous severe exacerbation (*eg*, intubation or ICU admission for asthma)
- Two or more hospitalizations for asthma in the past year
- Three or more ED visits for asthma in the past year
- Hospitalization or Ed visit for asthma in the past mo
- Using > 2 canisters of SABA per mo
- Difficulty perceiving asthma symptoms or severity of exacerbations

Social History
- Low socioeconomic status or inner city residence
- Illicit drug use
- Major psychosocial problems

Comorbidities
- Cardiovascular disease
- Other chronic lung disease
- Chronic psychiatric disease

Figure 1-23. Risk factors for death from asthma [1]. Specific factors help identify patients at increased risk of asthma-related death. These patients require aggressive treatment of exacerbations, and they also benefit from attention prior to the exacerbation with regard to intensive patient education, more frequent monitoring, and therapy carefully optimized to achieve control. These patients should be counseled to receive asthma care early in the course of an exacerbation and to utilize emergency service (*eg*, ambulance transport) to minimize threat to life from an acute exacerbation. ED—emergency department; ICU—intensive care unit; SABA—short-acting β_2-agonist. (*Adapted from* [1].)

REFERENCES

1. Expert Panel Report 3: *Guidelines for the Diagnosis and Management of Asthma*. Bethesda, MD: US Department of Health and Human Services; National Institutes of Health; National Heart Lung and Blood Institute; National Asthma Education and Prevention Program; 2007. NIH Publication Number 07-4051.

2. Pleis JR, Lethbridge-Cejku M: Summary health statistics for U.S. adults: National Health Interview Survey, 2005. *Vital Health Stat* 2006, 1–153.

3. Akinbami L: Asthma prevalence, health care use and mortality: United States, 2003–05. Accessible at http://www.cdc.gov/nchs/products/pubs/pubd/hestats/ashtma03-05/asthma03-05.htm. Accessed September 21, 2007.

4. Weiss KB, Sullivan SD: The health economics of asthma and rhinitis. I. Assessing the economic impact. *J Allergy Clin Immunol* 2001, 107:3–8.

5. Holgate ST, Polosa R: The mechanisms, diagnosis, and management of severe asthma in adults. *Lancet* 2006, 368:780–793.

6. James AL, Wenzel S: Clinical relevance of airway remodelling in airway diseases. *Eur Respir J* 2007, 30:134–155.

7. Saetta M, Turato G: Airway pathology in asthma. *Eur Respir J* 2001, 34:18s–23s.

8. Hing E, Cherry DK, Woodwell DA: National Ambulatory Medical Care Survey: 2004 summary. Advance data from vital and health statistics 2006;1–33.

9. McCaig LF, Nawar EW: National Hospital Ambulatory Medical Care Survey: 2004 emergency department summary. Advance data from vital and health statistics 2006; 1–29.

10. Minino AM, Heron MP, Smith BL: Deaths: preliminary data for 2004. *Natl Vital Stat Rep.* 2006, 54:1–49.

11. Moorman JE, Rudd RA, Johnson CA, *et al.*: National surveillance for asthma—United States, 1980–2004. *MMWR Surveill Summ* 2007, 56:1–54.

12. Mannino DM, Homa DM, Akinbami LJ, *et al.*: Surveillance for asthma—United States, 1980–1999. *MMWR Surveill Summ* 2002, 51:1–13.

13. Eder W, Ege MJ, von Mutius E: The asthma epidemic. *N Engl J Med* 2006, 355:2226–2235.

14. Wenzel SE, Szefler SJ, Leung DY, *et al.*: Bronchoscopic evaluation of severe asthma. Persistent inflammation associated with high dose glucocorticoids. *Am J Respir Crit Care Med* 1997, 156:737–743.

15. Busse WW, Lemanske RF Jr: Asthma. *N Engl J Med* 2001, 344:350–362.

16. Burrows B, Martinez FD, Halonen M, *et al.*: Association of asthma with serum IgE levels and skin-test reactivity to allergens. *N Engl J Med* 1989, 320:271–277.

17. Strunk RC, Bloomberg GR: Omalizumab for asthma. *N Engl J Med* 2006, 354:2689–2695.

18. Solway J, Irvin CG: Airway smooth muscle as a target for asthma therapy. *N Engl J Med* 2007, 356:1367–1369.

19. Beuther DA, Weiss ST, Sutherland ER: Obesity and asthma. *Am J Respir Crit Care Med* 2006, 174:112–119.

20. Beuther DA, Sutherland ER: Overweight, obesity, and incident asthma: a meta-analysis of prospective epidemiologic studies. *Am J Respir Crit Care Med* 2007, 175:661–666.

21. Holgate ST, Sewell JA, Payne DK: Asthma. In *Bone's Atlas of Pulmonary Medicine*. Edited by Crapo JD. Philadelphia, PA: Current Medicine; 2005.

22. Pellegrino R, Viegi G, Brusasco V, *et al.*: Interpretative strategies for lung function tests. *Eur Respir J* 2005, 26:948–968.

23. Crapo RO, Casaburi R, Coates AL, *et al.*: Guidelines for methacholine and exercise challenge testing—1999. *Am J Respir Crit Care Med* 2000, 161:309–329.

24. Eisner MD, Katz PP, Yelin EH, *et al.*: Risk factors for hospitalization among adults with asthma: the influence of sociodemographic factors and asthma severity. *Respir Res* 2001, 2:53–60.

25. Fuhlbrigge AL, Kitch BT, Paltiel AD, *et al.*: FEV_1 is associated with risk of asthma attacks in a pediatric population. *J Allergy Clin Immunol* 2001, 107:61–67.

26. Nathan RA, Sorkness CA, Kosinski M, *et al.*: Development of the asthma control test: a survey for assessing asthma control. *J Allergy Clin Immunol* 2004, 113:59–65.

27. Working Group Report on Managing Asthma During Pregnancy: *Recommendations for Pharmacologic Treatment*. Bethesda, MD: U.S. Department of Health and Human Services; National Institutes of Health; National Heart Lung and Blood Institute; National Asthma Education and Prevention Program; 2005. NIH Publication Number 05-5236.

SEVERE ASTHMA

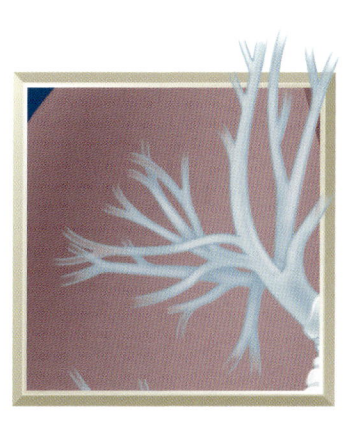
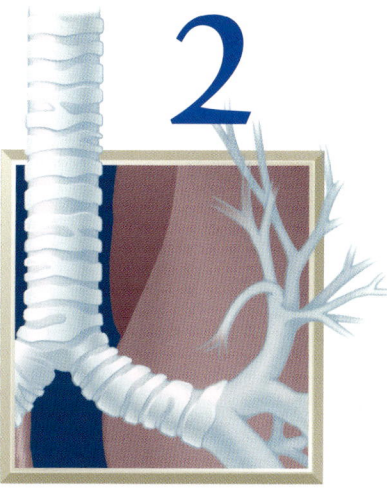
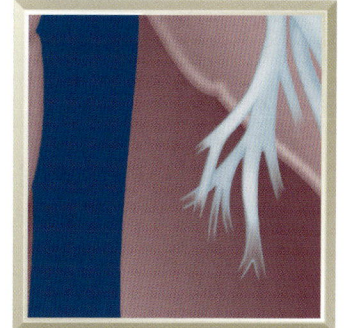

Adam L. Friedlander and Sally E. Wenzel

Severe asthma affects a small percentage of the asthma population, likely around 5%, but is responsible for a considerable portion of the costs associated with this disease, as well as with considerable morbidity. Traditionally, "refractory asthmatic" patients have been defined by their need for high medication levels to maintain good disease control and by their persistent symptoms, asthma exacerbations, or airflow obstructions despite considerable drug therapy [1]. Very little is understood regarding why these asthmatic patients are so much more difficult to treat than their milder asthmatic counterparts. However, it is likely that a combination of genetic, environmental, physiologic, and pathologic factors contribute to the severity of their cases. Furthermore, it is highly likely that severe asthma is not a single disease but rather a disease consisting of multiple phenotypes [2]. These distinctions allow for phenotypic characterization of individual asthmatics who are at increased risk for a near-fatal event, and it is hoped that they will also allow for tailored therapy to be created for those patients who suffer from difficult-to-control asthma. Finally, treatment of severe asthma remains highly problematic. Although corticosteroids, long-acting β_2-agonists, and leukotriene modifiers are all of reasonable efficacy for treating mild cases of the disease, the majority of severe asthma patients require frequent steroid bursts, if not continuous corticosteroids, and a percentage are poorly responsive or completely unresponsive to these agents.

DEFINITION AND EPIDEMIOLOGY

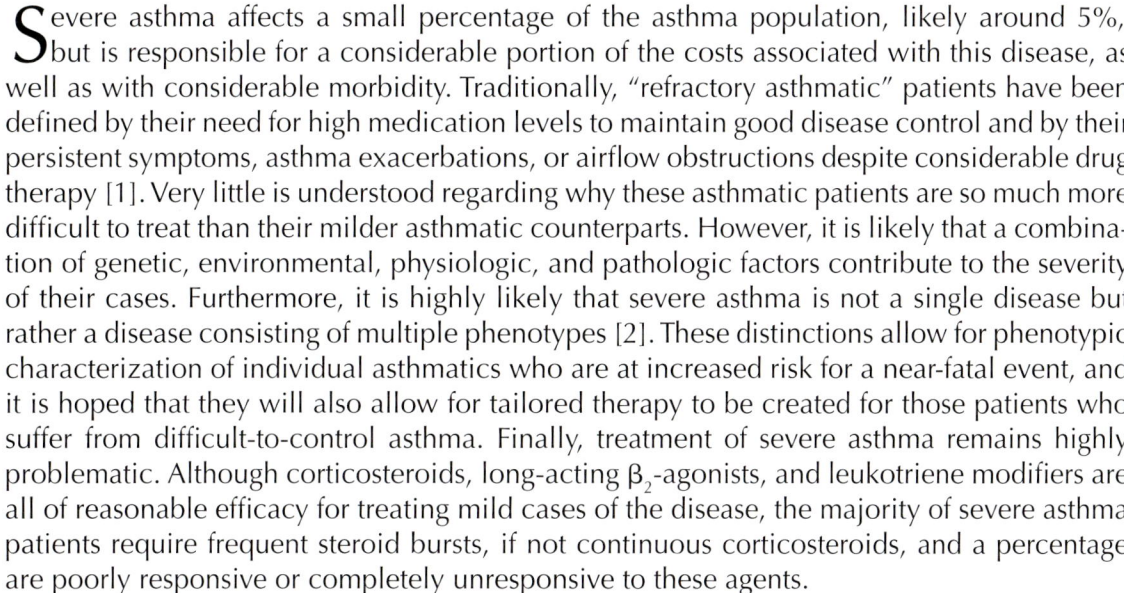

Figure 2-1. American Thoracic Society (ATS) definition of severe asthma. Severe asthma no longer describes only patients having fatal or near-fatal asthma; this term has come to encompass asthma subgroups previously described as refractory, steroid dependent and/or steroid resistant, difficult to control, poorly controlled, brittle, or irreversible [1]. This phenotypic diversity is reflected in the working definition of severe asthma established by the ATS, the details of which are contained in the figure. One of two major criteria must be met, and two of seven minor criteria must be fulfilled. FEV_1—forced expiratory volume in 1 second; FP—fluticasone propionate; PEF—peak expiratory flow. (*Adapted from* Wenzel et al. [1].)

Frequency of ATS Severity Criteria by Disease Severity

	Mild	Moderate	Severe
Major criteria			
OCSs for ≥ 50% of the year	< 1%	0%	32%
Continuous high-dose ICSs	0%	0%	98%
Minor criteria			
Daily 2nd controller medication	52%	79%	94%
Daily short-acting β_2-agonist	27%	44%	75%
Persistent airflow obstruction	0%	100%	78%
≥ 1 urgent care visit per year	16%	31%	54%
≥ 3 OCS bursts per year	5%	13%	54%
Deterioration with reduced steroids	32%	60%	78%
History of a near-fatal event	4%	6%	23%

Figure 2-2. Clinical features of asthma severity by American Thoracic Society (ATS) criteria. In an effort to better define the clinical, pathophysiologic, and biologic mechanisms that result in severe asthma, the Severe Asthma Research Program (SARP) prospectively characterized more than 400 subjects with variable phenotypic expression of the disease [3]. Just over a half of these subjects met the ATS criteria for severe asthma. The details of the clinical features of the severe asthma patients, in comparison with the mild and moderate subjects from the SARP study, are noted in the figure. Nearly 95% of the subjects with severe asthma were treated with a second long-term controller medication, suggesting that they remained symptomatic despite having been given appropriate maximal therapy for asthma. Over half of the severe asthma patients required more than one urgent care visit per year, which supports prior observations that this group requires high levels of health care despite appropriate therapy. Finally, almost a quarter of severe asthma subjects reported a history of a near-fatal event. ICS—inhaled corticosteroids; OCS—oral corticosteroids. (*Adapted from* Moore et al. [3].)

Potential Genetic Determinants of Asthma Severity

Related to allergy/atopy
- Polymorphisms in genes for IL-4, IL-4Rα, CD14

Related to fibrosis/remodeling
- Polymorphisms in TGF-β_1 (C-509T), MCP-1

Related to response to therapy
- Glucocorticoid and β-receptors (Arg/Arg)

Figure 2-3. Determinants of severe asthma: genetics. The genetics of asthma remain poorly understood, with those for severe asthma being even less clear. It is helpful to think about the genetics of severe asthma as falling into three broad categories: allergy/atopy, structural/remodeling, and response to therapy. In that regard, mutations in interleukin (IL)-4 have been linked to near-fatal events, whereas mutations in the receptor for IL-4 (which serves as a receptor for IL-4 and IL-13) have been associated with more rapid decline in lung function [4,5]. There is evolving evidence that a functional single-nucleotide polymorphism in the gene encoding CD14 may be a risk factor for allergic phenotypes, which varies with the level of endotoxin exposure and highlights the complex gene-environment interactions in determining asthma-related outcomes [6]. In the structural/remodeling category, transforming growth factor (TGF)-β_1, a prominent profibrotic factor, has been linked to worsened disease, whereas mutations in *ADAM33*, which are strong predictors of asthma, have also been linked to more severe airflow limitation [7]. Finally, no studies have suggested that mutations in the steroid pathway are linked to worsened asthma. However, studies on the β_2-adrenergic receptor have suggested that homozygosity for arginine at the 16 locus produces a long-term decline in lung function when β_2-agonists are used on a regular basis, as they often are in cases of severe asthma [8]. Although this observation gained support in a genotype-stratified, prospective randomized clinical trial [9], the clinical importance of the Arg/Arg variant remains unclear. Which, if any, of these described genetic mutations is most important is not at all clear. MCP—monocyte chemotactic protein.

Environmental Risk Factors for Severe Asthma

- Continued allergen exposure
- Infection (viral, chlamydial, mycoplasmal)
- Endotoxin
- Intercurrent rhinitis/sinusitis
- GERD
- Obesity
- Compliance

Figure 2-4. Determinants of severe asthma: environment. In addition to genetic elements, environmental and comorbid factors also contribute to asthma severity. Continued allergen exposure, primarily to indoor aeroallergens, is likely to contribute to day-to-day symptoms, and some data suggest that cockroach allergen exposure and sensitivity are particularly important factors [10]. Endotoxin has been reported to protect against the development of T-helper (Th2) responses, but in established cases of the disease, exposure to endotoxin may worsen asthma symptoms [11,12].

Intercurrent rhinitis and sinusitis often coexist with severe asthma [13]. Although it is commonly held that improvements in upper airway diseases will improve lower airway diseases as well, effective treatment of sinusitis is often difficult to achieve. Although gastroesophageal reflux disease (GERD) has also been associated with asthma symptoms, there are no studies that consistently show that treatment of reflux improves severe asthma.

The increasing prevalence of obesity in our population has led to the observation that many diseases may be caused or worsened by having an abnormally elevated body mass index (BMI). Asthma is certainly one such disease; an analysis of nearly 4800 patients with severe asthma reported that the average BMI of these patients was greater than 30 [14]. However, a causal relationship between obesity and asthma has yet to be proven.

Finally, compliance/adherence must always be addressed in cases of severe asthma. However, whether compliance rates are worse for patients with severe asthma than for those with mild asthma is not clear.

CLINICAL FEATURES

Differential Diagnosis of Severe Asthma

In children	In adults
Obliterative bronchiolitis	Cystic fibrosis
Bronchomalacia	Bronchiectasis
Inhaled foreign bodies	Inhaled foreign body
Cystic fibrosis	Tracheobronchomalacia
Congenital abnormalities of the upper airway	Tumors in or impinging on central airways
Immunoglobulin deficiencies	Recurrent aspiration
Primary ciliary dyskinesia	Chronic obstruction pulmonary disease
Part of the asthma spectrum of disease	Congestive heart failure
Allergic bronchopulmonary aspergillosis/mycosis	Obliterative or follicular bronchiolitis
Pulmonary eosinophilic syndromes (eg, Churg-Strauss syndrome)	Vocal cord dysfunction
	Bronchial amyloidosis

Figure 2-5. Differential diagnosis of severe asthma. Prior to labeling an asthmatic as "severe" or "refractory," care must be taken in certain clinical circumstances to exclude alternate diagnoses. In children, these include congenital and anatomical abnormalities (such as bronchomalacia), as well as the presence of inhaled foreign bodies. Inherited disorders, such as cystic fibrosis and primary ciliary dyskinesia, must also be considered if there is evidence of associated bronchiectasis. In adults, tumors that cause localized airway obstruction (eg, tracheal carcinoma or bronchial carcinoid) may mimic asthma. Finally, airway disease is often associated with a variety of connective tissue diseases, such as rheumatoid arthritis (obliterative bronchiolitis) and Sjögren's syndrome (follicular bronchiolitis). (*Adapted from Chung et al.* [15].)

Patients at High Risk for Life-Threatening Asthma

Underperceivers
Have abnormal response to airway narrowing, and/or
Do not sense worsening airflow limitation
Require ongoing monitoring of PEF

Brittle asthmatics
Characterized by tremendous variability in PEF
- Type 1: wide PEF variability (> 40% diurnal variability that occurs > 50% of time over a period exceeding 150 days, despite appropriate therapy)
- Type 2: sudden severe attacks on background of apparently good control (stable baseline peak flows); associated with high incidence of food allergies and aspirin sensitivity; should perform PEF monitoring twice daily

Morning dippers
Prone to life-threatening bronchospasm early in the morning
Episodes correlate with excessive diurnal variation in PEF (> 50%)

Aspirin sensitives
Defined by chronic rhinoconjunctivitis, nasal polyps, and asthma
Increased risk for severe, acute, and potentially fatal episodes
Cross-sensitive to all nonsteroidal anti-inflammatory drugs

Figure 2-6. Subgroups of asthmatics at high risk for a life-threatening event. Despite improved management over the past decade, asthma still accounts for over 4000 deaths in the United States annually [16]. Any attempt to prevent further asthma-related deaths or increased morbidity first requires identification of patients at highest risk for a near-fatal event. PEF—peak expiratory flow.

PHYSIOLOGY

Physiology of Severe Asthma

Ongoing airflow limitation with incomplete reversibility
Air trapping—increase in residual volume
Airway hyper-responsiveness/reactivity
Collapsibility

Figure 2-7. List of known physiologic changes in severe asthma.

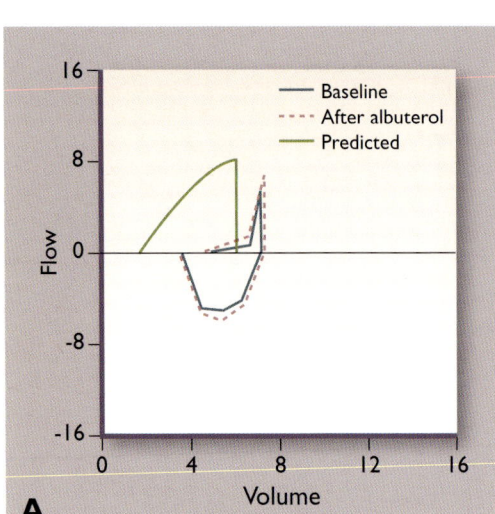

Study	Predicted	Baseline	Baseline Percent Predicted	After Albuterol	Postalbuterol Change in Baseline, %
Lung volume					
TLC, L	6.2	7.12	115	7.3	3
TGV, L	3.63	4.21	116	3.64	-14
RV, L	1.66	3.55	214	3.42	-4
Forced expiration					
FVC, L	4.53	2.04	45	2.9	42
FEV_1, L	3.18	0.95	30	1.46	54
FEV_1/FVC, %	4.53	47	67	50	6
SVC, L	70	3.56	79		
Additional studies					
Raw, cm H_2O/L/s	1.69	3.47	205	1.97	-43
sGaw, L/s/cm H_2O/L	0.16	0.05	31	0.11	120

Figure 2-8. Representative pulmonary function in a severe asthmatic. The flow-volume loop (**A**) and corresponding lung volumes (**B**) are a classic representation of physiologic abnormalities seen in severe asthma. There is a low starting forced expiratory volume at 1 second (FEV_1), which improves dramatically after bronchodilation, although it does not return to normal. There is evidence of air trapping, as shown by the increased residual volume (RV), but relatively little hyperinflation, as measured by total lung capacity (TLC) or thoracic gas volume (TGV). Finally, the flow-volume loop shows a rapid fall-off in flows early in expiration, which is suggestive of airway collapse. Similarly, there is a large difference between the forced (rapid) vital capacity (FVC) and the slow vital capacity (SVC) that is performed in a controlled ("nonforced") maneuver. When there is more than a 250 to 300 mL difference in these readings, some element of collapse is suggested [17]. Raw—airway resistance; sGaw—specific airway conductance.

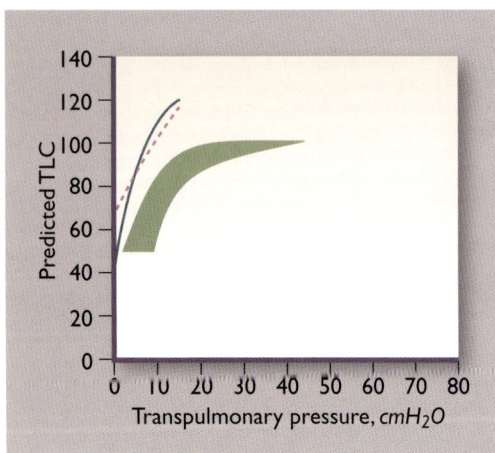

Figure 2-9. Representative pressure–volume curve for a patient with severe asthma. This patient's pressure–volume curve is shifted left as well as upward. This suggests a loss of lung elastic recoil, which means that much smaller changes in pressure are occurring in relation to volume than would normally be seen. This pattern is typically seen in patients with emphysema. The mechanisms that cause a loss of elastic recoil in a subgroup of patients with persistent asthma in the absence of emphysema remain elusive [18]. TLC—total lung capacity.

PATHOLOGY

Pathologic Explanations
Persistent eosinophilic inflammation
   "Steroid resistance"
Difference in underlying pathology
   Role of neutrophils
Structural changes in airways
   Airway remodeling
Difference in location of disease
   Small airways disease

Figure 2-10. List of potential pathologic explanations for severe asthma.

Persistent Eosinophilic Inflammation
Persistent eosinophilic inflammation *despite* steroids
   Only 50% of patients with severe asthma have eosinophilic inflammation [2,17,19]
   Eosinophilia may differ in childhood- vs adult-onset disease [2]
Poor response to standard medications
   "Steroid unresponsiveness"

Figure 2-11. Persistent eosinophilic inflammation. Only 50% of severe asthma patients have apparent persistent eosinophilia, with eosinophilia more common in late-onset disease as compared with early-onset disease [2,19,20]. These patients are representative of those whose eosinophilic inflammation responds poorly to or is "resistant" to corticosteroids. These observations suggest that there exists a noneosinophilic (neutrophil mediated) phenotype, and that allergic mechanisms may not be the only underlying mechanism for asthma. Because most treatment and prevention strategies are focused on allergic/eosinophilic asthma and allergen avoidance, the existence of a common noneosinophilic severe asthma phenotype has important consequences on future therapeutic strategies [19].

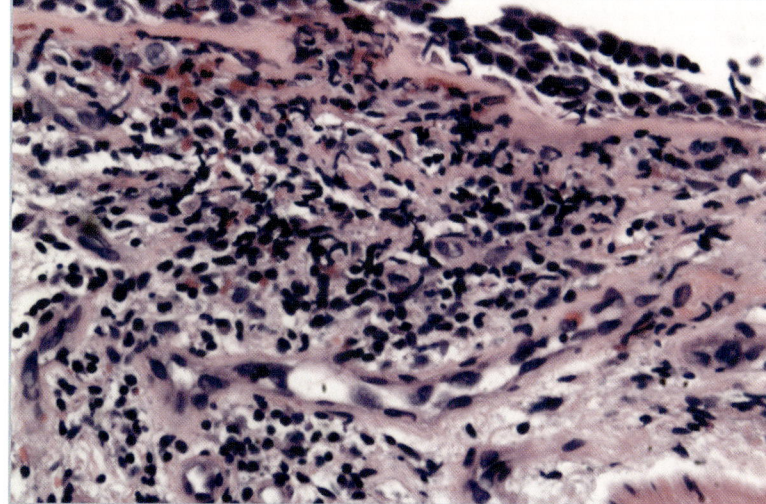

Figure 2-12. Eosinophilic inflammation. Severe asthma, even in the face of high-dose corticosteroids, may be associated with abundant eosinophils, just beneath the epithelium. (*Courtesy of Dr. Steve Groshong.*)

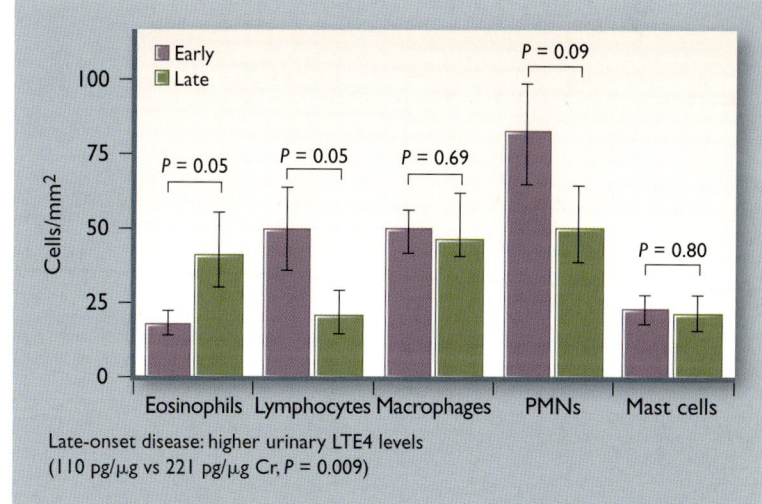

Late-onset disease: higher urinary LTE4 levels (110 pg/μg vs 221 pg/μg Cr, $P = 0.009$)

Figure 2-13. Graph of inflammatory cell types in early- versus late-onset disease. In 80 subjects with severe asthma, 30 developed disease at age 12 or later. Those patients had greater airway eosinophilia, as measured by lavage or endobronchial biopsy, than did severe asthmatic subjects who developed disease earlier in life. In contrast, there was more evidence for a lymphocytic—perhaps T helper (Th2)—type of process in subjects with early-onset disease, suggesting that these two subgroups, differentiated by age of onset, are pathologically different as well. LTE4—leukotriene E4; PMNs—polymorphonuclear neutrophils. (*Adapted from* Miranda *et al.* [2].)

Different Phenotype

Little inflammation and/or neutrophils seen [21,22]

 Neutrophil prominence—different disease? (eg, bronchiolitis obliterans)

Associated with increased MMP-9, perhaps less fibrosis and lower FEV_1

Not clear whether part of disease itself or caused by high-dose steroids' effect of prolonging neutrophil survival [23]

Figure 2-14. Possible difference in phenotype in severe asthma. In the 50% of patients without eosinophilia, there may be "no" inflammatory cell-based inflammation, or there may be an increase in neutrophils. This increase in neutrophils is associated with increases in matrix metalloproteinase (MMP) and a lower forced expiratory volume in 1 second (FEV_1). However, it is not clear whether the increase in neutrophils is a result of the disease itself or the high doses of corticosteroids (which enhance neutrophil survival) used in this population [23]. Further, it is not known whether some of these patients, particularly those with late-onset disease and no eosinophilia, are part of a subgroup that may be closer to bronchiolitis obliterans than to asthma [24].

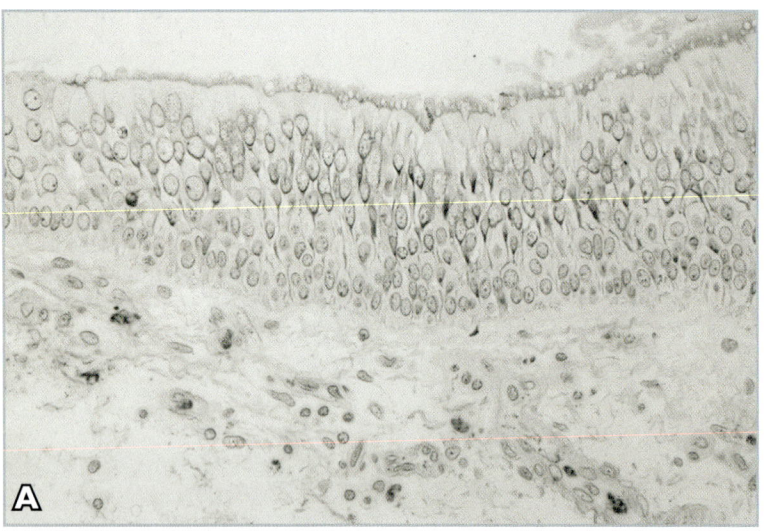
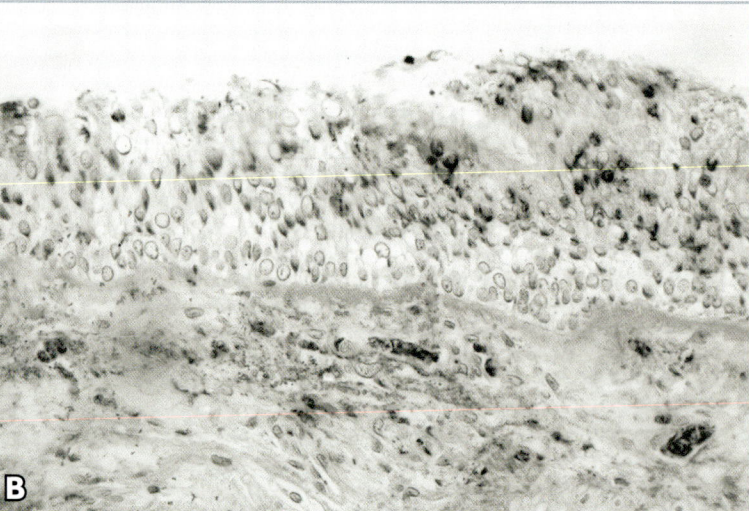

Figure 2-15. Matrix metalloproteinase-9 (MMP-9) is increased along with neutrophils; a normal subject (**A**) compared with a severe asthma patient (**B**). The MMP-9 appears to be selectively deposited in the subepithelial basement membrane. Increases in MMP-9 in severe asthma are also directly related to neutrophil presence [25,26]. An increased level of neutrophils has been reported in the sputum of severe asthmatics as compared with those with mild asthma and normal controls. Chemoattractants for these cells have been reported to be increased in severe asthma patients as well [21,22].

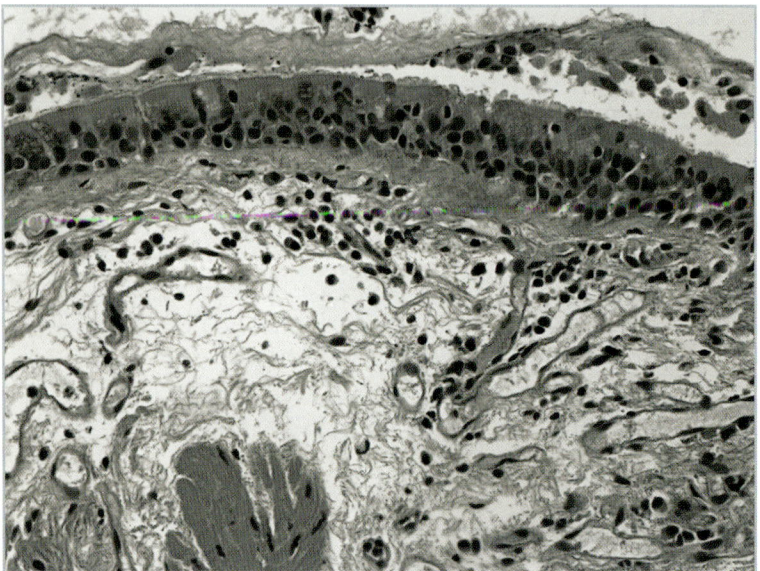

Figure 2-16. "Lack" of classic inflammation associated with some types of severe asthma. Minimal nonspecific cellular infiltrate, but with increased mucus production and edema, is present in the tissue [2].

Structural Changes

Chronic inflammation leads to structural changes ("remodeling")

Implicated structures include SBM, smooth muscles, nerves, epithelium, and vessels

Relationship of structure to function is poorly understood

Figure 2-17. Structural changes observed in severe asthma. It has long been suggested that chronic inflammation leads to structural changes in the airways, such as thickening of subepithelial basement membrane (SBM), increases in smooth muscle, changes in nerves, and alterations in the epithelium. However, how these changes relate to clinical severity or lung function is not clear.

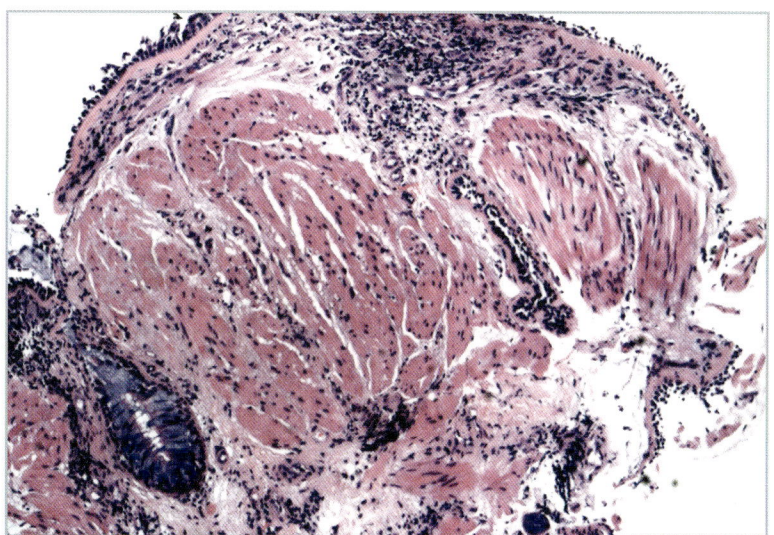

Figure 2-18. Endobronchial biopsy from a patient with severe asthma (40×). A thickened subepithelial basement membrane (SBM) is seen in association with high numbers of eosinophils. SBM thickening is likely related to increases in submucosal eosinophils. The SBM is thickest in severe asthmatics with eosinophilic inflammation as compared with normal subjects and asthmatics with milder disease. However, severe asthmatics without eosinophils do not have a significantly thicker SBM than do controls [17]. It is also not clear whether the SBM thickening has a functional effect on the airway or whether it is a marker for some other process. Smooth muscle hypertrophy, which may contribute to structural changes and airway remodeling seen in severe asthma, can also be appreciated. (*Courtesy of* Dr. Steve Groshong.)

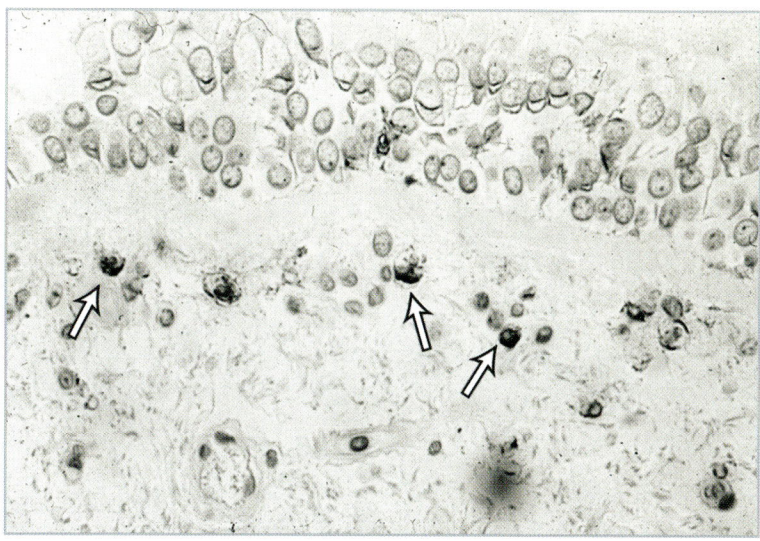

Figure 2-19. Transforming growth factor (TGF)-β (+) cells just beneath the subepithelial basement membrane (SBM) (*arrows*). The growth factor most closely associated with a thickened SBM is TGF-β [17,27]. Cells immediately below the SBM (eosinophils, neutrophils, and macrophages) express TGF-β, likely inducing collagen production from subepithelial fibroblasts to enhance thickness of the membrane [28].

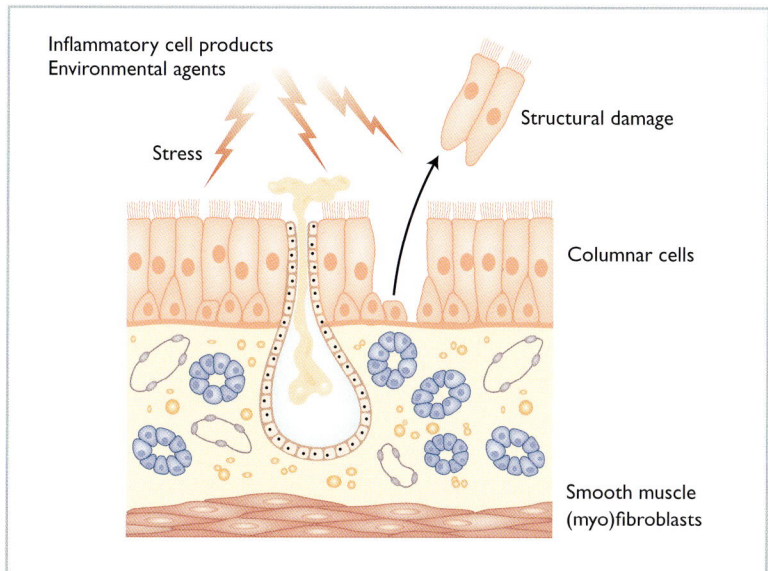

Figure 2-20. Epithelial remodeling. Epithelial cells are reported to be hyperplastic, metaplastic, transformed, and absent. Some differences may be related to endobronchial biopsy methodology [29]. However, increases in goblet cell–to–ciliated cell ratio are consistently reported [30]. In addition, epithelial cells, as the "first line" of defense in the air passages, may contribute both inflammatory and structural mediators that affect other parts of the airway.

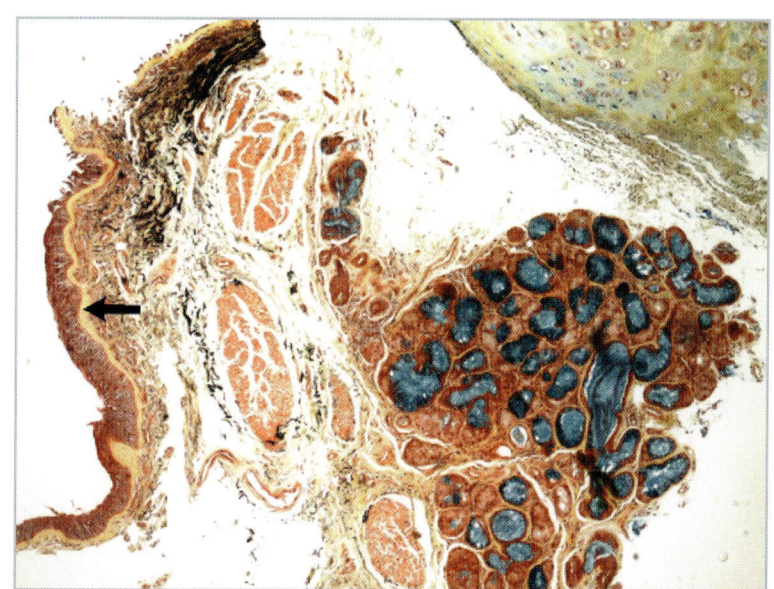

Figure 2-21. Endobronchial biopsy from a patient with severe asthma (pentachrome stain, 4×) demonstrating very distorted subepithelial elastin fiber architecture and organization. It is has been proposed that chronic inflammation and mechanical stretching in the air passages of some asthmatics lead to conformational alterations in the fibers of the elastic system, which is important in regulating airway patency and lung elastic recoil. This pattern of distorted elastin-fiber architecture is termed *elastosis*, and it is thought to contribute to airway remodeling in severe asthma [31]. Additionally, thickening of the subepithelial basement membrane (*arrow*) can be appreciated. (*Courtesy of* Dr. Steve Groshong.)

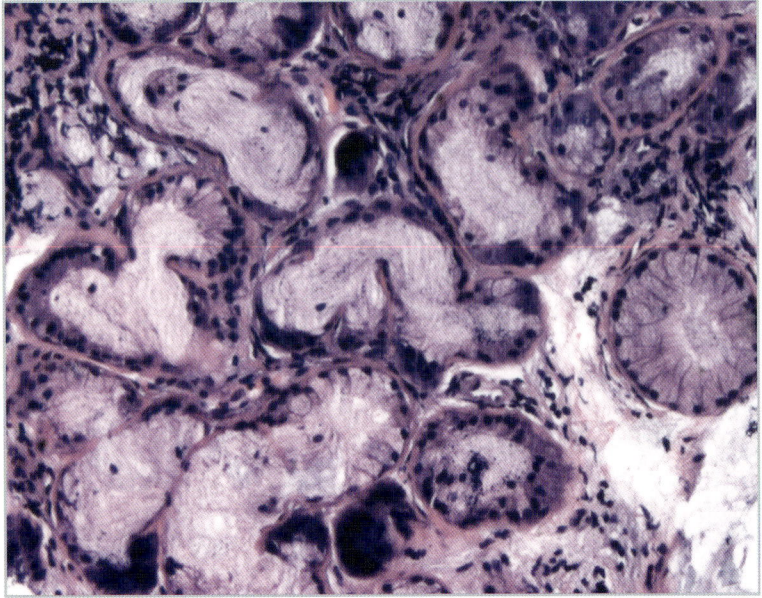

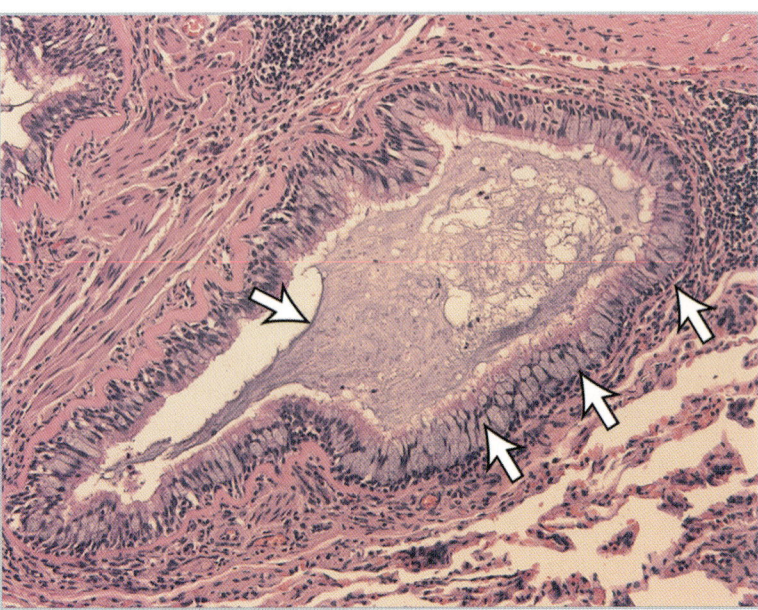

Figure 2-22. Mucus hypersecretion (100×) by the submucosal glands in a patient with severe asthma. Epithelial goblet cells and mucus-secreting submucosal glands are the major source of luminal mucus; goblet cell hyperplasia and submucosal gland hypertrophy are features relating to large airways in asthma patients [32]. These features cause many asthmatics to suffer from excessive mucus production, which, together with inflammatory exudates, form tenacious plugs that block the air passages. Mucus hypersecretion has clinically been more often observed in patients with severe steroid-dependent asthma as compared with milder disease, and it is closely correlated with bronchoalveolar lavage eosinophilia [33]. (*Courtesy of* Dr. Steve Groshong.)

Figure 2-23. Massive goblet cell hyperplasia in a patient who died from status asthmaticus. Ciliated goblet cells are largely replaced by goblet cells (*arrows*) and mucus-filled airway lumen.

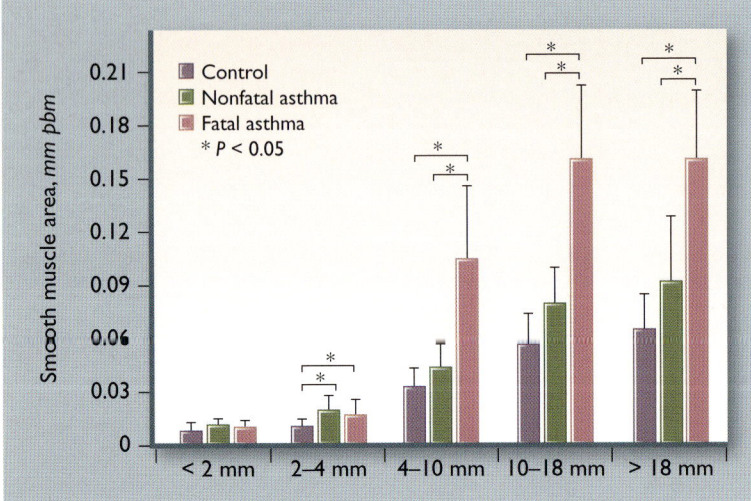

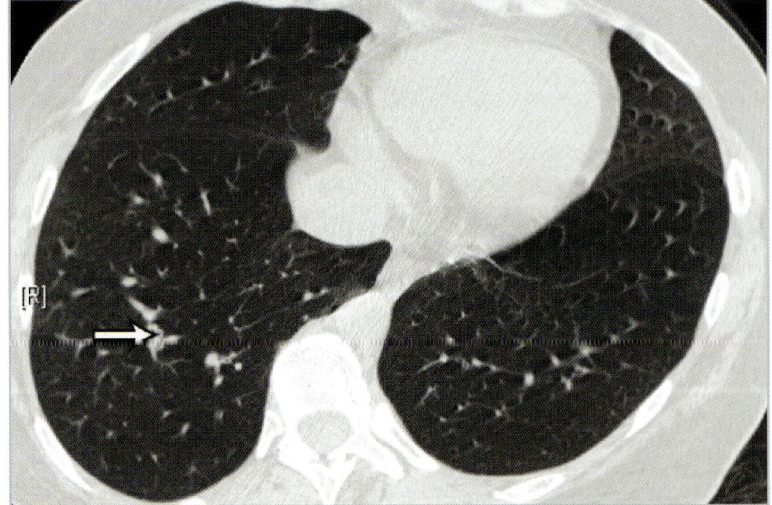

Figure 2-24. Smooth muscle cell changes. An increase in smooth muscle area (as part of the overall airway) has been noted in cases of severe asthma [34]. Other studies have suggested that the smooth muscle cells are larger (hypertrophic; *see* Fig. 2-20) in severe asthma [35]. Still others have suggested that the smooth muscle cells are normal, but that the matrix surrounding them in severe asthma is abnormal [36]. pbm—basement membrane perimeter. (*Adapted from* Carroll *et al.* [34].)

Figure 2-25. Axial cut from a high-resolution computed tomography (HRCT) scan of the chest in a subject with documented severe asthma. The inspiratory HRCT image demonstrates generalized hyperlucency throughout both the lower lobes, as well as the right-middle lobe and lingula, suggesting significant air trapping. Note the marked thickening of smaller peripheral air passages (*arrow*) in the right-lower lobe. Physiologic and radiographic studies suggest that asthma, particularly severe asthma, involves small airways. However, because of the paucity of distal lung samples available for study, it has been difficult to confirm the link between small-airways disease and severe asthma. (*Courtesy of* Dr. John Newell.)

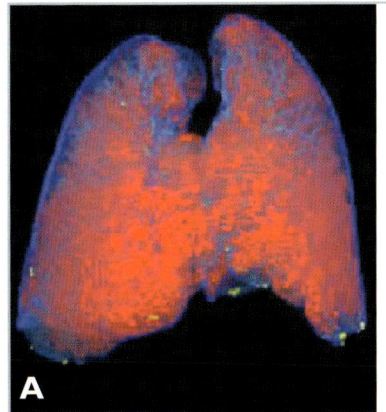 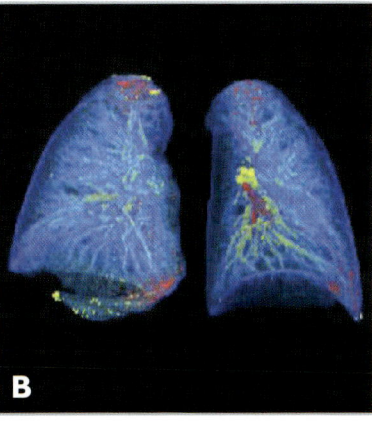

Figure 2-26. **A,** Three-dimensional reconstruction of contiguous multichannel high-resolution computed tomography (HRCT) done at functional residual capacity (expiratory) in the same subject with severe asthma shown in Figure 2-25. Areas that are less than 856 Hounsfield units (HU), and thus less dense, correspond to increased air trapping and are coded in *red*. Areas that are more than 856 HU (more dense) are coded in *blue*. **B,** By comparison, a normal subject without asthma illustrates that the marked air trapping from small-airways disease suspected in severe asthma can be visualized using advanced imaging techniques. Vessels are coded *yellow*. (*Courtesy of* Dr. John Newell.)

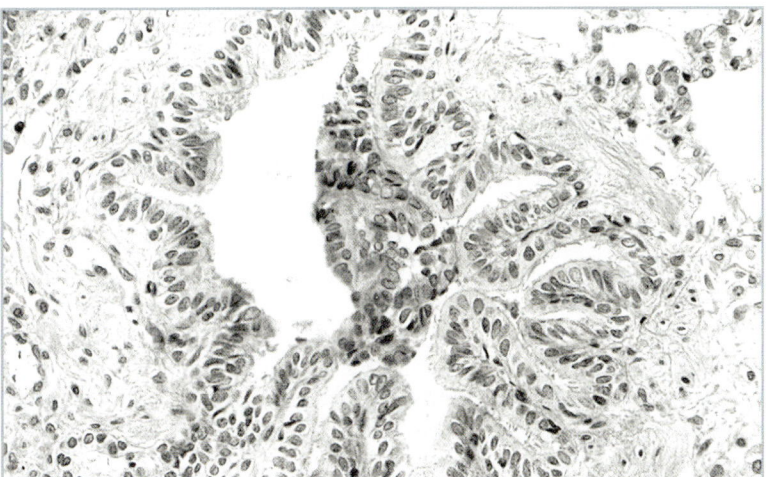

Figure 2-27. Thickened small airway in severe asthma.

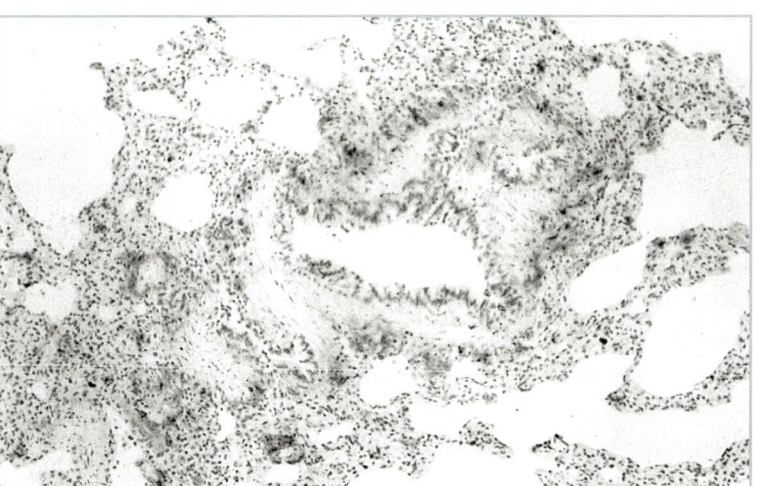

Figure 2-28. Distal airway mast cells positively stained for the mast cell protease tryptase. In addition to thickened airways and evidence of inflammation, there is evidence to suggest that the pattern of inflammatory cells is likely to be different as well. Mast cells become progressively more abundant in small airways, particularly the outer wall, than in the larger airways, making them the most abundant inflammatory cell in the peripheral airways.

TREATMENT

Therapy for Severe Asthma

- Refractory asthma: shift dose response to corticosteroids
  - Very few completely "resistant"
- High potency ICS still best therapy to decrease need for oral steroids
- Most current *inhaled* forms may not reach distal lungs

Figure 2-29. Implications for therapy. In the absence of large-scale clinical trials, high-potency inhaled and systemic corticosteroids remain the most effective therapy [37]. When compliance/adherence is a concern, corticosteroids may be injected. In individuals with small airway/peripheral disease (as assessed by high-resolution computed tomography and/or physiologic testing), one of the reasons for poor response may be relatively low peripheral deposition of most inhaled corticosteroids (ICS).

Alternative Approaches

- Anti-LT therapy [37]
- Anti-IgE therapy
- Methotrexate, gold, cyclosporin
  - Reported to work, but response modest
  - Studies not done with phenotypes in mind
- LABA: often not helpful in very severe disease [38]
  - Studies not done with phenotype in mind

Figure 2-30. Alternative approaches. As a large percentage of severe asthma is asthma sensitive, a trial with a leukotriene (LT) modifier, particularly a 5-lipoxygenase inhibitor, is often indicated [38]. In select patients with elevated serum IgE and refractory disease despite corticosteroids, a trial of anti-IgE therapy (omalizumab) is warranted and has been shown to allow tapering of oral steroids in this population [39]. However, the effect of anti-IgE on disease severity or exacerbations is not clear. Long-acting β_2-agonists (LABA) may not be as efficacious in this population as it is in subjects with moderate asthma [40]. Other approaches, including anti-tumor necrosis factor (TNF)-α, await larger-scale clinical trials.

Continued on the next page

Figure 2-30. *(Continued)* Treatment of 10 severe asthmatics with entanercept, the soluble TNF-α receptor, was shown to improve forced expiratory volume at 1 second (FEV$_1$), bronchial hyperresponsiveness, and quality of life [41]. A larger (300 patient) clinical trial of a monoclonal antibody to TNF-α failed in its primary purpose of improving exacerbations or FEV$_1$. However, evaluation of the subgroup with documented bronchodilator reversibility determined a significant response in time to first exacerbation, as well as number of exacerbations [42]. At this point, it is best to proceed with caution, because treatment with anti-TNF-α has been associated with an increased risk for severe infections and possibly for malignancy. Further attempts at determining a responder phenotype for many (if not all) of these newer, more expensive, and broadly immune-modulating approaches is highly desirable.

REFERENCES

1. Wenzel SE, Fahy JV, Irvin CG, et al.: Proceedings of the ATS workshop on refractory asthma: current understanding, recommendations, and unanswered questions. *Am J Respir Crit Care Med* 2000, 162:2341–2351.

2. Miranda C, Busacker A, Balzar S, et al.: Distinguishing severe asthma phenotypes: role of age of onset and eosinophilic inflammation. *J Allergy Clin Immunol* 2004, 113:101–108.

3. Moore WC, Bleecker ER, Curran-Everett D, et al.: Characterization of the severe asthma phenotype by the National Heart, Lung, and Blood Institute's Severe Asthma Research Program. *J Allergy Clin Immunol* 2007, 119:405–413.

4. Burchard EG, Silverman EK, Rossenwasser LJ, et al.: Association between a sequence variation in the IL-4 gene promoter and FEV$_1$ in asthma. *Am J Respir Crit Care Med* 1999, 160:919–922.

5. Sandford AJ, Chagani T, Zhu S, et al.: Polymorphisms in the IL4, IL4RA, and FCERIB genes and asthma severity. *J Allergy Clin Immunol* 2000, 106:135–140.

6. Martinez FD: CD14, endotoxin, and asthma risk: actions and interactions. *Proc Am Thorac Soc* 2007, 4:221–225.

7. Jongepier H, Boezen HM, Dijkstra A, et al.: Polymorphisms of the ADAM33 gene are associated with accelerated lung decline in asthma. *Clin Exp Allergy* 2004, 34:757–760.

8. Israel E, Drazen JM, Liggett SB, et al.: Effect of polymorphisms of the β$_2$-adrenergic receptor on response to regular use of albuterol in asthma. *Int Arch Allergy Immunol* 2001, 124:183–186.

9. Israel E, Chinchilli VM, Ford JG, et al.: Use of regularly scheduled albuterol treatment in asthma: genotype-stratified, randomized, placebo-controlled cross-over trial. *Lancet* 2004, 364:1505–1512.

10. Rosentreich DL, Eggleston P, Kattan M, et al.: The role of cockroach allergy and exposure to cockroach allergen in causing morbidity among inner-city children with asthma. *N Engl J Med* 1997, 336:1356–1363.

11. Martinez FD, Holt PG: Role of microbial burden in aetiology of allergy and asthma. *Lancet* 1999, 354:SII12–15.

12. Prescott SL, Macaubas C, Smallacombe T, et al.: Development of allergen-specific T-cell memory in atopic and normal children. *Lancet* 1999, 353:196–200.

13. Peters S: The impact of comorbid allergic disease on asthma: clinical expression and treatment. *J Asthma* 2007, 44:149–161.

14. Dolan CM, Fraher KE, Bleecker ER, et al.: Design and baseline characteristics of the epidemiology and natural history of asthma: Outcomes and Treatment Regimens (TENOR) study: a large cohort of patients with severe or difficult-to-treat asthma. *Ann Allergy Asthma Immunol* 2004, 92:32–39.

15. Chung KF, Godard P, Adelroth E, et al.: Difficult/therapy-resistant asthma: the need for an integrated approach to define clinical phenotypes, evaluate risk factors, understand pathophysiology and find novel therapies. ERS Task Force on Difficult/Therapy-Resistant Asthma. *Eur Respir J* 1999, 13:1198–1208.

16. Centers for Disease Control and Prevention: Asthma prevalence and control characteristics by race/ethnicity- United States, 2002. *MMWR Morb Mortal Wkly Rep* 2004, 53:145–148.

17. Wenzel SE, Schwartz LB, Langmack EL, et al.: Evidence that severe asthma can be divided pathologically into two inflammatory subtypes with distinct physiologic and clinical characteristics. *Am J Respir Crit Care Med* 1999, 160:1001–1008.

18. Gelb AF, Zamel N: Unsuspected pseudophysiologic emphysema in chronic persistent asthma. *Am J Respir Crit Care Med* 2000, 162:1778–1782.

19. Douwes J, Gibson P, Pekkanen J, et al.: Non-eosinophilic asthma: importance and possible mechanisms. *Thorax* 2002, 57:643–648.

20. Louis R, Lau LC, Bron AO, et al.: The relationship between airways inflammation and asthma severity. *Am J Respir Crit Care Med* 2000, 161:9–16.

21. Wenzel SE, Szefler SJ, Leung DY, et al.: Bronchoscopic evaluation of severe asthma. Persistent inflammation associated with high dose glucocorticoids. *Am J Respir Crit Care Med* 1999, 156:737–743.

22. Jatakanon A, Uasuf C, Maziak W, et al.: Neutrophilic inflammation in severe persistent asthma. *Am J Respir Crit Care Med* 1999, 160:1532–1539.

23. Cox G: Glucocorticoid treatment inhibits apoptosis in human neutrophils. Separation of survival and activation outcomes. *J Immunol* 1995, 154:4719–4725.

24. Jenkins HA, Cherniak R, Szefler SJ, et al.: A comparison of the clinical characteristics of children and adults with severe asthma. *Chest* 2003, 124:1318–1324.

25. Cundall M, Sun Y, Miranda C, et al.: Neutrophil-derived matrix metalloproteinase-9 is increased in severe asthma and poorly inhibited by glucocorticoids. *J Allergy Clin Immunol* 2003, 112:1064–1071.

26. Wenzel SE, Balzar S, Cundall M, et al.: Subepithelial basement membrane immunoreactivity for matrix metalloproteinase 9: association with asthma severity, neutrophilic inflammation, and wound repair. *J Allergy Clin Immunol* 2003, 111:1345–1352.

27. Minshall EM, Hogg JC, Hamid QA: Cytokine mRNA expression in asthma is not restricted to the large airways. *J Allergy Clin Immunol* 1998, 101:386–390.

28. Chu HW, Trudeau JB, Balzar S, et al.: Peripheral blood and airway tissue expression of transforming growth factor β by neutrophils in asthmatic subjects and normal control subjects. *J Allergy Clin Immunol* 2000, 106:1115–1123.

29. Ordonez C, Ferrando R, Hyde DM, et al.: Epithelial desquamation in asthma: artifact or pathology? *Am J Respir Crit Care Med* 2000, 162:2324–2329.

30. Ordonez CL, Khashayar R, Wong HH, et al.: Mild and moderate asthma is associated with airway goblet cell hyperplasia and abnormalities in mucin gene expression. *Am J Respir Crit Care Med* 2001, 163:517–523.

31. Mauad T, Xavier AC, Saldiva PH, et al.: Elastosis and fragmentation of fibers of the elastic system in fatal asthma. *Am J Respir Crit Care Med* 1999, 160:968–975.

32. Jeffery PK: Remodeling in asthma and chronic obstructive lung disease. *Am J Respir Crit Care Med* 2001, 164:S28–S38.

33. Tanizaki Y, Kitani H, Okazaki M, et al.: Mucus hypersecretion and eosinophilia in bronchoalveolar lavage fluid in adult patients with bronchial asthma. *J Asthma* 1993, 30:257–262.

34. Carroll N, Elliot J, Morton A, et al.: The structure of large and small airways in nonfatal and fatal asthma. *Am Rev Respir Dis* 1993, 147:405–410.

35. Benayoun L, Druilhe A, Dombret MC, et al.: Airway structural alterations selectively associated with severe asthma. *Am J Respir Crit Care Med* 2003, 167:1360–1368.

36. Wang L, McParland BE, Pare PD: The functional consequences of structural changes in the airways: implications for airway hyperresponsiveness in asthma. *Chest* 2003, 123:356S–362S.

37. Noonan M, Chervinsy P, Busse WW, et al.: Fluticasone propionate reduces oral prednisone use while it improves asthma control and quality of life. *Am J Respir Crit* Care Med 1995, 152:1467–1473.

38. European Network for Understanding Mechanisms of Severe Asthma: The ENFUMOSA cross-sectional European multicentre study of the clinical phenotype of chronic severe asthma. *Eur Respir J* 2003, 22:470–477.

39. Walker S, Monteil M, Phelan K, et al.: Anit-IgE for chronic asthma in adults and children. *Cochrane Database Syst Rev* 2006, CD003559.

40. Nightingale JA, Rogers DF, Barnes PJ: Comparison of the effects of salmeterol and formoterol in patients with severe asthma. *Chest* 2002, 121:1401–1406.

41. Berry MA, Hargadon B, Shelley M, et al.: Evidence of a role of tumor necrosis factor alpha in refractory asthma. *New Engl J Med* 2006, 354:697–708.

42. Wenzel S, Bleecker E, et al.: Phase 2, multicenter, double-blind study of CNTO 148, a human monoclonal anti-tumor necrosis factor antibody, in symptomatic patients with severe persistent asthma. *European Respiratory Society*. Stockholm, Sweden; September 15–19, 2007.

CHRONIC OBSTRUCTIVE PULMONARY DISEASE

Peter J. Barnes

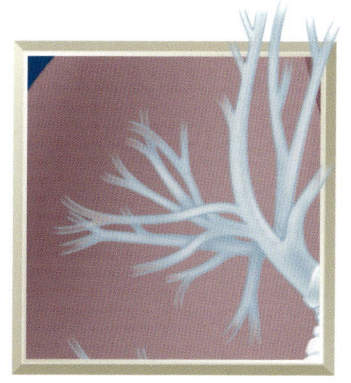
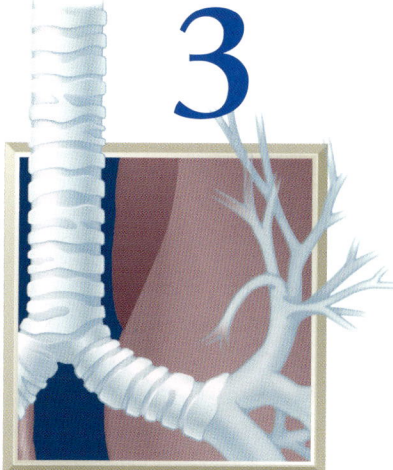
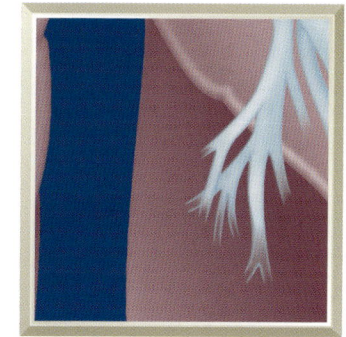

Chronic obstructive pulmonary disease (COPD) is a major and increasing global health problem and is predicted to become the third most common cause of death and the fifth most common cause of disability in the world by 2020 [1]. Despite the prevalence of COPD, this devastating disease has been neglected by health care professionals, pharmaceutical companies, and politicians [2]. Although there have been major advances in the understanding and management of asthma, there are no therapies in current use to reduce the inevitable progression of COPD. COPD is poorly recognized and often inappropriately treated [3]. However, because of the enormous burden of this disease and the escalating health care costs, there is renewed interest in the underlying cellular and molecular mechanisms and a search for new therapies, which has resulted in a reevaluation of the disease [4].

COPD is characterized by slow progressive development of airflow limitation that is marginally reversible, in sharp contrast to asthma, where there is variable airflow obstruction that is usually reversible spontaneously or with treatment. COPD has been defined by the Global Initiative on Obstructive Lung Disease (GOLD) as "a preventable and treatable disease with some significant extrapulmonary effects that may contribute to the severity in individual patients. Its pulmonary component is characterized by airflow limitation that is not fully reversible. The airflow limitation is usually progressive and associated with an abnormal inflammatory response of the lung to noxious particles or gases" [5]. This definition stresses the progressive nature of COPD, encompasses the idea that it is a chronic inflammatory disease, and also emphasizes that there are systemic components of the disease that are increasingly recognized as playing a key role in prognosis.

COPD includes chronic obstructive bronchitis with fibrosis and obstruction of small airways, and emphysema with enlargement of air spaces and destruction of lung parenchyma, loss of lung elasticity, and closure of small airways. Chronic bronchitis, by contrast, is characterized by a productive cough of more than 3 months' duration for more than 2 successive years; this reflects mucous hypersecretion and is not necessarily associated with airflow limitation. Most patients with COPD display all three pathologic mechanisms (chronic obstructive bronchitis, emphysema, and mucus plugging) that are induced by smoking but may differ in the proportion of emphysema and obstructive bronchitis. In developed countries cigarette smoking is by far the leading cause of COPD, but there are several other risk factors, including air pollution (particularly indoor pollution from burning fuels), poor diet, and occupational exposure. COPD is characterized by acceleration of the normal decline of lung function seen with age. The slowly progressive airflow limitation leads to disability and premature death from respiratory failure and is quite different from the variable airway obstruction and symptoms of asthma, which rarely progresses in severity and does not lead to respiratory failure. Although COPD and asthma both involve inflammation of the respiratory tract, there are marked differences in the nature of the inflammatory process, including differences in inflammatory cells, mediators, response to inflammation, anatomical distribution, and response to anti-inflammatory therapy [6]. Some patients appear to show characteristics of both COPD and asthma, however. Rather than this representing a graded spectrum of disease, it is more likely that these patients have both of these common diseases at the same time.

There have been important advances in understanding the cellular and molecular mechanisms of COPD. The inflammatory response differs from that of asthma in terms of a marked increase in numbers of macrophages in the alveoli, neutrophils in air spaces, and cytotoxic CD8+ lymphocytes in small airways and alveoli [7]. In some way this inflammatory process leads to the characteristic fibrosis and narrowing of small airways and alveolar destruction or emphysema, which together lead to airflow limitation and hyperinflation. The inflammation in lungs appears to be an amplification of the low-grade inflammation normally seen in cigarette smokers or in relation to exposure to other inhaled irritants. It is often stated that only 10% to 20% of smokers are susceptible to COPD, but now that smokers survive longer because they are less likely to die of other causes, the proportion of smokers developing airflow limitation is greater. It seems likely that the susceptibility of smokers to COPD is determined by genetic factors, although which genes confer this susceptibility is currently unknown [8]. Another characteristic of COPD that distinguishes it from asthma is its insensitivity to corticosteroids. The molecular basis of steroid resistance in COPD is now better understood and appears to be linked to the amplification of inflammation [9]. Better understanding of the inflammatory response in COPD patients may lead to more effective therapies in the future, and particularly to the development of treatments that may slow the progression of the disease and prevent its exacerbation.

COPD is still underdiagnosed in clinical practice, and spirometry, which is needed to confirm the diagnosis, is still not widely available [10,11]. The prevalence of COPD in population studies is much higher than previously recognized [12]. However, there is now a growing awareness of COPD and general recognition that it differs in important clinical respects from asthma and should therefore be managed differently. In contrast to asthma, there is a slow but relentless progression of COPD with increasing severity over time, eventually leading to respiratory failure and death [13]. The medical costs of COPD now far exceed those of asthma, as hospital stays are much longer [11].

There have been important advances in the management of COPD with the introduction of treatment guidelines in many countries. Smoking cessation is so far the only known way to reduce the progression of the disease, and the earlier smoking is stopped the greater the benefit [14]. The mainstay of medical management is bronchodilator therapy and long-acting bronchodilators, including long-acting β_2-agonists and anticholinergics, are superior to short-acting bronchodilators [5]. Bronchodilators produce symptomatic benefit in COPD patients, although the increase in forced expiratory volume in 1 second (FEV_1) and peak expiratory flow is very small. The major effect of bronchodilators is to reduce hyperinflation, resulting in more comfortable breathing and improved exercise tolerance. However, bronchodilators do not appear to reduce the progression of the disease, so new treatments will be needed in the future. Inhaled corticosteroids are widely used in the management of COPD, but their use has been controversial. There is no evidence that these treatments suppress the inflammatory response in COPD, in contrast to their striking effectiveness in asthma patients. This probably explains why inhaled corticosteroids fail to reduce the progression of COPD, even in patients with mild disease. Recent evidence suggests that the high inhaled doses used in COPD may increase pneumonia risk [15]. However, inhaled corticosteroids reduce the number of exacerbations in patients with severe COPD [16], so they are now recommended in patients with FEV_1 less than 50% predicted who have two or more exacerbations a year. Other treatments that are used in COPD include antileukotrienes, but there is no evidence that these treatments are effective. Mucolytics used to be popular, but there is no convincing evidence that they are effective in mucus hypersecretion, although systematic reviews of small studies suggest that N-acetylcysteine appears to reduce exacerbations, possibly because it is also an antioxidant. However, a large controlled trial of N-acetylcysteine in COPD patients showed that it did not reduce either exacerbations or disease progression [17]. Long-term oxygen therapy is indicated in patients who develop respiratory failure, but because of the high expense of administering this therapy careful assessment of patients is required before this treatment is used.

Nonpharmacologic treatments are also important in the management of COPD. Pulmonary rehabilitation, which includes education and graded exercises, has been shown to be beneficial in improving health status and reducing hospitalization length [18]. It is also cost-effective. There is debate about which regime is most effective and how frequently it should be administered. Surgery is an option in patients with severe COPD. Lung volume reduction surgery is indicated in some patients with predominantly upper zone emphysema, but surgical mortality is relatively high and patients need to be carefully selected. There is increasing interest in nonsurgical lung volume reduction by bronchoscopic valve insertion, but no long-term studies using this approach have yet been reported.

It is now recognized that there are important systemic features of COPD, including cachexia, skeletal muscle wasting, anemia, and depression, which may also require treatment [19]. Therapy for cachexia with nutritional supplementation has not been proven to be effective, and a better understanding of mechanism is needed for development of rational therapies. In addition, there are often comorbid diseases with COPD, particularly cardiovascular disease and lung cancer, which are often the cause of death [20].

There is increasing interest in COPD in view of its rising global prevalence and major impact on health costs. No therapies have been shown to significantly reduce the progression of the disease, probably because none has an impact on the underlying chronic inflammatory process. Research into the underlying cellular and molecular mechanisms of COPD is expanding in an effort to identify new targets so that effective anti-inflammatory therapies may be developed [21]. Several new drugs are currently in clinical development, the most advanced being phosphodiesterase-4 inhibitors, which appear to have a broad spectrum of anti-inflammatory effects appropriate for COPD, with inhibitory effects on neutrophils, macrophages, monocytes, and T lymphocytes. It is assumed that anti-inflammatory treatments can reduce the progression of the disease and prevent exacerbations, although this will be known only when an effective anti-inflammatory therapy becomes available.

Why only a minority of smokers develop COPD is not certain, but this is likely explained by differences in genetic susceptibility [8]. However, the identity of the susceptibility genes is not yet known, and there are now intensive research efforts to identify polymorphisms of known and novel genes. COPD is likely a complex polygenic disease, so it will be difficult to identify susceptibility genes and how they interact with environmental factors such as cigarette smoke, but in the future it may be possible to predict which smokers will develop COPD at a much earlier stage. Profiling the expression of genes using gene array analysis and of different proteins by means of proteomics is of potential value in identifying abnormal expression patterns in COPD. This may allow more effective focusing of smoking cessation and risk reduction strategies, or perhaps the early use of anti-inflammatory therapies. Identification of susceptibility genes may also reveal new targets that could help in the development of new treatments.

COPD is a heterogeneous disease with variable contributions of emphysema, small airway disease, and mucus hypersecretion. Since cigarette smoking induces all these processes, they usually occur together, but in some patients one aspect may be predominant. This means that different treatment strategies may be needed. Currently it is difficult to distinguish these separate aspects of the disease. Emphysema may be quantified by high-resolution computed tomography (CT) and more crudely by transfer factor, but small airway disease is difficult to measure with existing techniques.

Clinical trials for COPD are difficult, as any improvement is small and in view of the variability of measurements large numbers of patients may be needed [22]. Because progression of the disease is so slow, any treatment must be assessed over at least 3 years, which poses a major problem for new classes of drugs whose long-term safety is unknown. There is a search for biomarkers of disease activity that may predict clinical efficacy and several potential biomarkers of disease activity are being investigated in sputum, exhaled breath, and blood [23].

COPD is now emerging from the shadows as a very important and growing global disease that deserves much more attention, with needs for improved diagnosis, better management, and new and more effective therapies.

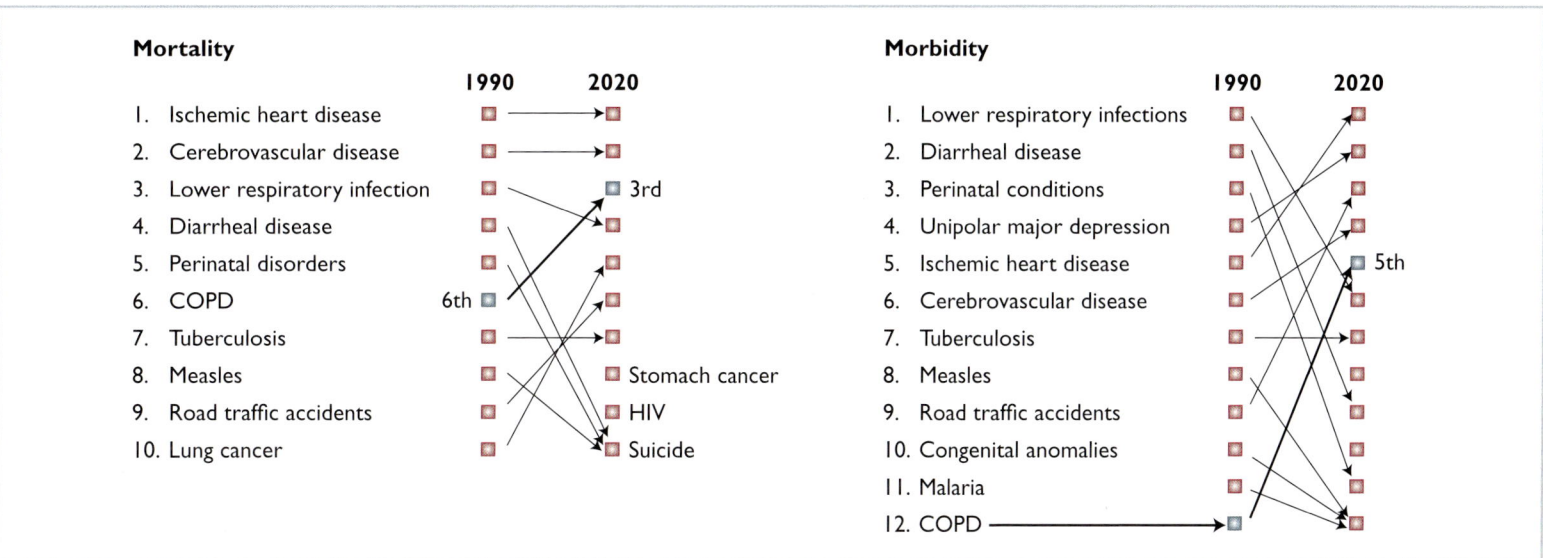

Figure 3-1. The rising global burden of chronic obstructive pulmonary disease (COPD). There has been an increase in COPD prevalence and mortality, even in industrialized countries, and COPD now represents a major worldwide health problem. The World Health Organization/World Bank analysis of the global impact of disease predicts that COPD will rise from the sixth to the third most common cause of death by 2020 [24]. In the United States COPD is the fourth most common cause of death and the only common cause of death that is rising. COPD is also an increasing cause of morbidity (measured by disability-adjusted life years, DALY), expected to rise from its current ranking of 12th most prevalent disease worldwide to the fifth position by 2020. Reasons for the dramatic increase in COPD include reduced mortality from other causes, such as cardiovascular diseases in industrialized countries and infectious diseases in developing countries, with a marked increase in cigarette smoking and environmental pollution in developing countries. There is also increased survival, so that more smokers live to develop COPD.

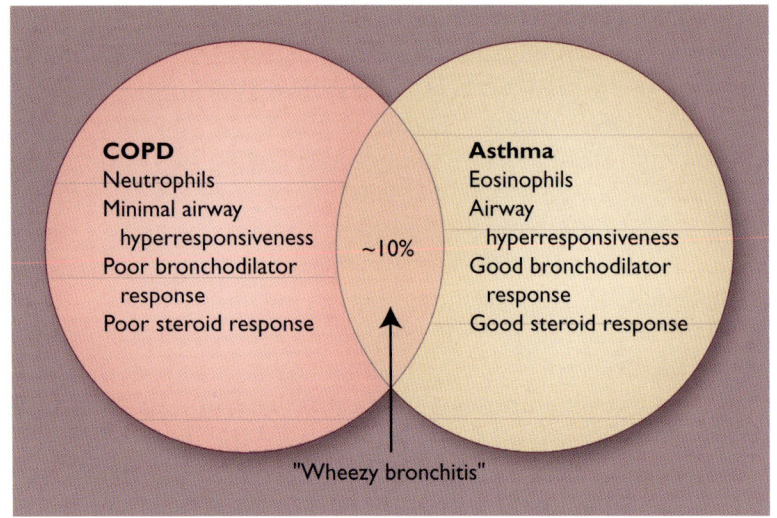

Figure 3-2. Overlap between chronic obstructive pulmonary disease (COPD) and asthma. Asthma and COPD are different diseases, but some patients have features of both diseases, which some have suggested represents a spectrum of a single disease (this is the essence of the "Dutch hypothesis"). Approximately 10% of patients with COPD have asthma and will share inflammatory features between these diseases. This overlap group may be termed "wheezy bronchitis." It is important to recognize these patients, as they may require treatment for both diseases to optimize symptom control.

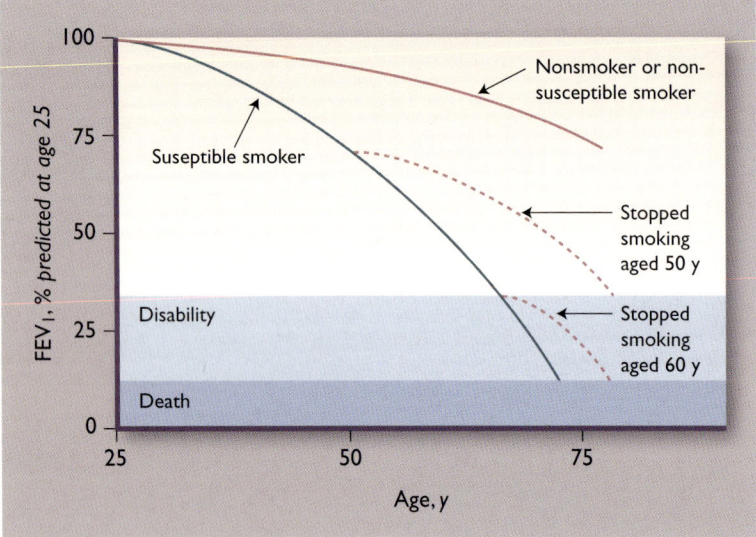

Figure 3-3. Natural history of chronic obstructive pulmonary disease (COPD). Annual decline in airway function showing accelerated decline in susceptible smokers and effects of smoking cessation. Patients with COPD usually show an accelerated annual decline in forced expiratory volume in 1 second (FEV_1), often greater than 50 mL/y, compared with the normal decline of approximately 20 mL/y, although this is variable between patients. The classic studies of Fletcher and Peto [25] established that 10% to 20% of cigarette smokers are susceptible to this rapid decline. However, with longer follow-up more smokers may develop COPD. The propensity to develop COPD among smokers is only weakly related to the number of cigarettes smoked, and this suggests that other factors play an important role in determining susceptibility. Most evidence points to genetic factors, although the genes determining susceptibility have not yet been determined. Long-term studies show that a greater proportion of smokers develop COPD when they are followed for longer periods.

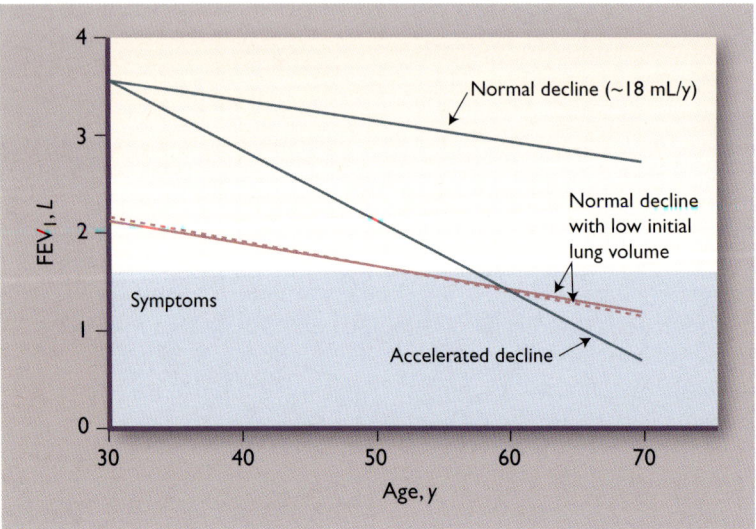

Figure 3-4. Annual decline in lung function. Patients with chronic obstructive pulmonary disease (COPD) may develop airway obstruction following an accelerated rate of decline or a normal rate of decline starting from low initial lung function. However some patients may have small lungs because of impaired fetal development, so that even a normal decline in lung function may lead to symptoms. Passive smoke inhalation during childhood may also impair lung growth and predispose one to develop COPD in later life.

Risk Factors in Chronic Obstructive Pulmonary Disease

Environmental	Endogenous
Cigarette smoking	Genetic factors (eg, α_1-AT deficiency)
Air pollution (indoor, outdoor)	Atopy, airway hyperresponsiveness?
Occupational exposure	Low birth weight
Diet (low antioxidants)	

Figure 3-5. Risk factors for chronic obstructive pulmonary disease (COPD). In industrialized countries cigarette smoking accounts for most cases of COPD, but in developing countries other environmental pollutants, such as particulates (wood smoke) associated with cooking with biomass fuels in confined spaces, are important causes. It is likely that there are important interactions between environmental factors and a genetic predisposition to develop the disease. Air pollution (particularly sulfur dioxide and particulates), exposure to certain occupational chemicals such as cadmium, and passive smoking may all be risk factors. The role of airway hyperresponsiveness and allergy as risk factors for COPD is still uncertain. Atopy, serum IgE, and blood eosinophilia are not important risk factors, but the Lung Health Study showed that airway responsiveness to inhaled methacholine was a predictor of accelerated decline in lung function over 5 years [26]. However, this is not necessarily the same type of abnormal airway responsiveness that is seen in asthma. Low birth weight is also a risk factor for COPD, probably because poor nutrition in fetal life results in small lungs, so that decline in lung function with age starts from a lower peak value (see Fig. 3-4).

Genetic Factors Implicated in Chronic Obstructive Pulmonary Disease

Candidate Genes	Risk
α_1-Antitrypsin	ZZ genotype, high risk
	MZ, SZ genotype, small risk
α_1-Chymotrypsin	Associated in some populations
MMP-1, -9, -12	Associated in some studies
Microsomal epoxide hydrolase	Increased risk
Glutathione S transferase	Increased risk
SERPINE 2	Increased risk
Heme oxygenase-1	Small risk
Vitamin D binding protein	Inconsistent
TNF-α promoter	Inconsistent
Interleukin-13	Small risk

Figure 3-6. Some of the genetic factors implicated in chronic obstructive pulmonary disease (COPD). Several linkages between COPD and candidate genes have been described [8]. These linkages are often weak and not confirmed by studies in other populations. This suggests that there are multiple genetic determinants of COPD, and it is likely that combinations of susceptibility genes are responsible for the increased risk of COPD among smokers. Powerful genome-wide association studies are now under way to identify these genes.

Figure 3-7. Mechanisms of airflow limitation in chronic obstructive pulmonary disease (COPD). The airway in normal subjects is distended by alveolar attachments during expiration, allowing alveolar emptying and lung deflation. In COPD these attachments are disrupted because of emphysema, which contributes to airway closure during expiration, trapping gas in the alveoli and resulting in hyperinflation [27]. Peripheral airways are also obstructed and distorted by inflammation and peribronchiolar fibrosis (chronic obstructive bronchiolitis) and by occlusion of the airway lumen by inflammatory exudate and mucus secretions, which may be trapped in the airways because of poor mucociliary clearance.

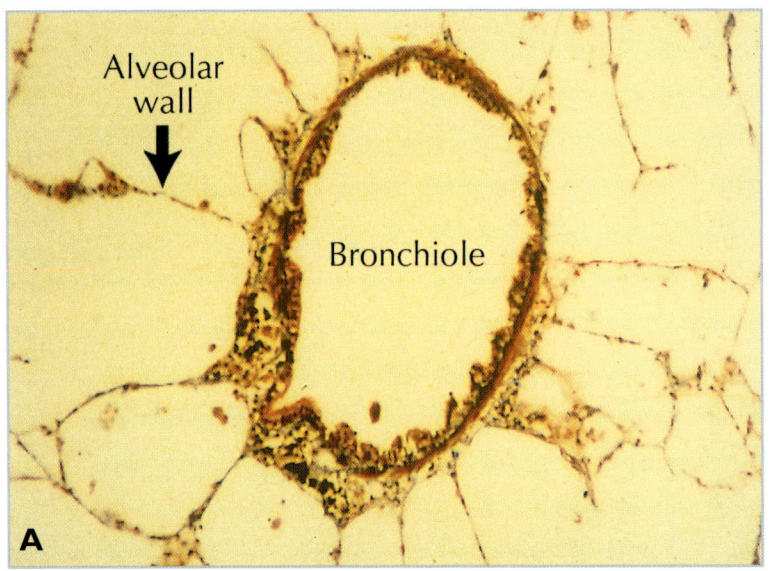
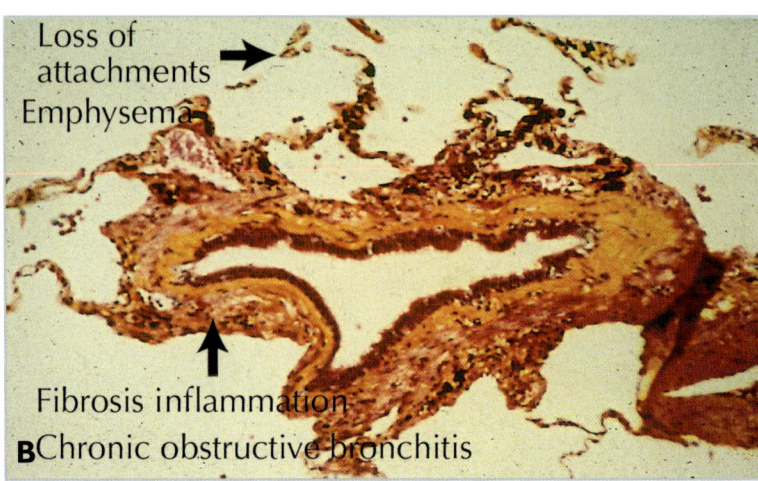

Figure 3-8. Peripheral lung pathology of chronic obstructive pulmonary disease (COPD). **A**, Peripheral airway of a normal subject with alveolar attachments intact. **B**, Thickening and distortion of a small airway with loss of alveolar attachments as a result of emphysema. (*Courtesy of* Dr. Manuel Cosio.)

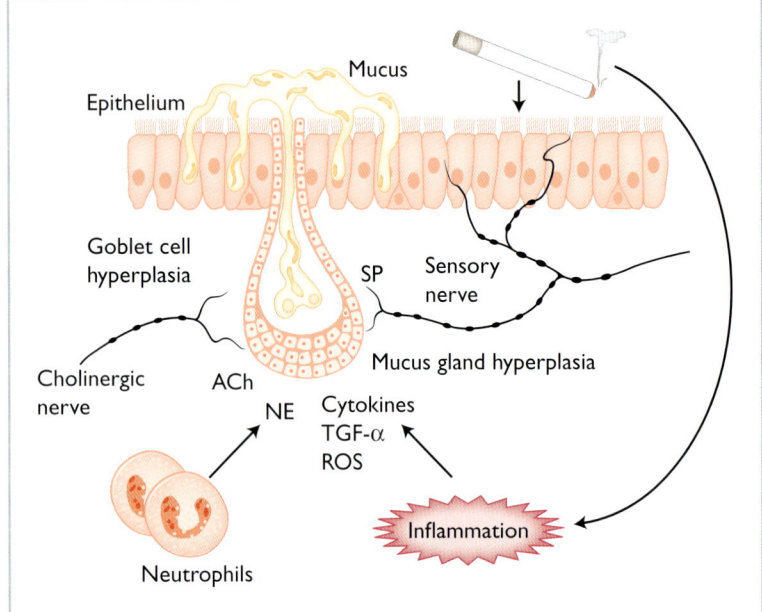

Figure 3-9. Mucus hypersecretion in chronic obstructive pulmonary disease (COPD). Mucus gland secretion may be stimulated via neural mechanisms and the release of acetylcholine (ACh) from cholinergic nerves and of substance P (SP) from sensory nerves [28]. Probably the most important stimulants of mucus secretion are neutrophil elastase (NE) from activated neutrophils and epithelial growth factor (EGF) receptor ligands such as transforming growth factor-α (TGF–α). Several stimulants of mucus hypersecretion, such as cigarette smoke and reactive oxygen species (ROS), also appear to activate EGF receptors [29].

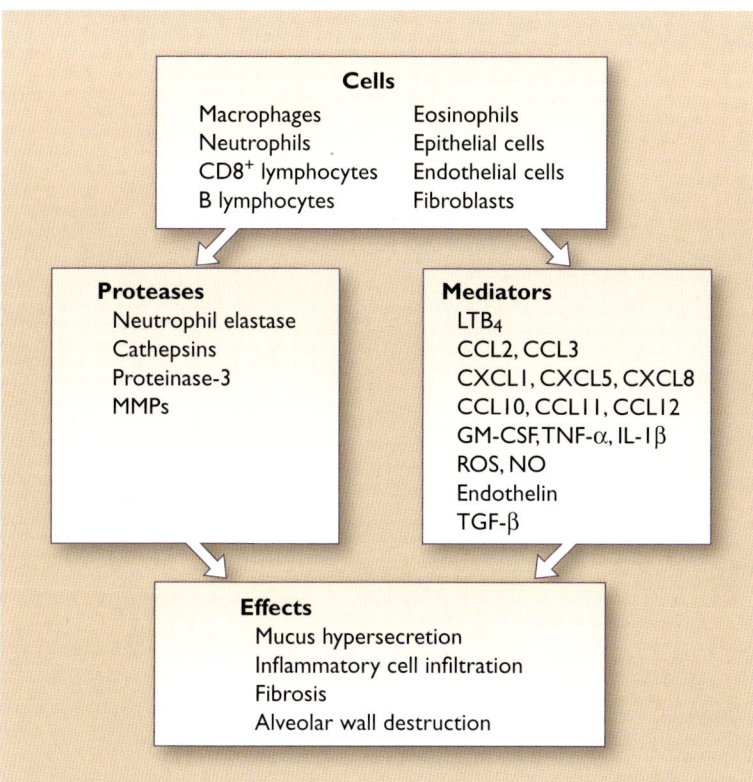

Figure 3-10. Inflammation in chronic obstructive pulmonary disease (COPD) is complex, with many activated inflammatory and structural cells that release multiple mediators [30], including lipid mediators such as the following:
- Leukotriene B_4 (LTB_4), which is a chemoattractant for neutrophils
- Chemokines such as
  - CCL2 and CCL3, which attract monocytes
  - CXCL8, CXCL1, and CXCL5, which attract neutrophils and monocytes
  - CXCL10, CXCL11, and CXCL12, which attract $CD8^+$ cells
- Reactive oxygen species (ROS) and nitric oxide (NO)
- Granulocyte-macrophage colony-stimulating factor (GM-CSF), which prolongs neutrophil survival
- Tumor necrosis factor (TNF)-α and interleukin (IL)-1β, which amplify inflammation by switching on multiple inflammatory genes and may also account for some of the systemic effects of the disease
- Endothelin and transforming growth factor-β (TGF-β), which induce fibrosis

In addition, multiple proteases are released that result in elastolysis, including the serine proteinases neutrophil elastase and proteinase C, cathepsins, and matrix metalloproteinases (MMPs). This combination of mediators that attract and activate inflammatory cells, and proteases that cause elastolysis and mucus hypersecretion, result in the typical pathophysiology of COPD.

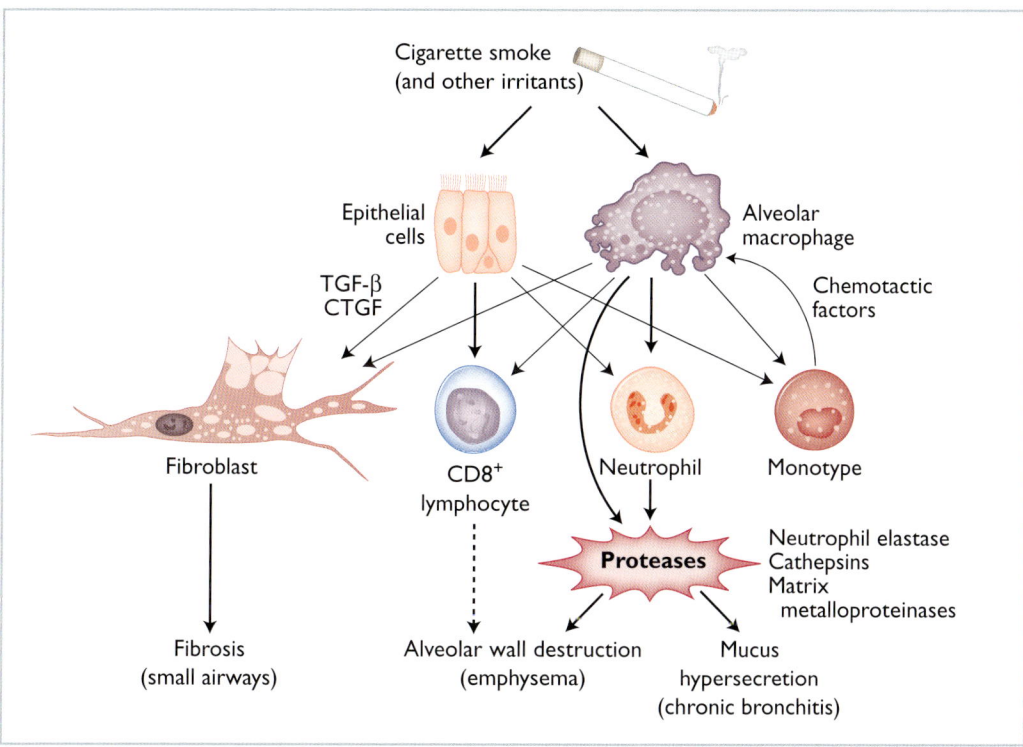

Figure 3-11. Inflammatory mechanisms in chronic obstructive pulmonary disease (COPD). Cigarette smoke and other inhaled irritants activate macrophages and epithelial cells in the respiratory tract to cause the release of multiple chemotactic factors, including chemokines and leukotriene B_4 (LTB_4), which recruit inflammatory cells (monocytes, neutrophils, and T lymphocytes) from the circulation into airways and lung parenchyma. These calls also release fibrogenic factors, such as transforming growth factor-β (TGF-β) and connective tissue growth factor (CTGF), that stimulate fibroblasts to cause fibrosis. Several cells release proteases that break down connective tissue in the lung parenchyma (particularly elastin), resulting in emphysema, and also stimulate mucus hypersecretion. Recruited cytotoxic T cells ($CD8^+$) may be involved in alveolar wall destruction through induction of apoptosis in type I pneumocytes.

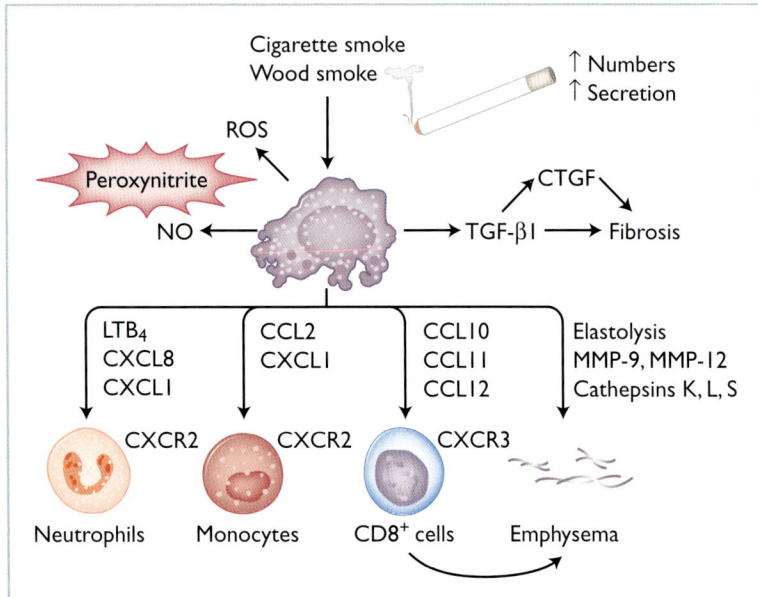

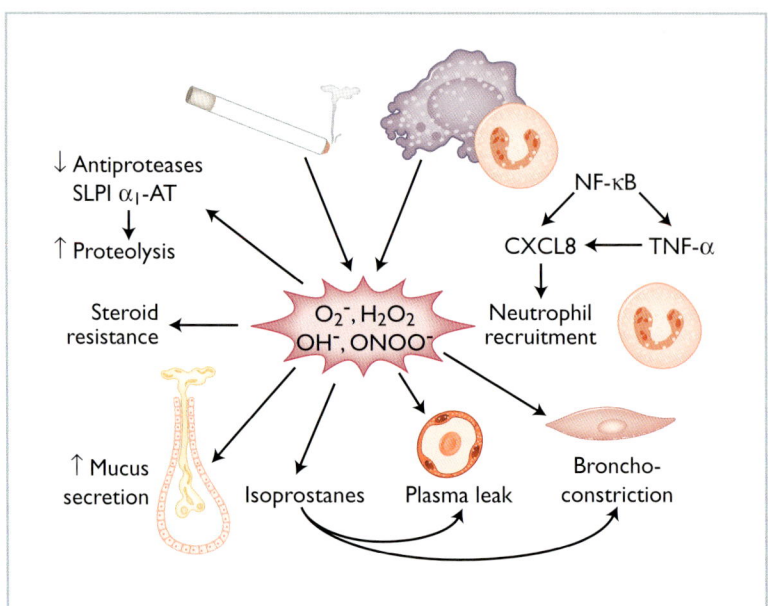

Figure 3-12. Macrophages in chronic obstructive pulmonary disease (COPD). Macrophages may play a pivotal role in COPD, as they are activated by cigarette smoke extract and secrete many inflammatory proteins that may orchestrate the inflammatory process in COPD. Neutrophils may be attracted by CXCL1, CXCL8, and leukotriene B_4 (LTB_4); monocytes by CCL2 and CXCL1; and $CD8^+$ lymphocytes by CCL10, CCL11, and CCL12. Release of elastolytic enzymes including matrix metalloproteinases (MMPs) and cathepsins cause elastolysis and release of transforming growth factor (TGF)-β1 and connective tissue growth factor (CTGF). Macrophages also generate reactive oxygen species (ROS) and nitric oxide (NO), which together form peroxynitrite and may contribute to steroid resistance.

Figure 3-13. Oxidative stress in chronic obstructive pulmonary disease (COPD). Oxidative stress plays a key role in the pathophysiology of COPD and amplifies the inflammatory and destructive process [31]. Reactive oxygen species from cigarette smoke or from inflammatory cells (particularly macrophages and neutrophils) produce several damaging effects in COPD, including decreased antiprotease defenses such as $α_1$-antitrypsin (AT) and secretory leukoprotease inhibitor (SLPI); activation of nuclear factor-κB (NF-κB), resulting in increased secretion of the cytokines interleukin-8 (IL-8) and tumor necrosis factor-α (TNF-α); increased production of isoprostanes; and direct effects on airway function. In addition, recent evidence suggests that oxidative stress induces steroid resistance [9].

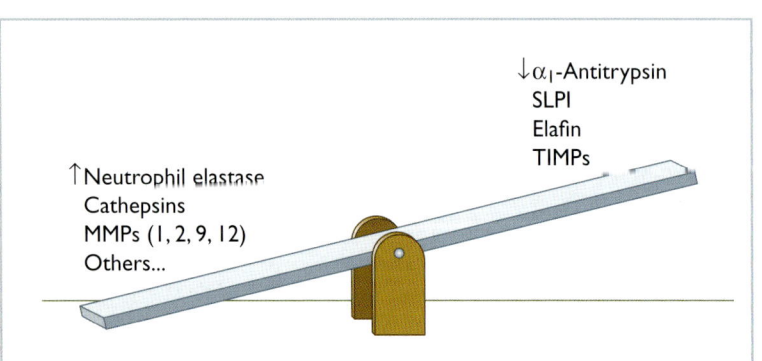

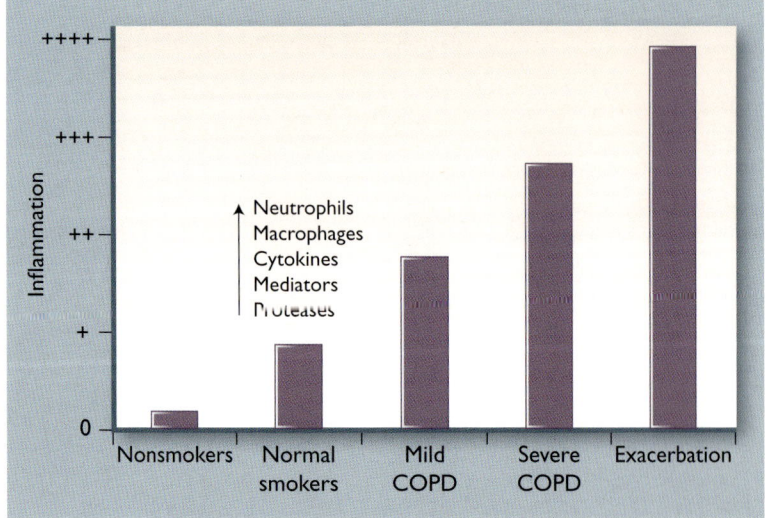

Figure 3-14. Protease-antiprotease imbalance in chronic obstructive pulmonary disease (COPD). In COPD the balance appears to be tipped in favor of increased proteolysis, either because of an increase in proteases, including neutrophil elastase, cathepsins, and matrix metalloproteinases (MMPs), or a deficiency in antiproteases, which may include $α_1$-antitrypsin, elafin, secretory leukoprotease inhibitor (SLPI), and tissue inhibitors of matrix metalloproteinases (TIMPs).

Figure 3-15. Amplification of lung inflammation in chronic obstructive pulmonary disease (COPD). Normal smokers have a mild inflammatory response, which represents the normal reaction of the respiratory tract to chronic inhalation of irritants. In COPD this same inflammatory response is markedly amplified, and this amplification increases as the disease progresses. It is further increased during exacerbations triggered by infective organisms. The molecular mechanisms of this amplification are currently unknown, but may be determined by genetic factors or possibly latent viral infection. Oxidative stress is an important amplifying mechanism and may increase the expression of inflammatory genes through impairing the activity of histone deacetylase 2 (HDAC2), which is needed to switch off inflammatory genes [9].

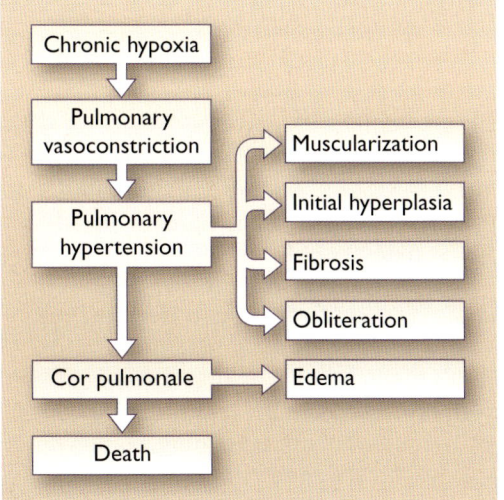

Figure 3-16. Vascular changes in chronic obstructive pulmonary disease (COPD). Chronic hypoxia results in hypoxic pulmonary vasoconstriction and over time leads to structural changes, resulting in secondary pulmonary hypertension. Over time this may lead to right heart failure (cor pulmonale), which has a poor prognosis, most patients surviving only 6 to 12 months.

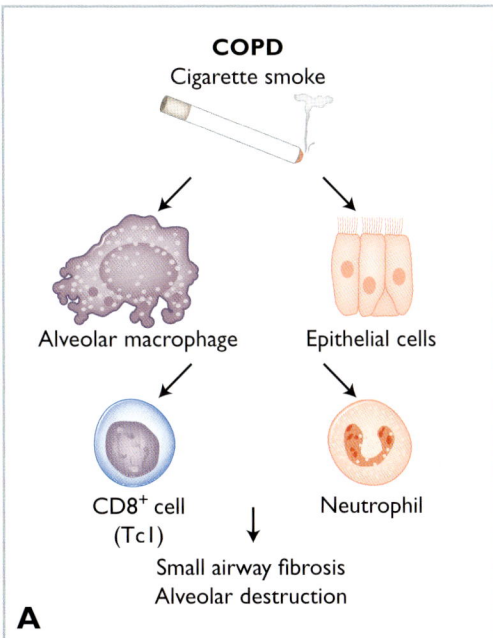
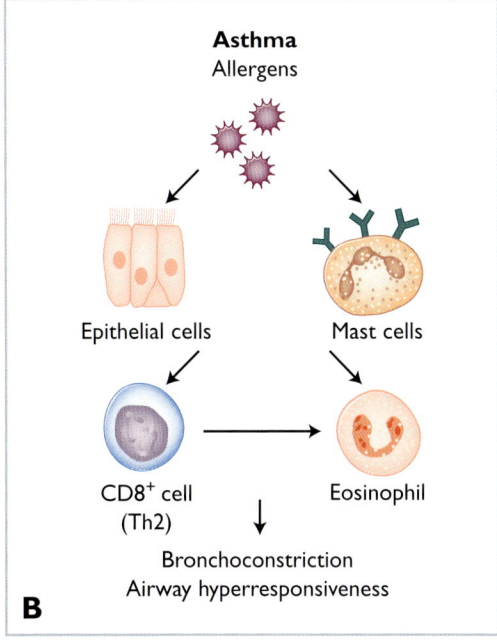

Figure 3-17. Chronic obstructive pulmonary disease (COPD) versus asthma. The pattern of inflammation differs markedly between COPD and asthma, and this underlies the different symptoms, clinical presentations, and responses to treatment of these diseases [32]. In COPD (**A**) the predominant inflammatory cells are neutrophils, macrophages, and $CD8^+$ (Tc1) lymphocytes, whereas in asthma (**B**) eosinophils, mast cells, and $CD4^+$ (Th2) lymphocytes predominate. In COPD this inflammatory pattern leads to slowly progressive airflow limitation, whereas in asthma the inflammation results in variable bronchoconstriction and airway hyperresponsiveness.

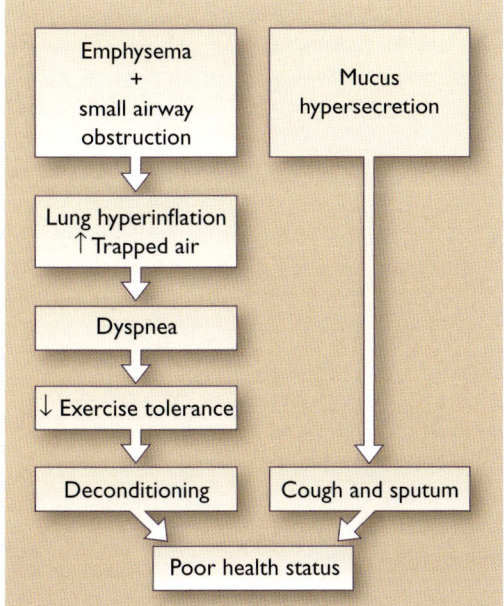

Figure 3-18. Symptoms of chronic obstructive pulmonary disease (COPD). The most prominent symptom of COPD is dyspnea, which is largely due to hyperinflation of the lungs as a result of small airway collapse due to emphysema and narrowing due to fibrosis, so that the alveoli are not able to empty. Hyperinflation induces an uncomfortable sensation and reduces exercise tolerance. This leads to immobility and deconditioning and results in poor health status. Other common symptoms of COPD are cough and sputum production as a result of mucus hypersecretion, although not all patients have these symptoms and many smokers with these symptoms do not have airflow obstruction (simple chronic bronchitis).

| Chronic Obstructive Pulmonary Disease |

Investigation of Chronic Obstructive Pulmonary Disease Patients

Indication	Test
Routine	FEV_1, FEV_1/FVC
	Bronchodilator response
	Chest radiograph
	TL_{CO}/K_{CO}
Moderate/severe COPD	Lung volumes
	SaO_2 and/or blood gases
	ECG
	Hemoglobin
Persistent purulent sputum	Sputum culture/sensitivity
Emphysema at young age	α_1-Antitrypsin, genotype if low
Assessment of bullae	CT scan
Disproportionate breathlessness	Exercise test
Suspected asthma	Trial of steroids
	PEF monitoring
	Airway responsiveness
Suspected sleep apnea	Nocturnal sleep study

Figure 3-19. Investigation of chronic obstructive pulmonary disease (COPD) patients. Spirometry is important for initial diagnosis and assessment of severity, but less useful in assessing disability during routine follow-up as it is poorly related to symptoms. A chest radiograph should be obtained at the initial assessment. A bronchodilator test is also important; typically COPD patients have less than a 12% (or <200 mL) increase after a short-acting bronchodilator. However, if the bronchodilator response is pronounced, this usually signifies concomitant asthma and predicts a better response to steroid therapy. Often there is no bronchodilator response, yet these patients still benefit symptomatically from bronchodilators as a result of the reduction in hyperinflation and residual volume. In more severe patients it may be useful to measure lung volume, particularly total lung capacity and residual volume. Inspiratory capacity is more closely related to symptoms than is forced expiratory volume in 1 second (FEV_1). Checking arterial blood gases is also indicated in more severe patients and is critical in assessing the need for supplementary oxygen therapy. Other tests may be indicated if there is suspected asthma or sleep apnea. A course of oral steroids is very useful in identifying an asthmatic component. ECG—electrocardiogram; FVC—forced vital capacity; PEF—peak expiratory flow.

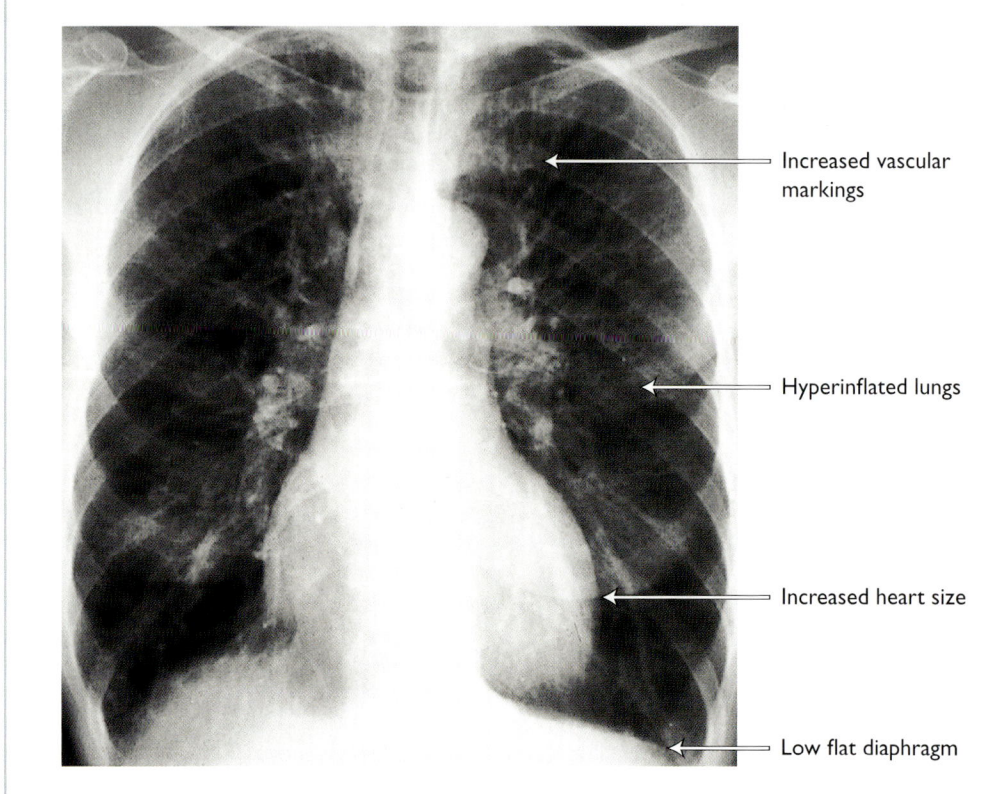

Figure 3-20. Chest radiograph of patient with chronic obstructive pulmonary disease (COPD). The lungs are hyperinflated, the diaphragm is flattened, vascular markings are increased, and the heart size is marginally increased. A chest radiograph is also useful in identifying pulmonary infections and pneumothorax during acute exacerbations. A chest radiograph is also used to detect lung cancer and should be performed if there is a change in the usual symptoms because COPD patients are at increased risk of lung cancer.

Atlas of Pulmonary Medicine

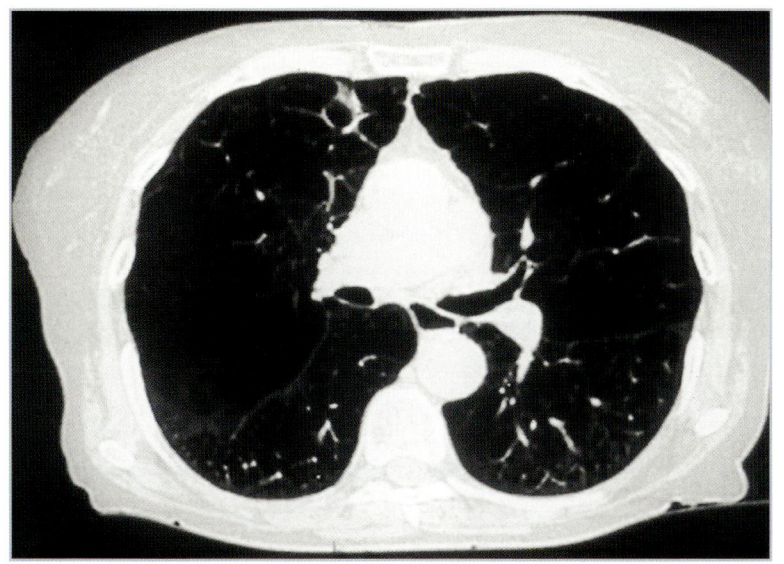

Figure 3-21. High-resolution computed tomography (CT) scan of emphysema. There is reduced density of the lungs with enlarged air spaces. A high-resolution CT scan is useful to confirm a diagnosis of emphysema, to identify bullae, to assess the distribution of emphysema before lung surgery, and to detect concomitant bronchiectasis, which may account for excessive purulent mucus production. It is also useful for detecting lung cancer.

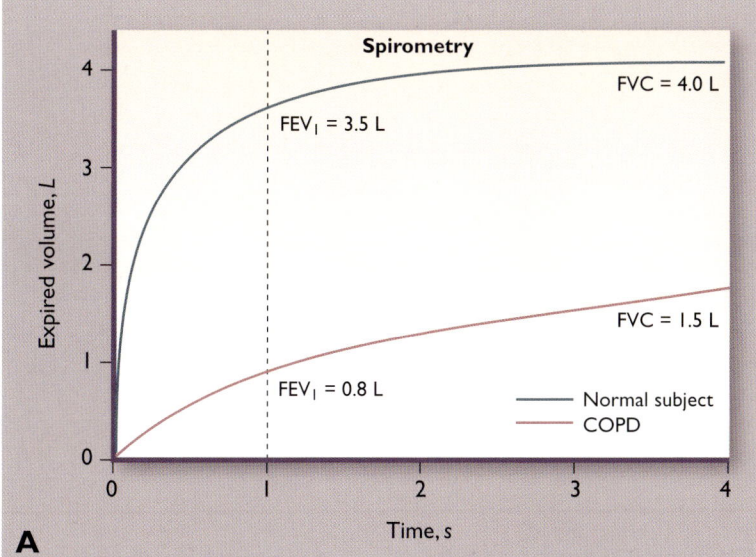
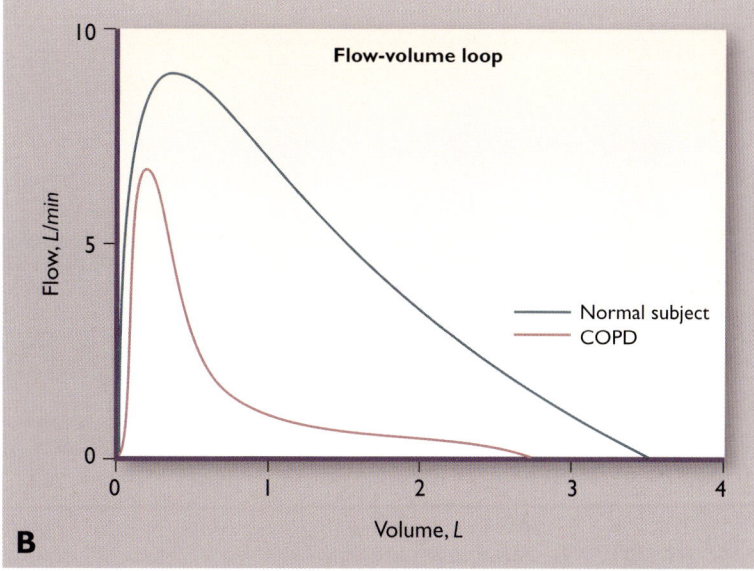

Figure 3-22. Lung function in chronic obstructive pulmonary disease (COPD). **A**, Spirometry shows a marked reduction in forced expiratory volume in 1 second (FEV_1), forced vital capacity (FVC), and FEV_1/FVC ratio (<70%) in COPD patients. Severity of COPD is defined by the percent predicted FEV_1. **B**, Flow-volume curve showing a marked reduction in expiratory flow with a relatively preserved peak expiratory flow in COPD patients.

Severity of Chronic Obstructive Pulmonary Disease

Lung Function Test	Result
FEV_1, L	Decreased
FVC, L	Decreased
FEV_1/FVC ratio, %	Decreased
Peak expiratory flow, L/min	Decreased
Total lung capacity, L	Increased
Inspiratory capacity, L	Decreased
Functional residual capacity, L	Increased
Residual volume, L	Increased
Specific airway conductance, $cm\ H_2O^{-1} \times sec^{-1}$	Decreased
Transfer factor, mL/min/mm Hg	Decreased
Transfer coefficient, mL/min/mm Hg/L	Decreased

Figure 3-23. Severity of chronic obstructive pulmonary disease (COPD). The severity of COPD is based on spirometry, and the divisions between different grades of severity are arbitrary and differ between different guidelines. The figure shows the divisions of severity based on the Global Initiative for Chronic Obstructive Lung Disease (GOLD) guidelines [5], which are useful in determining the progression of therapy. Severity progresses slowly in most patients, necessitating more intense therapy with time. FEV_1—forced expiratory volume in 1 second; FVC—forced vital capacity.

Lung Function in Chronic Obstructive Pulmonary Disease

Severity	Signs
I Mild	± Chronic symptoms (cough, sputum)
	$FEV_1/FVC < 70\%$, $FEV_1 > 80\%$ predicted
II Moderate	Chronic symptoms (cough, sputum, dyspnea)
	$FEV_1/FVC < 70\%$, $FEV_1 < 80\%$; 50% predicted
III Severe	Chronic symptoms (cough, sputum, dyspnea)
	$FEV_1/FVC < 70\%$, $FEV_1 < 50\%$; 30% predicted
IV Very severe	Chronic symptoms (cough, sputum, dyspnea)
	$FEV_1 < 30\%$ predicted
	Or respiratory insufficiency/right heart failure

Figure 3-24. Lung function in chronic obstructive pulmonary disease (COPD). Spirometry is useful in establishing the diagnosis and severity of COPD but does poorly in relation to symptoms. Plethysmography measurements show an increase in total lung capacity (TLC), functional residual capacity (FRC), and residual volume (RV), reflecting lung hyperinflation. This results in a reduced inspiratory capacity that can be measured by spirometry and correlates better with symptoms. Plethysmography also shows an increase in airway resistance and a reduction in specific airway conductance. Gas diffusion measurements show a reduction in total lung transfer of carbon monoxide (TL_{CO}) and TL_{CO} corrected for alveolar volume (K_{CO}), which reflect the extent of emphysema. FEV_1—forced expiratory volume in 1 second; FVC—forced vital capacity.

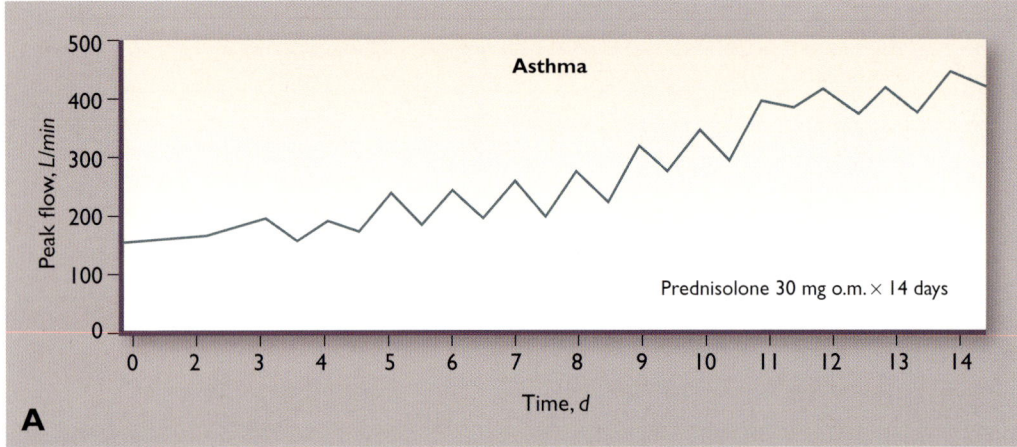

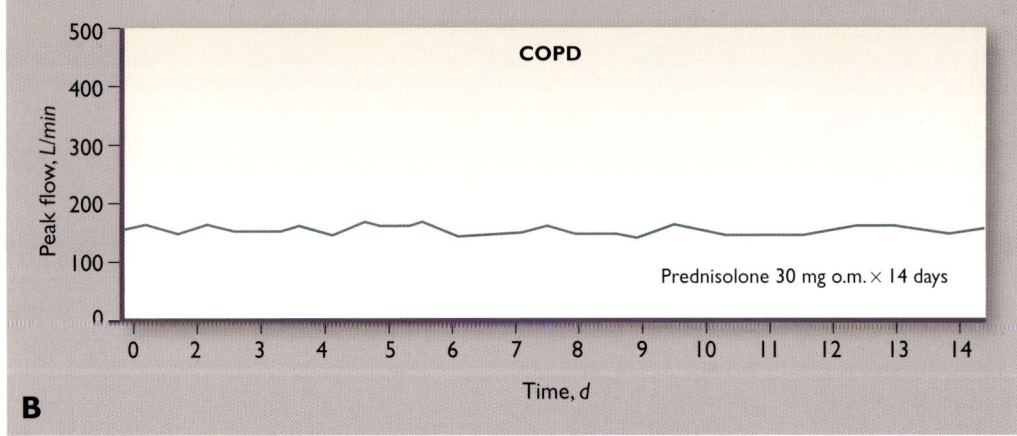

Figure 3-25. Trial of steroids. Oral prednisone (30 mg daily for 14 days) produces a marked improvement in patients with asthma (**A**) but has no effect on lung function in patients with chronic obstructive pulmonary disease (COPD) (**B**). This is a useful test to assess the degree of associated asthma and is a useful predictor of response to inhaled steroids.

Systemic Features of Chronic Obstructive Pulmonary Disease

Systemic Feature	Possible Mechanism
Cachexia	TNF-α, IL-6, leptin
Muscle wasting	Apoptosis of skeletal muscle due to TNF-α?
Polycythemia	Chronic hypoxia
Anemia (normocytic)	TNF-α?
Depression	TNF-α, IL-6
Cardiovascular abnormalities	CRP, fibrinogen?
Osteoporosis	Effect of corticosteroid therapy; effect of cytokines

Figure 3-26. Systemic features of chronic obstructive pulmonary disease (COPD). Patients with severe COPD may develop systemic features that include weight loss (cachexia), lassitude, muscle wasting with apoptosis of skeletal muscles, polycythemia (secondary to hypoxia), anemia (usually normochromic normocytic anemia of chronic disease) and depression [19]. Some of these changes are due to release of cytokines, such as tumor necrosis factor (TNF)-α and interleukin (IL)-6 in the systemic circulation. Cardiovascular abnormalities are also common in severe disease and may be due to cigarettes smoking, but also to mediators such as C-reactive protein (CRP) and fibrinogen. Patients who develop systemic features have a poor prognosis, with survival usually less than 12 months.

Aims of Therapy

- Prevent disease progression
- Reduce symptoms
- Improve exercise tolerance
- Improve health status
- Prevent and treat exacerbations
- Prevent mortality

Figure 3-27. Aims of therapy. In managing chronic obstructive pulmonary disease (COPD) there are several aims of therapy.

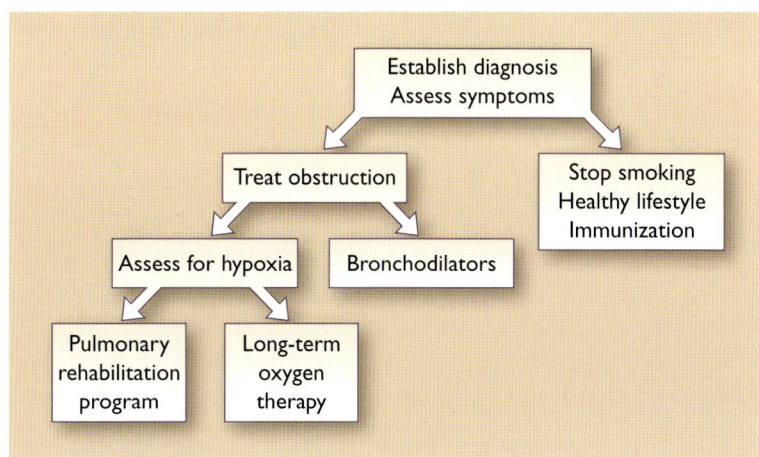

Figure 3-28. Treatment strategy in chronic obstructive pulmonary disease (COPD). All patients should be encouraged to stop smoking and should also receive influenza and pneumococcal vaccinations. The mainstay of treatment is the use of bronchodilators to reduce symptoms. Bronchodilators may improve symptoms by deflating the lungs, even without any significant change in spirometry. In more severe patients pulmonary rehabilitation may be very helpful in improving health and reducing hospitalization stays. For patients with respiratory failure or right heart failure long-term oxygen therapy is indicated.

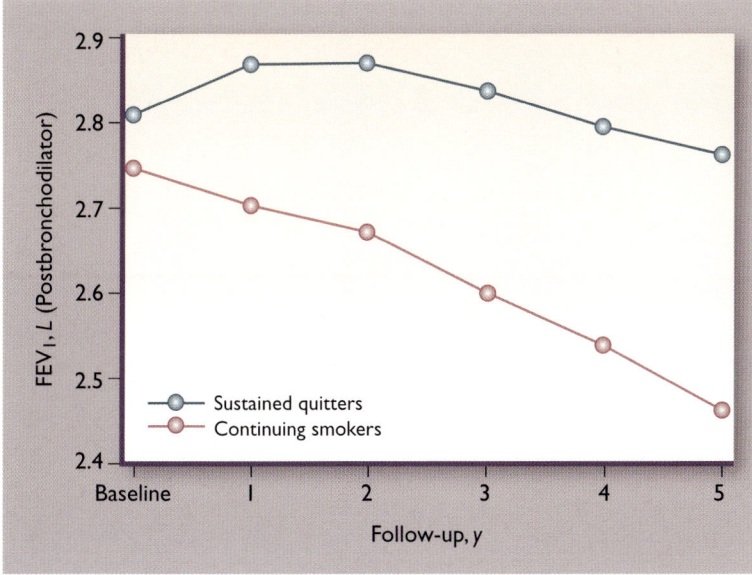

Figure 3-29. Smoking cessation. Stopping smoking is the single most beneficial management strategy and the only intervention that reduces the rate of decline in lung function [33]. Nicotine addiction is the problem, and treatment should be directed at dealing with this addictive state. The major approaches have involved behavioral modification and nicotine replacement therapy, but the overall rates of quitting are low (5%–15%). Abrupt cessation is more successful that gradual reduction, but even after an intensive smoking cessation program, over 75% of smokers are still smoking 1 year later. There are several ways to encourage smoking cessation. Psychological counseling and smoking reduction clinics may be useful; advice from doctors, structured interventions from nurses, and individual and group counseling are all effective. Group therapy may help some patients. Nicotine replacement therapy doubles long-term (6–12 months) abstinence rates. Several treatment forms are available, all of which have some effect. Nicotine chewing gum is the most widely used but the least effective, and skin patches are more successful. Hypnosis and acupuncture may be helpful in some patients, but controlled trials have demonstrated that they are ineffective. Bupropion is an atypical antidepressant that is similar in efficacy to nicotine replacement therapies, but sustained quit rates at 12 months are only about 15% in chronic obstructive pulmonary disease (COPD) patients. Varenicline is a new partial $\alpha_4\beta_2$ nicotinic agonist that appears to be the most effective antismoking therapy, with 1 year quit rates around 25%, and is relatively well tolerated [34].

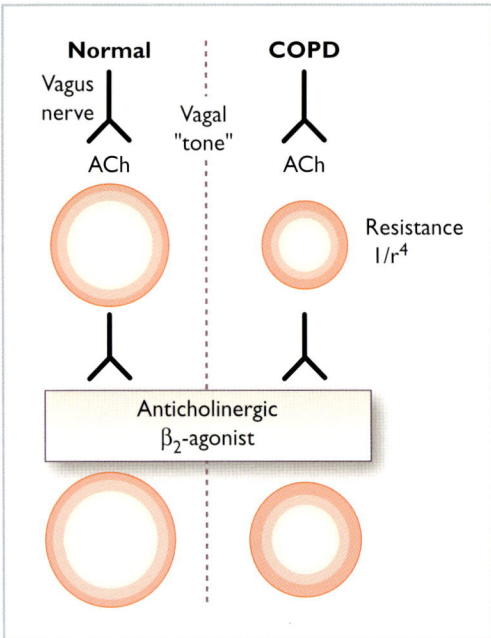

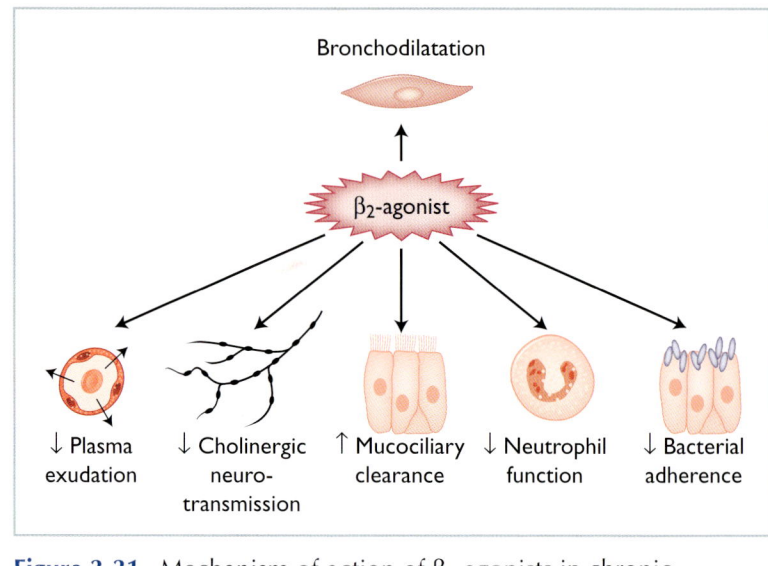

Figure 3-30. Rationale for anticholinergics in chronic obstructive pulmonary disease (COPD). Normally there is a certain amount of cholinergic tone, but this has little effect on airway resistance. The effect of this tone is exaggerated in COPD because of geometric factors related to the fixed narrowing of the airways, so that airway resistance improves to a greater extent than in a normal airway with an anticholinergic drug. Cholinergic tone is the only reversible component of COPD, and anticholinergic bronchodilators have a comparable or even greater effect than β_2-agonists. β_2-Agonists are also effective in reversing the effects of cholinergic tone, as they are functional antagonists. Anticholinergics may have some beneficial effect in reducing mucus hypersecretion. ACh—acetylcholine.

Figure 3-31. Mechanism of action of β_2-agonists in chronic obstructive pulmonary disease (COPD). Although their primary action is likely to be on airway smooth muscle, these agonists are associated with several additional effects that may be beneficial in COPD, including reduction in plasma exudation, inhibition of cholinergic tone, inhibition of neutrophils, stimulation of mucociliary clearance, and inhibitory effects on bacterial adhesion.

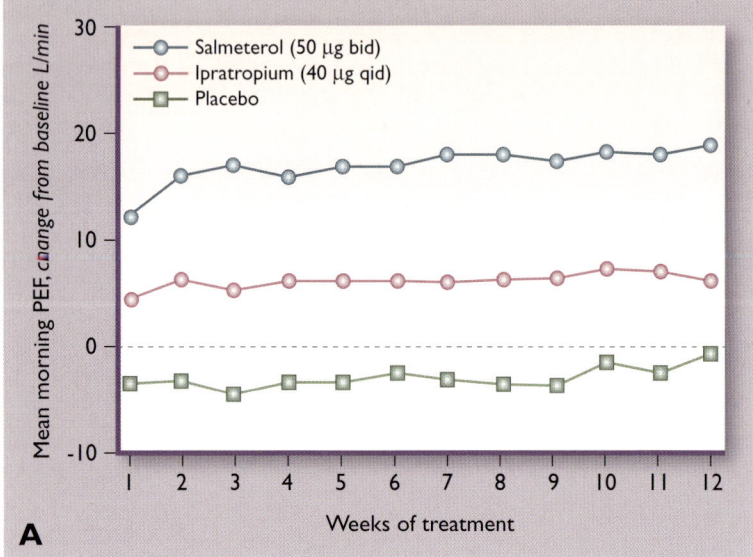

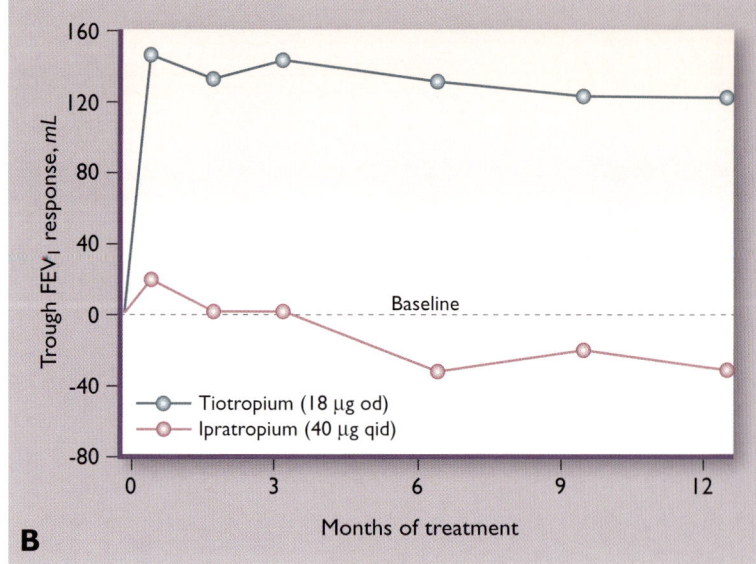

Figure 3-32. Long-acting bronchodilators. Long-acting bronchodilators are more effective than regular short-acting bronchodilators and are now the bronchodilators of choice. **A**, The superior effect of the long-acting β_2-agonist salmeterol compared with the short-acting ipratropium bromide [35]. **B**, The effect of the long-acting anticholinergic drug tiotropium bromide compared with ipratropium bromide [36]. b/l—baseline; bid—twice a day; FEV_1—forced expiratory volume in 1 second; od—once a day; PEF—peak expiratory flow; qid—four times a day.

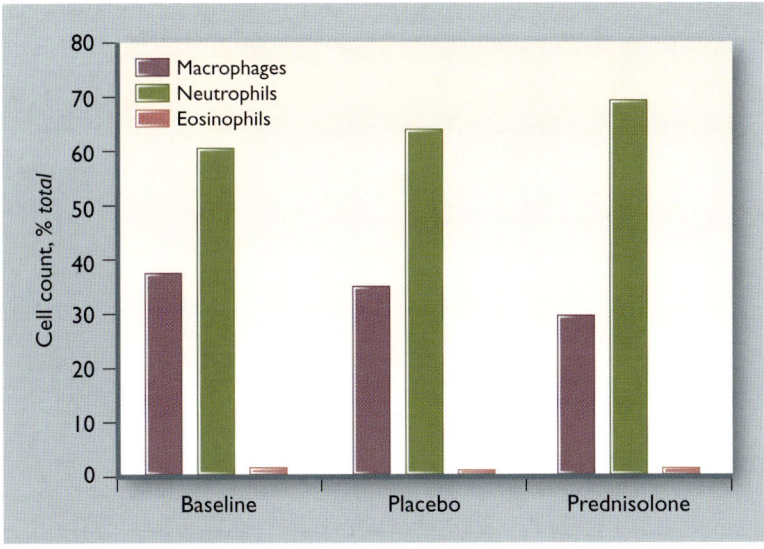

Figure 3-33. Ineffectiveness of oral steroids on inflammation in chronic obstructive pulmonary disease (COPD). Oral prednisolone (30 mg for 14 days) or high doses of inhaled steroids have no effect on inflammatory cells in induced sputum of patients with COPD [37]. Inhaled corticosteroids also have no effect on cytokines, chemokines, or proteases that would normally be inhibited by corticosteroids, which indicates that there is an active resistance to steroids in COPD patients. This is seen even at the level of single cells, such as alveolar macrophages, which are resistant to the effects of corticosteroids in vitro [38]. This may explain why inhaled corticosteroids showed no effect on the annual decline in lung function in four large studies over a 3-year period in patients with mild and moderate COPD [39].

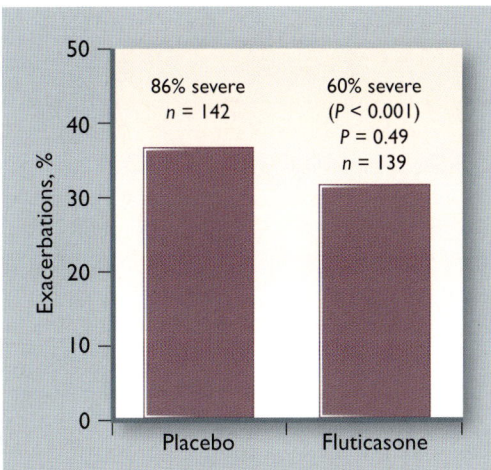

Figure 3-34. Effect of an inhaled corticosteroid on exacerbations of chronic obstructive pulmonary disease (COPD). Fluticasone propionate (500 µg twice a day) is overall effective in reducing exacerbations of COPD, but in patients with severe COPD there is a significant reduction [40]. This has led to the recommendation that inhaled corticosteroids may be added to bronchodilator therapy in patients with severe COPD who have frequent (>2/y) exacerbations.

Recommendations for Long-term Oxygen Therapy

Absolute indications: COPD, hypoxemia, edema

FEV_1 < 1.5 L, FVC < 2 L

PaO_2 < 55 mm Hg (7.3 kPa); $PaCO_2$ > 45 mm Hg (6 kPa)

Stability demonstrated over 2 wk

As above, without edema or $PaCO_2$ > 45 mm Hg

Palliation

Figure 3-35. Long-term oxygen therapy (LTOT). Because LTOT is expensive, patients should be carefully assessed before this therapy is recommended. The recommendations for LTOT are shown in the figure. LTOT should be given for at least 15 hours a day to achieve benefit. It is most efficiently provided by an oxygen concentrator or by a liquid oxygen supply and nasal prongs set at a flow of 2 to 4 L/min. Patients on LTOT should be reassessed regularly. LTOT can improve quality of life and is the only therapy so far shown to reduce chronic obstructive pulmonary disease (COPD) mortality. FEV_1—forced expiratory volume in 1 second; FVC—forced vital capacity.

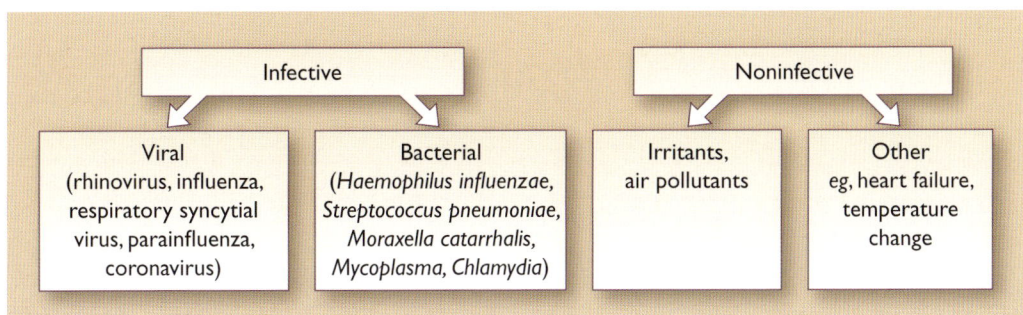

Figure 3-36. Acute exacerbations of chronic obstructive pulmonary disease (COPD). Acute exacerbations may be due to bacterial or viral infections, or to noninfective causes, such as air pollution and temperature change, that are poorly understood [41]. Acute exacerbations are associated with an increase in airway inflammation, resulting in increased purulence of sputum, worsened symptoms (dyspnea, cough), and reduced health status that may last several weeks. They account for a large proportion of the health care costs of COPD, and prevention of exacerbations an important goal of treatment.

Management of Acute Exacerbations

- Controlled oxygen therapy (24% or 28%)
- Nebulized bronchodilators
- Antibiotics
- Oral corticosteroids
- Noninvasive positive pressure ventilation
- Chest physiotherapy?

Figure 3-37. Management of acute exacerbations. Oxygen (24% or 28% via Venturi mask) should be given to achieve a PaO_2 of at least 50 mm Hg (6.6 kPa) without a fall in pH to less than 7.26 (indicating an acute change) and blood gases checked within 1 hour of starting oxygen therapy. Oxygen saturation by pulse oximetry may be used to monitor response providing that $PaCO_2$ and pH are normal. Bronchodilators (ipratropium bromide, 0.25–0.5 mg, plus salbutamol, 2.5–5 mg) should be given by nebulization four to six times an hour and continued for 24 to 48 hours. If there is no response, intravenous aminophylline should be added (0.5 mg/kg/h). Antibiotics should be started if indicated (as above). In severe exacerbations sputum culture should be done to check for antibiotic sensitivity. Oral corticosteroids are indicated for a severe exacerbation (prednisolone, 30 mg daily for 7–14 days). A course of oral steroids in the first 72 hours speeds recovery and reduces hospital stay. However, side effects may be a problem, and there is no evidence of any long-term benefit. Noninvasive positive pressure ventilation is useful in treating respiratory failure associated with acute exacerbations and reduces the need for intubation and reduces mortality. Diuretics are indicated if there is peripheral edema. Chest physiotherapy may be useful (but there is no evidence from controlled studies that it improves recovery).

Surgical Intervention and the NETT Trial

Surgical Intervention	NETT Trial
Lung transplantation	1218 patients
SLT	Mortality
Bilateral sequential SLT	16% -
Heart-lung transplantation	FEV_1 < 20% +
Bullectomy	Homogenous disease
Lung volume reduction surgery	or TL_{CO} < 20%
	Remainder
	UZ emphysema & < 25W (RR 0.47)
	Non-UZ & > 24W (F) > 40W (M) (RR 2.06)
	Exercise
	Increase by 10W at 2 years
	Surgery 16%
	Medical 3%

Figure 3-38. Surgical intervention. Originally heart-lung transplantation was used in patients with end-stage emphysema, but more recently single lung transplantation (SLT) has become the favored technique in view of the difficulty of obtaining donor organs and improvements in lung preservation and anesthetic management [42]. There is a severe limitation related to the availability of donor lungs. Because of problems with residual infection in the remaining lung and of hyperinflation of the existing lung if there is extensive bullous disease, heart-lung transplantation or preferably bilateral sequential SLT is used in patients with these complications. There is still controversy over the indications for bullectomy, and good results depend on careful patient selection. The ideal patient is young with a large bulla and minimal airway obstruction. In patients with chronic obstructive pulmonary disease (COPD) the problem is that surgical removal of one bulla leads to growth of other bullae as the emphysematous lung expands.

Lung volume reduction surgery has become popular for the treatment of severe emphysema. This involves resection of peripheral portions of both lungs to remove severely affected areas, which allows the remaining lung tissue to ventilate more effectively. This results in an increase in forced expiratory volume in 1 second (FEV_1) and a reduction in residual volume, with decreased dyspnea, improved exercise tolerance, and improved quality of life. Careful patient selection is essential, and patients with predominantly upper lobe involvement appear to do best.

The recent National Emphysema Treatment trial (NETT) showed the best effects in patients with upper zone (UZ) emphysema and impaired exercise performance, and a high mortality in patients with poor lung function and homogeneous disease [43]. Bronchoscopic lung volume reduction is currently under investigation using special valve implants to occlude airways as an alternative to surgical resection and has a lower mortality [44]. F—female; M—male; TL_{CO}—total lung transfer of carbon monoxide; W—watts.

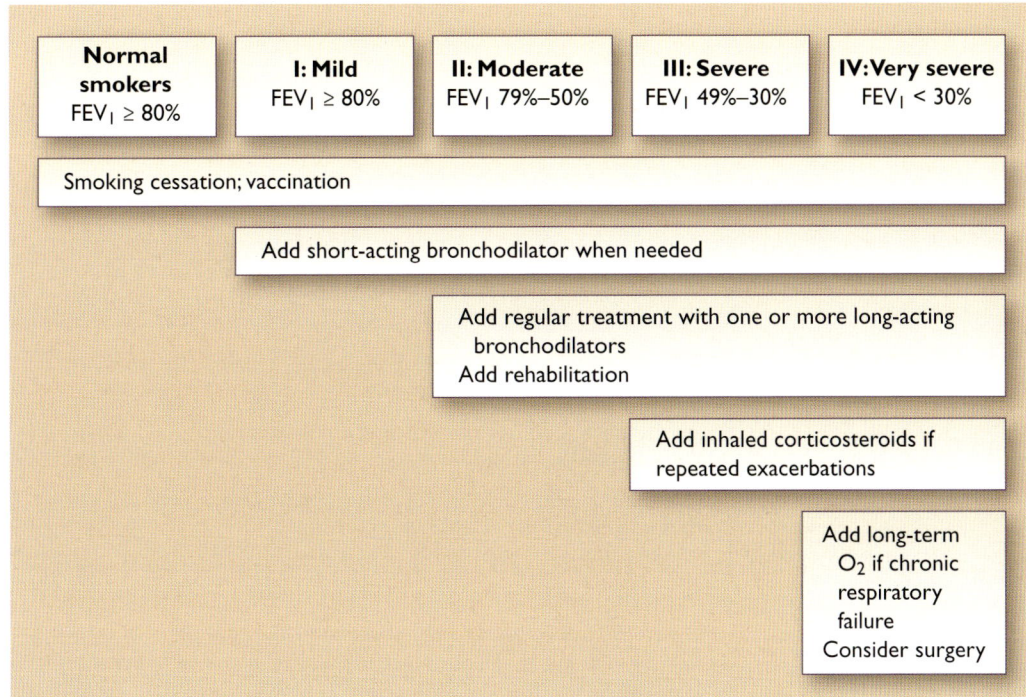

Figure 3-39. Stepwise approach to chronic obstructive pulmonary disease (COPD) therapy. Management of COPD involves increasing the intensity of treatment depending on the increasing severity of the disease [5]. Long-acting bronchodilators are indicated in patients with moderate disease who are symptomatic, together with pulmonary rehabilitation. In severe disease an inhaled steroid may be added if there are frequent exacerbations, and this is conveniently given as a combination inhaler containing a long-acting β_2-agonist and corticosteroid. Long-term oxygen therapy and surgery are considerations in patients with very severe disease. FEV_1—forced expiratory volume in 1 second.

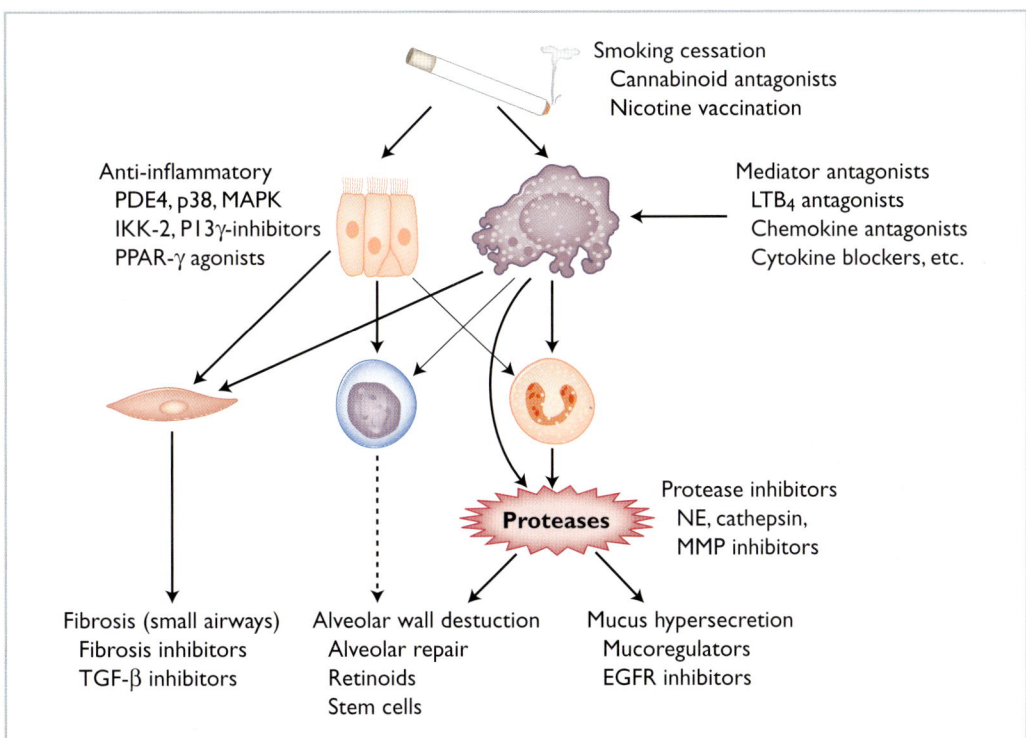

Figure 3-40. New treatments for chronic obstructive pulmonary disease (COPD). Many new treatments for COPD are now in development based on logical targets revealed by a better understanding of cellular and molecular mechanisms involved in disease pathogenesis [21,45]. More effective smoking cessation drugs are needed. Antagonists of specific mediators, such as leukotriene B_4 (LTB_4), and chemokine receptors, such as CXCL2, are in clinical trial but may be too specific. Inhibition of specific cytokines is currently being evaluated, but blocked tumor necrosis factor (TNF)-α has not been effective. Other approaches include inhibiting proteases (elastases) such as neutrophil elastase, cathepsins, or matrix metalloproteinases. Drugs with a broader spectrum of anti-inflammatory effects, such as phosphodiesterase (PDE)-4 inhibitors or inhibitors of signal transduction pathways, such as inhibitors of nuclear factor-κB kinase (IKK2), p38 mitogen activated protein kinase (MAPK), or phosphoinositide-3-kinase (PI3K), are promising. Drugs that inhibit transforming growth factor-β (TGF-β) may inhibit the fibrosis in small airways. There are also approaches to repair emphysema using retinoids (which are effective in rodent lungs) and stem cells. CACC—calcium-activated chloride channel; EGFR—epidermal growth factor receptor.

REFERENCES

1. Lopez AD, Shibuya K, Rao C, *et al.*: Chronic obstructive pulmonary disease: current burden and future projections. *Eur Respir J* 2006, 27:397–412.

2. Barnes PJ: Chronic obstructive pulmonary disease: a growing but neglected epidemic. *PLoS Med* 2007, 4:e112.

3. Chapman KR, Mannino DM, Soriano JB, *et al.*: Epidemiology and costs of chronic obstructive pulmonary disease. *Eur Respir J* 2006, 27:188–207.

4. Barnes PJ: New concepts in COPD. *Ann Rev Med* 2003, 54:113–129.

5. Rabe KF, Hurd S, Anzueto A, *et al.*: Global strategy for the diagnosis, management, and prevention of COPD: 2006 update. *Am J Respir Crit Care Med* 2007, 176:532–555.

6. Saetta M, Turato G, Maestrelli P, *et al.*: Cellular and structural bases of chronic obstructive pulmonary disease. *Am J Respir Crit Care Med* 2001, 163:1304–1309.

7. Barnes PJ, Shapiro SD, Pauwels RA: Chronic obstructive pulmonary disease: molecular and cellular mechanisms. *Eur Respir J* 2003, 22:672–688.

8. Silverman EK: Progress in chronic obstructive pulmonary disease genetics. *Proc Am Thorac Soc* 2006, 3:405–408.

9. Barnes PJ: Reduced histone deacetylase in COPD: clinical implications. *Chest* 2006, 129:151–155.

10. Calverley PM, Walker P: Chronic obstructive pulmonary disease. *Lancet* 2003, 362:1053–1061.

11. Chapman KR, Mannino DM, Soriano JB, *et al.*: Epidemiology and costs of chronic obstructive pulmonary disease. *Eur Respir J* 2006, 27:188–207.

12. Mannino DM, Bist AS: Global burden of COPD: risk factors, prevalence, and future trends. *Lancet* 2007, 370:765-773.

13. Barnes PJ: Chronic obstructive pulmonary disease. *New Engl J Med* 2000, 343:269–280.

14. Scanlon PD, Connett JE, Waller LA, *et al.*: Smoking cessation and lung function in mild-to-moderate chronic obstructive pulmonary disease: the Lung Health Study. *Am J Respir Crit Care Med* 2000, 161:381–390.

15. Ernst P, Gonzalez AV, Brassard P, Suissa S: Inhaled corticosteroid use in chronic obstructive pulmonary disease and the risk of hospitalization for pneumonia. *Am J Respir Crit Care Med* 2007, 176:162–166.

16. Burge PS, Calverley PMA, Jones PW, *et al.*: Randomised, double-blind, placebo-controlled study of fluticasone propionate in patients with moderate to severe chronic obstructive pulmonary disease: the ISOLDE trial. *Br Med J* 2000, 320:1297–1303.

17. Decramer M, Rutten-van Molken M, Dekhuijzen PN, *et al.*: Effects of N-acetylcysteine on outcomes in chronic obstructive pulmonary disease (Bronchitis Randomized on NAC Cost Utility Study, BRONCUS): a randomised placebo-controlled trial. *Lancet* 2005, 365:1552–1560.

18. Troosters T, Casaburi R, Gosselink R, Decramer M: Pulmonary rehabilitation in chronic obstructive pulmonary disease. *Am J Respir Crit Care Med* 2005, 172:19–38.

19. Agusti A. Chronic obstructive pulmonary disease: a systemic disease. *Proc Am Thorac Soc* 2006, 3:478–481.

20. Sevenoaks MJ, Stockley RA: Chronic obstructive pulmonary disease, inflammation and co-morbidity: a common inflammatory phenotype? *Respir Res* 2006, 7:70.

21. Barnes PJ, Hansel TT: Prospects for new drugs for chronic obstructive pulmonary disease. *Lancet* 2004, 364:985–996.

22. Calverley PM, Rennard SI: What have we learned from large drug treatment trials in COPD? *Lancet* 2007, 370:774–785.

23. Barnes PJ, Chowdhury B, Kharitonov SA, *et al.*: Pulmonary biomarkers in chronic obstructive pulmonary disease. *Am J Respir Crit Care Med* 2006, 174:6–14.

24. Lopez AD, Murray CC: The global burden of disease, 1990–2020. *Nat Med* 1998, 4:1241–1243.

25. Fletcher C, Peto R: The natural history of chronic airflow obstruction. *Br Med J* 1977, 1:1645–1648.

26. Tashkin DP, Altose MD, Connett JE, *et al.*: Methacholine reactivity predicts changes in lung function over time in smokers with early chronic obstructive pulmonary disease: the Lung Health Study Research Group. *Am J Respir Crit Care Med* 1996, 153:1802–1811.

27. Hogg JC: Pathophysiology of airflow limitation in chronic obstructive pulmonary disease. *Lancet* 2004, 364:709–721.

28. Rogers DF, Barnes PJ: Treatment of airway mucus hypersecretion. *Ann Med* 2006, 38:116–125.

29. Nadel JA, Burgel PR: The role of epidermal growth factor in mucus production. *Curr Opin Pharmacol* 2001, 1:254–258.

30. Barnes PJ: Mediators of chronic obstructive pulmonary disease. *Pharm Rev* 2004, 56:515–548.

31. Rahman I: Oxidative stress in pathogenesis of chronic obstructive pulmonary disease: cellular and molecular mechanisms. *Cell Biochem Biophys* 2005, 43:167–188.

32. Barnes PJ: Mechanisms in COPD: differences from asthma. *Chest* 2000, 117:10S–14S.

33. Anthonisen NR, Connett JE, Kiley JP, *et al.*: Effects of smoking intervention and the use of an inhaled anticholinergic bronchodilator on the rate of decline of FEV1. *JAMA* 1994, 272:1497–1505.

34. Reus VI, Obach RS, Coe JW, *et al.*: Varenicline: new treatment with efficacy in smoking cessation. *Drugs Today (Barc)* 2007, 43:65–75.

35. Mahler DA, Donohue JF, Barbee RA, *et al.*: Efficacy of salmeterol xinafoate in the treatment of COPD. *Chest* 1999, 115:957–965.

36. Vincken W, van Noord JA, Greefhorst AP, *et al.*: Improved health outcomes in patients with COPD during 1 yr's treatment with tiotropium. *Eur Respir J* 2002, 19:209–216.

37. Keatings VM, Jatakanon A, Worsdell YM, Barnes PJ: Effects of inhaled and oral glucocorticoids on inflammatory indices in asthma and COPD. *Am J Respir Crit Care Med* 1997, 155:542–548.

38. Culpitt SV, Rogers DF, Shah P, *et al.*: Impaired inhibition by dexamethasone of cytokine release by alveolar macrophages from patients with chronic obstructive pulmonary disease. *Am J Respir Crit Care Med* 2003, 167:24–31.

39. Yang IA, Fong KM, Sim EH, *et al.*: Inhaled corticosteroids for stable chronic obstructive pulmonary disease. *Cochrane Database Syst Rev* 2007, CD002991.

40. Paggiaro PL, Dahle R, Bakran I, *et al.*: Multicentre randomised placebo-controlled trial of inhaled fluticasone propionate in patients with chronic obstructive pulmonary disease. *Lancet* 1998, 351:773–780.

41. Celli BR, Barnes PJ: Exacerbations of chronic obstructive pulmonary disease. *Eur Respir J* 2007, 29:1224–1238.

42. Meyers BF, Patterson GA: Chronic obstructive pulmonary disease. 10: Bullectomy, lung volume reduction surgery, and transplantation for patients with chronic obstructive pulmonary disease. *Thorax* 2003, 58:634–638.

43. Fishman A, Martinez F, Naunheim K, *et al.*: A randomized trial comparing lung-volume-reduction surgery with medical therapy for severe emphysema. *N Engl J Med* 2003, 348:2059–2073.

44. Toma TP, Hopkinson NS, Hillier J, *et al.*: Bronchoscopic volume reduction with valve implants in patients with severe emphysema. *Lancet* 2003, 361:931–933.

45. Barnes PJ, Stockley RA: COPD: current therapeutic interventions and future approaches. *Eur Respir J* 2005, 25:1084–1106.

CYSTIC FIBROSIS

*Raymond D. Coakley,
Richard C. Boucher,
Stanley B. Fiel, and
Daniel V. Schidlow*

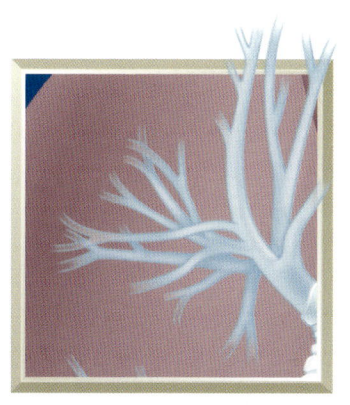
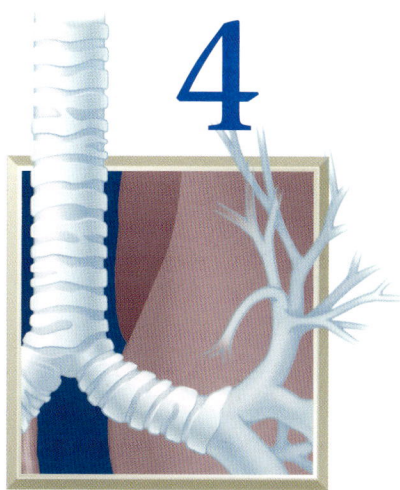
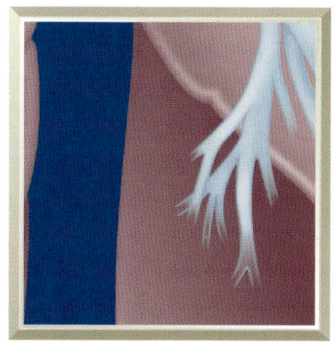

> "Woe to that child which when kissed on the forehead tastes salty.
> He is bewitched and soon must die."
> —*Adage from* northern European folklore referring to the salty sweat that characterizes cystic fibrosis, circa 1705

Cystic fibrosis (CF) is the most common fatal inherited disease among whites [1]. Approximately 1000 new cases are diagnosed each year in the United States, and some 30,000 Americans live with the disease [2,3].

The diverse clinical manifestations of CF, including the salty brow to which the opening adage refers, are caused by mutations in the gene that encodes the cystic fibrosis transmembrane conductance regulator (CFTR) protein. The CFTR protein is a plasma membrane protein that plays an essential role in regulating the movement of electrolytes and liquid across epithelial membranes. Defective electrolyte transport in CF promotes depletion of airway surface liquid and dehydration of the mucus layer lining the airway epithelium. As a consequence, viscous secretions impair mucociliary clearance, and mucus accumulation in airways results. The chronic infection of thickened mucus and inflammation that ensues characteristically causes bronchiectasis and progressive respiratory failure. This syndrome ultimately leads to death in 90% of patients. Disease in CF is not confined to the lung. Secretory epithelia throughout the body are affected, contributing to endocrine and exocrine pancreatic insufficiency (in 80%–90% of patients), rhinosinusoidal disease, intestinal obstruction, biliary tract disease, and congenital bilateral absence of the vas deferens (CBAVD), a cause of infertility in almost all men with CF.

Reported cases of steatorrhea and pancreatic insufficiency date to the mid-17th century [4]. However, the first description of CF as a clinical entity did not appear until the 1930s, when the disease was characterized as a genetic disorder of the pancreas and lung [5–8]. By 1953 an elevated concentration of chloride in sweat had been established as a diagnostic feature of the disease [9]. This advance led to the development of the sweat test [10], which is still one of the cornerstones of diagnosis. The reason for abnormal electrolyte concentrations in sweat remained obscure for 30 more years, until investigators identified a defect in chloride conductance in the epithelial cells of sweat glands [11] and airways [12]. It is now clear that the defect in chloride conductance occurs in secretory epithelial cells throughout the body and reflects a defect in chloride channel activity of the CFTR protein itself. CFTR dysfunction produces a change in the electrical potential of ion transport in all epithelial cells, including the cells lining the airways, such as in the nose. Increasing proficiency in the measurement of the change in this parameter in the nose using nasal potential difference (NPD) suggests that this test can serve as another useful diagnostic tool for CF. In the future, NPD may also be used to measure the level of correction in ion transport obtained in the course of clinical trials of new CF treatments.

Neonatal screening suggests that CF occurs in approximately 1 in 3500 births in whites [13,14]. The incidence is lower among African-Americans, Native Americans, Hispanics (1 in 8000–9000) and Asians [15–19] (*see* Fig. 4-1).

Over the last half of the 20th century, advances in supportive care improved the quality of life for thousands of patients and extended their lives by several decades. An increasingly sophisticated understanding of the pathophysiology of the condition promises novel future therapies with the potential for disease prevention or even cure.

EPIDEMIOLOGY AND GENETICS

Epidemiology, Survival, and Lung Function of Cystic Fibrosis in the United States

Age, y	Patients, %
0–17	57
≥ 18	43
Average Lung Function, FEV_1, % predicted	
6–12	95.1
13–17	87.4
18–30	86
≥ 18	62.8
≥ 30	54
Ethnicity	
White	97.7
Hispanic	3.2
African American	2.7
Other	0.4
Gender	
Male	54
Female	46

Data from the 2000 Cystic Fibrosis Foundation registry.

Figure 4-1. Cystic fibrosis: Epidemiology, survival, and lung function of patients. FEV_1—forced expiratory volume in 1 second.

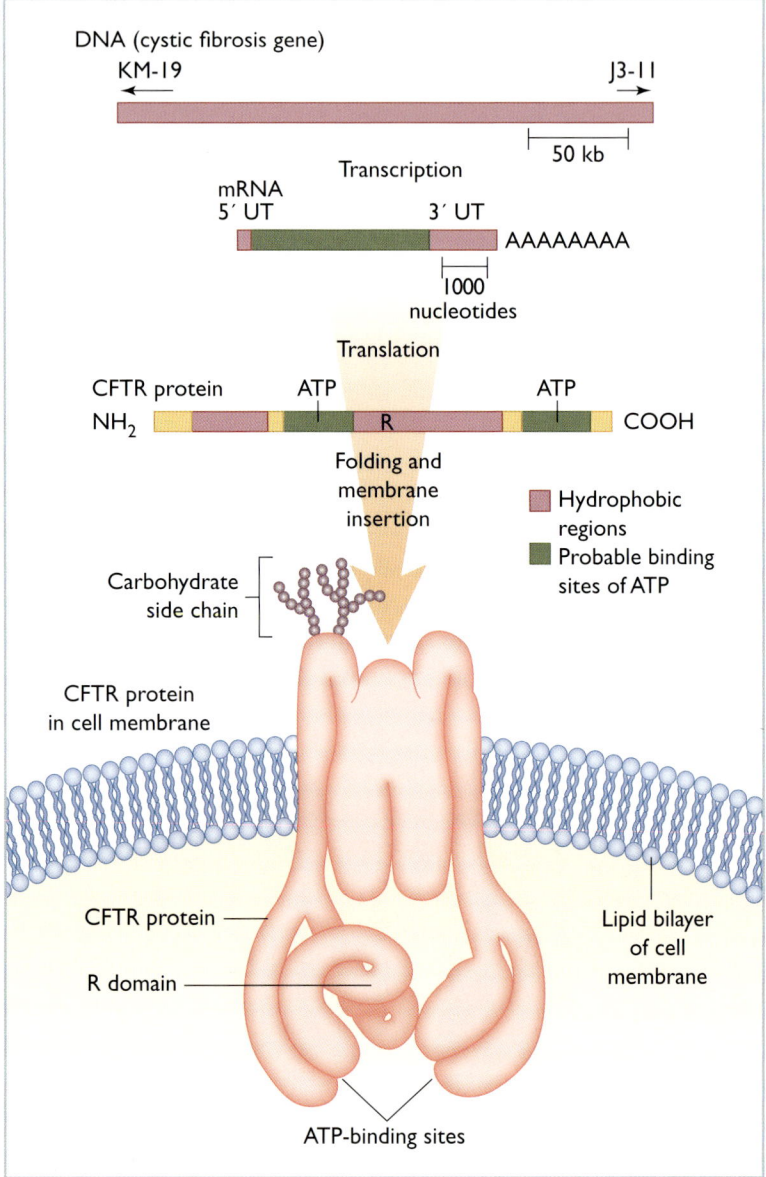

Figure 4-2. Predicting the structure of the cystic fibrosis transmembrane conductance regulator (CFTR) protein. The CFTR gene, located on chromosome 7, was first cloned and sequenced in 1989 [20–22]. The gene consists of 250 kb of genomic DNA containing 27 exons. Introns within the CFTR gene contain information that allows for alternative splicing. The clinical significance of alternative splicing in vivo is incompletely understood. The messenger RNA transcript (approximately 6129 bp) encodes a glycosylated protein containing 1480 amino acids. Structurally, the protein comprises two hydrophobic membrane-spanning domains, two nucleotide-binding folds (NBF1 and NBF2), and an intracellular regulatory (R) domain with many phosphorylation sites. The CFTR protein plays a critical role in electrolyte transport, serving not only as a chloride channel [23], but also as a regulator of other transepithelial ion channels, most notably epithelial Na^+ channels [24]. CFTR is a low-abundance protein, expressed primarily in the apical membrane of many epithelia. (*Adapted from* Cutting [25].)

| Atlas of Pulmonary Medicine |

CFTR Mutations

Class	Genotype examples	Frequency, %	Disease severity (phenotype)	Mechanism	Defect
I	G542X	2.4	Severe (PI)	Mutations produce premature termination signals and result in defective production of CFTR before the protein reaches the endoplasmic reticulum	No CFTR protein
	621+1 GτT	0.6			No cell surface chloride transport
	W1282X	1.5			
	R553X	0.9			
	1717-1 GτA	0.5			
	3905 ins T				
II	ΔF5008	66	Severe (PI)	Mutations result in failure to correctly traffic the protein to the apical membrane	Defective CFTR processing
	N1303K	1.2			Defective CFTR trafficking
	(P574H)				No cell surface chloride transport
	(A455E)				
III	G551D	1.8	Severe (usually) (PI)	Mutations result in abnormal protein regulation and a net decrease in Cl-secretion	Defective CFTR channel regulation
	G551S	0.1			Reduced surface chloride conductance
IV	R117H	0.3	Mild (PS)	Mutations impair the conductance of chloride through the CFTR channel pore	Reduced chloride conductance
	R347P	0.2			Reduced cell surface chloride transport
	R334W	0.1			
	R314E				
	P574H				
V	3849+10kb	0.6	PS	Defined by splicing defects; the result is synthesis of full-length CFTR, but at reduced amounts	CFTR channels normal but reduced in number
	CτT	0.3			Reduced cell surface chloride transport
	2789+5 GτA	0.1			
	3272-26 AτT				
	A455E				
	3120+1 GτA				
	1811+1.6kb				
	AτG				

Figure 4-3. Mutations that disrupt cystic fibrosis transmembrane conductance regulator (CFTR) function. **A**, Thus far, investigators have described the mechanisms by which five classes of cystic fibrosis mutations disrupt protein function. Recently, investigators [26,27] have proposed that identified mutants that impair regulation of other types of ion channels should be labeled as class VI. Others [28] have suggested that C-terminal truncations in CFTR, which lead to accelerated degradation of CFTR, should comprise class VI mutations.

Continued on the next page

Classes of Cystic Fibrosis Mutations

Class I

Mutations produce premature termination signals and result in defective production of CFTR before the protein reaches the endoplasmic reticulum for posttranslational processing. This category includes nonsense, splice-site, and frameshift mutations, all of which are predicted to eliminate channel function. These mutations are associated with severe disease.

Class II

Mutations result in failure to traffic the protein to the correct cellular location. In the well-known case of DF508, the CFTR protein does not meet the apical membrane and is localized largely in the endoplasmic reticulum. These mutations are associated with severe disease.

Class III

Mutations impair protein regulation, resulting in a net decrease in Cl- channel activity. Most, but not all, mutations in this class are associated with severe disease.

Class IV

Mutations impair conduction of Cl- through the CFTR channel pores. At least three mutations in this class are associated with mild disease. R117H is associated with two different phenotypes. Some men with the R117H genotype have CBAVD and pulmonary disease, whereas others have only CBAVD. This anomaly is the focus of some attention.

Class V

Defined by defects in splicing and production of the full-length normal CFTR, these mutations lead to a deficit of normal CFTR and a reduction in cell surface chloride transport, despite the presence of normal CFTR channels. Researchers concur that 10% wild-type CFTR expression represents the critical point for disease. Commonly, these patients will be pancreatic sufficient. Several genotypes are associated with this class, including 3849 + 10 kb C → T; 2789 + 5 G → A; 3272-26 A → G; A455E, and others. In addition, there is controversy regarding the inclusion of an intron variant, 5T, which renders different levels of expression of a normal CFTR [21].

Figure 4-3. *(Continued)* **B**, The relationship between specific CFTR gene mutations and clinical manifestations of the disease are much more complex than was previously thought [25,26]. In general, classes I, II, and III are associated with the more severe phenotypic expression of the CFTR gene, and classes IV and V are associated with less severe clinical consequences. Although most of the reported mutations in CFTR are rare and unclassified, it may be possible to use genotype–phenotype correlations to gain prognostic insights for individual patients. CBAVD—congenital bilateral absence of the vas deferens; CFTR—cystic fibrosis transmembrane conductance regulator.

Types of Non-ΔF508 Mutations

Mutation	Example	Description
Missense	G551D	Substitution of glycine (G) at codon 551 by aspartic acid (D)
Nonsense	G542X	Substitution of glycine (G) at codon 542 by a stop signal (X)
Frameshift	3095 insT	Insertion of thymine (T) after nucleotide 3905 in exon 20
Splice-site	621+1G→T	Substitution of thymine (T) for guanine (G) immediately after nucleotide 621 (last base in exon 4)

Figure 4-4. Four major types of non-ΔF508 mutations. More than 1000 mutations have been identified. The most common mutation, ΔF508, is carried by more than 70% of the affected chromosomes worldwide. This mutation reflects the deletion of three nucleotides, which leads to the loss of phenylalanine at position 508 of the gene product [3]. This mutation may have first appeared in Europe more than 50,000 years ago [29]. Examples of four other common mutation types are provided in the figure. Many of the mutations reported to date are rare, appearing in only one family. Others are concentrated in a particular ethnic group. For example, the stop codon mutation W1282X, which constitutes only 2% of all cystic fibrosis mutations worldwide, is carried by approximately 50% of the cystic fibrosis chromosomes in Ashkenazi Jews, whereas the frequency of ΔF508 is relatively low (40%) in this population [29] and G542X is relatively common (12%). Furthermore, the mutation 3120+1 GτA uniquely accounts for 12% of CFTR mutations in African-American patients [30].

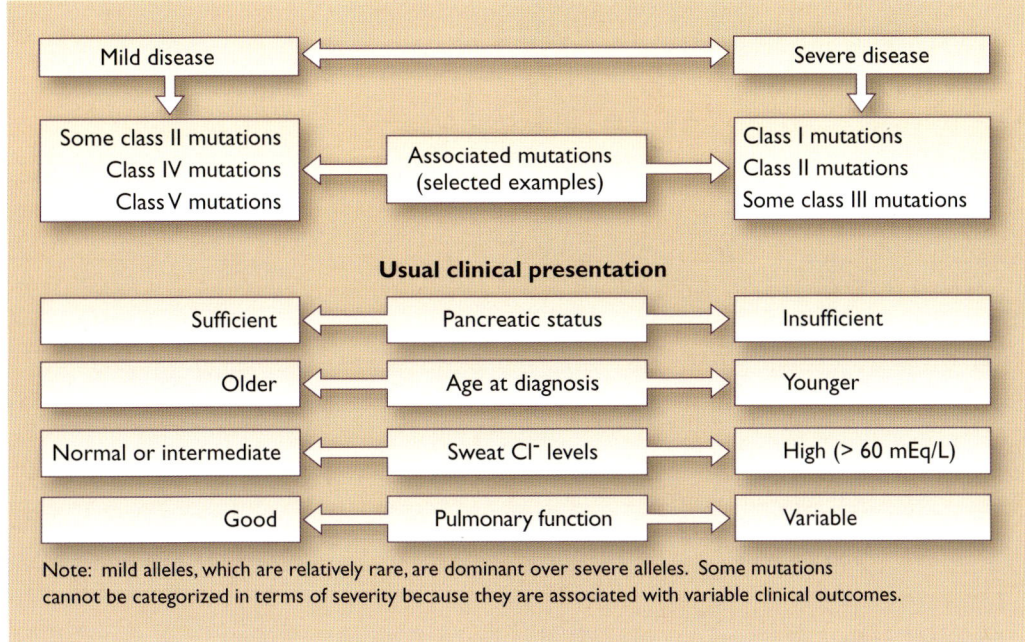

Figure 4-5. Genotype–phenotype relationships. Phenotypic severity bears some relationship to genotype [25,31]. However, the relationship between genotype and clinical expression is complicated and remains poorly understood. Investigators have studied the impact of genotype on the severity of pancreatic and pulmonary disease and the occurrence of congenital bilateral absence of the vas deferens (CBAVD). The incidence of CBAVD among men with cystic fibrosis is high though not invariant, and the condition also occurs in men with few or no other manifestations of the disease. CBAVD is unrelated to disease severity. Although the relationship is not invariant, pancreatic status is linked to particular classes of mutations, and cystic fibrosis phenotypes have traditionally been classified as "mild" or "severe" on the basis of pancreatic function. Many mutations, including ΔF508, are associated with pancreatic insufficiency (ie, dependence on pancreatic enzymes), whereas a much smaller number are associated with pancreatic sufficiency. The severity and course of pulmonary disease are predicted less reliably by genotype. Some mutations are common among patients with "mild" lung disease, but variability is high among patients with "severe" mutations [32,33]. Variability in pulmonary disease may be due, in part, to polymorphisms or mutations of other genes, as well as environmental factors.

PATHOPHYSIOLOGY

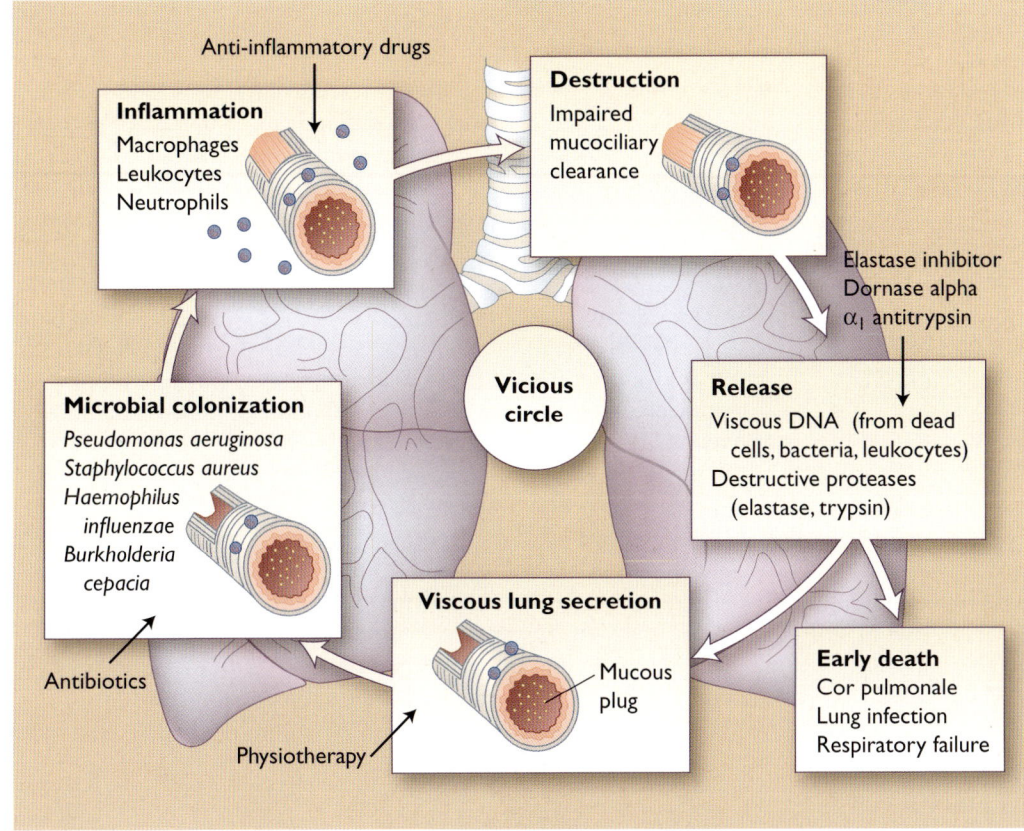

Figure 4-6. The "vicious circle" of lung disease in cystic fibrosis. Cystic fibrosis is a genetic form of chronic bronchitis characterized by a vicious circle of obstruction, infection, and inflammation related to impaired local host defense mechanisms. This produces progressive bronchiectasis and, ultimately, respiratory failure. Despite the identification of the *CFTR* gene and characterization of its role as an ion channel, intense efforts are still under way to understand how defective transepithelial electrolyte transport leads to the devastating consequences seen throughout the airways.

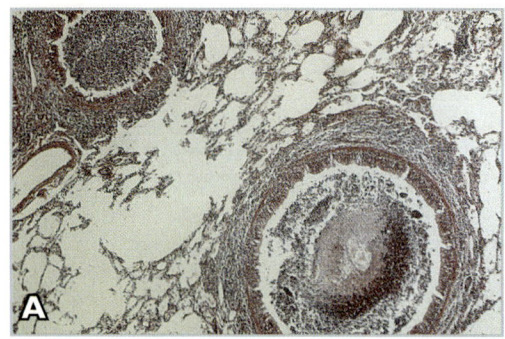
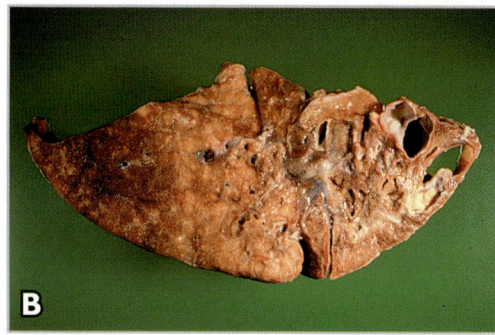

Figure 4-7. Airway obstruction. Airway obstruction is rooted ultimately in CFTR dysfunction. It is thought that defective electrolyte transport dehydrates the airway surface, impairing the viscoelastic properties of mucus and reducing its ability to clear microorganisms from the respiratory tract [34]. DNA deposited by neutrophils that flood cystic fibrotic airways in response to bacterial infection further increases the viscosity of airway secretions.

A, Pathology of early lung disease. Thickened mucus plaques and plugs adhere to airway mucosal surfaces, leading to occlusion of the lumen with viscous secretions and cellular debris in an infant 5 months of age. **B**, Advanced lung disease. The disease has spread from the small airways to larger airways. Bronchiectasis, cystic changes, diffuse mucus plugging, and fibrosis are visible.

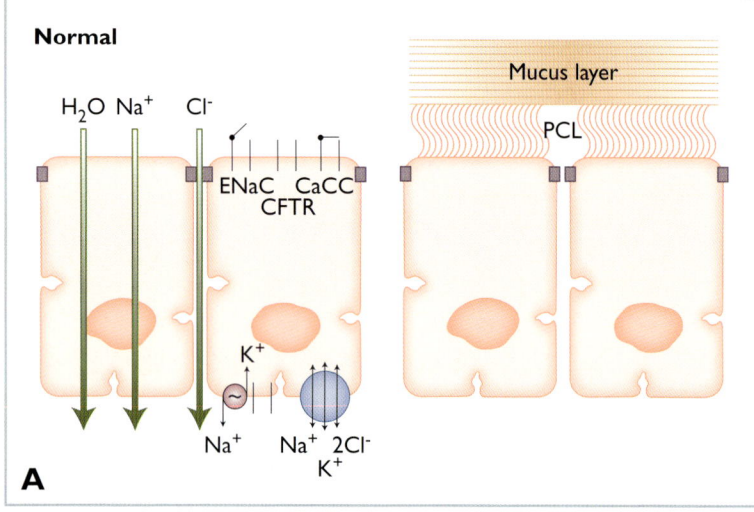
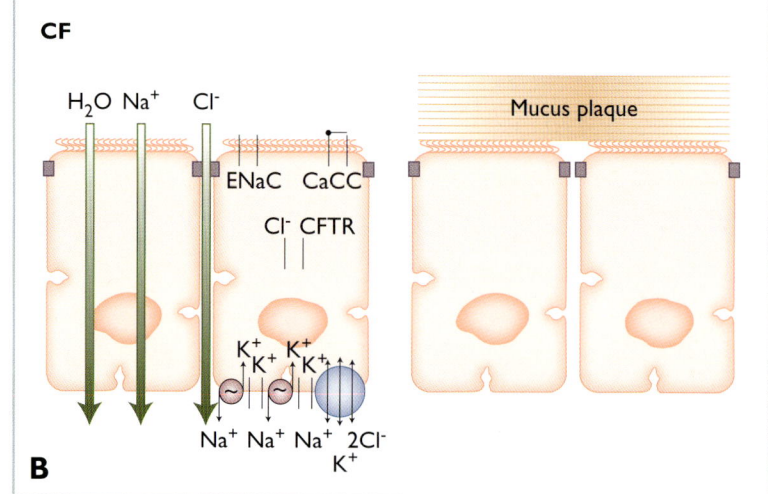

Figure 4-8. Defects in airway defenses against bacterial infection. Several theories have emerged to explain why airway defenses against bacterial infection are defective in cystic fibrosis (CF). The characteristic bacterial flora in CF led some researchers to focus on bacterial binding to airway epithelial surfaces [35] or abnormal clearance of locally deposited bacteria by cystic fibrosis transmembrane conductance regulator (CFTR) attachment site–mediated epithelial phagocytosis [36]. In contrast, the striking inflammation that characterizes the CF airway prompted others to propose innate dysregulation of airway inflammation due to intraepithelial cell accumulation of mutant CFTR protein [37,38] as opposed to a mere response to persistent airway infection.

Others have attempted to link epithelial ion transport abnormalities to the colonization and infection of airways with bacteria. Proponents of a "high salt" theory suggested that defective CFTR function results in elevated airway surface liquid tonicity and thus inactivation of defensins, host molecules with innate antimicrobial properties [39]. However, accumulating in vitro and in vivo evidence appears to favor a contrasting "airway surface liquid hydration" hypothesis of CF pathogenesis. This theory is based on the premise that airway surface liquid is isotonic and that salt is actively transported across airway epithelium, with water following passively. It is thought that defective CFTR function is associated with both impaired chloride secretion and hyperabsorption of sodium across airway epithelia. These combined defects are postulated to result in depletion of airway surface liquid, accumulation and adherence of mucus to airway epithelial surfaces, impaired mucociliary and cough clearance, and, ultimately, chronic bacterial infection of the accumulated intraluminal mucus [40–42]. This hypothesis is presented in the figure. **A**, The major active ion transport processes of normal airway epithelium. Adequate hydration of airway surface liquid depends on a balance between Na^+ absorption via epithelial Na^+ channels (ENaC) and anion secretion via CFTR. Calcium-activated chloride channels (CaCC) are also present, but their activity appears to be insufficient to adequately hydrate airway surfaces in the absence of CFTR. **B**, In CF, Na^+ absorption is increased compared with normal, reflecting the absence of CFTR-mediated inhibition, and chloride secretion via CFTR is absent. These defects produce a marked reduction in the volume (height) of the periciliary liquid (PCL) layer, as well as a concentration of mucus and its adhesion to epithelial surfaces.

Continued on the next page

| Atlas of Pulmonary Medicine |

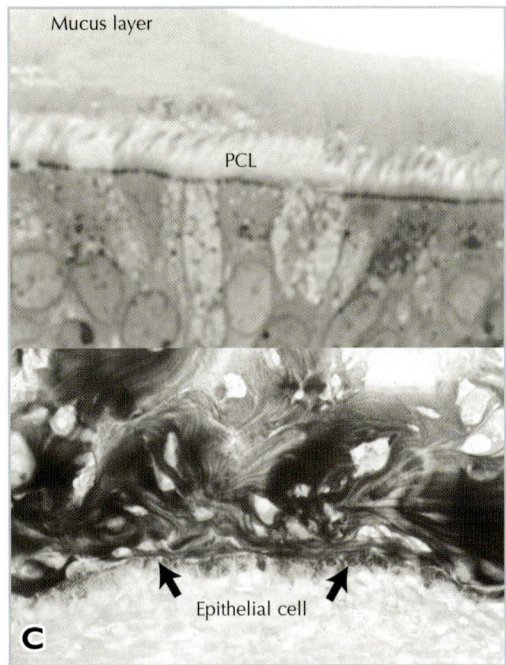

Figure 4-8. *(Continued)* **C**, Light microscopic images of normal (*upper image*) and CF (*lower image*) airway epithelium. In the normal tissue, the periciliary liquid layer is preserved, whereas in the CF tissue, the periciliary liquid layer is absent and a large mucus plaque adheres to the apical epithelial surface.

Further experimental data suggest that the low oxygen tension within these abnormal mucus plaques provides a favorable environment for bacterial proliferation and, in particular, pseudomonal biofilm formation [43]. These hypoxic niches may also provide an appropriate environment for the growth of anaerobic bacteria, which would not be detected under conventional sputum culture conditions. Thus, a complex, mixed aerobic–anaerobic flora may contribute to the pathogenesis of the condition.

Finally, a putative role for CFTR in transepithelial secretion of bicarbonate into the airway lumen has been proposed in several extrapulmonary secretory epithelia. More recently, a similar defect has been examined in airway epithelium, and this might lead to abnormally acidified airway surface liquid in CF, which could also interfere with local host defense [44,45].

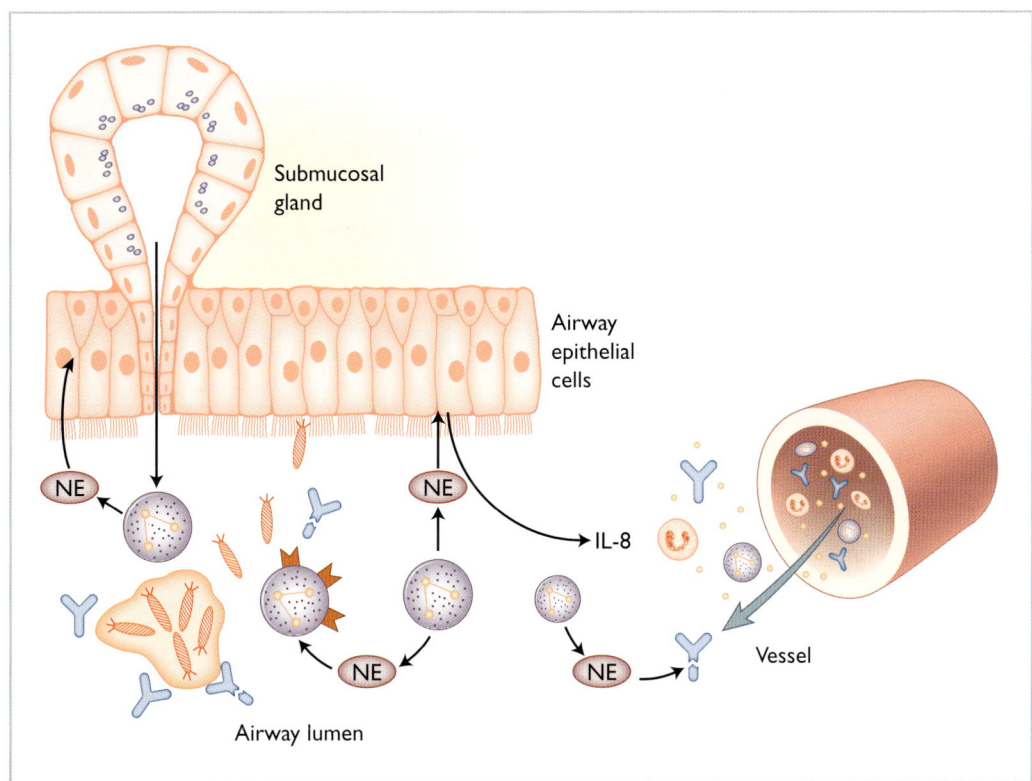

Figure 4-9. Airway inflammation mediated by neutrophils and neutrophil products. Though cystic fibrosis (CF) airways are infiltrated with mononuclear cells, the inflammatory response in the condition is characteristically dominated by polymorphonuclear neutrophils and their destructive products, which perpetuate and amplify lung damage. Once recruited to the site of inflammation and primed by interleukin-8 (IL-8) and other cytokines [46], neutrophils release an arsenal of proteases, oxidative radicals (including H_2O_2), and other inflammatory mediators that stimulate mucus hypersecretion and exacerbate the pathologic process [47–51]. The most damaging of the products to flood the cystic airways is neutrophil elastase (NE), an "omnivorous" serine protease. Under normal circumstances, NE is complexed and inactivated by α_1-antitrypsin and secretory leukoprotease inhibitor. In cystic fibrosis, however, the relentless influx of neutrophils that reflects the failure to eliminate bacteria contained within the mucus produces a persistent source of NE [52]. This high rate of elastase release exceeds the capacity of local antiproteases to complex it, and therefore, unopposed in its action, NE contributes to progressive pulmonary damage by 1) directly injuring the cellular and matrix components of the airways, 2) impairing antibody- and complement-mediated opsonophagocytosis, 3) stimulating mucus secretion, 4) reducing ciliary beat frequency, and 5) inducing epithelial cell production of IL-8, which further perpetuates the process. Chronic neutrophil-dominated inflammation and impaired anti-NE neutralization have been reported in children with CF as young as 1 year [46–53]. Decaying neutrophils release DNA into the airways, where it accumulates, further increasing the viscosity and adhesiveness of mucus. (*Adapted from* Marshall [34]).

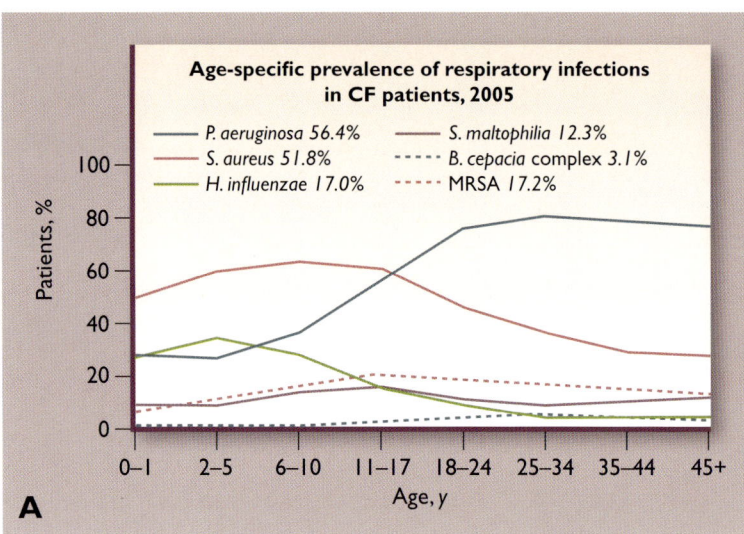

B	Organisms and Infection Rates	
Organism		**Infection Rate, %**
Pseudomonas aeruginosa (patients < 18 y)		40.1
P. aeruginosa (patients ≥ 18 y)		75.9
Methicillin-resistant *Staphylococcus aureus*		18.9
P. aeruginosa reported as mucoid type		65.9
P. aeruginosa reported as multiply antibiotic resistant		16
Burkholderia cepacia complex		2.9
Stenotrophomonas maltophilia		12.7

Figure 4-10. A, Age-specific frequencies of five common airway pathogens. *Pseudomonas aeruginosa* usually supersedes *Staphylococcus aureus* to become the predominant pathogen by the end of the first decade of life. The high prevalence of *P. aeruginosa* in this population is likely related to a growth advantage conferred on the organism by the abnormal airway surface microevironment in cystic fibrosis (CF) (eg, hypoxia). However, it may also be a consequence of selection associated with increased life expectancy and aggressive antibiotic treatment [24,43,48–58]. It has also been proposed that *Pseudomonas* pili appear to bind avidly to sialylated CF cells, perhaps contributing to the puzzling affinity of this pathogen in CF airways [55]. Once established in CF airways, *P. aeruginosa* is difficult or impossible to eradicate. Initial infection is usually by nonmucoid, piliated organisms; however, the nonmucoid form often switches to a mucoid variant in the airway. Alginate gel is produced in response to anaerobic conditions, and this modification, coupled with biofilm physiology, protects PsA against host defenses and manufactures a broad range of virulent proteases, toxins, and antigenic agents. Antibiotic selection has also likely contributed to an increased incidence of newer pathogens and resistant strains (eg, methicillin-resistant *S. aureus*).

The new pathogens of greatest concern are members of the *Burkholderia cepacia* complex, which are transmissible by close person-to-person contact. Infection with *B. cepacia* is frequently associated with an indolent but nonetheless relentless decline in lung function. However, some colonized patients exhibit more rapidly accelerated lung destruction or even succumb to acute systemic infection. In contrast, some others show no change in clinical status. Pulmonary colonization by *B. cepacia* may occur 2 years before it is detectable by routine culturing [59]. Nine genomovars of the *B. cepacia* complex known to be present in patients with CF in the United States have been identified [59,60]. In addition, multiple novel species have been identified that have not been associated with human colonization or infection thus far. The designation *B. cepacia* is reserved for genomovar I. Members of this group also include *Burkholderia multivorans* (genomovar II), *Burkholderia cenocepacia* (genomovar III), *Burkholderia stabilis* (genomovar IV), *Burkholderia vietnamiensis* (genomovar V), *Burkholderia dolosa* (genomovar VI), *Burkholderia ambifaria* (genomovar VII), *Burkholderia anthia* (genomovar VIII), and *Burkholderia pyrrocinia* (genomovar IX). In addition, another species, *Burkholderia gladioli*, although not a member of the *B. cepacia* complex, has been recovered from CF sputum. It is hoped that these efforts to confirm species identification will be informative regarding infection transmissibility and virulence, leading to infection control consensus.

The clinical significance of *Stenotrophomonas (Xanthomonas) maltophilia* and *Alcaligenes xylosoxidans* in patients with CF is becoming clearer. There is evidence to suggest that colonization with *S. (Xanthomonas) maltophilia* does not alter the course of CF but is associated with an increased use of antibiotics [61,62]. Improved surveillance may account for some of the apparent increase in prevalence of these pathogens [63]. *Mycobacterium tuberculosis*, although rare in patients with CF [64], may be associated with an increase in disease progression.

The pathogenicity of nontuberculous mycobacteria (NTM) in CF is increasingly recognized. They are cultured from the sputa of approximately 13% of CF patients, the species most frequently recovered being *Mycobacterium avium* complex (72%) and *Mycobacterium abscessus* (16%) [65,66]. Positive cultures for NTM are associated with older age, higher forced expiratory volume in 1 second (FEV_1), and reduced frequency of infection with *Pseudomonas*. Symptoms of persistent low-grade fever, weight loss, and increased cough, coupled with radiologic evidence of nodular pulmonary infiltrates in a "tree and bud" pattern and cavitary lung lesions on computed tomographic imaging, are considered consistent with active infection.

Although invasive aspergillus disease is rare in CF, allergic bronchopulmonary aspergillosis is not, occurring in 5% to 15% of CF adults [67]. A diagnosis of the latter is considered in the presence of asthma, pulmonary infiltrates, central bronchiectasis, positive immediate skin reactivity to *Aspergillus fumigatus*, peripheral blood eosinophilia, serum IgE levels greater than 1000 mg/mL, and elevated serum IgE and IgG levels of anti–*A. fumigatus* antibodies. There are no current data to suggest that *Candida* spp play a role in the pathogenicity of CF lung disease.

There is a paucity of data relating to the role of respiratory tract viruses in CF, although influenza and respiratory syncytial virus infection may be associated with significant pulmonary deterioration [68]. (*Data from* the Cystic Fibrosis Foundation patient registry report, 2005 [http://www.cff.org/research/clinical research/patient registry report/].)

B, Organisms and infection rates. (*Data from* the 2006 Cystic Fibrosis Foundation registry.)

CLINICAL MANIFESTATIONS AND COMORBID CONDITIONS

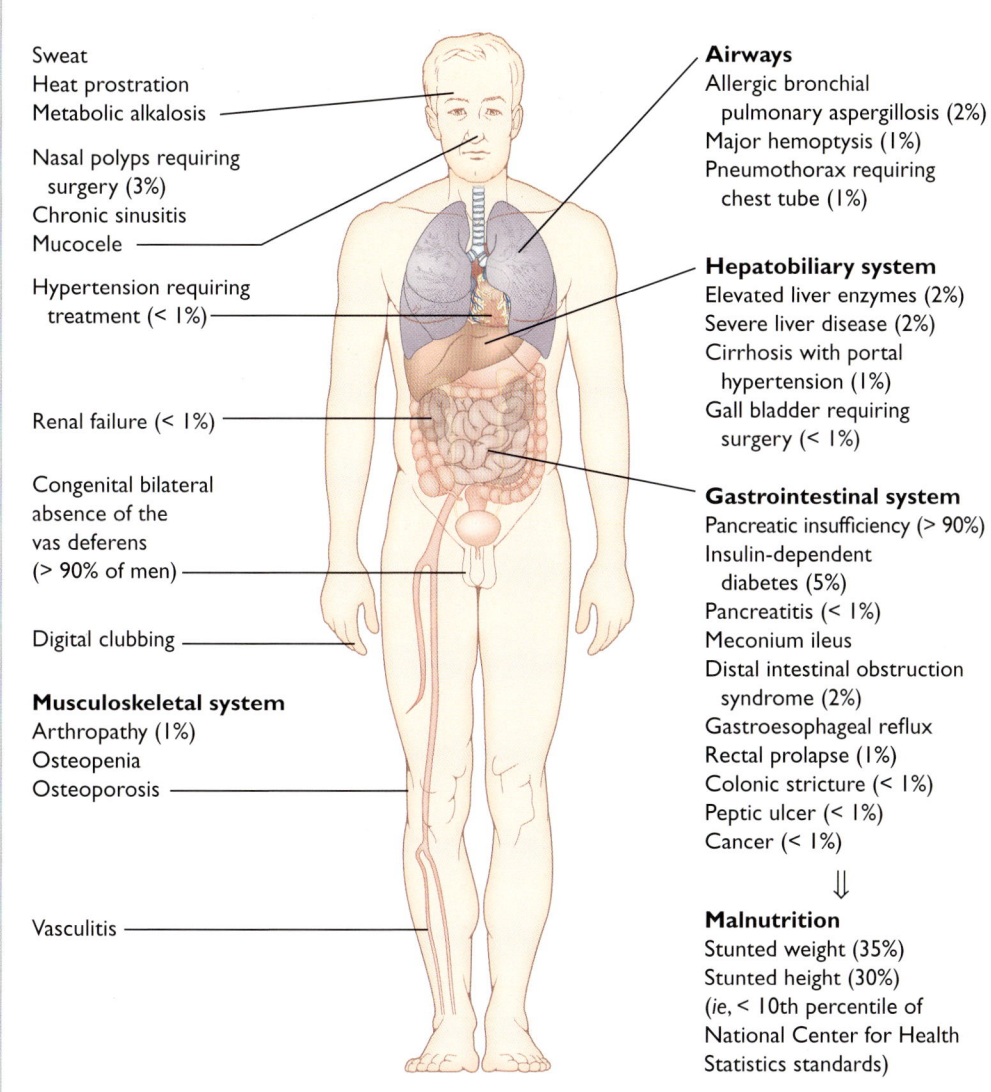

Figure 4-11. Clinical manifestations and comorbidity of cystic fibrosis. Cystic fibrosis (CF) is associated with numerous complications and comorbid conditions. As indicated in the figure, almost every patient with cystic fibrosis who lives long enough will eventually develop pulmonary symptoms. However, the age of onset, the rate of CF progression, and the incidence of comorbid conditions are extremely variable. The 1999 incidence of some of these manifestations and comorbid conditions, obtained from the Cystic Fibrosis Foundation Registry, are provided in parentheses. It is important to note that the incidence of most of these conditions increases significantly with age and disease progression. Thus, the prevalence of some conditions (eg, liver disease and diabetes mellitus) in a clinical setting that includes adolescents and young adults may be significantly higher than these figures suggest.

Cystic fibrosis transmembrane conductance regulator (CFTR) is expressed in the biliary tract cells, and at least one third of patients have abnormal liver function tests. Fatty infiltration of the liver is seen in up to 70% of older patients, and this may progress to biliary cirrhosis in 10% of this group. A small, poorly functioning gallbladder is present in up to 30% of patients with cystic fibrosis, and gallstones are noted in 10%. Fecal loss of bile acids is associated with bile-salt pool depletion, and biliary lipid becomes lithogenic [69]. Ursodeoxycholic acid can correct abnormal liver function tests, although the impact of this strategy on progression to cirrhosis is not known with certainty. In those who do develop hepatic failure, liver transplantation is an option [69,70].

A review of the diagnosis and management of diabetes mellitus and osteopenia/osteoporosis complicating cystic fibrosis is beyond the scope of this chapter, but these issues are dealt with comprehensively elsewhere [71,72].

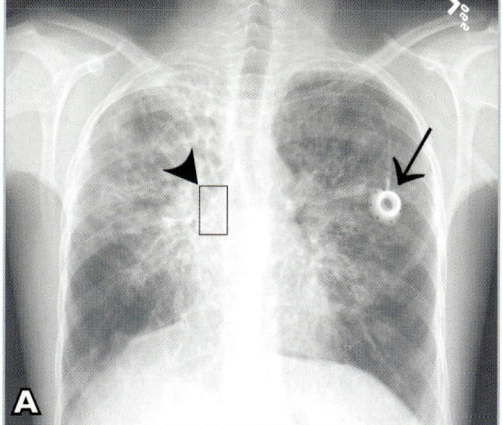
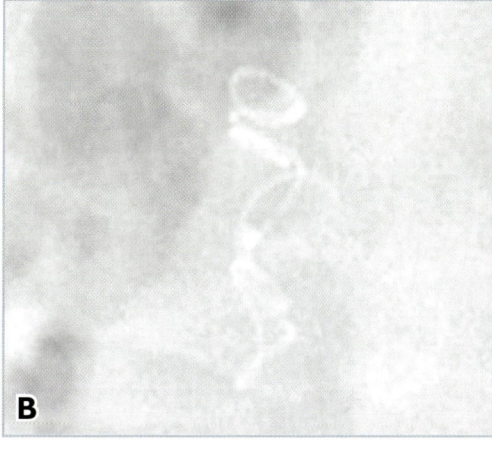

Figure 4-12. Advanced respiratory disease and pulmonary complications. Recurrent pulmonary infection is the principal cause of morbidity in patients with cystic fibrosis. Respiratory failure, defined by hypoxemia and hypercapnia, is the usual cause of death. Complications associated with advanced disease include pneumothorax, experienced by 16% to 20% of patients older than 18 years, and major hemoptysis. Guidelines on the management of pulmonary complications have been published [64,73]. **A**, Radiograph showing abnormalities typical of cystic fibrosis in a man aged 19 years with advanced disease. Ring shadows and tram-tracking are present bilaterally, in this case most prominently in the mid and upper zone of the right lung. These are secondary to bronchial thickening and dilation. The reservoir of an indwelling vascular access device (portacath) is seen overlying the left hemithorax (*arrow*). In addition, in the upper zone of the right lung, the *solid arrowhead* indicates the position of a coil placed during bronchial artery embolization for major hemoptysis. **B**, The area within the *box* in panel A is expanded for clearer visualization of the embolization coil. Occlusion of bronchial vessels using microspheres is also practiced.

Continued on the next page

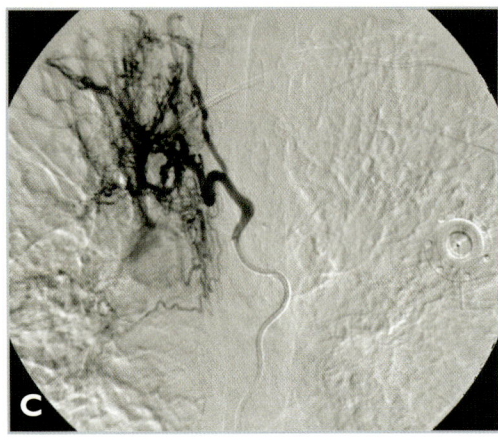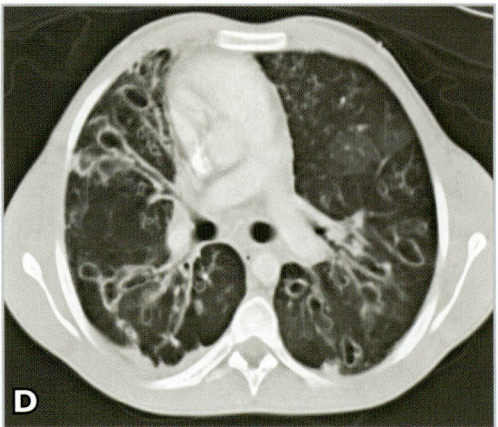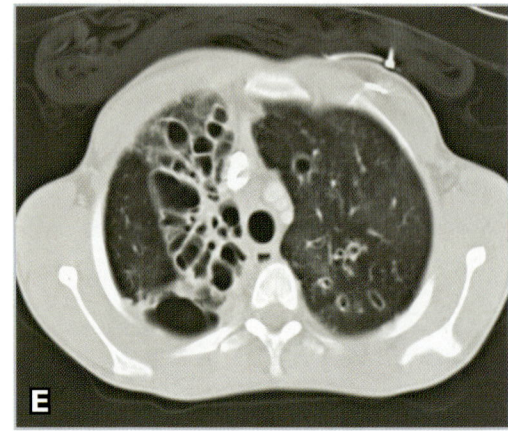

Figure 4-12. *(Continued)* **C,** Bronchial arteriogram from the same patient, performed at the time of major hemoptysis, demonstrating abnormal proliferation and ectasia of right upper lobe bronchial vessels. Again, the reservoir of the portacath is seen over the left hemithorax. **D,** Computed tomography (CT) scan with intravenous contrast of the lung showing severe bronchiectasis in the midlung zones from the same patient. Note the grossly dilated airways and cystic changes. **E,** CT scan with intravenous contrast of the lung from the same patient showing very advanced fibrocystic destruction of the upper lobe of the right lung.

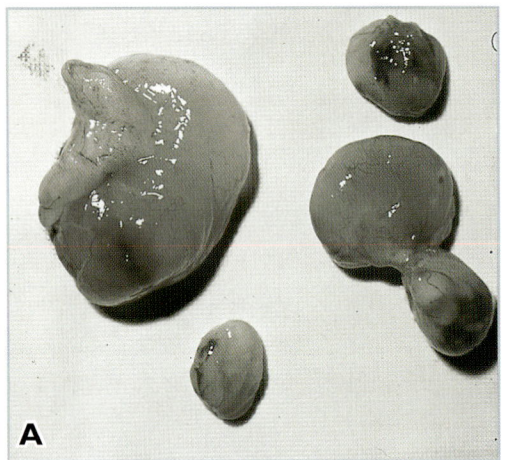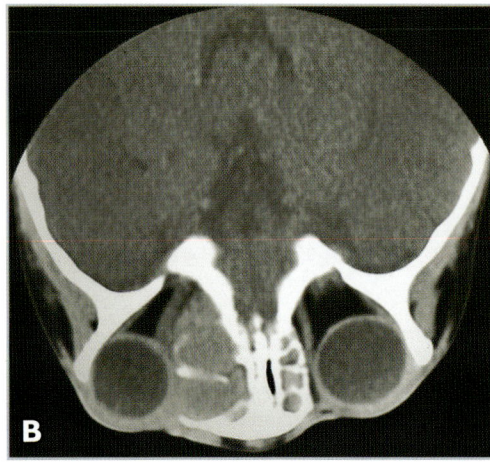

Figure 4-13. Other respiratory tract complications and manifestations in cystic fibrosis (CF). These complications and manifestations include persistent productive cough (a hallmark of CF pulmonary disease from infancy) and infectious exacerbations, which punctuate periods of clinical stability and are defined by increased cough, weight loss, increased sputum volume, low-grade fever, and decrements in pulmonary function [74]. Treatment-resistant sinus disease occurs in more than 90% of patients with CF and is associated with a high frequency of local complications [75]. Although some children are asymptomatic, a history of headache, postnasal drip, and nasal obstruction may often be elicited. There is considerable variation in the degree and type of sinus disease in patients with CF, but there does not seem to be a strong correlation between the severity of lung disease and the symptoms of sinus disease [75]. Thickening of the mucosal lining of the paranasal sinuses, fluid accumulation, and recurrent sinusitis are common. Opacification on sinus radiographs is so characteristic of CF that normal sinus radiographs should cast doubt on the diagnosis [76]. **A,** Nasal polyps, which originate in the paranasal sinuses, are present in up to 40% of patients with CF and tend to recur after resection. **B,** This CT scan shows a large mucocele arising from the ethmoid sinus, causing a mass effect into the right orbit. Mucoceles are slow-growing cysts that fill with mucoid secretions when sinus drainage is obstructed by inflammatory processes or other causes. The expanding mass can erode bone and compress adjacent structures [77]. Clinical manifestations of paranasal mucoceles include headache, eyelid ptosis, and limitation of eye movement. In children, paranasal sinus mucoceles are rare and occur almost exclusively in patients with CF [77]. However, routine imaging of the paranasal sinuses of patients with CF is not standard practice; thus, the prevalence of paranasal mucoceles may be higher than expected [76]. Treatment involves resection of the mucocele.

DIAGNOSIS

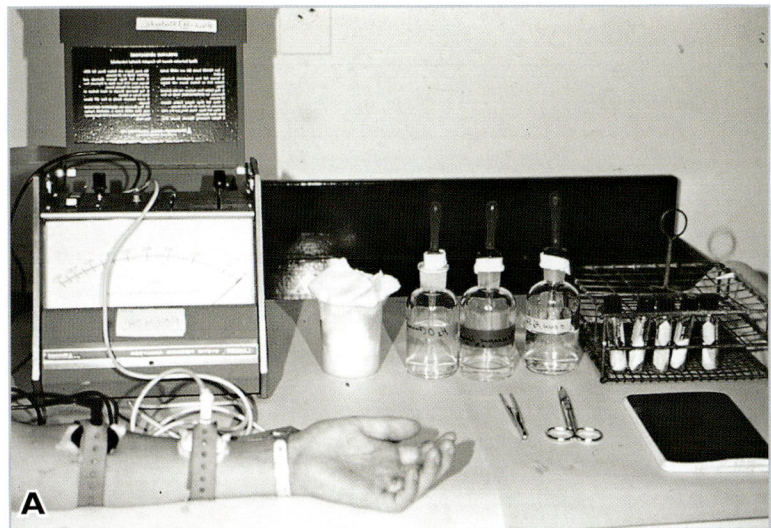

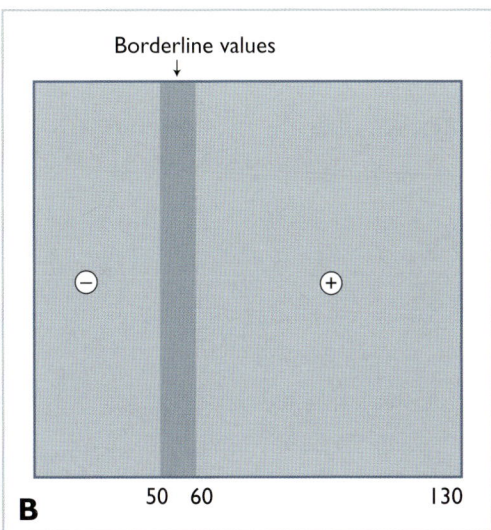

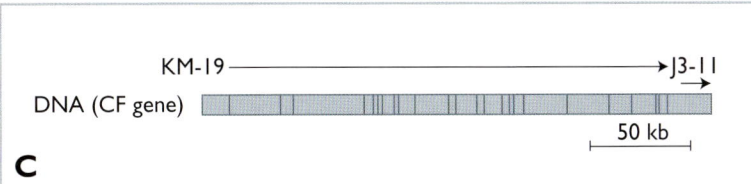

Figure 4-14. Sweat testing, genotyping, and measurement of nasal potential difference (nasal PD) are available to confirm or exclude the diagnosis of cystic fibrosis (CF). Other specialized diagnostic capabilities to rule out the diagnosis of CF include electron microscopic examination of bronchial biopsies for the immotile cilia syndromes and immunologic evaluation for various immune deficiencies that predispose patients to respiratory infections. The sweat test remains one of the cornerstones of the diagnosis and characterization of the CF syndrome, and it is helpful in confirming the diagnosis in patients with a suspicious clinical picture. Quantitative determinations of chloride concentrations in sweat obtained by the Gibson and Cooke pilocarpine iontophoresis method are highly reliable; errors are usually a consequence of sample contamination and technical inexperience. Subcutaneous edema and severe malnutrition can cause false-negative results. False-negative results are associated with hypothyroidism, hypoparathyroidism, and other rare metabolic disorders. False-positive results may be seen in pseudohypoaldosteronism. **A,** Sweat test administration. Indications for a sweat test include a history of CF in the immediate family, chronic pulmonary disease, or pancreatic insufficiency. Other indicators include nasal polyposis, cirrhosis in childhood, and clinical signs or symptoms suggesting a diagnosis. **B,** Borderline sweat chloride values (50–60 mmol/L). More than 98% of patients have abnormal chloride concentrations (*ie*, >60 mmol/L); however, some individuals present with borderline or normal values, which are usually associated with less common mutations of the CF gene and occur most frequently in adult patients.

C, The cystic fibrosis transmembrane regulator gene (CFTR) is located on the long arm of chromosome 7. When sweat chloride testing values are borderline, genetic testing can be useful in securing a diagnosis. Commercially available testing can identify more than 95 of the most common CFTR mutations. This will identify 90% to 95% of Caucasian CF patients; detection rates are lower for Hispanic and African-American patients (~75%). More limited genetic panels to detect CFTR mutations (20–30 mutations) are used in many centers. Thus, a percentage of CF patients will remain undiagnosed despite CFTR genetic testing. In exceptional circumstances, the CFTR gene may be fully sequenced to elucidate rare mutations, though more commonly, the clinical phenotype and sweat chloride testing values are correlated with findings of nasal potential difference testing in difficult cases.

The extension of genetic analysis to rare mutations in individual patients is often not practicable. The characteristic differences in nasal PD values from normal subjects and patients with CF can determine if a patient has CF in cases in which the sweat electrolyte test and genotyping tests are inconclusive [78,79]. As Na^+ and Cl^- ions move across airway cells, they generate an electrical potential difference that can be measured easily. Using a surface electrode to probe various regions of the nasal epithelium, the transepithelial potential in the airway epithelium is measured with respect to the interstitial fluid. The magnitude of the basal value for PD varies considerably between patients with CF and patients without CF, primarily reflecting hyperabsorption of Na^+ across the nasal airway epithelium in CF patients. With the perfusion of specific testing solutions (*eg*, blocking the Na^+ channel or activating the Cl^- channel), it is possible to determine whether the CFTR Cl^- channel is functional in a patient [80]. Nasal PD measurements also have other uses. Nasal PD can serve as a critical measure for the success of new therapies for CF (outcome measure), including intravenous, oral, or inhaled medications and gene therapy. In addition, nasal PD permits testing of the relationships between genotype and phenotype in terms of specific ion transport defects (Na^+ vs Cl^-) [80]. (*Panel C adapted from* Collins [81].)

TREATMENT

Routine Surveillance of Patients with Cystic Fibrosis
Minimum three monthly clinic visits, with clinical examination that includes evaluation for polyps
Spirogram on each visit (at least every 6 mo)
Sputum culture on each visit (at least annually)
Chest radiograph at least annually
Influenza vaccination at least annually
Arterial blood gases at least annually in patients with an FEV_1 < 40% of predicted values, including an assessment of need for nocturnal oxygen supplementation
Complete pulmonary function (lung volumes) at least annually
Review of chest physical therapy techniques and exercise regimen on each visit (at least annually)
Psychosocial assessment, including vocational aspects, annually
Nutritional assessment annually, including liver function analysis and assessment for diabetes
Fertility, pregnancy, and sexual issues discussed where appropriate
Bone density, risk factors for CF-related bone disease evaluated yearly; consider radiologic assessment of bone mineral density in "at-risk" patients

Figure 4-15. Suggestions for routine clinical surveillance from the Cystic Fibrosis Foundation of North America Guidelines Committee. These recommendations are not absolute and should be tailored to the needs of the individual patient.

Treatment of cystic fibrosis (CF) is directed toward alleviating symptoms and correcting organ dysfunction. Nutrition status in patients with CF is critical. Patients with poor nutrition status are more prone to chest infections than those with good nutrition status, and patients who have good nutrition status and normal fat absorption have a better prognosis than those who do not [82–84]. Acid-resistant microspheric pancreatic enzyme is useful in malabsorbing patients with CF. Oral caloric supplements and enteral feeding by nasogastric tube or gastrostomy tube are frequently adopted therapeutic interventions for malnourished patients. FEV_1—forced expiratory volume in 1 second.

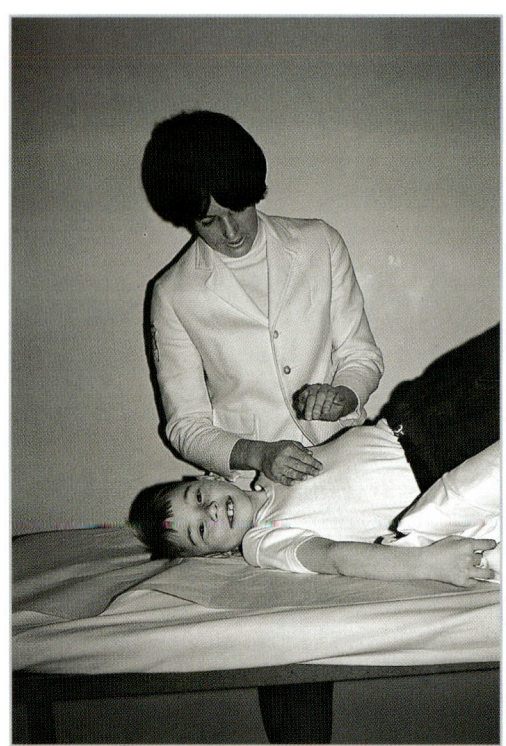

Figure 4-16. The cornerstones of pulmonary therapy for cystic fibrosis are clearance of airway secretions and treatment of pulmonary infections. For more than 50 years, the primary nonpharmacologic strategy for mobilizing viscous secretions and clearing them from the airways has been postural drainage and percussion with vibration [85].

Postural drainage percussion with vibration is still considered by many the gold standard of therapy, although several alternative airway clearance techniques (ACTs) exist, including 1) autogenic drainage, which can be performed independently by adolescents and adults; 2) positive expiratory pressure (PEP), which involves exhaling against expiratory resistance applied through a mask (PEP mask); and 3) active cycle of breathing technique, an independently performed breathing exercise. These three techniques are less demanding than postural drainage and percussion with vibration, and may be performed independently; thus, they are often preferred by patients. Newer ACTs (eg, high-frequency chest percussors and oral oscillators such as the flutter valve) are less time-consuming and promote independence, although patient compliance with these regimens has not been determined. Although the short-term effect of ACTs on lung function seems limited, lung function appears to deteriorate when they are discontinued. Exercise is considered an important adjunct to ACTs, not a replacement. Patients should be encouraged to incorporate ACTs and exercise into their lifestyles from the time cystic fibrosis is first diagnosed, even when they are asymptomatic. Clinical judgment is the best guide to selecting a regimen that will be most suitable for a particular patient of a given age and circumstance [85].

Physical exercise is beneficial in cystic fibrosis patients and should be a component of their therapeutic regimen. It increases lung function and sputum production as well as having a bronchodilator effect. It also improves cardiopulmonary fitness and inspiratory muscle strength [86–90]. There may also be a specific beneficial effect of exercise on mucociliary clearance and inhibition of Na^+ absorption [91], which is consistent with the notion that airway mucosal nucleotide release during exercise may activate alternative mechanisms of airway chloride secretion. A recently reported long-term clinical trial identified benefits from inhaling nebulizing hypertonic (7%) saline (4 mL) twice daily. This treatment was associated with approximately a 5% improvement in lung function over 1 year compared with subjects who inhaled normal (0.9%) saline. More important, inhalation of hypertonic saline was associated with a 50% reduction in the frequency of infective exacerbations requiring parenteral antibiotic therapy, as well as improvements in quality of life (in patients older than 14 years) and improved work/school attendance [92]. A second clinical trial of shorter duration demonstrated similar benefits in terms of lung function [93].

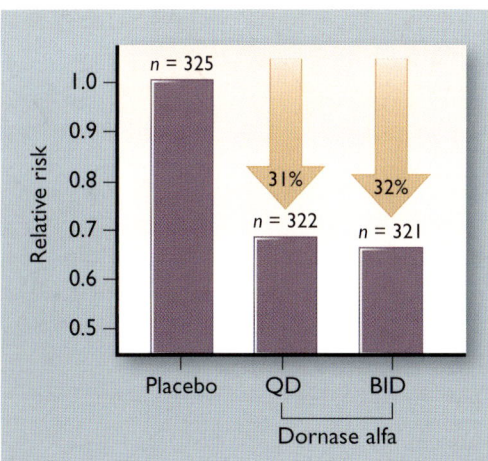

Figure 4-17. Therapies to alter mucus rheology and increase airway clearance. Traditional mucolytic therapies, such as N-acetylcysteine, confer little benefit by themselves in cystic fibrosis (CF) and are rarely used today. Two inhaled therapies have been shown to affect mucus clearance, improve lung function, and reduce exacerbations in CF patients: recombinant DNAase and hypertonic saline [94]. Aerosolized recombinant human deoxyribonuclease I (rhDNase, or Pulmozyme® [Genentech; South San Francisco, CA]) cleaves the DNA residue left by degenerating neutrophils. In doing so, it reduces sputum viscosity and enhances clearance [95]. The enzyme was approved by the US Food and Drug Administration in 1994 for use in CF patients after a clinical trial [96]. The Pulmozyme study enrolled 968 clinically stable patients older than 5 years from 51 CF centers in a randomized, double-blind, placebo-controlled study conducted in conjunction with usual therapy for CF [97]. Patients received 2.5 mg of rhDNase or a placebo once daily (QD) or twice daily (BID) for 24 weeks. Forced expiratory volume in 1 second (FEV_1) improved by approximately 6% in both dosage groups. As shown in the figure, the relative risk of pulmonary exacerbation was significantly reduced by rhDNase. Modest reductions in hospital days and days on parenteral antibiotics were also observed. Similar improvements have been observed in open-label studies, including a study conducted in the United Kingdom [98].

Because airway inflammation may be an important issue even in the youngest patients with CF, a follow-up study was initiated to examine the effects of treatment with dornase alfa of children 6 to 10 years of age with good lung function (ie, FEV_1 95%–96% predicted, forced vital capacity [FVC] 102% predicted) and good nutritional status [99]. In addition, approximately 20% of the study population had sinusitis, 10% in each of the two cohorts had daily sputum production, and nearly all subjects had pancreatic insufficiency. A total of 474 patients were enrolled in one of the two study cohorts: 235 patients receiving placebo and 239 patients receiving dornase alfa (2.5 mg daily). At week 96 of the study, patients receiving dornase alfa demonstrated an initial increase in FEV_1 of 3%, which was maintained over the course of the study. Force expired flow at 25% to 75% FVC (FEF 25–75) increased in the dornase alfa group by 8% over the placebo group, and was maintained throughout the study. When researchers looked at pulmonary exacerbations occurring during the study term, the group receiving dornase alfa demonstrated a 34% risk reduction of first exacerbation. These results suggest that early intervention and aggressive therapy in young, relatively healthy patients with CF may result in a substantial reduction in pulmonary exacerbations and a sustained benefit in lung function.

In vitro studies support the notion that osmotic extraction of water into poorly adherent mucus plaques on primary cultures of airway epithelium restores normal mucus transport. The effects of chronic inhalation of hypertonic saline were tested in CF patients in a multicenter double-blind, parallel-group trial. A total of 164 CF patients (age > 6 y) with stable lung disease were randomly assigned to inhale 4 mL of either 7% hypertonic saline or 0.9% (control) saline twice daily for 48 weeks. Hypertonic saline was associated with an absolute difference in lung function between groups ($P = 0.03$), significantly fewer pulmonary exacerbations (relative reduction of 56%; $P = 0.02$), and a significantly higher percentage of patients not experiencing an exacerbation. The beneficial effect on lung function and mucus transport was corroborated in another, single-center study.

Selective β_2-agonists and anticholinergic agents (eg, ipratropium bromide) may benefit CF patients who have symptoms of airway hyperresponsiveness due to asthma or other causes. Not all patients benefit from this treatment, however, and the clinical condition of some may even worsen. Thus, patients should be monitored carefully if bronchodilator or anticholinergic therapy is initiated. (*Adapted from* Fiel [100].)

Clinical Indications for Intravenous Antibiotic Therapy in Cystic Fibrosis

"CF-Pancreas"

Cough—increased

Fever

Pulmonary function—worsening

Appetite—decreased

Nutritional status—impaired

Complete blood count—leukocytosis with left shift

Radiograph—new infiltrates, overaeration, and mucus plugs

Examination—crackles, wheezes

Activity—decreased

Sputum—thicker, darker, and more abundant

Figure 4-18. Clinical indications for intravenous antibiotic therapy. Antibiotic therapy for patients with cystic fibrosis has been a cornerstone of treatment for five decades [101]. There is broad consensus regarding the value of intravenous antibiotics for acute pulmonary exacerbations and the indications for its administration. Appropriate antibiotic regimens and special therapeutic considerations for patients with cystic fibrosis are summarized in the figure. The selection of a route of administration (aerosol, oral, or intravenous) is generally tailored to the patient's clinical need. At this time, there is less agreement on the routine use of antibiotics for maintenance than on their use in treating pulmonary exacerbations (*see* Fig. 4-20). The prophylactic use of intravenous antibiotics, a practice that is advocated by Danish physicians, is uncommon in the United States and Canada. Aggressive antibiotic therapy may also have a role upon first positive culture for *Pseudomonas aeruginosa*, in an attempt to delay chronic colonization with this organism. (*Adapted from* Schidlow [102].)

A. Intravenous Antiobiotic Therapy for Common Cystic Fibrosis Pathogens: Bacterial

Organism	Primary Treatment	Alternative Treatment
Staphylococcus aureus	Oxacillin, nafcillin	First-generation cephalosporin, vancomycin, clindamycin
Methicillin-resistant S. aureus	Vancomycin	Linezolid, teicoplanin, fusidic acid
Haemophilus influenzae	Cefotaxime, ceftriaxone	Fluoroquinolone, trimethoprim sulfamethoxazole, carbapenem
P. aeruginosa	One agent from two of the following three groups (based on sensitivities): 1) Antipseudomonal penicillin, antipseudomonal third-generation cephalosporin, carbapenem, monobactam	2) Antipseudomonal aminoglycoside; 3) ciprofloxacin
Burkholderia cepacia complex	Ceftazidime, chloramphenicol, trimethoprim sulfamethoxazole, carbapenem, tetracyclines, and aminoglycosides (based on sensitivities)	

B. Intravenous Antibiotic Therapy for Common Cystic Fibrosis Pathogens: Nontuberculous Mycobacteria

Organism	Primary Treatment	Comments/Alternative Treatment
Mycobacterium avium complex	Clarithromycin, 30 mg/kg/d (max 1000 mg) po	12–18 mo therapy; also consider clofazimine, streptomycin, amikacin, ciprofloxacin
	Rifabutin, 5 mg/kg/d (max 300 mg) po	
	Ethambutol, 25 mg/kg/d po	
Mycobacterium abscessus	Cefoxitin, 200 mg/kg/d IV	
	Amikacin, 15 mg/kg/d IV every 12 h; aim for peak level of 18-24 µg/mL	
Mycobacterium fortuitum	Clarithromycin, 30 mg/kg/d (max 1000 mg po qd)	6–12 mo therapy
Mycobacterium kansasii	Isoniazid, 10–20 mg/kg/d po qd (max 300 mg) × 18 mo	18 mo therapy
	Rifampin, 10–20 mg/kg/d po qd (max 600 mg) × 18 mo	
	Ethambutol, 25 mg/kg/d po qd × 2 mo, then decrease to 15 mg/kg/d	

Figure 4-19. Antibiotic therapy for common cystic fibrosis pathogens. **A** and **B**, Bacteria and nontuberculous mycobacteria associated with pulmonary infection in patients with cystic fibrosis and appropriate intravenous treatments. Although intravenous (IV) aminoglycosides are active against *Pseudomonas aeruginosa*, the large doses that are required increase the risk of nephrotoxic and ototoxic effects, and appropriate monitoring of aminoglycoside levels is crucial. The choice of antibiotic therapy should be guided by current microbiologic sensitivities when possible. In patients with multidrug-resistant organisms (*ie*, organisms resistant to more than one class of antibiotic), resistance may be overcome by the synergistic effects of antibiotic combinations. The utility of two- or three-drug antibiotic synergy studies is being explored in some centers. Short-term, high-dose aerosol administration of tobramycin is an efficacious and safe treatment for endobronchial infection with *P. aeruginosa* in patients with clinically stable cystic fibrosis [103]. The practice of nebulizing tobramycin (300 mg twice daily) to cystic fibrosis patients every alternative month is widespread. The clinical usefulness of other inhaled antibiotics, such aztreonam, is currently being examined. Studies have confirmed that chronic trice weekly or daily oral azithromycin therapy is associated with improved lung function in CF patients infected with *P. aeruginosa*. Although the mechanism has not been established, this has also become a widespread therapy [104–106]. po—orally; qd—every day. (*Adapted from* Ramsey [24].)

Special Considerations in Antibiotic Treatment for Patients with Cystic Fibrosis

Goal	Return patient to baseline in terms of symptoms, sputum reduction, and lung function (forced expiratory volume in 1 s); eradication of *Pseudomonas aeruginosa* is impossible.
Target	Multiple organisms and multiple strains of *P. aeruginosa*, *Staphylococcus aureus*, *Haemophilus influenzae*, and *Burkholderia cepacia*
Dose	Dose must be significantly higher than for non-CF patients due to 1) altered pharmacokinetics in CF patients, 2) inactivation of some drugs (eg, tobramycin) that bind to free DNA, 3) coexistent strains of *P. aeruginosa* with varying susceptibility, and 4) presence of alginate strains of *P. aeruginosa*. Optimal dosing is based on monitoring of peak and trough serum concentrations.
Duration	2–3 wk or until return to clinical and pulmonary function baseline
Choice of drugs	Synergistic drug combinations can prevent or override resistance. Antipseudomonal combinations are generally comprised of aminoglycosides (eg, tobramycin, gentamicin) and β-lactams. Among the latter, cephalosporins (eg, ceftazidime) are preferred over the semisynthetic penicillins for their dosing convenience. Imipenem is not recommended for routine treatment because it readily induces resistance. Drug choice is based on sputum bacteriology and, when necessary, in vitro synergy testing.
IV drugs	IV drug delivery is used for moderate to severe exacerbations and subacute clinical or pulmonary deterioration. Home therapy, which is less disruptive to patients and less costly, may be considered if other traditional benefits of hospital care are unnecessary. Midline catheters and long-term indwelling venous catheters are useful alternatives for patients requiring frequent venous access; otherwise, arrangements must be made for placing an IV line at home or in the hospital.
Oral drugs	Oral drugs (primarily ciprofloxacin or other quinolones) are used for mild to moderate exacerbations and maintenance therapy. Quinolones are not approved for use in children < 18 y of age, but ciprofloxacin has been administered to > 1000 children on a compassionate basis with no clear increase in arthropathy. Broad-spectrum antibiotics may be useful against nonpseudomonal bacteria, and they may reduce the release of bacterial toxins, limiting inflammation.
Inhaled drugs	Aerosolized drugs (eg, tobramycin, colistin) are commonly used for maintenance therapy after chest physiotherapy. They are thought to provide high concentrations of drug and limited toxicity in the airways. High-dose tobramycin (300 mg twice daily) delivered by ultrasonic nebulizer improved lung function and decreased *P. aeruginosa* density in a multicenter double-blind crossover study. Decisions to use aerosolized drugs are made on a case-by-case basis.
Indications	See Fig. 4-18.
Monitoring	Careful monitoring is necessary to avoid renal or ototoxicity because aminoglycosides have a narrow therapeutic/toxic window at the high doses required in patients with CF (eg, peak and trough levels of 10–12 and 2 µg/mL, respectively). Ciprofloxacin is generally well tolerated, although arthropathy is sporadically reported. Intermittent use is desirable; long-term use is discouraged because drug resistance occurs after 3–4 wk of monotherapy.
Allergy	Desensitization may be necessary in cases of allergy to aminoglycosides or semisynthetic penicillins.
Multidrug resistance	Strategies for minimizing or overcoming multidrug resistance include 1) avoiding overuse, 2) avoiding monotherapy, 3) using in vitro synergy test results to guide drug choice, and 4) using high doses of drugs.
Maintenance therapy	Maintenance antibiotic therapy with oral or aerosolized agents to prevent a decline in lung function is common, but the effectiveness of this approach is being questioned [41,42,64] and the practice is coming under scrutiny for its possible role in the development of multidrug-resistant organisms [40,65].

Figure 4-20. Special considerations in antibiotic treatment for patients with cystic fibrosis (CF). IV—intravenous.

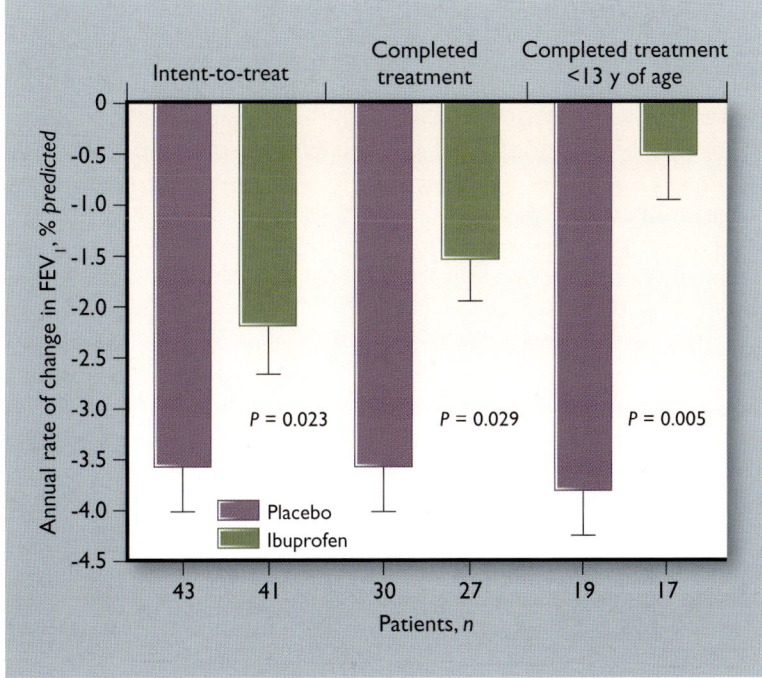

Figure 4-21. Effects of long-term anti-inflammatory therapy with ibuprofen on the annual rate of change in lung function. Unresolved safety issues with respect to the long-term use of steroids for patients with cystic fibrosis have heightened interest in the use of ibuprofen as a treatment for patients with mild lung disease. Ibuprofen is believed to reduce inflammation by decreasing neutrophil influx and reducing the stimulus for leukotriene B_4, a chemoattractant that is markedly elevated in the airway surface liquid of patients with cystic fibrosis. Because leukotriene B_4 promotes neutrophil adherence, aggregation, migration, degranulation, and superoxide release, inhibition of its production by ibuprofen would be predicted to inhibit inflammatory damage to the lung. The results of a 4-year, randomized, placebo-controlled, double-blind trial of high-dose ibuprofen in 85 cystic fibrosis patients with mild lung disease are shown in the figure [70]. Patients (aged 5 to 39 years) tolerated twice-daily treatment with 20 to 30 mg/kg. The authors concluded that high-dose ibuprofen, taken consistently, significantly slowed the progression of lung disease over the 4-year period without significant toxicity. Compared with placebo, ibuprofen decreased the annual rate of decline of pulmonary measures and Brasfield chest radiographic scores, and preserved the percentage of ideal body weight. For patients meeting the prospective criteria for completing the trial, the annual rate of decline in lung function, measured by the percent predicted forced expiratory volume in 1 second (FEV_1) was 59% lower for the ibuprofen-treated patients. Establishing the appropriate dose by pharmacokinetic studies in each patient is recommended, and monitoring for rare adverse effects is important. Administration of ibuprofen has been recommended, especially for patients aged 5 to 13 years who have mild disease.

Continued on the next page

Figure 4-21. *(Continued)* Several trials have confirmed the benefit of azithromycin therapy in cystic fibrosis. In the United States phase III clinical trial on the efficacy of azithromycin in cystic fibrosis, patients with *Pseudomonas aeruginosa* infection receiving azithromycin, 500 mg three times weekly, demonstrated improved FEV_1 (6.2%), higher body weight (0.8 kg), and fewer pulmonary exacerbations (40% reduction). *P. aeruginosa* density was reduced in the treatment group (0.2 $\log_{10}$ colony-forming units compared with a 0.3 $\log_{10}$ increase in the placebo group, although the significance of this difference is uncertain) [104]. The trial did not include patients colonized with *Burkholderia cepacia* complex or nontuberculous mycobacteria, or those with abnormal liver function, so data on efficacy or safety in these groups are lacking. Benefit was also documented in other trials [105,106]. It is currently not known with certainty if the beneficial effect of azithromycin is predominantly a manifestation of the immunomodulatory properties of macrolides or their antimicrobial effect [107,108]. (*Data from* Konstan *et al.* [109].)

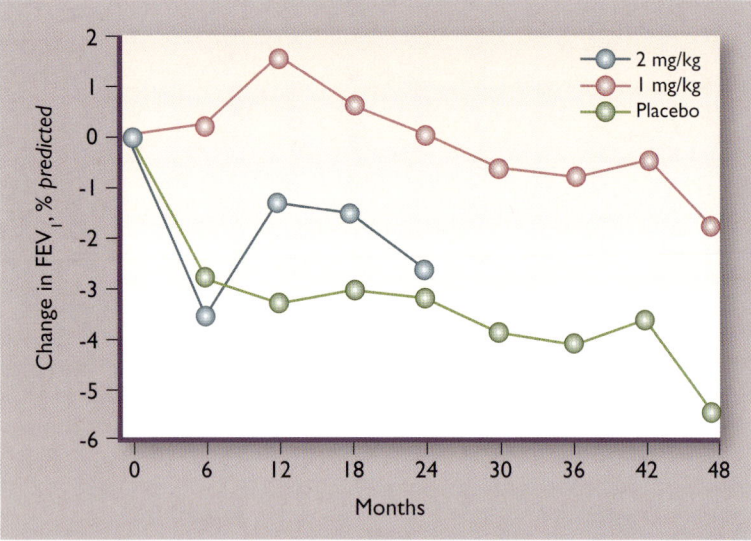

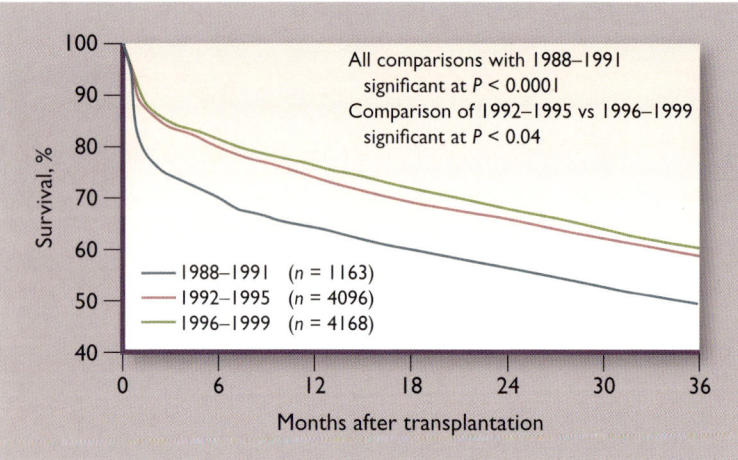

Figure 4-22. Effects of 4-year anti-inflammatory therapy with prednisone on lung function. Long-term therapy with prednisone is not widely practiced. Although the initial results of a 4-year double-blind trial of high-dose (2 mg/kg) alternate-day prednisone in 45 children younger than 12 years suggested that treatment was efficacious and without side effects [109], subsequent results were less promising. In the Cystic Fibrosis Foundation Prednisone Trial Group study [110], investigators randomized 285 children aged 6 to 14 years with mild to moderate lung disease to receive high-dose prednisone (2 mg/kg), low-dose prednisone (1 mg/kg), or placebo on alternate days. The results are represented in the figure. The high-dose group was terminated early because of growth retardation, glucose abnormalities, and cataract formation [109]. Results were modestly beneficial with respect to forced expiratory volume in 1 second (FEV_1) in the low-dose group by 6 months, but few other beneficial effects were seen. The mean FEV_1 of low-dose prednisone patients was not significantly different from baseline at 48 months. (*Adapted from* Eigen *et al.* [111].)

Figure 4-23. Lung transplantation and improved actuarial survival of patients with cystic fibrosis (CF). Despite treatment advances that have dramatically extended the life expectancy of patients with CF, most patients eventually die of progressive lung disease. Lung transplantation for end-stage CF, first performed in 1985, has altered this scenario for some patients. By 2007, almost 3000 CF patients had undergone lung transplantation (International Society of Heart and Lung Transplantation Registry Data, http://www.ishlt.org/registries/heartLungRegistry.asp). Approximately 150 lung transplants are performed on CF patients yearly [112] (United Network for Organ Sharing Database, www.unos.org).

The long-term implications of this technology for the CF community are unclear. Due to the acute shortage of donor organs, the option of transplantation is available only to a limited number of patients. In 2005 a new organ allocation system was introduced in the United States, replacing the previous system, where organs were allotted based strictly on time accrued on a lung transplant waiting list. In the new system patients are assigned a lung allocation score, which is based on functional status (*eg*, New York Heart Association functional status and 6-min walk distance) and physiologic parameters that have been shown to correlate with likelihood of death while awaiting transplantation (including pulmonary artery pressure, inspired oxygen/mechanical ventilation requirement, and forced vital capacity). Organ allocation is also influenced by blood group and the physical size of the recipient, which is matched to that of the donor. Of note, the score also takes into account the patient's actuarial likelihood of postoperative survival, which is increased in CF patients compared with patients transplanted for other conditions. The intention behind the new scoring system is to reduce the incidence of death while on the waiting list, although demand still exceeds organ availability. Consequently, close to 200 living-donor lobar transplants have been performed in CF patients. Timing of referral for transplantation is tailored to an individual patient's needs, although most centers judge a forced expiratory volume in 1 second below 30% in a patient receiving maximum medical treatment to be a good indicator for assessment for the procedure, with allowances being made for other extenuating circumstances, such as accelerated rate of decline in lung function. Although CF presents many additional management challenges once thought to be insurmountable, transplantation has prolonged survival and improved the quality of life for hundreds suffering from end-stage disease before surgery.

Further, the long-term survival of CF patients is excellent compared with that of other patients undergoing double-lung transplantation. Nonetheless, concern persists regarding transplantation of patients colonized with *Burkholderia cepacia* complex, particularly *Burkholderia cenocepacia* (genomovar III), which is more frequently associated with cepacia syndrome and thus is a heightened concern in the context of postoperative immunosuppression. These patients may be transplanted successfully, but survival is reduced compared with other CF patients [113]. For this reason, transplantation in this group is currently limited to a few centers worldwide [114,115].

Continued on the next page

Figure 4-23. *(Continued)* Despite the clinical challenges posed by their disease, CF patients make good transplantation candidates for a number of reasons, including 1) life-threatening manifestations are usually confined to the respiratory system, 2) patients are relatively young when considered for transplantation, and 3) patients have extensive experience in adhering to complex treatment regimens. Data from the International Society of Heart and Lung Transplantation Registry suggest that actuarial 1- and 5-year survival rates following lung transplantation in CF patients between 1990 and 2005 were ~80% and ~55%, respectively. *(Adapted from* Hosenpud et al. [116]*.)*

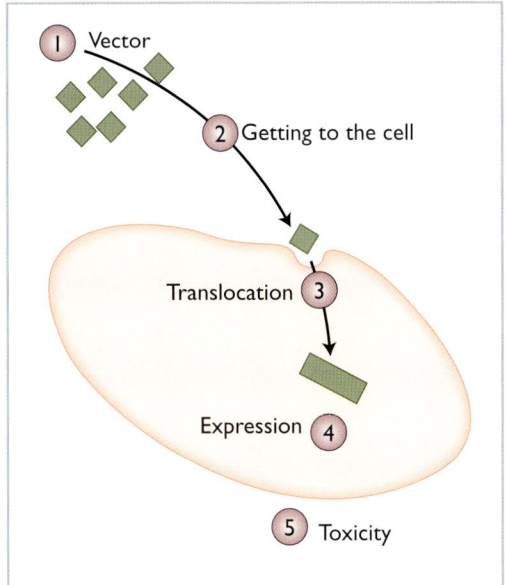

Figure 4-24. Gene therapy for cystic fibrosis (CF). Although therapeutic regimens have increased life expectancy and improved the quality of life for thousands of patients, traditional therapies target the signs and symptoms of CF while not addressing the basic molecular defect [117]. Conceptually, gene therapy is an attractive alternative. An intensive effort to develop gene therapy for CF has been under way since the gene was cloned in 1989. By mid-1995, 10 National Institutes of Health–approved CF gene therapy clinical trials were under way, representing more than half of the total trials approved for all inherited genetic diseases [118]. However, success has been elusive. Moreover, adverse outcomes in human gene therapy trials have led to more guarded optimism for gene therapy research in CF [118]. Trials have used viral or plasmid vectors, and even molecular conjugates designed to draw DNA molecules into cells by receptor-mediated endocytosis [119,120]. There are many hurdles to successful gene therapy in CF, including 1) selection of an effective vector, 2) delivery of the vector to the appropriate target cell, 3) translocation of the transgenic material to the site of expression (typically the nucleus), 4) successful gene expression and incorporation of cystic fibrosis transmembrane regulator gene (CFTR) protein in the apical membrane of target cells, and 5) absence of toxicity [121].

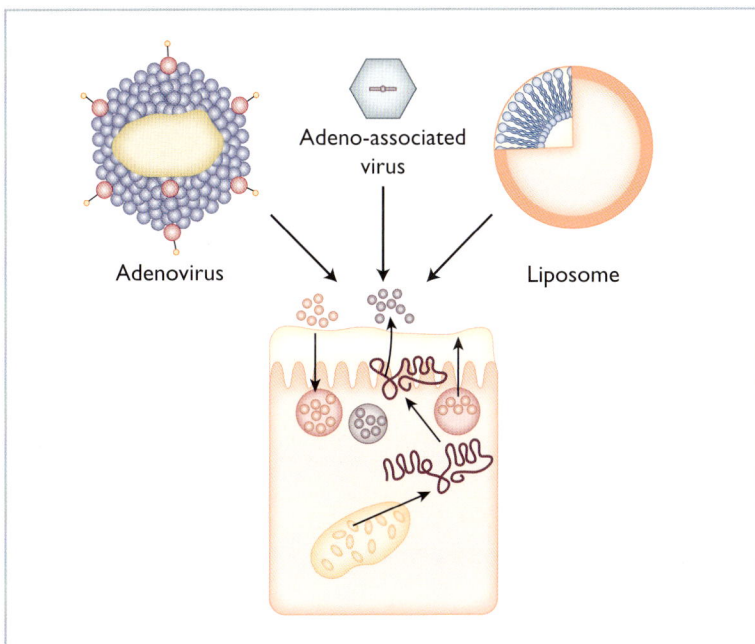

Figure 4-25. Approaches to gene therapy for cystic fibrosis. Three gene therapy strategies have been tested in human clinical trials. 1) Adenoviruses: Replication-deficient recombinant adenoviruses are the best-known and most widely studied of the viral vectors [122–130]. In animal models, adenoviruses elicit a cytotoxic T cell–mediated immune response, which is associated with transient lung inflammation after airway administration [124,128,129], and repetitive dosing stimulates production of neutralizing antibodies [131–133]. In clinical trials, efficacy was lower than expected, expression was transient, and molecular evidence of gene transfer did not necessarily predict or correlate with functional correction [134]. Moreover, significant inflammation has been noted in some patients [134,135]. Second- and third-generation vectors that are less easily recognized by the immune system are being developed. Some strategies attempt to disguise the virus by modifying its immunogenic epitopes; another approach is to coat the virus, creating a "stealth" vector [121]. 2) Adeno-associated virus: Recombinant adeno-associated virus (AAV) is a small, single-stranded DNA virus, barely large enough to accommodate the cystic fibrosis transmembrane conductance regulator (CFTR) expression cassette. Preclinical studies have shown that AAV does not integrate into the genome as readily as expected, making it likely that expression will be transient. Moreover, when integration occurs, it is not site specific, a problem that raises the specter of mutagenesis from random insertion of AAV genes into the host genome. Recombinant AAV vectors from serotype 2 have been used in clinical trials, but may not gain entry into target cells (*ie*, ciliated cells) as well as other serotypes, and thus may not result in functional correction [117]. Generation of antibodies to the viral vector proteins remains a concern. 3) Liposomes: An alternative, nonviral strategy uses plasmid CFTR complementary DNA complexed to a cationic lipid such as DOPE (dioleoylphosphatidylethanolamine). Lipid-mediated gene transfer avoids problems with immunogenicity and can transfect genes in animal models [136,137] and in human nasal epithelium [138]. However, it is much less efficient than the viral approach, and gene expression remains sufficiently low and transient to result in little therapeutic benefit. Investigators have attempted insertion of proteins analogous to viruses into their constructs in an effort to improve the yield [121]. An unexpected toxic property of plasmid-based therapy has been activation of toll receptor–mediated inflammation by CpG motifs in bacterial DNA [139]. Clinical trials for cystic fibrosis using lipid-mediated gene transfer have been undertaken in the United States without evidence of efficacy [117]. Further data are needed regarding the role of the CFTR defect in cystic fibrosis for researchers to determine the level of corrected CFTR expression that is required for effective treatment of the disease. Although hundreds of trials of gene therapies have been undertaken, no gene therapy has received approval by the US Food and Drug Administration (FDA). Perhaps the future rests with new vectors, with pseudotyped (retargeted) lentiviral and paramyxovirus vectors seeming novel candidates. *(Adapted from* Wilson [140]*.)*

Standard care	Recent strategies	Target	Investigational
		Genetic defect	← Gene therapy
		CFTR trafficking and processing	CPX Phenylbutyrate Genistein Milrinone Chemical chaperones Chemical CFTR correctors and potentiators
	Hypertonic saline →	Mucus dehydration	← Amiloride analogues (Na⁺ blocker) ← Nucleotide analogues (Cl⁻ channel agonist)
Oral antimicrobials → IV antimicrobials →	Aerosolized tobramycin → Azithromycin →	Bacterial infection	← Hyperimmune gammaglobulin ← Vaccines ← Magainins ← Inhaled aztreonam ← Inhaled amikacin
	Ibuprofen →	Inflammation	← Elastase inhibitors
	Dornase alfa →	Viscous mucus	← Gelsolin ← Thymosin B
Chest PT → Exercise → Bronchodilators →	Flutter → Vest →	Airway obstruction	
	Lung transplant →	Respiratory failure	

Figure 4-26. Current treatments for cystic fibrosis (CF). A broad range of supportive therapies are currently available to treat the pathologic manifestations of CF. However, it is hoped that advances in our understanding of CF pathogenesis will generate more effective therapies designed to target and treat the basic physiologic defect, rather than merely treat disease manifestations. Among the most promising in this regard are strategies to durably restore hydration to the epithelial surface and thus restore normal mucociliary clearance [94], correct the CFTR trafficking defect [141], achieve successful CFTR gene therapy, control excessive airway inflammation, and effectively kill harmful microorganisms by novel means. A comprehensive list of novel agents being assessed for utility in CF patients by the Cystic Fibrosis Foundation's Therapeutic Development Network is available at http://www.cff.org/research/DrugDevelopmentPipeline/. IV—intravenous; PT—physiotherapy.

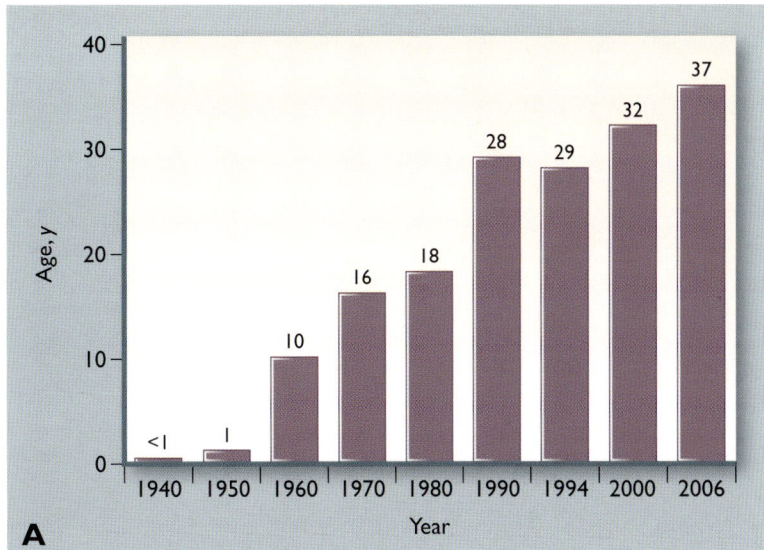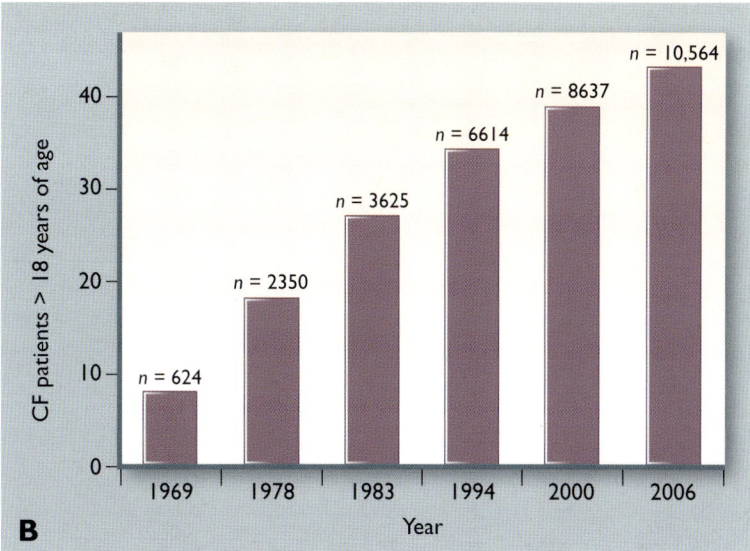

Figure 4-27. Developments in life expectancy of patients with cystic fibrosis (CF) linked to quality of care. **A** and **B**, The median survival age of patients with CF almost tripled between 1960 and 1994 (*panel A*). Data from the Cystic Fibrosis Foundation of North America registry suggests a further improvement in median age of survival to 37 by 2006. The number of patients older than 18 years has quadrupled since 1969 (*panel B*). The burgeoning number of adult patients constitutes a dramatic testimonial to the excellence of care provided by the network of CF clinics that serve pediatric patients throughout North America. Unfortunately, we are less equipped to meet the needs of adults with CF [142]. On reaching adulthood, the care of patients with CF should be transferred to adult programs staffed by personnel with the expertise to meet their special needs. However, many young adults are unable to find age-appropriate caregivers and, therefore, remain under the care of pediatric teams or drift away from the health care system altogether.

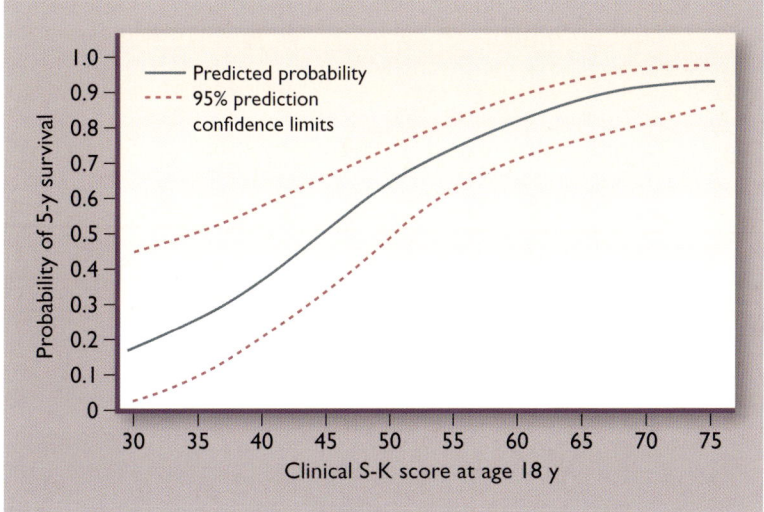

Figure 4-28. Using clinical scores to predict survival in young adults with cystic fibrosis. Median survival of patients with cystic fibrosis is approximately 32 years. Long-term follow-up of 110 young adults with cystic fibrosis identified factors that predicted 5-year survival. Stepwise logistic regression applied to 11 variables identified Shwachman and Kulczycki (S-K) scores at 18 years of age as the best predictor of survival to age 23 [143]. The S-K scoring system assesses general activity, physical findings, and nutritional status, with 25 points for each and a total of 75 points for normal findings [144]. Median duration of survival for patients with clinical scores of 65 to 75 (12 years) was more than double that of patients with clinical scores of 30 to 49 (5 years). Favorable prognostic factors for long-term survival (*ie*, beyond age 18) include good nutrition, good pulmonary function, high clinical scores, and absence of chronic respiratory colonization with multidrug-resistant organisms [137]. Specialized centers for adult patients with cystic fibrosis make it possible to collect longitudinal historical, physical, and laboratory data that will permit clinicians to respond promptly to subtle changes in any of these indicators; timely intervention is likely to slow disease progression and prolong survival. (*Adapted from* Huang *et al.* [143].)

ADULT PATIENTS: A NEW CLINICAL FRONTIER

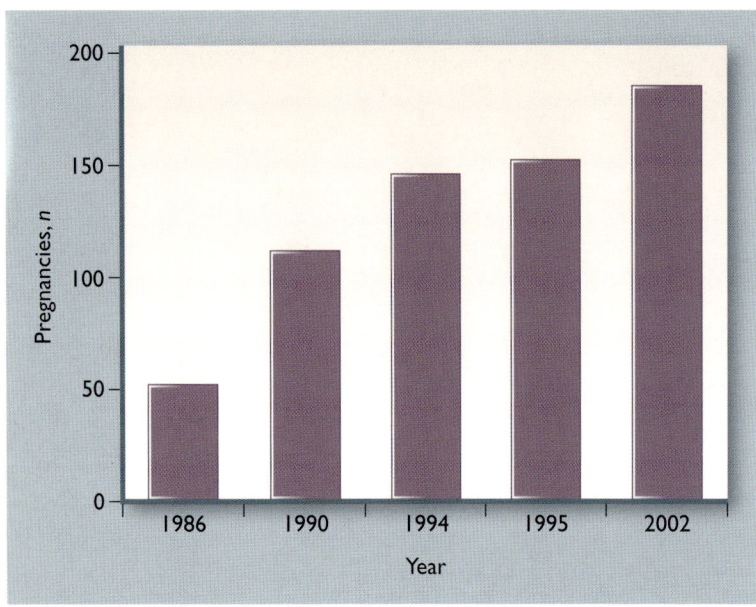

Figure 4-29. Reproductive issues of men and women with cystic fibrosis (CF). Clinical challenges associated with caring for adult patients with CF are not limited to increasing morbidity and the prospect of death. The number of pregnancies among women with CF has increased 10-fold over the past 30 years [145]. Most women with CF tolerate pregnancy well, despite earlier fears that pregnancy is inherently hazardous for them [146,147]. However, pregnancy may still be contraindicated in most patients with severely compromised pulmonary and pancreatic status. Pregnancy is only one of several issues that were once of little consequence to those who cared for pediatric patients but that are becoming increasingly relevant as the number of adults with CF escalates [148]. Infertility is nearly universal among men with CF as a consequence of congenital bilateral absence of the vas deferens. Options were limited to adoption and artificial insemination by a donor. However, microsurgical epididymal sperm aspiration in combination with in vitro fertilization has been performed successfully [149], and there is no reason to believe that the technology should not be effective among men with CF, provided that sperm count, morphology, and motility are normal.

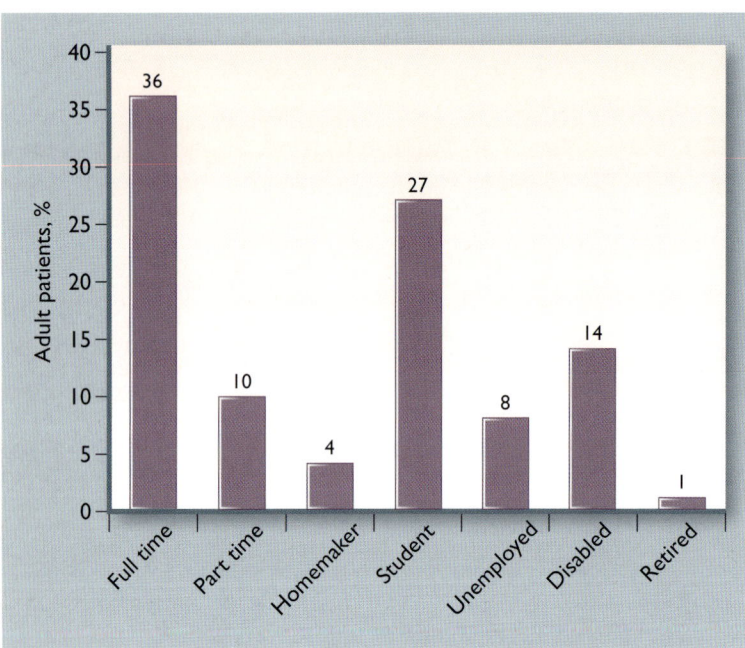

Figure 4-30. Employment status of adult patients with cystic fibrosis (CF), 2005. Adult patients with CF also present clinicians with complex psychosocial challenges. According to the Cystic Fibrosis Foundation (CFF) registry, approximately 50% of adult CF patients are employed full- or part-time and almost 20% are students. This demonstrates that many patients pursue their educational and vocational goals successfully in the face of daunting obstacles. The trend toward home-based intravenous therapy has facilitated these activities. However, the transition to independence is not always easy, or even possible. Almost 200 CF patients were reported as being pregnant in the 2005 CFF Registry Report. Not all patients are able to leave their family homes for college or paid employment, and many of those who become independent face diminished opportunities and a reduced earning capacity because of the constraints of their illness [150–152]. Many patients also face difficulties in obtaining health insurance. Although the resilience of most CF patients is remarkable, the psychosocial costs of decreased life expectancy are substantial. Thus, it is important to provide support services appropriate to their age and situation. The situation faced by young adults with CF represents a serious public policy issue. The health care system is not prepared to deal with the growing population of individuals with so-called childhood disorders who have achieved adulthood and are living to a relatively advanced age [142]. The problem is particularly acute for young adults who are not yet integrated into the workforce and who lack health insurance. Care for many young adults with CF—and others with chronic diseases—is seriously compromised. Our challenge as caregivers is to develop strategies and mechanisms to ensure that CF patients continue to receive the best possible care as they grow older. (*Adapted from* The New Insights Editorial Board [153].)

REFERENCES

1. Boat TF: Cystic fibrosis. In *Textbook of Respiratory Medicine*. Edited by Murray JF, Nadel JA. Philadelphia: WB Saunders; 1988:1126–1152.

2. Yankaskas JR, Marshall BC, Sufian JD, *et al.*: Cystic Fibrosis Adult Care Consensus Conference report. *Chest* 2004, 125:1S–39S.

3. Welsh MJ, Smith AE: Cystic fibrosis. *Sci Am* 1995, 273:52–59.

4. Taussig LM: Cystic fibrosis: an overview. In *Cystic Fibrosis*. Edited by Taussig LM. New York: Thieme-Stratton Inc; 1984:1–9.

5. Hess JH, Saphir O: Celiac disease: chronic intestinal digestion. *J Pediatr* 1935, 6:1–13.

6. Fanconi G, Uehlinger E, Knaver C: Coeliaksyndrom bei angeborener zystischer pankreas fibromatose und bronchiektasien. *Wien Med Wochenschr* 1936, 86:753–756. (Cited in Rosenfeld MA, Collins FS: Gene therapy for cystic fibrosis. *Chest* 1996, 109:241–252.)

7. Andersen DH: Cystic fibrosis of the pancreas and its relation to celiac disease. *Am J Dis Child* 1938, 56:344–399.

8. Andersen DH, Hodges RG: Celiac syndrome. V. Genetics of cystic fibrosis of the pancreas with a consideration of etiology. *Am J Dis Child* 1946, 72:62–80.

9. Di Sant'Agnese PA, Darling RC, Perera GA, *et al.*: Abnormal electrolytic composition of sweat in cystic fibrosis of the pancreas: clinical significance and relationship to the disease. *Pediatrics* 1953, 12:549–562.

10. Gibson LE, Cooke RE: A test for concentration of electrolytes in sweat in cystic fibrosis of the pancreas. *Pediatrics* 1959, 23:545–549.

11. Quinton PM: Chloride impermeability in cystic fibrosis. *Nature* 1983, 301:421–422.

12. Knowles MR, Stutts MJ, Spock A, *et al.*: Abnormal ion permeation through cystic fibrosis respiratory epithelium. *Science* 1983, 221:1067–1070.

13. Hammond KB, Abman SH, Sokol RJ, *et al.*: Efficacy of statewide neonatal screening for cystic fibrosis by assay of trypsinogen concentrations. *N Engl J Med* 1991, 325:765–774.

14. Gregg RG, Wilfond BS, Farrell PM, *et al.*: Application of DNA analysis in a population-screening program for neonatal diagnosis of cystic fibrosis (CF): comparison of screening protocols. *Am J Hum Genet* 1993, 52:616–626.

15. Hamosh A, Fitz-Simmons SC, Macek M, *et al.*: Comparison of the clinical manifestations of cystic fibrosis in black and white patients. *J Pediatr* 1998, 132:255–259.

16. Kulczycki LL, Schauf V: Cystic fibrosis in blacks in Washington, DC: incidence and characteristics. *Am J Dis Child* 1974, 127:64–67.

17. Grebe TA, Seltzer WK, DeMarchii J, *et al.*: Genetic analysis of Hispanic individuals with cystic fibrosis. *Am J Hum Genet* 1994, 54:443–446.

18. Grebe TA, Duane WW, Richter SF, *et al.*: Mutation analysis of the cystic fibrosis transmembrane regulator gene in Native American populations of the Southwest. *Am J Hum Genet* 1992, 51:736–740.

19. Powers CA, Potter EM, Wessel HU, *et al.*: Cystic fibrosis in Asian Indians. *Arch Pediatr Adolesc Med* 1996, 150:554–555.

20. Kerem BS, Rommens JM, Buchanan JA, *et al.*: Identification of the cystic fibrosis gene: genetic analysis. *Science* 1989, 245:1073–1080.

20a. Riordan JR, Rommens JM, Kerem B-S, *et al.*: Identification of the cystic fibrosis gene: cloning and characterization of complementary DNA. *Science* 1989, 245:1066–1073.

21. Rommens JM, Iannuzzi MC, Kerem B-S, *et al.*: Identification of the cystic fibrosis gene: chromosome walking and jumping. *Science* 1989, 245:1059–1065.

22. Anderson MP, Gregory RJ, Thompson S, *et al.*: Demonstration that CFTR is a chloride channel by alteration of its anion selectivity. *Science* 1991, 53:202–205.

23. Stutts MJ, Canessa JC, Olsen M, *et al.*: CFTR as a cAMP-dependent regulator of sodium channels. *Science* 1995, 269:847–850.

24. Ramsey BW: Management of pulmonary disease in patients with cystic fibrosis. *N Engl J Med* 1996, 335:179–188.

25. Cutting GR: Genotype defect: its effect on cellular function and phenotypic expression. *Sem Respir Crit Care Med* 1994, 15:356–363.

26. Schwartz M, Johansen HK, Koch C: Frequency of the delta F508 mutation on cystic fibrosis chromosomes in Denmark. *Hum Genet* 1990, 85:427–428.

27. Mickle JE, Cutting GR: Clinical implications of cystic fibrosis transmembrane conductance regulator mutations. In *Clinics in Chest Medicine—Cystic Fibrosis*, vol 19. Edited by Fiel SB. Philadelphia: WB Saunders; 1999:443–458.

28. Haardt M, Benharouga M, Lechardeur D, *et al.*: C-terminal truncations destabilize the cystic fibrosis transmembrane conductance regulator without impairing its biogenesis: a novel class of mutation. *J Biol Chem* 1999, 274:21873–21877.

29. Kerem B, Kerem E: The molecular basis for disease variability in cystic fibrosis. *Eur J Hum Genet* 1996, 4:65–73.

30. Macek M, Mackova A, Hamosh A, *et al.*: Identification of common cystic fibrosis mutations in African-Americans with cystic fibrosis increases the detection rate to 75%. *Am J Hum Genet* 1997, 60:1122–1127.

31. Mastella G: Relationships between gene mutations and clinical features in cystic fibrosis. *Pediatr Pulmonol* 1995, 11:63–65.

32. Burke W, Aitken ML, Chen S-H, Scott CR: Variable severity of pulmonary disease in adults with identical cystic fibrosis mutations. *Chest* 1992, 102:506–509.

33. Cystic Fibrosis Genotype-Phenotype Consortium: Correlation between genotype and phenotype in patients with cystic fibrosis. *N Engl J Med* 1993, 329:1308–1313.

34. Marshall BC: Pathophysiology of pulmonary disease in cystic fibrosis. *Sem Res Crit Care Med* 1994, 15:364–374.

35. Imundo L, Barasch J, Prince A, *et al.*: Cystic fibrosis epithelial cells have a receptor for pathogenic bacteria on their apical surface. *Proc Natl Acad Sci U S A* 1995, 92:3019–3023.

36. Pier GB, Grout M, Zaidi TS, *et al.*: Role of mutant CFTR in hypersusceptibility of cystic fibrosis patients to lung infections. *Science* 1996, 271:64–67.

37. Knorre A, Wagner M, Schaefer HE, *et al.*: DeltaF508-CFTR causes constitutive NF-kappaB activation through an ER-overload response in cystic fibrosis lungs. *Biol Chem* 2002, 383:271–282.

38. Chmiel JF, Berger M, Konstan MW: The role of inflammation in the pathophysiology of CF lung disease *Clin Rev Allergy Immunol* 2002, 23:5–27.

39. Smith JJ, Travis SM, Greenberg EP, *et al.*: Cystic fibrosis airway epithelia fail to kill bacteria because of abnormal airway surface fluid. *Cell* 1996, 85:229–236.

40. Matsui H, Grubb BR, Tarran R, *et al.*: Evidence for periciliary liquid layer depletion, not abnormal ion composition, in the pathogenesis of cystic fibrosis airways disease. *Cell* 1998, 95:1005–1015.

41. Jayaraman S, Song Y, Vetrivel L, *et al.*: Noninvasive in vivo fluorescence measurement of airway-surface liquid depth, salt concentration, and pH. *J Clin Invest* 2001, 107:317–324.

42. Knowles MR, Robinson JM, Wood RE, *et al.*: Ion composition of airway surface liquid of patients with cystic fibrosis as compared with normal and disease-control subjects. *J Clin Invest* 1997, 100:2588–2595.

43. Worlitzsch D, Tarran R, Ulrich M, *et al.*: Effects of reduced mucus oxygen concentration in airway *Pseudomonas* infections of cystic fibrosis patients. *J Clin Invest* 2002, 109:317–325.

44. Coakley RD, Grubb BR, Paradiso AM, *et al.*: Abnormal surface liquid pH regulation by cultured cystic fibrosis bronchial epithelium. *Proc Natl Acad Sci U S A* 2003, 100:16083–16088.

45. Reddy MM, Quinton PM: Control of dynamic CFTR selectivity by glutamate and ATP in epithelial cells. *Nature* 2003, 423:756–760.

46. Birrer P: Consequences of unbalanced protease in the lung: protease involvement in destruction and local defense mechanisms of the lung. *Agents Actions Suppl* 1993, 40:3–12.

47. Smith JJ, Travis SM, Greenberg EP, Welsh MJ: Cystic fibrosis airway epithelia fail to kill bacteria because of abnormal airway surface fluid. *Cell* 1996, 85:229–236.

48. Govan JRW, Nelson JW: Microbiology of cystic fibrosis lung infections: themes and issues. *J R Soc Med* 1993, 86(Suppl 20):11–18.

49. Ruef C, Jefferson DM, Schlegel SE, Suter S: Regulation of cytokine secretion by cystic fibrosis airway epithelial cells. *Eur Respir J* 1993, 6:1429–1436.

50. Sibille Y, Marchandise FX: Pulmonary immune cells in health and disease: polymorphonuclear neutrophils. *Eur Respir J* 1993, 6:1429–1443.

51. Warner JO: Immunology of cystic fibrosis. *Br Med Bull* 1992, 48:893–911.

52. Koch C, Høiby N: Pathogenesis of cystic fibrosis. *Lancet* 1993, 341:1065–1069.

53. McElvaney NG, Doujaiji B, Moan MJ, *et al.*: Pharmacokinetics of recombinant secretory leukoprotease inhibitor aerosolized to normals and individuals with cystic fibrosis. *Am Rev Respir Dis* 1993, 148:1056–1060.

54. Pier GB, Saunders JM, Ames P, *et al.*: Opsonophagocytic killing antibody to *Pseudomonas aeruginosa* mucoid exopolysaccharide in older noncolonized patients with cystic fibrosis. *N Engl J Med* 1987, 317:793–798.

55. Prince A, Saiman L: *Pseudomonas aeruginosa* pili bind to asialo GM1 which is increased on the surface of cystic fibrosis epithelial cells. *J Clin Invest* 1993, 92:1875–1880.

56. Stutman HR: Paper presented at the Ninth Annual North American Cystic Fibrosis Conference. Dallas, TX, October 11–15, 1995.

57. Beardsmore CS, Thompson JR, Williams A, *et al.*: Pulmonary function in infants with cystic fibrosis: the effects of antibiotic treatment. *Arch Dis Child* 1994, 71:133–137.

58. Jensen T, Pedersen SS, Hoiby N, *et al.*: Use of antibiotics in cystic fibrosis: the Danish approach. *Antibiot Chemother* 1989, 42:237–246.

59. Coenye T, Mahenthiralingam E, Henry D, *et al.*: Classification of *Burkholderia cepacia*–like biocontrol strains and strains isolated from CF patients as a new member of the *B. cepacia* complex [abstract]. *Pediatr Pulmonol* 2000, 20:289.

60. Bernhardt SA, Spilker T, Coffee T, *et al.*: *Burkholderia cepacia* complex in cystic fibrosis: frequency of strain replacement during chronic infection. *Clin Infect Dis* 2003, 37:780–785.

61. Demko CA, Stern RC, Doerchuk CF: *Stenotrophomonas maltophilia* in cystic fibrosis. *Pediatr Pulmonol* 1998, 25:304–308.

62. Goss CH, Otto K, Aitkin ML: Detecting *Stenotrophomonas maltophilia* does not reduce survival of patients with cystic fibrosis. *Am J Respir Crit Care Med* 2002, 166:356–361.

63. Saiman L. Epidemiology and management of Infection. In *Highlights*. Bethesda, MD: Cystic Fibrosis Foundation; 1995:26–28.

64. Cystic Fibrosis Foundation: Concepts in care: pulmonary complications of cystic fibrosis. *Consensus Conferences* 1991, II:Sect III.

65. Elbert DL, Olivier KN: Nontuberculous mycobacteria in the setting of cystic fibrosis. *Clin Chest Med* 2002, 23:655–663.

66. Olivier KN, Weber DJ, Wallace RJ, *et al.*: Nontuberculous mycobacteria. I: Multicenter prevalence study in cystic fibrosis. *Am J Respir Crit Care Med* 2003, 167:828–834.

67. Knutsen A, Slavin RG: Allergic bronchopulmonary mycosis complicating cystic fibrosis. *Semin Respir Infect* 1992, 7:179–192.

68. Conway SP, Simmonds EJ, Littlewood JM: Acute severe deterioration in cystic fibrosis associated with influenza A virus infection. *Thorax* 1992, 47:112–114.

69. Cystic Fibrosis Foundation. Consensus document: management of liver and biliary tract disease in cystic fibrosis. *Consensus Conferences* 1999, IX:Sect I.

70. Cheng K, Ashby D, Smyth R: Ursodeoxycholic acid for cystic fibrosis-related liver disease: *Cochrane Database Syst Rev* 2000, 2:CD000222.

71. Cystic Fibrosis Foundation. Consensus document: diagnosis, screening and management of cystic fibrosis related diabetes mellitus. *Consensus Conferences* 1990, IX:Sect II.

72. Cystic Fibrosis Foundation. Consensus document: guide to bone health and disease in cystic fibrosis. *Consensus Conferences* 2002, X:Sect IV.

73. Schidlow DV, Taussig LM, Knowles MR: Cystic Fibrosis Foundation Consensus Conference report on pulmonary complications of cystic fibrosis. *Pediatr Pulmonol* 1993, 15:187–198.

74. Boucher RC: Cystic fibrosis. In *Harrison's Principles of Internal Medicine*, edn 13. Edited by Isselbacher KI, Braunwald E, Wilson JD, *et al*. New York: McGraw-Hill; 1994:1194–1197.

75. Gentile VG, Isaacson G: Patterns of sinusitis in cystic fibrosis. *Laryngoscope* 1996, 106:1005–1009.

76. Sexauer W, Schidlow D, Fiel SB: Unusual manifestations of cystic fibrosis. *Sem Respir Crit Care Med* 1994, 15:375–382.

77. Zrada SE, Isaacson GC: Endoscopic treatment of pediatric ethmoid mucoceles. *Am J Otolaryngol* 1996, 17:197–201.

78. Knowles MR, Gatzy J, Boucher R: Increased bioelectric potential difference across respiratory epithelia in cystic fibrosis. *N Engl J Med* 1981, 305:1485–1495.

79. Alton EW, Currie D, Logan-Sinclair R, *et al.*: Nasal potential difference: a clinical diagnostic test for cystic fibrosis. *Eur Respir J* 1990, 3:922–926.

80. Hofmann T, Böhmer O, Bittner P, *et al.*: Conventional and modified nasal potential difference measurement: clinical use in cystic fibrosis. *Am J Respir Crit Care Med* 1997, 155:1908–1913.

81. Collins FS: Cystic fibrosis: molecular biology and therapeutic implications. *Science* 1992, 256:774–779.

82. Farrell PM, Kosorok MR, Rock MJ, *et al.*: Early diagnosis of cystic fibrosis through neonatal screening prevents severe malnutrition and improves long-term growth. *Pediatrics* 2001, 107:1–13.

83. Gaskin K, Gurwitz D, Durie P, *et al.*: Differences in resting energy expenditure between male and female children with cystic fibrosis. *J Pediatr* 1982, 100:857–862.

84. Corey M, McLaughlin FJ, Williams M, *et al.*: A comparison of survival, growth, and pulmonary function in patients with cystic fibrosis in Boston and Toronto. *J Clin Epidemiol* 1988, 41:583–591.

85. Davidson G, McIlwaine M: Airway clearance techniques in cystic fibrosis. *New Insights into Cystic Fibrosis* 1995, 3:6–11.

86. Scheiderman-Walker J, Pollock SL, Corey M, *et al.*: A randomized controlled trial of a three-year home exercise program in cystic fibrosis. *J Pediatr* 2000, 136:304–310.

87. Baldwin DR, Hill AL, Peckham DG, et al.: Effect of addition of exercise to chest physiotherapy on sputum expectoration and lung function in adults with cystic fibrosis. *Respir Med* 1994, 88:49–53.

88. Alison JA, Donnelly PM, Lennon M, *et al.*: The effect of a comprehensive, intensive inpatient treatment program on lung function and exercise capacity in patients with cystic fibrosis. *Phys Ther* 1994, 74:583–591.

89. Orenstein DM, Franklin BA, Doershuk CF, *et al.*: Exercise conditioning and cardiopulmonary fitness in cystic fibrosis: the effects of a three-month supervised running program. *Chest* 1981, 80:382–398.

90. Sawyer EH, Clanton TL: Improved pulmonary function and exercise tolerance with inspiratory muscle conditioning in children with cystic fibrosis. *Chest* 1993, 104:1490–1497.

91. Salzano FA, Manola M, Tricarico D, *et al.*: Mucociliary clearance after aerobic exertion in athletes [in Italian]. *Acta Otorhinolaryngol Ital* 2000, 20:171–176.

92. Bye P, Elkins MR, Robinson M, *et al.*: Long-term inhalation of hypertonic saline in patients with cystic fibrosis: a randomized clinical trial. *Pedatr Pulmonol* 2004, 27(Suppl):A402.

93. Donaldson SH, Bennet W, Zeman K, *et al.*: A pilot study of amiloride and hypertonic saline in cystic fibrosis. *Pediatr Pulmonol* 2004, 27(Suppl):A325.

94. Tarran R, Grubb B, Parsons D, *et al.*: The CF salt controversy: in vivo observations and therapeutic approaches. *Mol Cell* 2001, 8:149–158.

95. Elkins MR, Robinson M, Rose BR, et al.: A controlled trial of long-term inhaled hypertonic saline in patients with cystic fibrosis. *N Engl J Med* 2006, 354:229–240.

96. Donaldson SH, Bennett WD, Zeman KL, et al.: Mucus clearance and lung function in cystic fibrosis with hypertonic saline. *N Engl J Med* 2006, 354:241–250.

97. Fuchs HJ, Borowitz DS, Christiansen DH, et al.: The effect of aerosolized recombinant DNase on respiratory exacerbations and pulmonary function in patients with cystic fibrosis. *N Engl J Med* 1994, 331:637–642.

98. Shah PL, Scott SF, Fuchs HJ, et al.: Medium-term treatment of stable stage cystic fibrosis with recombinant human DNase I. *Thorax* 1995, 50:333–338.

99. Konstan MW, Tiddens HA, Quan JM, et al.: A randomized, placebo-controlled trial of two years' treatment with dornase alfa (Pulmozyme®) in cystic fibrosis patients aged 6–10 years with early lung disease [abstract]. *Pediatr Pulmonol* 2000, 20:299.

100. Fiel SB: Clinical management of pulmonary disease in cystic fibrosis. *Lancet* 1993, 341:1070–1074.

101. Di Sant'Agnese PEA, Andersen DH: Celiac syndrome: IV. Chemotherapy in infections of the respiratory tract associated with cystic fibrosis of the pancreas: observations with penicillin and drugs of the sulfonamide group, with special reference to penicillin aerosol. *Am J Dis Child* 1946, 72:17–61.

102. Schidlow DV: Cystic fibrosis. In *A Practical Guide to Pediatrics*. Edited by Schidlow DV, Smith DSS. Philadelphia: Hanley and Belfus; 1994:75–81.

103. Ramsey BW, Dorkin HL, Eisenberg JD, et al.: Efficacy of aerolised tobramycin in patients with cystic fibrosis. *N Engl J Med* 1993, 328:1740–1746.

104. Saiman L, Marshall BC, Mayer-Hamblett N, et al.: Azithromycin in patients with cystic fibrosis chronically infected with *Pseudomonas aeruginosa*: a randomized controlled trial. *JAMA* 2003, 290:1749–1756.

105. Equi A, Balfour-Lynn IM, Bush A, et al.: Long-term azithromycin in children with cystic fibrosis: a randomised, placebo-controlled crossover trial. *Lancet* 2002, 390:978–984.

106. Wolter J, Sweeny S, Bell S, et al.: Effect of long-term treatment with azithromycin on disease parameters in cystic fibrosis: a randomised trial. *Thorax* 2002, 57:212–216.

107. Saiman L, Chen Y, Gabriel PS, et al.: Synergistic activities of macrolide antibiotics against *Pseudomonas aeruginosa*, *Burkholderia cepacia*, *Stenotrophomonas maltophilia*, and *Alcaligenes xylosoxidans* isolated from patients with cystic fibrosis. *Antimicrob Agents Chemother* 2002, 46:1105–1107.

108. Ren CL: Use of modulators of airways inflammation in patients with CF. *Clin Rev Allergy Immunol* 2002, 23:29–39.

109. Konstan MW, Byard PJ, Hoppel CL, Davis PB: Effect of high-dose ibuprofen in patients with cystic fibrosis. *N Engl J Med* 1995, 332:848–854.

110. Auerbach HS, Williams M, Kirkpatrick JA, Colten HR: Alternate-day prednisone reduces morbidity and improves pulmonary function in cystic fibrosis. *Lancet* 1985, 2:686–688.

111. Eigen H, Rosenstein BJ, FitzSimmons S, Schidlow DV: A multicenter study of alternate-day prednisone therapy in patients with cystic fibrosis. *J Pediatr* 1995, 126:515–523.

112. Cryz SJ Jr, Wedgwood J, Lang AB, et al.: Immunization of noncolonized cystic fibrosis patients against *Pseudomonas aeruginosa*. *J Infect Dis* 1994, 169:1159–1162.

113. Aris RM, Routh JC, LiPuma JJ, et al.: Transplantation for cystic fibrosis patients with *Burkholderia cepacia* complex: Survival linked to genomovar type. *Am J Respir Crit Care Med* 2001, 164:2102–2106.

114. Egan TM, Detterback FC, Mill MR, et al.: Long-term results of lung transplantation for cystic fibrosis. *Eur J Cardiothorac Surg* 2002, 22:602–609.

115. De Soyza A, Corris PA: Lung transplantation and the *Burkholderia cepacia* complex. *J Heart Lung Transplant* 2003, 22:954–958.

116. Hosenpud JD, Bennett LE, Keck BM, et al.: The Registry of the International Society for Heart and Lung Transplantation Seventeenth Official Report. 2000, 19(10):909–931.

117. Rosenfeld MA, Collins FS: Gene therapy for cystic fibrosis. *Chest* 1996, 109:241–252.

118. Balter M: Gene therapy on trial. *Science* 2000, 288:951–957.

119. Curiel DT, Agarwal S, Romer MU, et al.: Gene transfer to respiratory epithelial cells via the receptor-mediated endocytosis pathway. *Am J Respir Cell Mol Biol* 1992, 6:247–252.

120. Gao L, Wagner E, Cotten M, et al.: Direct in vivo gene transfer to airway employing adenovirus-polylysine-DNA complexes. *Hum Gene Ther* 1993, 4:17–24.

121. Crystal RG: Gene therapy for cystic fibrosis: lessons learned and hurdles to success. Paper presented at the Ninth Annual North American Cystic Fibrosis Conference. Dallas, TX: October 11–15, 1995.

122. Rosenfeld MA, Yoshimura K, Trapnell B, et al.: In vivo transfer of the human cystic fibrosis transmembrane conductance regulator gene to the airway epithelium. *Cell* 1992, 68:143–155.

123. Rosenfeld MA, Chu CS, Seth P, et al.: Gene transfer to freshly isolated human respiratory epithelial cells in vitro using a replication-deficient adenovirus containing the human cystic fibrosis transmembrane conductance regulator cDNA. *Hum Gene Ther* 1994, 5:331–342.

124. Englehardt JF, Simon RH, Yang Y, et al.: Adenovirus-mediated transfer of the CFTR gene to lung of nonhuman primates: biological efficacy study. *Hum Gene Ther* 1993, 4:759–769.

125. Englehardt JF, Yang Y, Stratford-Perricaudet LD, et al.: Direct gene transfer of human CFTR into human bronchial epithelia of xenografts with E1-deleted adenoviruses. *Nat Genet* 1993, 4:27–34.

126. Mastrangeli A, Danel C, Rosenfeld MA, et al.: Diversity of airway epithelial cell targets for in vivo recombinant adenovirus-mediated gene transfer. *J Clin Invest* 1993, 91:225–234.

127. Rich DP, Couture LA, Cardoza LM, et al.: Development and analysis of recombinant adenoviruses for gene therapy of cystic fibrosis. *Hum Gene Ther* 1993, 4:461–476.

128. Yang Y, Nunes FA, Berencsi K, et al.: Inactivation of E2a in recombinant adenoviruses improves the prospect for gene therapy for cystic fibrosis. *Nat Genet* 1994, 7:362–369.

129. Zabner J, Petersen DM, Puga AP, et al.: Safety and efficacy of repetitive adenovirus-mediated transfer of CFTR cDNA to airway epithelia of primates and cotton rats. *Nat Genet* 1994, 6:75–83.

130. Zabner J, Couture LA, Smith AE, Welsh MJ: Correction of cAMP-stimulated fluid secretion in cystic fibrosis airway epithelia: efficiency of adenovirus-mediated gene transfer in vivo. *Hum Gene Ther* 1994, 5:585–593.

131. Wilson JM: Cystic fibrosis: strategies for gene therapy. *Sem Respir Crit Care Med* 1994, 15:439–445.

132. Wilson JM: Gene therapy for cystic fibrosis lung disease with recombinant adenoviruses: host-vector interactions. *Pediatr Pulmonol* 1994, 10:155.

133. Johnson LG: Gene therapy for cystic fibrosis. *Chest* 1995, 107:77S–82S.

134. Knowles MR, Hohneker KW, Zhou Z, et al.: A controlled study of adenoviral-vector-mediated gene transfer in the nasal epithelium of patients with cystic fibrosis. *N Engl J Med* 1995, 333:823–831.

135. Crystal RG, McElvaney NG, Rosenfeld MA, et al.: Administration of an adenovirus containing the human CFTR cDNA to the respiratory tract of individuals with cystic fibrosis. *Nat Genet* 1994, 8:42–51.

136. Alton EW, Middleton PG, Caplen NJ, et al.: Non-invasive liposome-mediated gene delivery can correct the ion transport defect in cystic fibrosis mutant mice. *Nat Genet* 1993, 5:135–142.

137. Hyde SC, Gill DR, Higgins CF, et al.: Correction of the ion transport defect in cystic fibrosis transgenic mice by gene therapy. *Nature* 1993, 362:250–255.

138. Caplen NJ, Alton RW, Middleton PG, et al.: Liposome-mediated CFTR gene transfer to the nasal epithelium of patients with cystic fibrosis. *Nat Med* 1995, 1:39–46.

139. Schwartz DA, Quinn TJ, Thorne PS, et al.: CpG motifs in bacterial DNA cause inflammation in the lower respiratory tract. *J Clin Invest* 1997, 100:68–73.

140. Wilson JM: Prospects for human gene therapy. In *Highlights*. Bethesda, MD: Cystic Fibrosis Foundation; 1995:20–22.

141. Yang H, Shelat AA, Guy RK, et al.: Nanomolar affinity small molecule correctors of defective Delta F508-CFTR chloride channel gating. *J Biol Chem* 2003, 278:35079–35085.

142. Schidlow DV, Fiel SB: Life beyond pediatrics: transition of chronically ill adolescents from pediatric to adult health care systems. *Med Clin North Am* 1990, 74:1113–1120.

143. Huang NN, Schidlow DV, Szatrowski TE, et al.: Clinical features, survival rate, and prognostic factors in young adults with cystic fibrosis. *Am J Med* 1987, 82:871–879.

144. Shwachman H, Kulczycki LL: Long-term study of one hundred five patients with cystic fibrosis. *Am J Dis Child* 1958, 96:6–15.

145. Fiel SB, Tullis E: What are the key issues associated with cystic fibrosis in adulthood? In *Highlights*. Bethesda, MD: Cystic Fibrosis Foundation; 1995:17–19.

146. Canny HJ, Corey M, Livingston RA, et al.: Pregnancy and cystic fibrosis. *Obstet Gynecol* 1991, 77:850–853.

147. FitzSimmons SC, Winnie G, Fiel S, et al.: Effect of pregnancy on women with cystic fibrosis: a one to six year follow-up study. *Am J Respir Crit Care Med* 1995, 151:A742.

148. Kotloff RM: Reproductive issues in patients with cystic fibrosis. *Sem Respir Crit Care Med* 1994, 15:402–413.

149. Hirsh AV, Mills C, Bekir J, et al.: Factors influencing the outcome of in-vitro fertilization with epididymal spermatozoa in irreversible obstructive azoospermia. *Hum Reprod* 1994, 9:1710–1716.

150. Aitken ML: Managing cystic fibrosis in adults. *New Insights into Cystic Fibrosis* 1995, 3:7–11.

151. Aspin AJ: Psychological consequences of cystic fibrosis in adults. *Br J Hosp Med* 1991, 45:368–371.

152. Blair C, Cull A, Freeman CP: Psychosocial functioning of young adults with cystic fibrosis and their families. *Thorax* 1994, 49:798–802.

153. New Insights Editorial Board: A look at the national CF patient registry. *New Insights into Cystic Fibrosis* 1996, 3:1–6.

BRONCHIOLAR DISORDERS

*Thomas V. Colby,
Gary R. Epler, and
James F. Gruden*

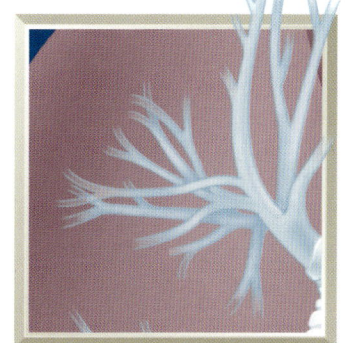
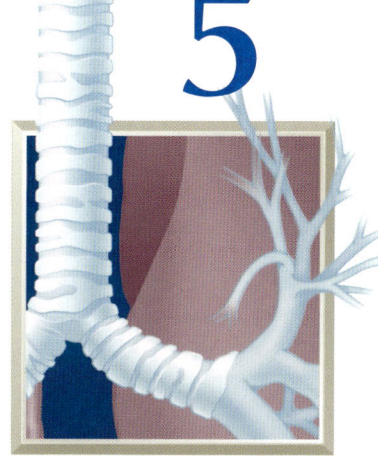
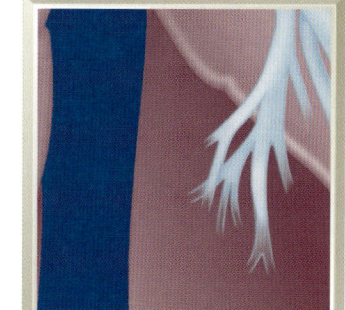

Pathologic changes in the bronchioles are found in many lung diseases[1,2]. They may represent the primary finding and the cause of the clinical and radiologic findings, or they may be an incidental finding in some other process such as a chronic interstitial pneumonia. The term *small airways* generally refers to airways less than 2 mm in diameter, and for practical purposes this primarily pertains to bronchioles, although some small bronchi are also included under this definition [1].

This chapter will illustrate the clinical, radiologic, and pathologic spectrum of small airway pathology, excluding that associated with well-defined clinical entities such as asthma (in which individuals with predominant small airway involvement may actually have more severe disease [3]) and chronic obstructive pulmonary disease (COPD), where small airways are the major site of airway obstruction [4]. The bronchiolar disorders will be covered using a conceptual approach based on the various pathologic changes that may affect the bronchioles and the resulting clinical and radiologic syndromes. The terms *bronchiolitis obliterans, obliterative bronchiolitis, constrictive bronchiolitis,* and *bronchiolitis obliterans organizing pneumonia (BOOP)* will be clarified and put into historical perspective.

The term *bronchiolitis obliterans* was originally used by Lange to describe the histologic finding of intraluminal polyps in the small airways (*see* Fig. 5-1) [5–20]. This is now recognized as a common reaction in the setting of organizing pneumonia (from any of a variety of causes) [1,2]. The term *BOOP,* or *bronchiolitis obliterans organizing pneumonia* (or *bronchiolitis obliterans with intraluminal polyps*), has also been used for this lesion; when this is seen in the clinical setting of an interstitial pneumonia, the term *organizing pneumonia* is now preferred [21]. Even though the term *bronchiolitis obliterans* was originally used to describe a histologic finding, it has also become used to describe airflow obstruction due to pathology in the small airways, and the term is commonly used in that context today. In the setting of transplantation, the synonym *obliterative bronchiolitis (OB)* is sometimes preferred, and the clinical term *bronchiolitis obliterans syndrome (BOS),* a finding based on forced expiratory volume in 1 second (FEV_1) is frequently used for clinical (nonbiopsy) diagnosis [22].

In pathology the term *bronchiolitis obliterans* (obliterative bronchiolitis) has also been used to describe luminal narrowing and obliteration in the small airways (in contrast to the original reference to intraluminal polyps), and this is the histologic lesion that is associated with the clinical and radiologic finding of airflow obstruction and hyperinflation [1,2]. The term *constrictive bronchiolitis* is now used to describe this subset of cases to avoid the confusion that has been encountered with the term *bronchiolitis obliterans* [1,2,23,24].

HISTORICAL BACKGROUND

Historical Milestones in Bronchiolar Disorders

1901	Bronchiolitis obliterans [5]
1902	Fume-related bronchiolitis obliterans [6]
1904	Postinfectious bronchiolitis obliterans [7,8]
1977	Connective tissue disease–related bronchiolitis obliterans [9]
1977	Drug-related bronchiolitis obliterans [9]
1982	Bone marrow transplantation bronchiolitis obliterans [10]
1983	Diffuse panbronchiolitis [11]
1984	Heart-lung transplantation bronchiolitis obliterans [12]
1985	Idiopathic BOOP [13]
1987	Respiratory bronchiolitis-interstitial lung disease [14,15]
1989	Neuroendocrine cell hyperplasia with airflow obstructions [16–18]
1992	Neuroendocrine cell hyperplasia [17]
1995	*Sauropus androgynus*–related bronchiolitis obliterans [19]
1996	Diacetyl-associated bronchiolitis obliterans [20]

Figure 5-1. Historical milestones in bronchiolar disorders. Modern understanding of bronchiolar diseases began when Lange described two patients in 1901 [5]. Fume-related and postinfectious causes were described during the next 3 years [6–8]. Eventually, obliterative bronchiolar lesions were described in relation to connective tissue disorders, after bone marrow transplantation, and after lung transplantation [9–11]. Obliterative bronchiolitis has been described in association with neuroendocrine cell hyperplasia in bronchiolitis [16–18]. This disorder has also been described as resulting from the ingestion of *Sauropus androgynus,* a leafy vegetable used for its alleged effects of reducing body weight and controlling blood pressure [19]. Bronchiolitis obliterans has recently been described among workers in a microwave popcorn factory who were exposed to volatile butter-flavoring ingredients, including diacetyl [20]. From the historical background of the bronchiolar diseases, it is apparent that bronchiolar pathology may be associated with what are considered obstructive diseases as well as with conditions considered interstitial diseases. This list also includes some conditions in which the pathology in the small airways is associated with what is clinically interpreted as interstitial lung disease. Idiopathic BOOP (cryptogenic organizing pneumonitis) and respiratory bronchiolitis–associated interstitial lung disease (RBILD) are examples [1,21]. BOOP—bronchiolitis obliterans organizing pneumonia.

ANATOMY OF THE AIRWAYS

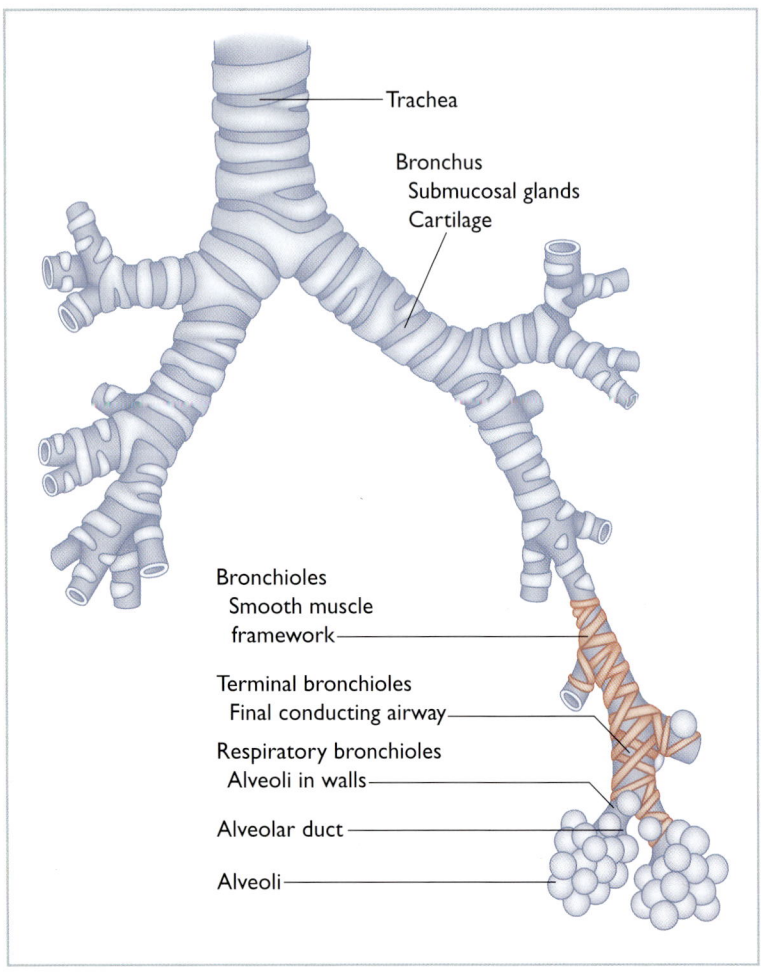

Figure 5-2. Anatomy of the airways. Bronchioles are small airways up to 1 to 2 mm in diameter without cartilage or submucosal glands [25]. An estimated 28,000 bronchioles, with a diameter of 0.6 mm, form the final conducting bronchioles at the 16th generation. The 224,000 respiratory bronchioles are distinguished from the terminal bronchioles by the alveolar sacs in their walls. The respiratory bronchioles terminate at the 13.8 million alveolar ducts and 300 million alveoli.

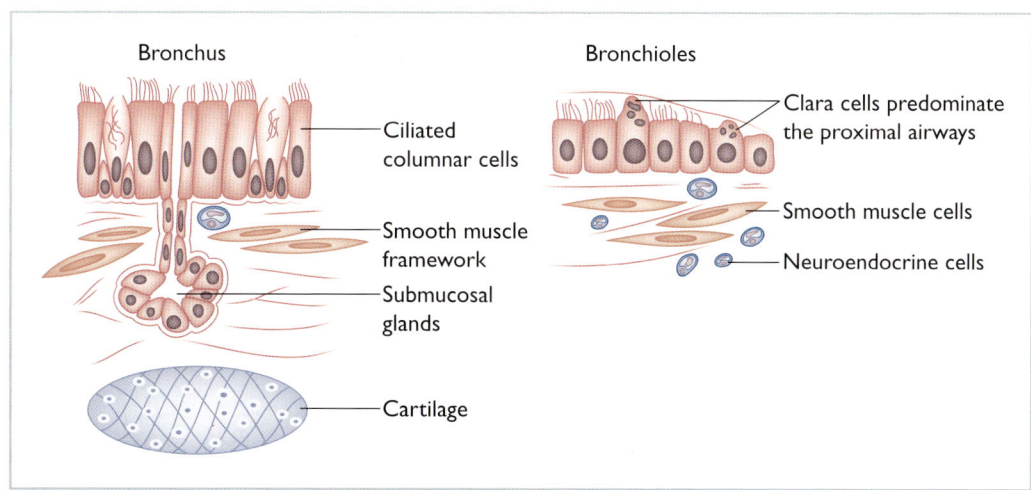

Figure 5-3. Normal airway histology. Ciliated cells predominate on the surface of the epithelium of the proximal airways, whereas Clara cells constitute the majority of cells in the bronchiolar mucosa [25,26]. Apically, Clara cells contain membrane-bound secretory granules that are probably active in the secretion of proteins and may be active in surfactant secretion. Neuroendocrine cells reach maximal density in the proximal bronchioles and are rarely found in the terminal bronchioles. These cells occur individually and in clusters, and tend to be concentrated at the bifurcations of the conducting airways. They are thought to be a source of bioactive secretory products, including bombesin-like activity (gastrin-releasing peptide), somatostatin, endothelin, serotonin, and calcitonin.

OVERVIEW OF BRONCHIOLAR DISORDERS BASED ON PATHOLOGIC REACTION PATTERNS

Cellular and Mesencymal Components of Small Airways Inflammation

A. Cellular/exudative reaction dominates

B. Mesenchymal reaction predominates
1. Organization with intraluminal polyps (terms: bronchiolitis obliterans, bronchiolitis obliterans within luminal polyps, organizing pneumonia, bronchiolitis obliterans organizing pneumonia/BOOP)
2. Subepithelial fibrosis and scarring with partial or complete luminal compromise (terms: constrictive bronchiolitis, bronchiolitis obliterans, obliterative bronchiolitis)
3. Peribronchiolar scarring with preservation of luminal patency (terms: peribronchiolar metaplasia, Lambertosis, bronchiolarization)

C. Mixed patterns

Combination/overlap of the above changes with mixed pathological, clinical, and radiologic features

Figure 5-4. Inflammation in the small airways, as elsewhere in the body, includes both a cellular and a mesenchymal component. These are summarized in this figure and covered in detail below. Most examples of bronchiolar pathology include both a cellular and a mesenchymal reaction, but the extent of these reactions varies considerably from case to case. To aid in understanding the clinical and radiologic findings associated with bronchiolar disorders, Figures 5-5 through 5-11 illustrate these reactions as if they were separate and relatively pure. This approach allows one to appreciate the diversity of clinical and radiologic findings in this group of conditions. BOOP—bronchiolitis obliterans organizing pneumonia.

CLINICAL, PATHOLOGIC, AND RADIOLOGIC OVERVIEW OF BRONCHIOLAR DISORDERS

Cellular/Exudative Reaction Predominates

Clinical Aspects

Common findings in viral bronchitis/bronchiolitis and many other conditions. Respiratory syncytial virus is the most common cause of cellular and exudative bronchiolitis in infants [27]. Adenovirus, influenza, parainfluenza, and herpes viral infections may cause adult cellular bronchiolitis. Diffuse panbronchiolitis (discussed below) and many other infections (such as *Mycobacterium avium* complex infection) are also characterized primarily by a cellular bronchiolitis/exudative reaction. The clinical features include a nonproductive cough occurring for several weeks with normal chest radiograph and normal pulmonary function tests. Treatment is with a cough suppressant or a brief course of corticosteroid therapy for disabling symptoms.

Pathologic Findings

The cellular infiltrate may include acute inflammatory cells, chronic inflammatory cells, or lymphoid hyperplasia (follicular bronchiolitis). Granulomas may be part of the infiltrate. The airway lumen may contain cells, inflammatory exudate, or mucus. The additive effect of these pathologic changes may be sufficient to produce opacities radiologically and may make the lung stiff or produce airflow obstruction if the lumen is compromised.

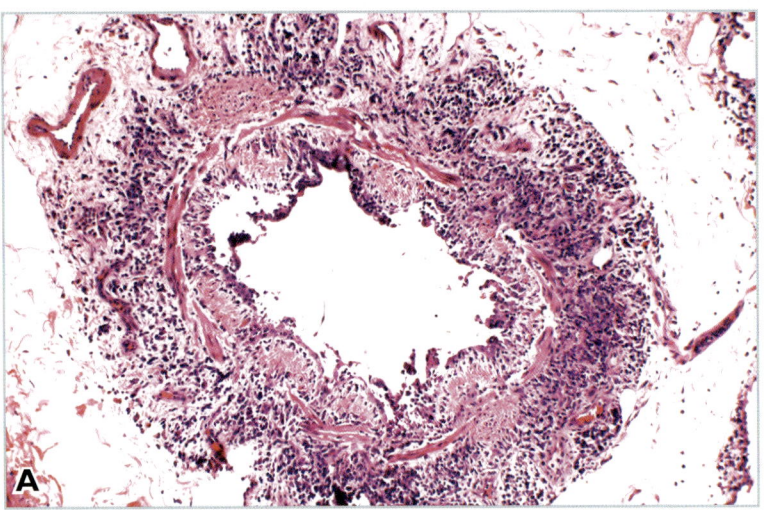
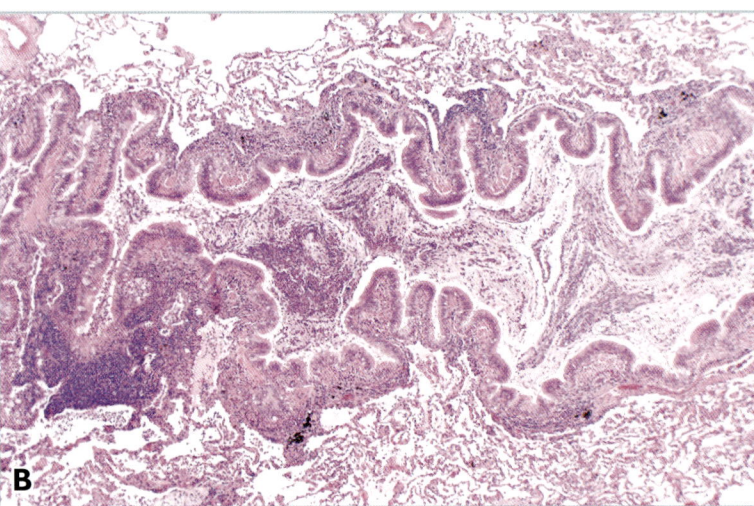

Figure 5-5. A, Cellular bronchiolitis from respiratory syncytial virus infection. There is a chronic inflammatory infiltrate. **B,** Cellular bronchiolitis associated with primary ciliary dyskinesia (PCD). PCD is a predisposing factor to recurrent infections that lead to acute and chronic cellular bronchiolitis with acute luminal exudate and inflammatory cells and mural inflammation of chronic inflammatory cells, here shown in a longitudinal section.

Radiologic Findings

Thickening and impaction of the peripheral bronchioles result in branching, nodular structures ("tree-in-bud" or "jacks") visible on high-resolution computed tomography (HRCT) [28,29]. These characteristic features reflect the significant intraluminal component of the inflammation and/or infection. Cellular bronchiolitis without a significant intraluminal component typically results in small centrilobular nodules of ground glass attenuation occult to chest radiographs but clearly visible on HRCT.

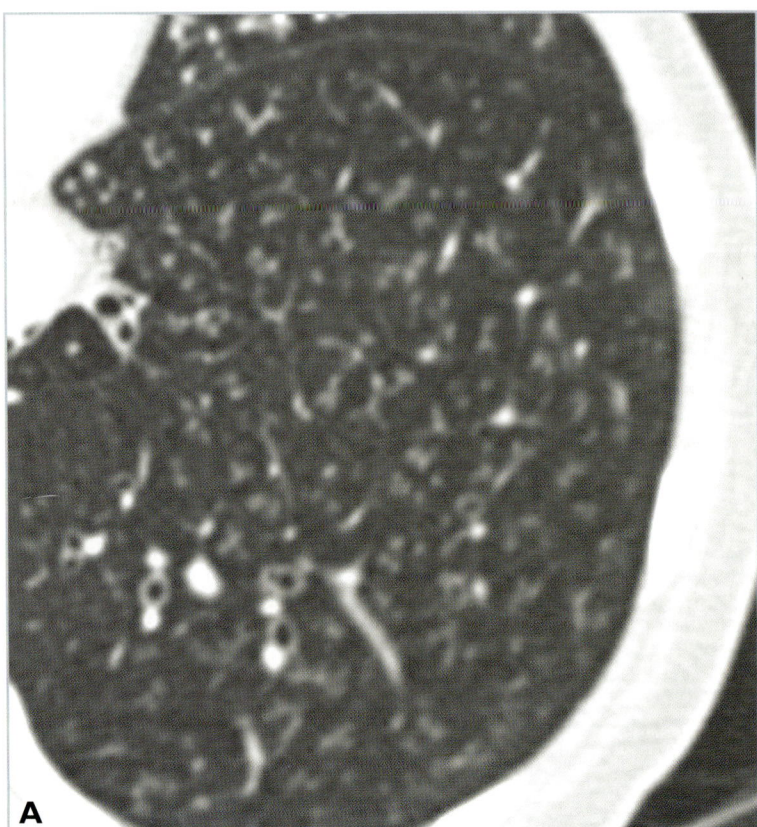
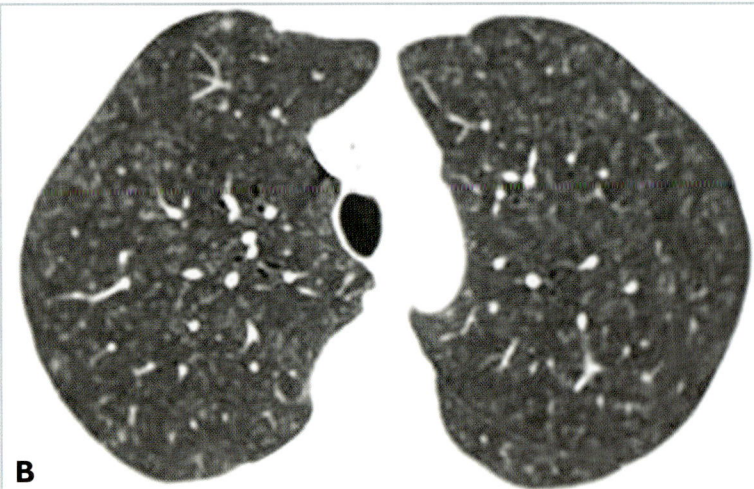

Figure 5-6. A, Magnified high-resolution computed tomography (HRCT) image of the left lower lobe shows branching, nodular structures representing impacted bronchioles in this patient with the immotile cilia syndrome. **B,** Axial HRCT image through the upper lobes in a patient with subacute hypersensitivity pneumonitis related to inhalation of *Mycobacterium avium* complex ("hot tub lung"). There are innumerable small nodules of ground glass attenuation surrounding the visible pulmonary arteries in cross-section. These centrilobular nodules are characteristic of cellular bronchiolitis in which the intraluminal inflammatory component is lacking or minimal.

Mesenchymal Reaction Predominates with Air Space Organization

Clinical Aspects

The cause may be idiopathic or associated with the connective tissue diseases, immunologic diseases, infectious pneumonia, medications, or organ transplantation. When the condition is idiopathic, patients have a subacute clinical course with a febrile illness and nonproductive cough for several days. Shortness of breath occurs later. Examination indicates bilateral end-inspiratory crackles in most patients. The illness may subside without treatment, but corticosteroid therapy is generally utilized at a beginning dose of 40 to 60 mg of prednisone and continuing at lower doses for several months. The prognosis is good, with 65% to 85% of patients being cured, and mortality is less than 5% [13].

Pathologic Findings

Organization with intraluminal polyps is usually associated with a similar intraluminal organizing reaction in the more distal alveolar ducts and alveoli. The net effect of this tissue is to produce an opacity radiologically and also to make the lung stiff (*ie*, restrictive). Despite the apparent luminal compromise by the intraluminal polyps in the bronchioles, airflow obstruction is not a prominent feature with this pattern.

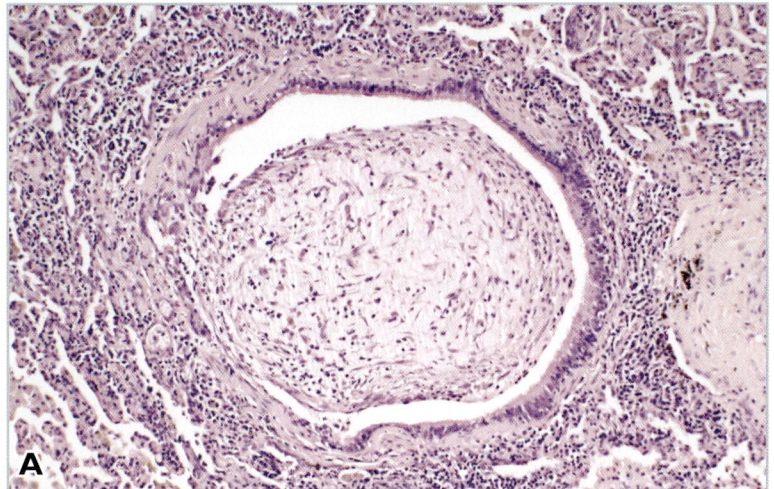
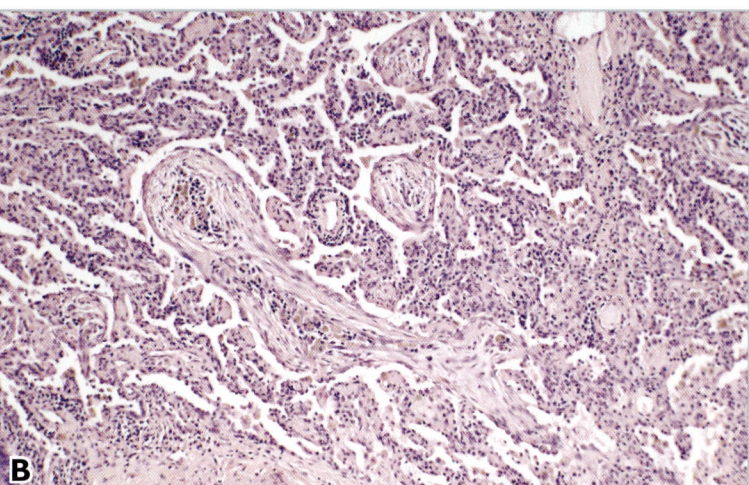

Figure 5-7. A, Organization with intraluminal polyps (bronchiolitis obliterans organizing pneumonia). There is polypoid myxoid tissue within the lumen of a bronchiole without associated significant scarring of the bronchiole or the surrounding lung.

B, The more distal parenchyma shows intraluminal organization within alveolar ducts. The organizing intraluminal polyp of granulation is cut longitudinally in an alveolar duct extending from right to left.

Radiologic Findings

The air space component obscures any associated bronchiolar abnormalities. The radiographic findings include consolidation, often peripheral, that often migrates over time from one part of the lung to another. The distribution is patchy, and portions of the lung appear totally normal. High-resolution computed tomography shows an unusual pattern of relatively normal lung surrounded by consolidation, possibly due to the tendency of the process to clear from the center to the periphery.

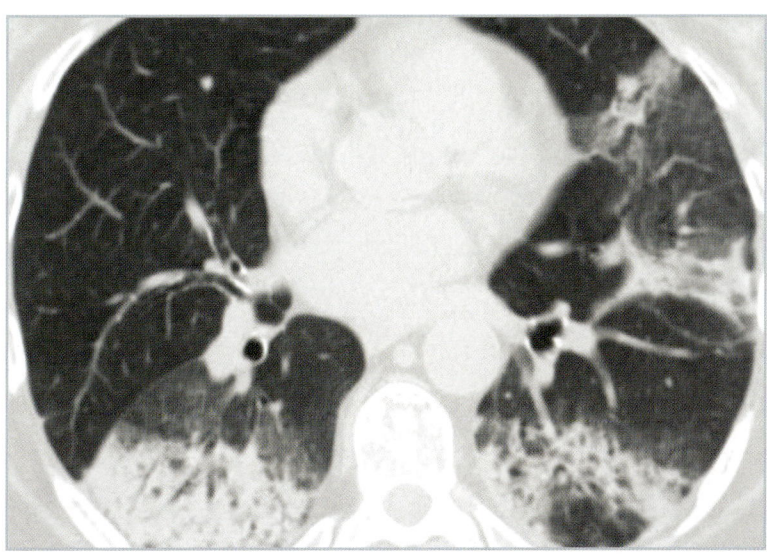

Figure 5-8. Idiopathic bronchiolitis obliterans organizing pneumonia, also known as cryptogenic organizing pneumonia. High-resolution computed tomography typically shows patchy peripheral consolidation. Note the typical central lucent zone of spared parenchyma in the center of the left lower lobe posterior consolidation.

Mesenchymal Reaction Predominates with Constrictive Bronchiolitis

Clinical Aspects

This is an irreversible airflow obstructive disease with a variable rate of progression. The process occurs after lung transplantation as a form of chronic rejection. It also occurs in chronic graft versus host disease in patients who have undergone allogenic bone marrow transplantation. This is rarely idiopathic and may occur after exposure to toxic acid fumes, infections, connective tissue diseases, and certain medications. Patients develop shortness of breath as the major clinical symptom. Physical findings may include bilateral early inspiratory crackles or sometimes "squeaks." Adrenergic bronchodilator agents may be helpful in some patients. Because this is a fibrotic lesion, corticosteroid therapy is not beneficial, although it may be useful for exacerbations. When the condition is progressive, the prognosis is poor, and lung transplantation is appropriate for life-threatening disabling disease.

Pathologic Findings

Subepithelial fibrosis and scarring with partial or complete luminal compromise. When this change is widespread, the clinical and radiologic findings are typically those of obstruction in the small airways.

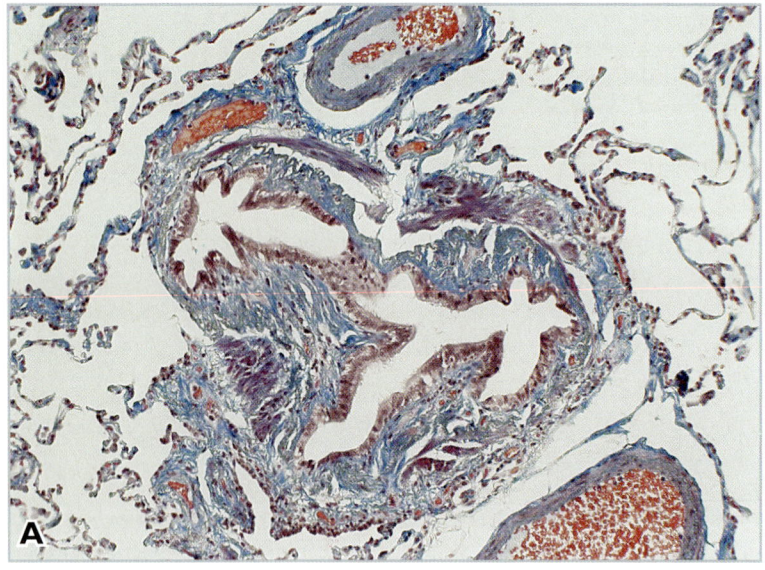
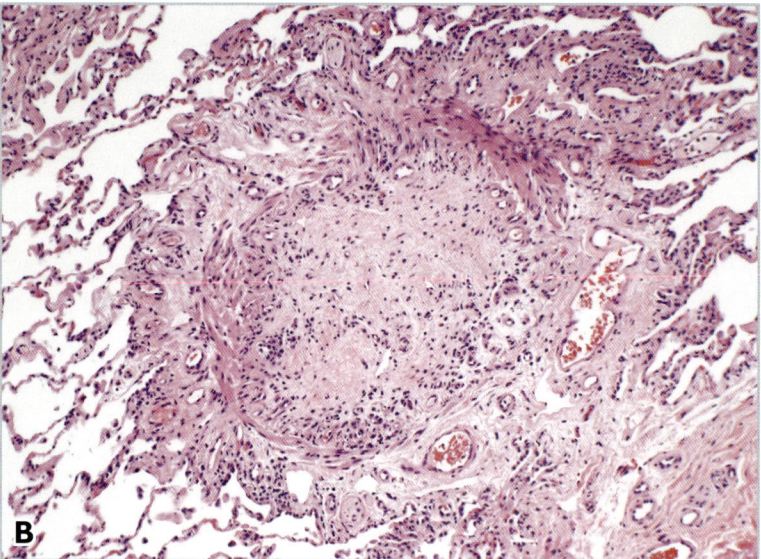

Figure 5-9. **A,** Constrictive bronchiolitis with subepithelial scarring and luminal compromise. In a case of chronic asthma with fixed obstruction, trichrome stain shows a layer of dense blue-staining collagen in between the rust-staining smooth muscle and the overlying epithelium. The resulting lumen is distorted and significantly compromised. **B,** In a case of idiopathic constrictive bronchiolitis there is complete luminal loss.

Radiologic Findings

Chest radiographs are typically normal or may depict large lung volumes due to the obstructive physiology. High-resolution computed tomography (HRCT) shows heterogeneous lung attenuation, or the "mosaic" pattern of attenuation or perfusion. This pattern refers to areas of apparent ground glass attenuation alternating with more lucent zones. The dark zones are abnormal lung, dark because of air trapping distal to areas of bronchiolar obstruction and because of the subsequent reflex vasoconstriction and reduced blood flow that occurs as the lung attempts to maintain ventilation and perfusion matching. Therefore, the visible pulmonary arteries are larger in the areas of ground glass attenuation (the normal, hyperperfused lung) than in the darker, more lucent abnormal segments. These changes may be subtle and are accentuated on expiratory HRCT scanning. The more central airways may be thickened and slightly dilated in advanced cases, which is likely the result of increased inspiratory pressure as breathing becomes labored.

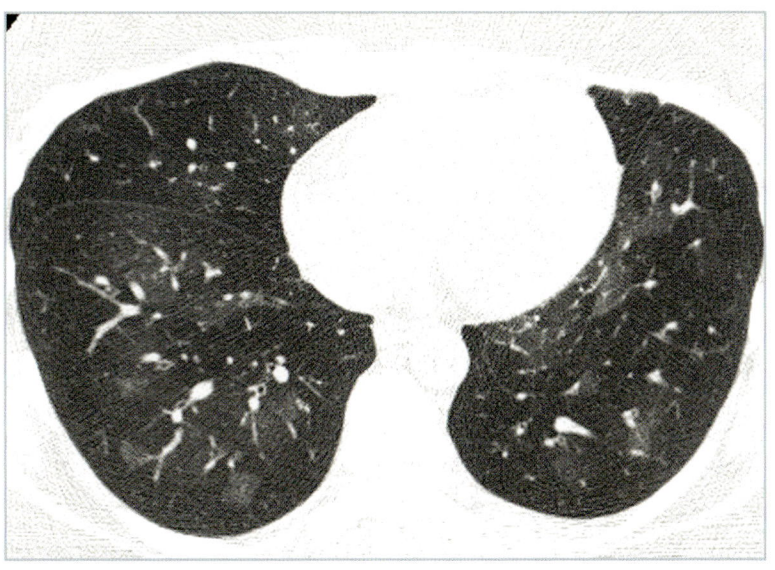

Figure 5-10. Constrictive bronchiolitis ("bronchiolitis obliterans") as a manifestation of chronic graft versus host disease several years after allogenic bone marrow transplant. High-resolution computed tomography (HRCT) shows a patchy pattern of mosaic attenuation. The arterial branches are larger in the areas of increased lung density and the vessels are inconspicuous in the more lucent zones. The HRCT findings reflect the underlying pathology and are secondary to the patchy areas of bronchiolar obstruction and the physiologic response of the lung.

MESENCHYMAL REACTION PREDOMINATES WITH PERIBRONCHIOLAR SCARRING AND METAPLASIA

Clinical Aspects

The clinical findings associated with this pathologic lesion as a primary process include a female predominance with symptoms of cough and shortness of breath. Some patients have associated connective tissue diseases. Physiology shows patterns of airflow obstruction, a restrictive pattern, or a combined restrictive and obstructive pattern. The prognosis is relatively favorable [30].

Pathologic Findings

Peribronchiolar scarring with preservation of luminal patency. There is a net increase in tissue that may be sufficient to produce radiologic opacities. The presence of scar tissue along the length of the small airway may be sufficient to produce a stiff lung (*ie*, restriction).

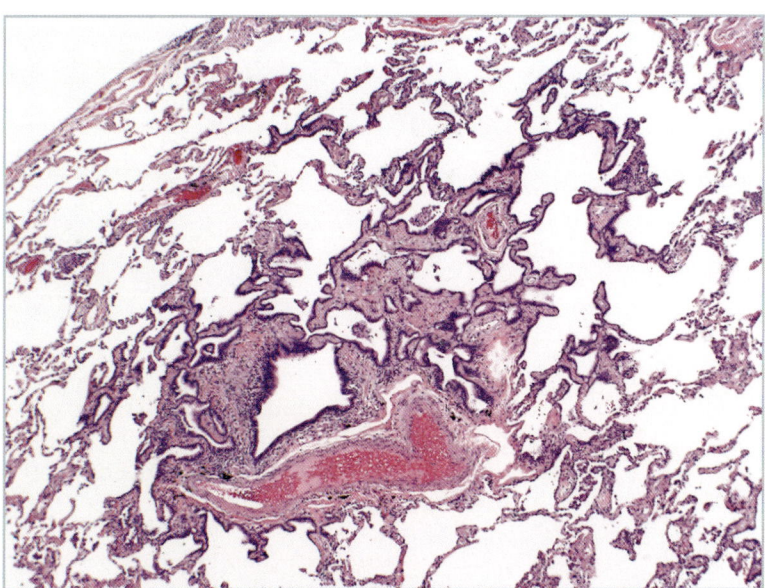

Figure 5-11. In peribronchiolar metaplasia the luminal patency of the bronchiole (*at 7 o'clock*) is maintained, but the peribronchiolar alveoli show thickening and fibrosis and are covered by metaplastic bronchiolar epithelium.

Radiologic Findings

Limited radiologic data are available for this group of patients and consistent abnormalities have not been noted. In the report by Fukuoka et al. [30] the findings include interstitial streaking, mosaic attenuation pattern, patchy subpleural ground glass opacity, "minimal fibrosis," "mild findings suggesting edema," "minimal abnormalities consistent with bronchiolitis," and "multiple opacities." The findings were described as diffuse in all cases.

Common Causes/Associations of the Pathologic Reaction Patterns in Figure 5-4

A. Cellular/exudate reaction

1. **Acute bronchiolitis (neutrophils predominate)**
   - Infections: bacterial and viral
   - Acute fume/toxic exposure
   - Acute aspiration
   - Component of bronchopneumonia

2. **Acute and chronic bronchiolitis (acute and chronic inflammatory cells present)**
   - Infections: all types
   - Distal to bronchiectasis
   - Allergic reactions
   - Inflammatory bowel disease
   - Diffuse panbronchiolitis
   - Connective tissue diseases
   - Aspiration
   - Transplant-associated
   - Idiopathic

3. **Chronic bronchiolitis (chronic inflammatory cells predominate)**
   - Distal to bronchiectasis
   - Connective tissue disease
   - Inflammatory bowel disease
   - Asthma
   - Transplant-associated
   - Immunodeficiency states
   - Respiratory bronchiolitis
   - Langerhans' cell histiocytosis
   - Diffuse panbronchiolitis
   - Chronic aspiration
   - Idiopathic

4. **Follicular bronchiolitis (lymphoid hyperplasia with germinal centers prominent)**
   - Immunodeficiency states: congenital and acquired
   - Connective tissue diseases
   - Hypersensitivity reactions
   - Distal to bronchiectasis
   - Middle lobe syndrome
   - Diffuse panbronchiolitis
   - Component of diffuse lymphoid hyperplasia
   - Idiopathic

B. Mesenchymal reaction

1. **Organization with intraluminal polyps (BOOP pattern/organizing pneumonia pattern)**
   - Organizing diffuse alveolar damage
   - Organizing infectious pneumonias
   - Organization distal to obstruction
   - Organizing aspiration pneumonia
   - Organizing fume/toxic exposures
   - Connective tissue diseases
   - Hypersensitivity pneumonitis
   - Eosinophilic pneumonia
   - Transplant-associated (especially lung or heart-lung)
   - Reaction distal to chronic airway disease (eg, bronchiectasis)
   - Idiopathic (cryptogenic organizing pneumonitis)

2. **Constrictive bronchiolitis**
   - Healed infections
   - Healed fume/toxin exposures
   - Connective tissue diseases, especially RA
   - Transplant-associated
   - Drug reactions
   - Inflammatory bowel disease
   - Diffuse idiopathic pulmonary neuroendocrine cell hyperplasia
   - Complication of asthma
   - Complication of hypersensitivity pneumonitis
   - Idiopathic (cryptogenic obliterative bronchiolitis)

3. **Peribronchiolar metaplasia**
   - Healed bronchiolitis: regardless of cause
   - Distal to bronchiectasis
   - Chronic hypersensitivity pneumonitis
   - Idiopathic

Figure 5-12. Common causes/associations of the pathologic reaction patterns seen in Figure 5-4. BOOP—bronchiolitis obliterans organizing pneumonia; RA—rheumatoid arthritis.

CLINICAL PATHOLOGIC SYNDROMES

Diffuse Panbronchiolitis

This disorder was initially reported in Japan [11] and has also been reported in China, Korea, Europe, the United States, and Latin America [31]. It has been associated with human leukocyte antigen (HLA) Bw54; a major susceptibility gene for diffuse panbronchiolitis has been located on the HLA-B locus on the chromosome 6p21.3 [31]. Patients present in the second to fifth decade with cough, sputum, and eventually dyspnea. Over 80% also have a history of chronic sinusitis. As symptoms progress, recurrent infections develop. In late stage, refractory pseudomonas infections are common. Prior to the use of erythromycin therapy (400–600 mg for at least 6 months) the prognosis was poor, with 5- and 10-year survival rates of approximately 62% and 33%. Following the institution of erythromycin therapy, 10-year survival is greater than 90% [31,32].

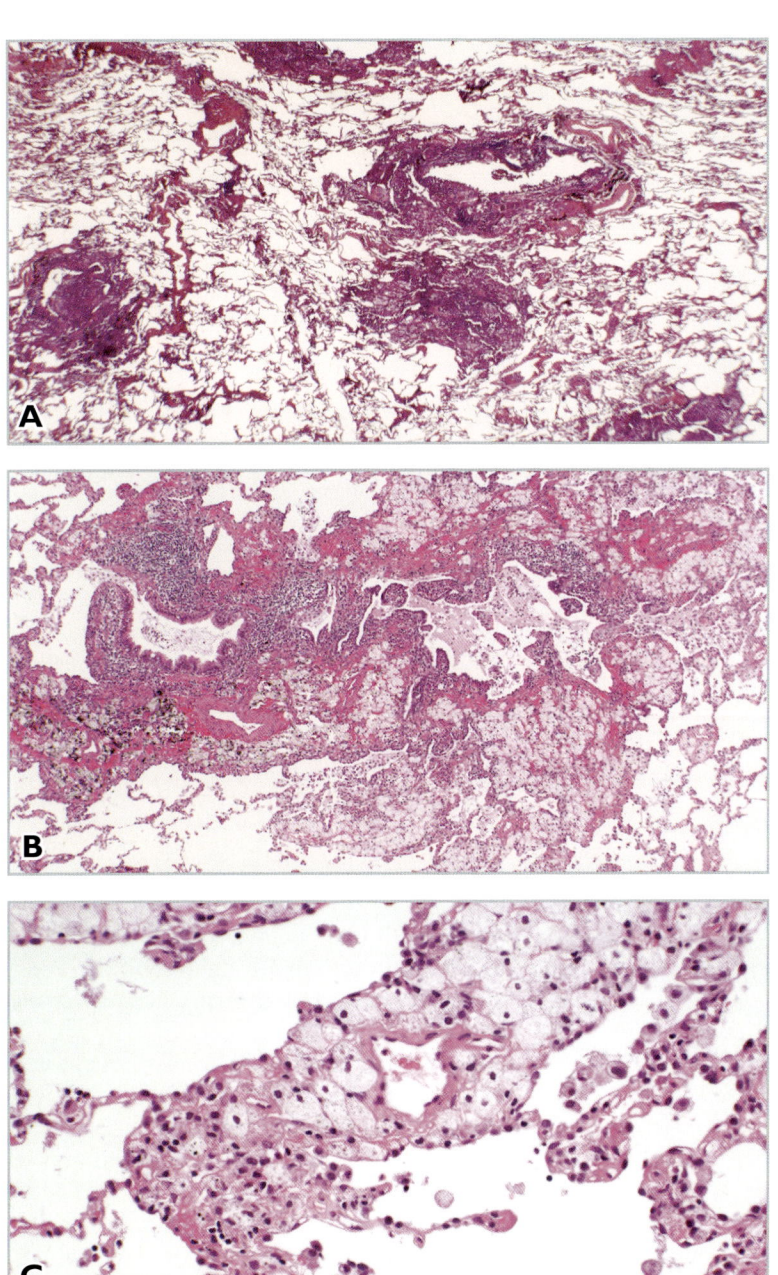

Figure 5-13. Diffuse panbronchiolitis. Scanning power microscopy of a case at autopsy shows nodules which represent markedly inflamed bronchioles (**A**). Surgical lung biopsy from another case shows transmural cellular inflammation, high chronic inflammatory cells (**B**), some luminal exudate, and prominent foamy macrophages in the interstitium of the immediately surrounding alveoli (**C**).

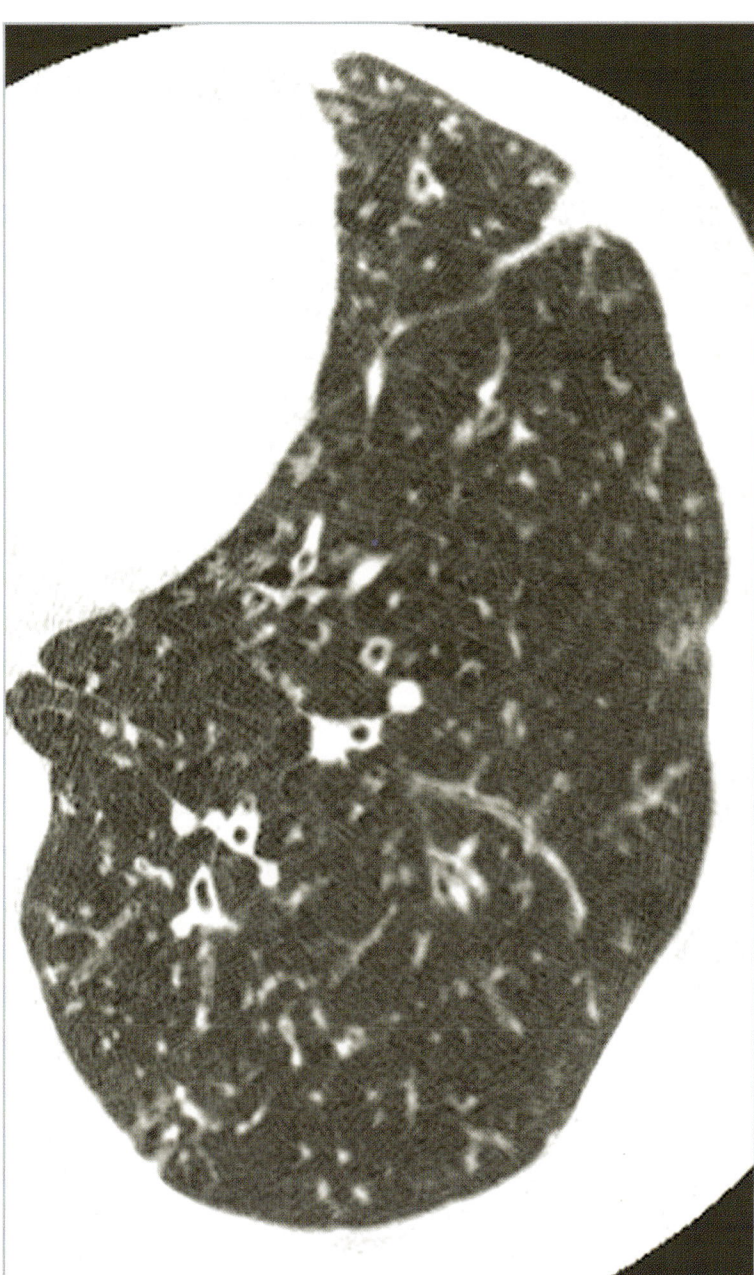

Figure 5-14. Diffuse panbronchiolitis. Magnified high-resolution computed tomography (HRCT) of the lingula and left lower lobe shows multiple small branching nodules in the lower lobe typical of bronchiolar impaction and intraluminal inflammation. Mild bronchiectasis is also noted more anteriorly in the lingula. The HRCT features are not specific for this entity but reflect the underlying pathology. (*Courtesy of* H. Sumikawa MD, Osaka, Japan.)

Cryptogenic Organizing Pneumonia/Idiopathic Bronchiolitis Obliterans Organizing Pneumonia

This condition is included among bronchiolar disorders because the small airways are involved pathologically in this condition with organization and intraluminal polyps in bronchioles, ie, "bronchiolitis obliterans" (see Fig. 5-4). The clinical and radiologic aspects are summarized in Figure 5-8.

Postinfectious Constrictive Bronchiolitis

This condition is rare in adults, although it may occur after a viral or mycoplasmal infection [33]. It is more common in children, especially after infection with respiratory syncytial virus or adenovirus [1,2]. Swyer-James syndrome is a clinical-radiologic variant of postinfectious constrictive bronchiolitis that usually develops after a pulmonary infection in infancy or early childhood [34]. The histology in this condition shows constrictive bronchiolitis and radiologic findings are summarized in Figure 5-10.

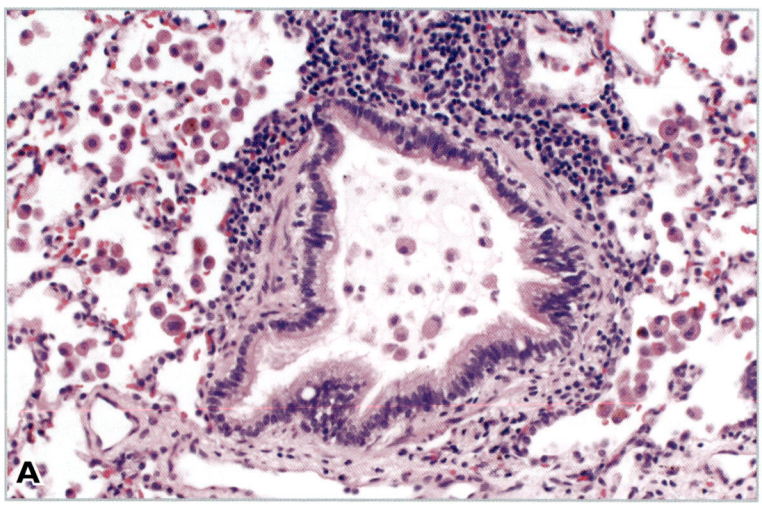
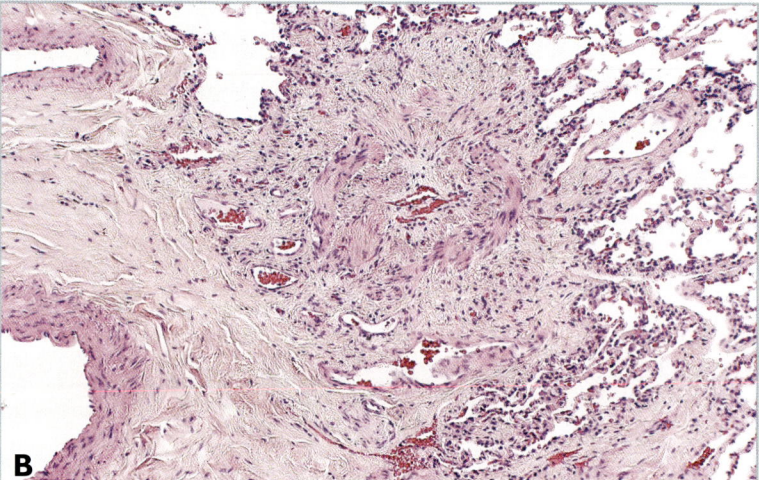

Figure 5-15. Constrictive bronchiolitis following severe mycoplasma pneumonia. **A,** Some of the airways show cellular bronchiolitis with mild distortion of the bronchiolar contour and stasis of mucin in cells within the lumen. **B,** Other bronchioles show complete obliteration with replacement of the bronchiole by scar tissue.

Fume-Related Constrictive Bronchiolitis

Toxic-Fume Bronchiolitis Obliterans

Event	Time	Lesion
Latent period	—	Probably early Inflammation
No symptoms or clinical findings		
Acute respiratory failure	4–6 h	Diffuse alveolar damage
Pulmonary edema pattern seen radiographically		
Progressive chronic respiratory failure	Days–weeks	Constrictive bronchiolitis and bronchiolitis obliterans
Early inspiratory crackles		
Normal chest radiograph		
Severe airflow obstruction		

Figure 5-16. Toxic-fume bronchiolitis obliterans may occur after exposure to nitrogen dioxide (NO_2), sulfur dioxide (SO_2), or other acid-based fumes. The events are summarized in the figure. An example of fume-related bronchiolitis obliterans was described in a 39-year-old truck driver who delivered fly ash. He developed acute respiratory failure requiring hospitalization [35]. His chest radiograph showed bilateral infiltrates. This episode improved rapidly with corticosteroid therapy. After 2 weeks, however, he returned with severe dyspnea. His forced vital capacity (FVC) was normal at 5.44 L (102% predicted), but his forced expiratory volume in 1 second (FEV_1) had decreased to 2.13 L (52% predicted) and his FEV_1/FVC ratio had fallen markedly to 39%. It is unknown whether the patient's condition was a result of the direct effect of the fly ash particles or toxic agents such as NO_2 or SO_2 adsorbed to the fly ash particles.

Smoke inhalation bronchiolitis obliterans was described in a 23-year-old man who was sleeping in his newly constructed house when it caught fire [36]. The synthetic structural materials used to build his house produced gases that contained acrolein, formaldehyde, acetaldehyde, NO_2 and SO_2 when burned. Smoke inhalation bronchiolitis obliterans was also described as resulting from the burning of synthetic construction materials in a wood-burning stove [37]. Two workers in a lithium battery factory were accidentally exposed to thionyl chloride, and one of them developed a prolonged clinical course and findings consistent with bronchiolitis obliterans [38]. Thionyl chloride is an acidic compound used in the lithium battery manufacturing process and produces SO_2 and hydrogen chloride fumes when in contact with water.

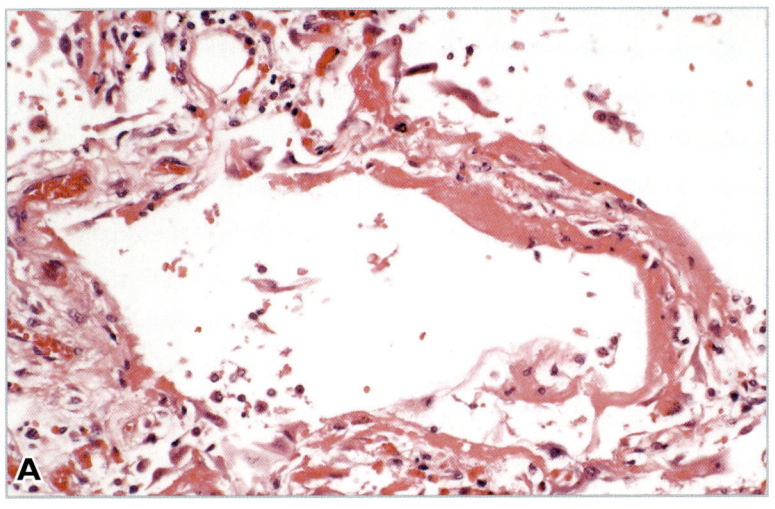
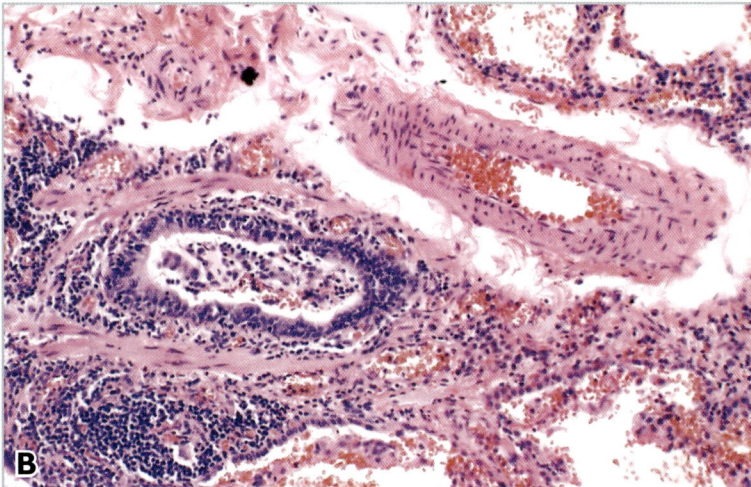
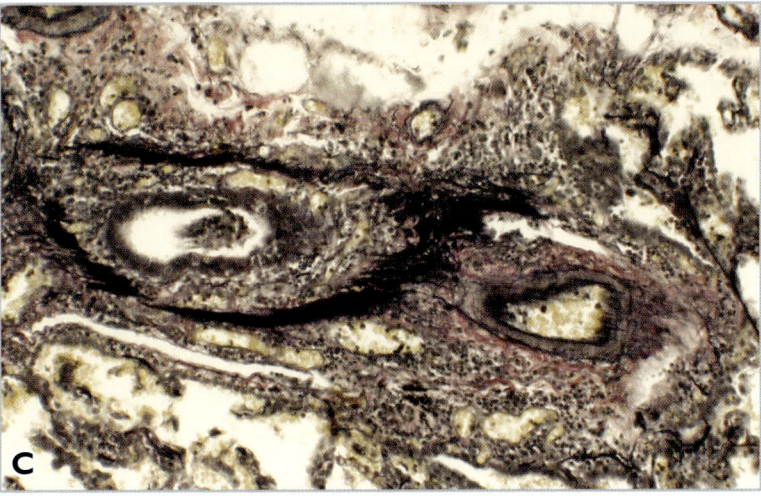

Figure 5-17. Fume inhalation associated with fires. In the acute phase there is severe acute injury with diffuse alveolar damage with hyaline membranes (**A**). In more chronic cases there is evidence of constrictive bronchiolitis with transmural inflammation of the bronchioles and luminal narrowing (**B**), which is highlighted with elastic tissue staining (**C**). The elastic tissue stain illustrates the deposition of fibrosis between the mucosa and the darkly stained elastica. Normally the mucosa would be sitting on the elastica.

Drug-related Constrictive Bronchiolitis

Drugs have been implicated only occasionally in constrictive bronchiolitis. The best known are Penacillamine and CCNU (lomustine) [39]. Some of the penacillamine-associated cases have been in patients with rheumatoid arthritis, and separating rheumatoid arthritis–related constrictive bronchiolitis from penacillamine-related constrictive bronchiolitis may be problematic.

Transplant-Associated Constrictive Bronchiolitis: Bone Marrow Transplantation

Risk Factors Associated with Bone Marrow Transplantation in Bronchiolitis Obliterans

- Allogeneic transplantation
- Graft-versus-host disease
- Late onset, indicating a poor prognosis
- Severe airflow obstruction, indicating a poor prognosis

Figure 5-18. Several risk factors have been identified for the development of bronchiolitis obliterans after bone marrow transplantation. The lesion may be preceded by findings typical of graft versus host (GVH) disease, including skin rash, mucositis, sicca, and angiitis, usually occurring within 3 months after transplantation. Six months later the patient develops a cough, then progressive dyspnea. At this late stage, the chest radiograph is normal in 80% of patients; however, the forced expiratory volume in 1 second is severely reduced, and no improvement is seen after bronchodilator inhalation. Response to therapy is poor once severe airflow obstruction has been established. Those with late onset and severe airflow obstruction have the worst prognosis. For these patients, therapy is directed at controlling chronic GVH disease and preventing infection. On the basis of a review of lung biopsy specimens taken from bone marrow transplant recipients and showing GVH disease, Yousem [40] classified observed morphologic changes into four categories: diffuse alveolar damage, lymphocytic bronchitis/bronchiolitis with interstitial pneumonitis, bronchiolitis obliterans organizing pneumonia, and constrictive bronchiolitis obliterans. The histologic findings for five patients with constrictive bronchiolitis indicated that the airway lumina had been obliterated by dense fibrous scar tissue; the atretic airways could be identified only by their location adjacent to arterioles. All patients had cough and shortness of breath, two died from bronchiolitis obliterans, one was alive with disease by the end of the study, and two had double-lung transplantations. It was noted that this lesion may reflect irreversible pulmonary GVH disease. An example of the pathology is shown in Figure 5-19A.

Continued on the next page

Figure 5-18. *(Continued)* Stem cell transplantation bronchiolitis obliterans occurs in less than 2% of patients. Among 6275 adult recipients of human leukocyte antigen (HLA)-identical sibling-matched hematopoietic stem cell transplantation for leukemia, 76 were found to have obliterative bronchiolitis with an incidence rate of 1.7% at 2 years after transplantation [41]. Known risk factors include an episode of acute graft versus host disease and busulfan-based conditioning regimen, and this study added four additional risk factors, including peripheral blood-derived stem cell, duration of 14 months or more to transplant, female donor to male recipient, and a prior episode of interstitial pneumonitis [41]. Among a group of 369 patients who received allogenic stem cell transplantation, 61 of them (16.5%) developed pulmonary complications, and 13 (3.5%) developed obliterative bronchiolitis occurring at a late stage with a median of 203 days [42]. In a review of 22 stem cell transplantation studies, Soubani and Uberti reported that bronchiolitis obliterans is one of the most challenging pulmonary complications for the clinician caring for stem cell transplantation recipients [43].

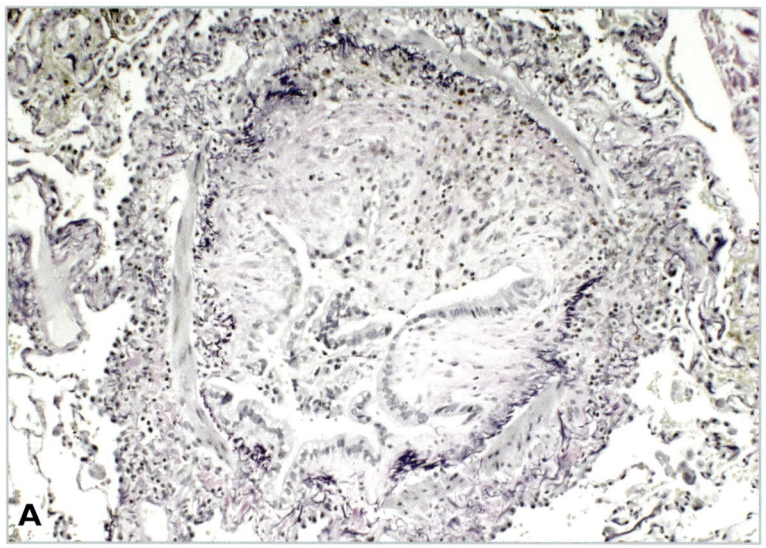 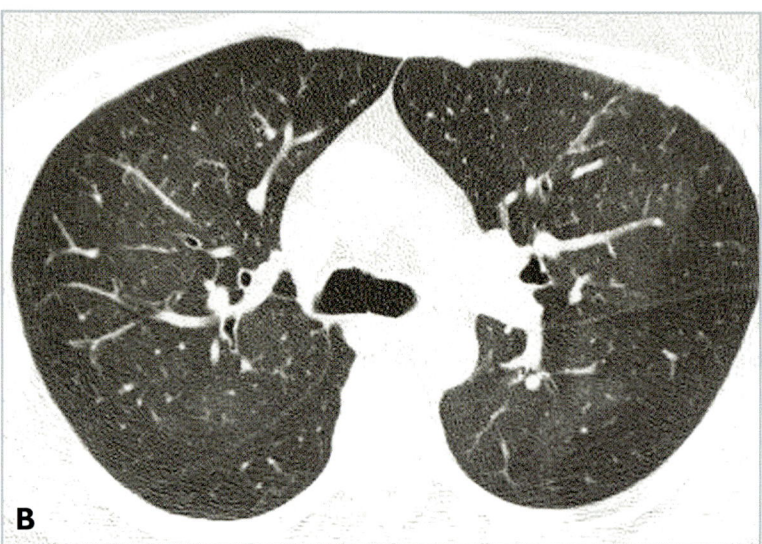

Figure 5-19. **A,** Constrictive bronchiolitis associated with bone marrow transplantation. There is eccentric subepithelial deposition of collagen that markedly separates the mucosa from the underlying dark-staining elastica. **B,** Constrictive bronchiolitis after marrow transplantation (same patient as in Fig. 5-10). High-resolution computed tomography shows the mosaic attenuation pattern with typical vascular caliber differences between the dense and lucent zones.

Transplant-Associated Constrictive Bronchiolitis: Lung Transplantation

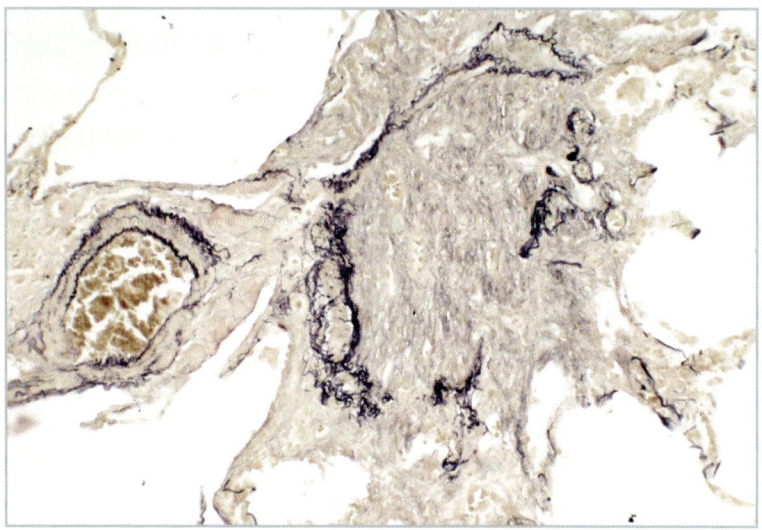

Figure 5-20. Constrictive bronchiolitis associated with lung transplantation (bronchiolitis obliterans syndrome). Elastic tissue staining highlights complete obliteration.

The 1-year survival rate of lung transplant recipients has improved to more than 75%, yet bronchiolitis obliterans continues to be a serious cause of morbidity and mortality [44–48]. The cumulative risk of bronchiolitis obliterans may be 60% to 80% from 5 to 10 years after transplantation. The major risk factor appears to be acute rejection; the more frequent and the more severe the rejection, the higher the risk. Factors not correlated with bronchiolitis obliterans include the age and sex of the recipient and donor and the recipient's underlying disease. The degree of human leukocyte antigen mismatch between donor and recipient also appears to predispose recipients to the development of severe bronchiolitis obliterans [44]. Recipients who have onset before 12 months with progressive deterioration have a poor prognosis; those with onset after more than 30 months have lower mortality. Expiratory chest computed tomography (CT) films are often helpful for diagnosis of transplant-related bronchiolitis obliterans; however, a study of seven patients indicated that thin section CT had limited accuracy in diagnosing early bronchiolitis obliterans [45]. Measurements of ventilation distribution can detect obliterative bronchiolitis in transplant recipients better than conventional pulmonary function testing [46]. Regarding treatment, the bronchiolitis obliterans lesion in these patients may be corticosteroid resistant, so cytolytic immunosuppression must be used. Treatment with a cytolytic drug such as OKT3 antithymocyte globulin or antilymphocyte globulin has been used [47]. Lung retransplantation for bronchiolitis obliterans has had some success, with 4- to 5-year survival rates comparable to those of primary lung transplantation [48]. It is thought that the best way to prevent this complication is to eliminate or change clinical events before, during, or after transplantation in a manner that will decrease the development of obliterative bronchiolitis [47].

Miscellaneous Causes of Constrictive Bronchiolitis

Neuroendocrine cells are a normal component of the airway mucosa. In rare circumstances these cells proliferate and when confined to the bronchiole, the term *diffuse idiopathic neuroendocrine cell hyperplasia* (DIPNECH) is used [49]. When the proliferation goes beyond the confines of the airway the term (carcinoid) *tumorlet* is used. A minority of cases in which neuroendocrine cell hyperplasia in airways is identified pathologically have signs and symptoms of constrictive bronchiolitis were the typical clinical and radiologic findings [16,17]. This is an exceptionally rare cause of constrictive bronchiolitis. Occasional cases have undergone lung transplantation [18].

Sauropus androgynus is a plant in Asia that was used as a dietary supplement to aid in weight loss. It was taken as a tea and a small epidemic of constrictive bronchiolitis was identified and some patients required lung transplantation for irreversible obstructive lung disease [19,50].

Recently, diacetyl, a compound used in the butter flavoring of microwave popcorn, was implicated a cause of constrictive bronchiolitis among factor workers exposed to this material in the production of microwave popcorn [20].

Bronchiolar Pathology in Connective Tissue Diseases

Bronchiolitis of various forms occurs in patients with connective tissue disease. Women with rheumatoid arthritis are most commonly affected, although patients with other connective tissue disorders, including scleroderma, lupus erythematosus, ankylosing spondylitis, and Sjögren's syndrome, can be affected also [1,2,51]. The full spectrum of findings illustrated in Figures 5-5 through 5-11 may be encountered. Follicular bronchiolitis is a characteristic histologic finding.

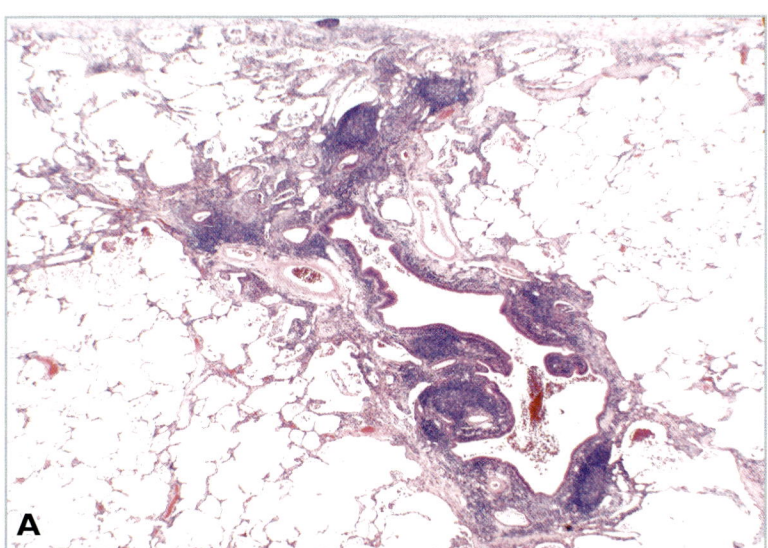
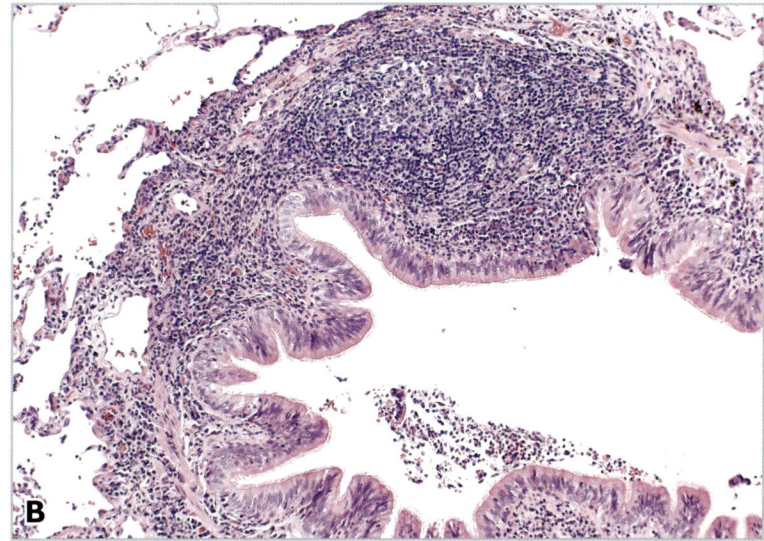

Figure 5-21. Follicular bronchiolitis associated with rheumatoid arthritis. **A,** There is a cellular infiltrate along a bronchiole associated with scattered lymphoid follicles containing germinal centers. **B,** At higher power the germinal center in this field is seen to reside in a submucosal position.

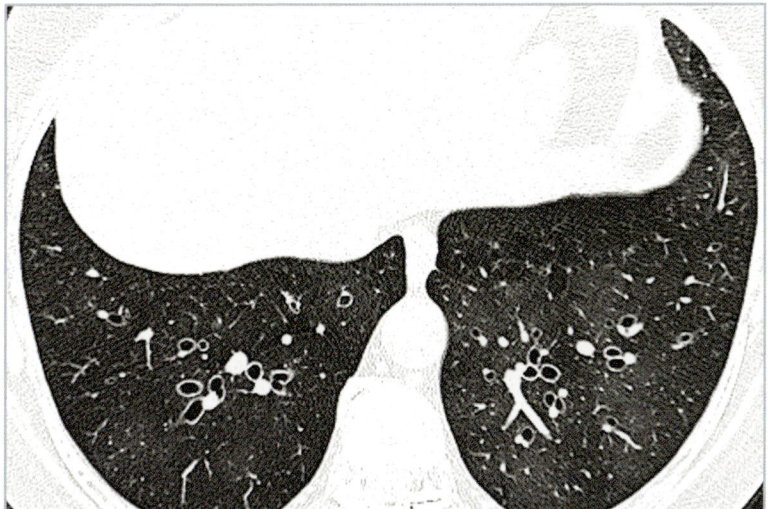

Figure 5-22. Constrictive bronchiolitis ("bronchiolitis obliterans") in a 53-year-old woman with recently diagnosed rheumatoid arthritis and progressive dyspnea. High-resolution computed tomography shows the mosaic attenuation pattern, typical vascular caliber differences between lucent and dense lung zones, and some thickening and mild dilation of the central airways.

Bronchiolar Disorders

Bronchiolar Pathology in Inflammatory Bowel Disease

Airway disease is an uncommon but well known intrathoracic complication of inflammatory bowel disease [51–53]. Purulent bronchitis and bronchiectasis are the best known manifestations but bronchiolitis also occurs. There is a spectrum of histologic involvement from cellular bronchiolitis to constrictive bronchiolitis and the clinical and radiologic manifestations parallel those findings as noted in Figures 5-5 through 5-11.

Bronchiolar Pathology of Unknown Cause

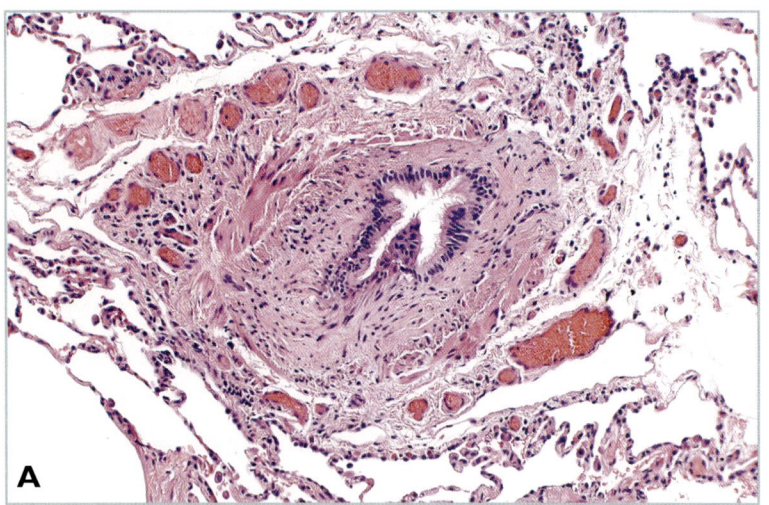
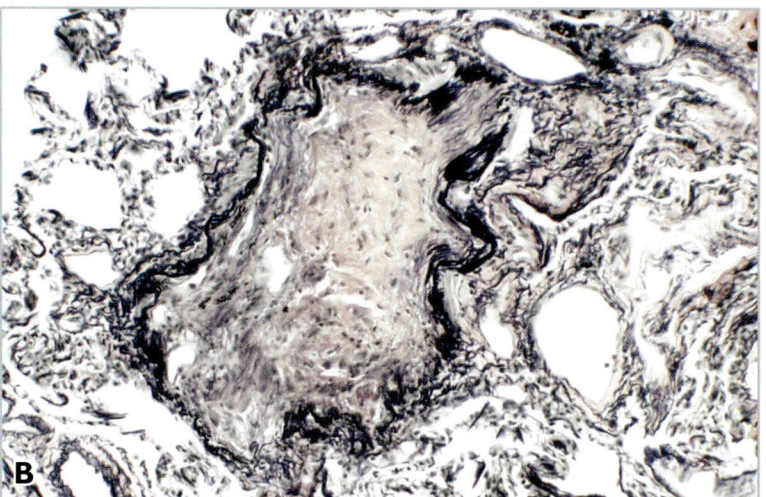

Figure 5-23. Idiopathic constrictive bronchiolitis. **A,** There is marked luminal compromise by subepithelial collagen deposition separating the mucosa from the smooth muscle fascicles. **B,** The same patient also had occasional bronchioles that showed complete obliteration, with elastic tissue staining highlighting the original elastica and the lumen replaced by fibrous tissue.

Any of the various patterns of bronchiolar pathology noted in Figure 5-4 may occasionally be histologic findings in patients who have an idiopathic process [1,2,30,54–57]. Depending on the histology, names for these cases have included idiopathic BOOP/cryptogenic organizing pneumonitis, bronchiolitis in adults, cryptogenic constrictive bronchiolitis, cryptogenic obliterative bronchiolitis, peribronchiolar metaplasia–associated interstitial lung disease, and others.

REFERENCES

1. Colby TV: Bronchiolitis. *Am J Clin Pathol* 1998, 109:101–109.

2. Travis WD, Colby TV, Koss MN, et al.: Bronchiolar disorders. In *Non-neoplastic Disorders of the Lower Respiratory Tract*, 1st Series, Fascicle 2. Washington, DC: American Registry of Pathology and the Armed Forces Institute of Pathology; 2002:351–380.

3. Ueda T, Niimi A, Matsumoto H, et al.: Role of small airways in asthma: investigation using high-resolution computed tomography. *J Allergy Clin Immunol* 2006, 118:1019–1025.

4. Hogg JC: State of the art: bronchiolitis in chronic obstructive pulmonary disease. *Proc Am Thorac Soc* 2006, 3:489–493.

5. Lange W: Ueber eine eigenthumliche erkrankung der kleinen bronchien und bronchilen [in German]. *Dtsch Arch Klin Med* 1901, 70:342–364.

6. Fraenkel A: Ueber bronchiolitis fibrosa obliterans, nebst bemerkungen uber lungenthy-peramie und indurirende pneumonia. *Dtsch Arch Klin Med* 1902, 73:484–512.

7. Hart C: Anatomische untersuchungen uber die bei masern vorkommenden lungenerkrankungen. *Dtsch Arch Klin Med* 1904, 79:108–128.

8. Jochmann G: Moltrecht, uber seltenere erkrankungsformen der bronchien nach masern und keuchhusten. *Beitrage zur Pah Anat zur Allgemeinen Path* 1904, 36:340–352.

9. Geddes DM, Corrin B, Brewerton DA, et al.: Progressive airway obliteration in adults and its association with rheumatoid disease. *Q J Med* 1977, 46:427–444.

10. Roca J, Granena A, Rodriguez-Roisin R, et al.: Fatal airway disease in an adult with chronic graft-versus-host disease. *Thorax* 1982, 37:77–78.

11. Homma H, Yamanaka A, Shinichi T, et al.: Diffuse panbronchiolitis: a disease of the transitional zone of the lung. *Chest* 1983, 83:63–69.

12. Burke CM, Theodore J, Dawkins KD, et al.: Post-transplant obliterative bronchiolitis and other late lung sequelae in human heart-lung transplantation. *Chest* 1984, 86:824–829.

13. Epler GR, Colby TV, McLoud TC, et al.: Bronchiolitis obliterans organizing pneumonia. *N Engl J Med* 1985, 312:152–158.

14. Myers JF, Veal CF, Shin MS, et al.: Respiratory bronchiolitis causing interstitial lung disease: a clinicopathologic study of six cases. *Am Rev Respir Dis* 1987, 135:880–884.

15. McGregor CGA, Dark JH, Hilton CJ, et al.: Early results of single lung transplantation in patients with end-stage pulmonary fibrosis. *J Thorac Cardiovasc Surg* 1989, 98:350–354.

16. Aguayo SM, Miller YE, Waldron JA, et al.: Idiopathic diffuse hyperplasia of pulmonary neuroendocrine cells and airways disease. *N Engl J Med* 1992, 327:1285–1288.

17. Miller RR, Muller NL: Neuroendocrine cell hyperplasia and obliterative bronchiolitis in patients with peripheral carcinoid tumors. *Am J Surg Pathol* 1995, 19:653–658.

18. Sheerin N, Harrison NK, Sheppard MN, et al.: Obliterative bronchiolitis caused by multiple tumorlets and microcarcinoids successfully treated by single lung transplantation. *Thorax* 1995, 50:207–209.

19. Lai RS, Chiang AA, Wu MT, et al.: Outbreak of bronchiolitis obliterans associated with consumption of *Sauropus androgynus* in Taiwan. *Lancet* 1996, 348:83–85.

20. Kreiss K, Gomaa A, Kullman G, et al.: Clinical bronchiolitis obliterans in workers at a microwave-popcorn plant. *N Engl J Med* 2002, 347:330–338.

21. American Thoracic Society/European Respiratory Society international multidisciplinary consensus classification of the idiopathic interstitial pneumonias. *Am J Respir Crit Care Med* 2002, 165:277–304.

22. Estenne M, Maurer JR, Boehler A, et al.: Bronchiolitis obliterans syndrome 2001: an update of the diagnostic criteria. J Heart Lung Transplant 2002, 21:297–310.

23. Wright JL, Cagle P, Churg A, et al.: Diseases of the small airways. *Am Rev Respir Dis* 1992, 146:240–262.

24. Ryu JH, Myers JL, Swensen SJ: Bronchiolar disorders. *Am J Respir Crit Care Med* 2003, 168:1277–1292.

25. Popper HH: Bronchiolitis: an update. *Virchows Arch* 2000, 437:471–481.

26. Thompson AB, Robbins RA, Romberger DJ, et al.: Immunological function of the pulmonary epithelium. *Eur Respir J* 1995, 8:127–149.

27. Johnson JE, Gonzales RA, Olson SJ, et al.: The histopathology of fatal untreated human respiratory syncytial virus infection. *Mod Pathol* 2007, 20:108–119.

28. Gruden JF, Webb WR, Warnock M: Centrilobular opacities in the lung on HRCT: diagnostic considerations and pathologic correlation. *AJR Am J Roentgenol* 1994, 162:569–574.

29. Gruden JF, Webb WR: Identification and evaluation of centrilobular opacities on high-resolution CT. *Semin Ultrasound CT MRI* 1995, 16:435–449.

30. Fukuoka J, Franks TJ, Colby TV, et al.: Peribronchiolar metaplasia: a common histologic lesion in diffuse lung disease and a rare cause of interstitial lung disease: clinicopathologic features of 15 cases. *Am J Surg Pathol* 2005, 29:948–954.

31. Poletti V, Casoni G, Chilosi M, et al.: Diffuse panbronchiolitis. *Eur Respir J* 2006, 28:862–871.

32. Kudoh S, Azuma A, Yamamoto M, et al.: Improvement of survival in patients with diffuse panbronchiolitis treated with low-dose erythromycin. *Am J Respir Crit Care Med* 1998, 157:1829–1832.

33. Chan E, Kalayanamit T, Lynch DA, et al.: *Mycoplasma pneumoniae*-associated bronchiolitis causing severe restrictive lung disease in adults. *Chest* 1999, 115:1188–1194.

34. Daniel TL, Woodring JH, MacVandiviere HM, Wilson HD: Swyer-James syndrome: unilateral hyperlucent lung syndrome. *Clin Pediatr* 1984, 23:393–397.

35. Boswell RT, McCunney RJ: Bronchilitis obliterans from exposure to incinerator fly ash. *J Occup Environ Med* 1995, 37:850–855.

36. Tasaka S, Kanasawa M, Mori M, et al.: Long-term course of bronchiectasis and bronchiolitis obliterans as late complications of smoke inhalation. *Respiration* 1995, 62:40–42.

37. Janigan DT, Toomas K, Michael R, McCleave JJ: Bronchiolitis obliterans in a man who used his wood-burning stove to burn synthetic construction materials. *CMAJ* 1997, 156:1171–1173.

38. Konichezky S, Schattner A, Ezri T, et al.: Thionyl-chloride-induced lung injury and bronchiolitis obliterans. *Chest* 1993, 104:971–973.

39. Myers JL, El-Zammar O: Pathology of drug-induced lung disease. In *Katzenstein and Askin's Surgical Pathology of Non-neoplastic Disease*, edn 4. Edited by Katzenstein ALA. Philadelphia: Saunders Elsevier.

40. Yousem SA: The histological spectrum of pulmonary graft-versus-host disease in bone marrow transplant recipients. *Hum Pathol* 1995, 26:668–675.

41. Tomas LHS, Loberiza FR, Klein JP, et al.: Risk factors for bronchiolitis obliterans in allogeneic hematopoietic stem-cell transplantation for leukemia. *Chest* 2005, 128:153–161.

42. Huisman C, van der Straaten HM, Canninga-van Dijk MR, et al.: Pulmonary complications after T-cell depleted allogenic stem cell transplantation: low incidence and strong association with acute graft-versus-host disease. *Bone Marrow Transplant* 2006, 38:561–566.

43. Soubani AO, Uberti JP: Bronchiolitis obliterans following hematopoietic stem cell transplantation. *Eur Respir J* 2007, 29:1007–1019.

44. Chalermskulrat W, Neuringer I, Schmitz JL, et al.: Human leukocyte antigen mismatches predispose to the severity of bronchiolitis obliterans syndrome after lung transplantation. *Chest* 2003, 123:1825–1831.

45. Lee ES, Gotway MB, Reddy GP, et al.: Early bronchiolitis obliterans following lung transplantation: accuracy of expiratory thin-section CT for diagnosis. *Radiology* 2000, 216:472–477.

46. Estenne M, Van Muylem A, Knoop C, Antoine M: Detection of obliterative bronchiolitis after lung transplantation by indexes of ventilation distribution. *Am J Respir Crit Care Med* 2000, 162:1047–1051.

47. Paradis I: Bronchiolitis obliterans: pathogenesis, prevention, and management. *Am J Med Sci* 1998, 315:161–178.

48. Brugiere O, Thabut G, Castier Y, et al.: Lung transplantation for bronchiolitis obliterans syndrome: long-term follow-up in a series of 15 recipients. *Chest* 2003, 123:1832–1837.

49. Travis WD, Brambilla E, Muller-Hermelink HK, Harris CC: *WHO Classification of Tumors: Tumors of the Lung, Pleura, Thymus, and Heart.* Lyon: IARC Press; 2004.

50. Yeh-Leong C, Yao Y-T, Wang N-S, Lee Y-C: Segmental necrosis of small bronchi after prolonged intakes of *Sauropus androgynus* in Taiwan. *Am J Respir Crit Care Med* 1998, 157:594–598.

51. Travis WD, Colby TV, Koss MN, et al.: Connective tissue and inflammatory bowel diseases. In *Non-neoplastic Disorders of the Lower Respiratory Tract*, 1st Series, Fascicle 2. Washington, DC: American Registry of Pathology and the Armed Forces Institute of Pathology; 2002:291–320.

52. Camus P, Colby TV: Respiratory manifestations in ulcerative colitis. *Eur Respir Mon* 2006, 34:168–183.

53. Colby TV, Camus P: Pathology of pulmonary involvement in inflammatory bowel disease. *Eur Respir Mon* 2007, 39:199–207.

54. Turton CW, Williams G, Green M: Cryptogenic obliterative bronchiolitis in adults. *Thorax* 1981, 36:805–810.

55. Kindt GC, Weiland JE, Davis WB, et al.: Bronchiolitis in adults. *Am Rev Respir Dis* 1989, 140:483–492.

56. Pletti V, Zompatori M, Boaron M, et al.: Cryptogenic constrictive bronchiolitis imitating imaging features of diffuse panbronchiolitis. *Monaldi Arch Chest Dis* 1995, 50:116–117.

57. Kraft M, Mortenson RL, Colby TV, et al.: Cryptogenic constrictive bronchiolitis: a clinicopathologic study. *Am Rev Respir Dis* 1993, 148:1093–1101.

SLEEP DISORDERED BREATHING

Michelle Cao, Nelly Huynh, and Christian Guilleminault

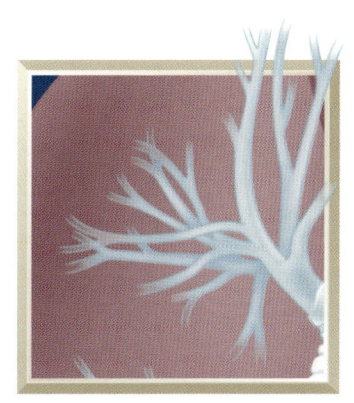
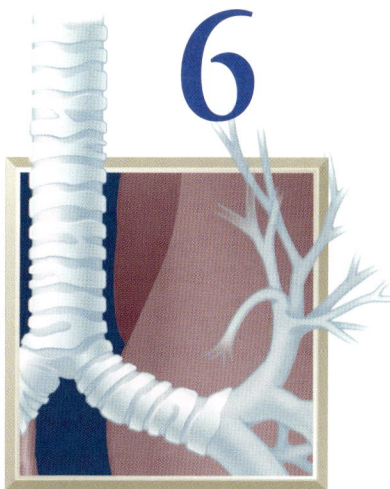
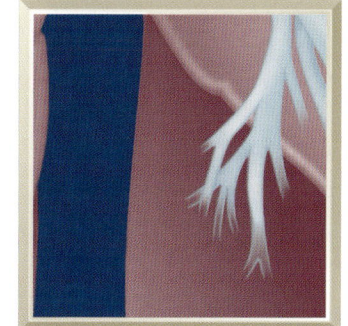

The spectrum of sleep-disordered breathing includes obstructive sleep apnea-hypopnea syndromes and central sleep apnea syndromes.

Approximately 7% of Caucasians and between 15% and 17% of Far-East Asians are affected by obstructive sleep apnea. Symptoms include snoring, gasping, choking, disrupted nocturnal sleep, and witnessed apneic episodes during sleep. Perhaps the most common reason that patients seek treatment is that a bed partner cannot sleep through loud snoring. Excessive daytime sleepiness and insomnia are also common causes of referral. The syndrome is characterized by recurrent episodes of partial or complete upper airway obstruction with significant decrease or complete cessation in airflow in the presence of ongoing respiratory effort. The obstruction causes recurrent electroencephalogram (EEG) arousals associated with or without clear oxygen desaturations during sleep.

In contrast to obstructive sleep apnea, central apnea is defined by a lack of respiratory effort during cessation of airflow. The clinical consequences of both syndromes include not only excessive daytime sleepiness or hypersomnolence and—particularly in women—insomnia, but also chronic fatigue, neurocognitive deficits, parasomnias such as sleepwalking, sleep terror, bruxism, morning headache, gastroesophageal reflux during sleep, and sexual dysfunction. Obstructive and central sleep apnea syndromes are associated with increased risk of cardiovascular, pulmonary, and metabolic dysfunction including hypertension, stroke, coronary artery disease, cardiac arrhythmias, congestive heart failure, cor pulmonale, and diabetes mellitus.

A comprehensive sleep history and upper airway physical examination are necessary in order to make appropriate referrals for polysomnography. The Epworth sleepiness scale is commonly used in the office setting to evaluate the severity of daytime sleepiness (a score of > 10 out of 24 is associated with symptoms of daytime sleepiness). Polysomnography is the "gold standard" test for the diagnosis of a sleep-related breathing disorder. The overnight study consists of multiple physiologic signals (EEG, electro-oculogram [EOG], electrocardiogram, and electromyogram; sensors of airflow with nasal cannula and oral pressure transducer; and sensors of respiratory efforts) that are continuously monitored in a sleeping patient. Standards have been created for the classification of disordered breathing events. An apnea is defined as cessation of airflow for at least 10 seconds, and a hypopnea is defined as reduction in airflow of a certain magnitude for at least 10 seconds in duration; both are associated either with an arousal or with oxygen desaturation. An oxygen desaturation of 3% to 4% and specific EEG criteria for arousals are commonly accepted in the literature. More recently, attention has been drawn toward abnormality of the contour of the nasal cannula waveform. Several patterns—particularly the flattening of the curve—have been described and have been shown to affect sleep. The sleep disturbances have been demonstrated by the presence of short EEG arousals, as well as disturbance of sleep continuity with presence of non–rapid eye movement (REM) sleep instability as demonstrated by cyclic alternating pattern (CAP) analysis or computerized EEG analysis. Respiratory effort may be abnormal and esophageal pressure monitoring may be needed to demonstrate this occurrence. In young and slim individuals, the first indication of abnormal breathing during sleep will be the presence of tachypnea that allows maintenance of minute ventilation despite some reduction in tidal volume. Starting at two years of age, maximum respiratory rate during non-REM sleep is 18 breaths per minute, and 20 breaths per minute during REM sleep.

Signs and Symptoms of Sleep Disordered Breathing

Adults	Children
Snoring	Snoring
Witnessed apnea during sleep	Restless sleep
Gasping/choking during sleep	Frequent agitated arousals
Coughing during sleep	Parasomnias
Excessive movements during sleep	Nightsweats
Frequent awakenings	Coughing during sleep
Parasomnias	Nocturnal enuresis
Nightsweats	Sleeping in unusual postures such as on hands and knees
Morning dry mouth	
Unrefreshed upon waking in the morning	Daytime sleepiness
Morning headaches	Daytime mouth breathing
Excessive daytime sleepiness	Swallowing difficulties
Daytime fatigue	Poor speech articulation
Drowsiness with driving	Hyperactivitiy disorder
Insomnia	Behavior disturbance
Neurocognitive deficits	Emotional disturbance
Disorientation	Poor school performance
Frequent or multiple daytime naps that are unrefreshing	Failure to thrive
Cold hands and feet	Developmental delay
Orthostatic hypotension	High blood pressure in an adolescent (rare)
High blood pressure (especially refractory to treatment)	

Figure 6-1. Signs and symptoms of sleep disordered breathing in adults and children.

Predisposing Factors to Sleep Disordered Breathing

Narrowing of the upper airway
- A. Excessive bulk of tissue
- B. Hereditary or acquired craniofacial abnormalities
- C. Hypertrophied tonsils and adenoids (more common in children)

Nasal obstruction

Micrognathia

Retrognathia

Macroglossia

High-arched hard palate

Pregnancy

Postmenopausal state

Hypothyroidism

Acromegaly

Obesity

Sedative and narcotic use

Underlying abnormality of neurologic control of upper airway musculature

Underlying abnormality of control of ventilation

Specific neurological lesion affecting control of ventilation or musculature

Figure 6-2. Predisposing factors to sleep disordered breathing.

Atlas of Pulmonary Medicine

Common Terms and Definitions in Adults and Children With Sleep Disordered Breathing

Term	Definition
Adults	
Obstructive apnea	Absence of airflow at the nose and mouth for at least 10 sec in duration with persistent respiratory effort as measured by thoracic and abdominal sensors; these events typically last 20–40 seconds and rarely can last for up to 2 min; they are more commonly seen in stages 1 & 2 sleep and are usually more severe in REM sleep
Hypopnea	Reduction in airflow ≥ 30% of baseline at the nasal cannula for at least 10 sec associated with an oxygen desaturation of ≥ 4% OR Reduction in airflow ≥ 50% of baseline at the nasal cannula for at least 10 sec associated with an oxygen desaturation of ≥ 3% and/or an arousal
Abnormal respiratory effort	Increased effort shown on Pes signal associated with a reduction in nasal flow of less than 30% with flattening of nasal cannula signal (flow limitation) and a decrease in the mouth signal (thermistor)
Respiratory event-related arousals (RERAs)	Patterns of progressive increase in snoring noise or (better study) negative inspiratory Pes terminated by end of snoring or (better) both a sudden change in pressure to a less negative level as well as an arousal event lasting 10 sec or more; this event does not meet criteria for an apnea or a hypopnea
Pes crescendo	Sequences of four or more breaths that show increasingly negative peak-end inspiratory Pes; may be seen with flow limitation on the nasal cannula
Pes reversal	Termination of abnormal increase in respiratory effort measured with Pes with abrupt switch to a less negative peak end inspiratory esophageal pressure
Continuous sustained respiratory effort	Repetitive, abnormally negative peak-end inspiratory Pes, ending at the same negative inspiratory Pes without a crescendo pattern. It is associated with discrete flow limitation on the nasal cannula pressure transducer signal, with flattening of the wave contour for at least four successive breaths
Central apnea	Absence of airflow at oral and nasal cannula as well as absence of thoracoabdominal movements for at least 10 sec
Central hypopnea	Reduction of airflow of at least 30% with oral and nasal cannula, as well as a 30% reduction in amplitude of thoracoabdominal movement contour for at least 10 sec or a decrease in respiratory effort measured with Pes compared to normal respiratory effort
Mixed apnea	An event meeting criteria for central apnea at the initial portion of the event, followed by resumption of inspiratory effort meeting criteria for an obstructive apnea; in a patient taking opoids, a mixed apnea may be reversed: presentation of an obstructive apnea followed by a central apnea
Children	
Obstructive apnea	Absence of airflow at the nose and mouth for longer than two breaths with sustained respiratory effort as measured by thoracic and abdominal sensors, independent of desaturation or change in EEG
Hypopnea	Reduction of at least 30% in nasal flow signal amplitude for a minimum of two breaths, and associated with an EEG arousal, an awakening, or ≥ 3% oxygen desaturation
Central apnea	Absence of airflow at the nasal or mouth cannula as well as absence of inspiratory effort for at least 20 sec, or an event lasting for at least 2 breaths and associated with an EEG arousal, an awakening, or a ≥ 3% oxygen desaturation
Tachypnea	Increase in respiratory rate, above that seen during quiet unobstructed breathing, by a minimum of 3 breaths/min in non-REM sleep or 4 breaths/minute in REM sleep for 30 sec or more; no changes in oxygen saturation, Pes, or EEG are required; after 24 mo of age, normal respiratory rate is a maximum of 16 to 18 breaths/min in non-REM sleep and 17 to 19 breaths/min in REM sleep; tachypnea may be the only sign of abnormal breathing during sleep, particularly in overweight children

Figure 6-3. Common terms and definitions used in studying adults and children with sleep disordered breathing. EEG—electroencephalogram; Pes—esophageal pressure; REM—rapid eye movement.

Sleep Disordered Breathing

Cyclic Alternating Pattern Definition

CAP	Periodic EEG activity characterized by abrupt shifts in amplitude and/or frequency of background EEG (phase A) from the sleep EEG background activity (phase B); this signifies instability of breathing during sleep and has been associated with daytime symptoms
Phase A	
Phase A1: Phase A consisting exclusively of synchronized EEG patterns (intermittent alpha rhythm in stage 1; sequences of k-complexes or of delta bursts in the other non-REM stages) Phase A2: Phase A consisting of desynchronized EEG patterns preceded by slow high-voltage waves (*ie*, k-complex sequences with alpha and beta activities, k-alpha) Phase A3: Phase A with desynchronized EEG patterns alone (ASDA arousals; fast activities)	
Phase B	
Phase B: EEG background activities according to each sleep state	
ASDA arousal	
Abrupt EEG shift toward fast activity, such as 8–13 Hz (alpha) or > 16 Hz (beta) Duration: lasting more than 3 and less than 15 sec	
CAP sequence	
Sequences of two phasic EEG events alternating with EEG background activities; each CAP sequence: at least two CAP cycles in succession	
CAP cycle	
Each CAP cycle includes Phase A (phasic events) + Phase B (recurring periods of EEG background activities)	

Figure 6-4. The definition of cyclic alternating pattern (CAP). *See* Figure 6-23 on CAP scoring. ASDA—American Sleep Disorders Association; EEG—electroencephalogram.

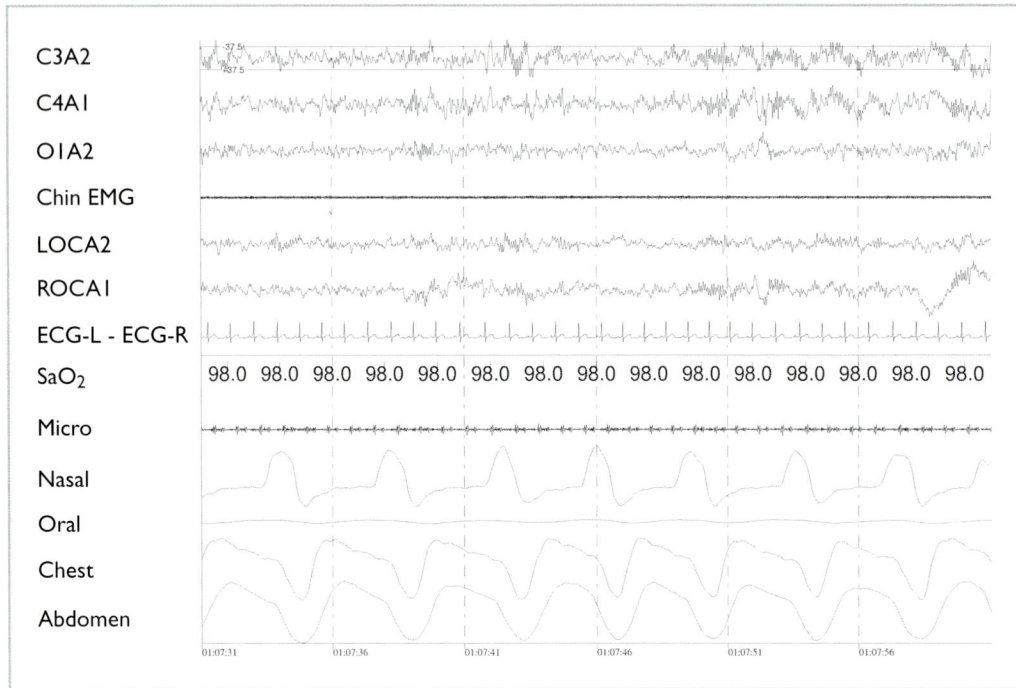

Figure 6-5. Normal airflow. This is an epoch (30 sec) from an overnight polysomnogram showing normal airflow by nasal transducer during non–rapid eye movement (REM) sleep. Recording from a nasal cannula pressure transducer is used to score breathing abnormalities. A mouth thermistor will demonstrate the presence of mouth breathing, which is abnormal during sleep. The shape of the nasal cannula pressure transducer is important because it allows for an analysis of each breath. With this equipment, a round contour waveform is seen in normal breathing. By convention, inspiration begins with an upslope of the wave contour, and expiration begins near the midpoint of the downslope of the wave contour. Investigation of the breath can also show abnormalities in inspiration and expiration timing. Respiratory rate can be calculated from a 30-second epoch in a normal adult and varies depending on the sleep stage. It peaks between 16 to 18 breaths per minute during non-REM sleep and 17 to 19 breaths per minute during REM sleep. Abdomen—abdominal respiratory effort; C4A1, C3A2—central electroencephalogram; Chest—chest respiratory effort; Chin EMG—chin electromyogram; ECG—electrocardiogram; LOCA2—left electro-oculogram; Micro—snore microphone; Nasal—nasal airflow; O1A2—occipital electroencephalogram; Oral—oral airflow; ROCA1—right electro-oculogram; SaO_2—oxygen saturation.

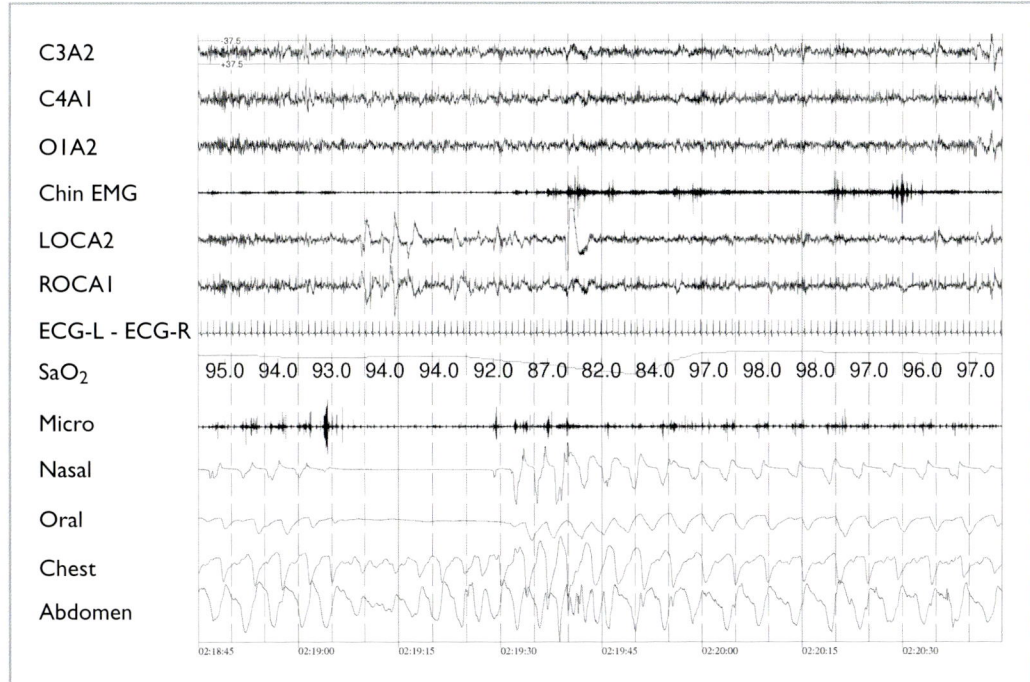

Figure 6-6. Obstructive sleep apnea during phasic rapid eye movement (REM) sleep. This is an epoch (120 sec.) from an overnight polysomnogram showing an obstructive apnea event during phasic REM sleep as indicated by rapid eye movement. Nasal and oral airflow are evidently absent but sustained chest and abdominal efforts are noticeable. The obstructive event is followed by a significant fall in oxygen saturation as measured by pulse oximetry. The event ends with an electroencephalogram arousal and a burst of electromyogram activity, and then snoring resumes. Despite the return to breathing with the return of sleep, the presence of airflow limitation is associated with snoring, as indicated by the abnormal wave contour on the nasal cannula. Abdomen—abdominal respiratory effort; C4A1, C3A2—central electroencephalogram; Chest—chest respiratory effort; Chin EMG—chin electromyogram; ECG—electrocardiogram; LOCA2—left electro-oculogram; Micro—snore microphone; Nasal—nasal airflow; O1A2—occipital electroencephalogram; Oral—oral airflow; ROCA1—right electro-oculogram; SaO$_2$—oxygen saturation.

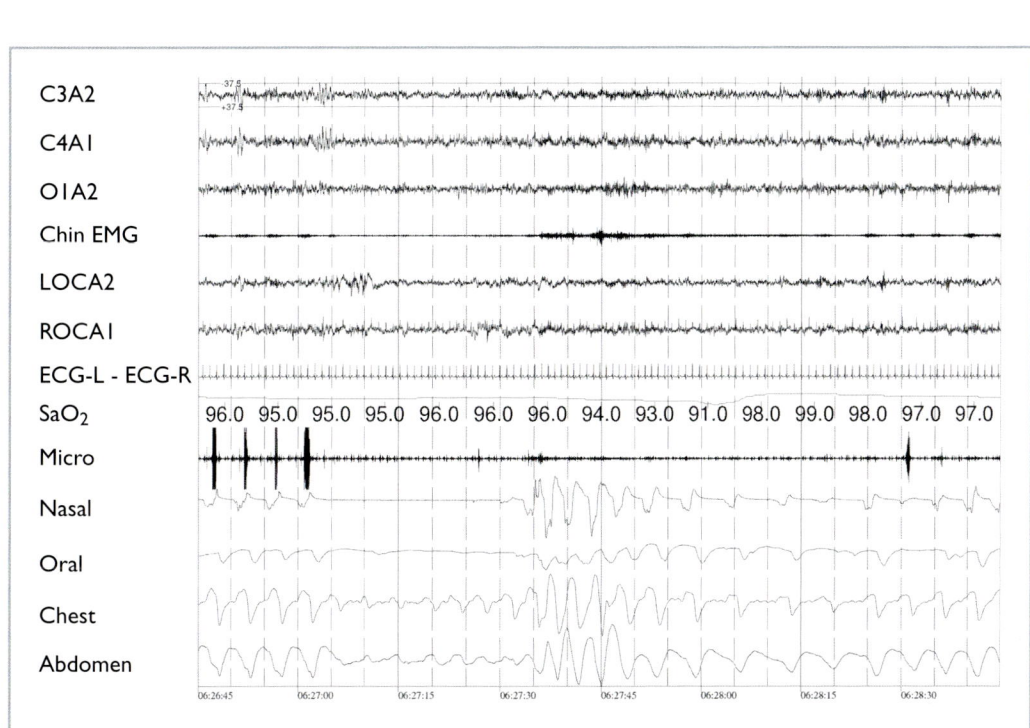

Figure 6-7. Obstructive sleep apnea during non–rapid eye movement (REM) sleep. This is an epoch (120 sec) from an overnight polysomnogram showing an obstructive apnea event during non-REM sleep. Nasal and oral airflow are absent, but sustained chest and abdominal efforts can be seen. There is a progressive increase of respiratory effort as indicated by an increase in swing of chest and abdominal signals. Snoring is terminated during the obstructive event. A 5% drop in oxygen saturation follows the obstructive event. An electroencephalogram arousal and an increase in electromyogram activity occur at the termination of the event. Abdomen—abdominal respiratory effort; C4A1, C3A2—central electroencephalogram; Chest—chest respiratory effort; Chin EMG—chin electromyogram; ECG—electrocardiogram; LOCA2—left electro-oculogram; Micro—snore microphone; Nasal—nasal airflow; O1A2—occipital electroencephalogram; Oral—oral airflow; ROCA1—right electro-oculogram; SaO$_2$—oxygen saturation.

Sleep Disordered Breathing

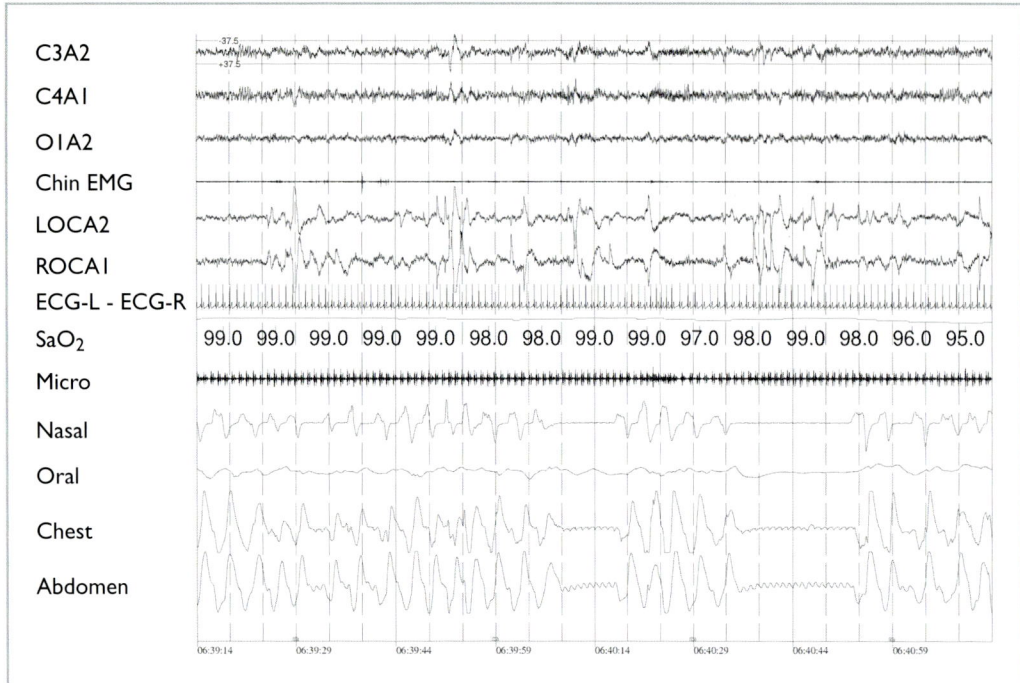

Figure 6-8. Central apneas during phasic rapid eye movement (REM) sleep. This is an epoch (120 sec) from an overnight polysomnogram showing two central apneas during phasic REM sleep. Chest and abdominal efforts are absent during the events. Electrocardiogram (ECG) artifact can be seen in chest and abdominal sensors during these events. Visualization of ECG artifact is a good indicator of a central event. There is no change in electromyogram (EMG) signal, and the absence of an increase in EMG signal during repetitive central apnea events forbid scoring the presence of any arousals. Abdomen—abdominal respiratory effort; C4A1, C3A2—central electroencephalogram; Chest—chest respiratory effort; Chin EMG—chin electromyogram; LOCA2—left electro-oculogram; Micro—snore microphone; Nasal—nasal airflow; O1A2—occipital electroencephalogram; Oral—oral airflow; ROCA1—right electro-oculogram; SaO_2—oxygen saturation.

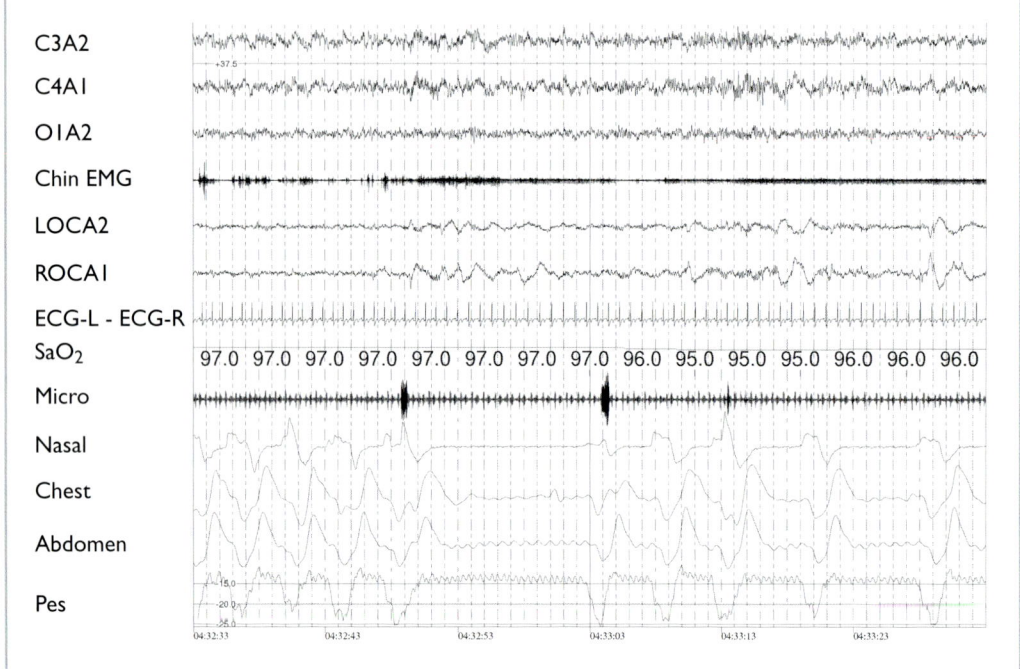

Figure 6-9. Central apnea with esophageal pressure (Pes) sensor. This epoch (120 sec) from an overnight polysomnogram shows a central apnea event during stage 1 sleep. Chest and abdomen sensors show an absence of respiratory effort, as complimented by the Pes monitor. Electrocardiogram (ECG) artifact can be seen in all three respiratory effort sensors. Pes is the best sensor for investigation of diaphragmatic (central) apnea. The ECG artifact can also be seen also on Pes recording, as in the case of this patient. Abdomen—abdominal respiratory effort; C4A1, C3A2—central electroencephalogram; Chest—chest respiratory effort; Chin EMG—chin electromyogram; LOCA2—left electro-oculogram; Micro—snore microphone; Nasal—nasal airflow; O1A2—occipital electroencephalogram; Oral—oral airflow; ROCA1—right electro-oculogram; SaO_2—oxygen saturation.

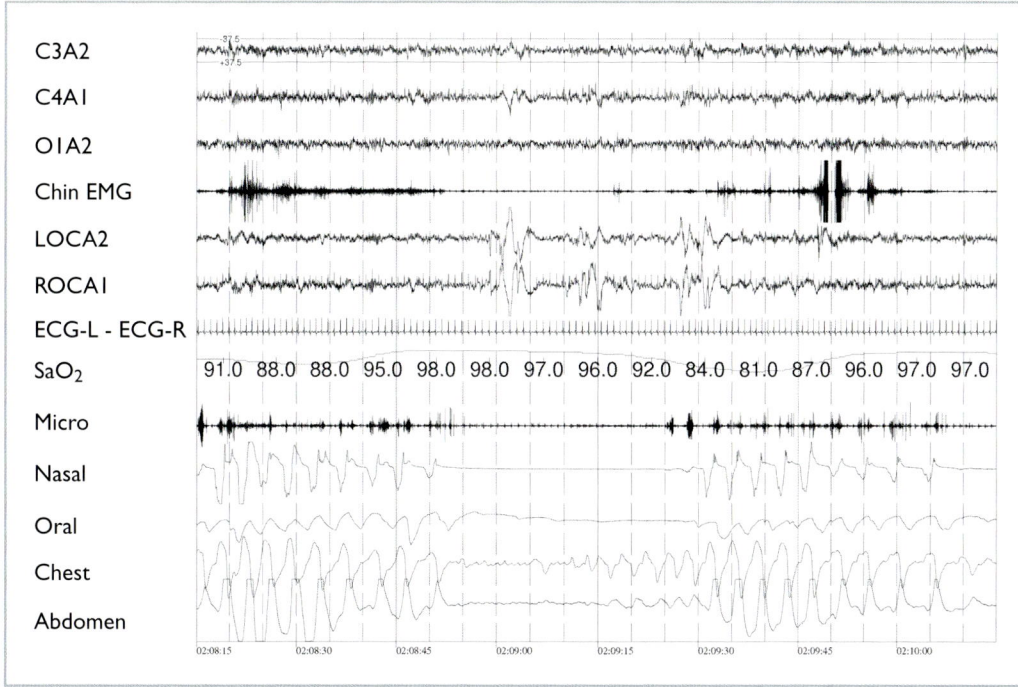

Figure 6-10. Mixed obstructive and central apnea during phasic rapid eye movement (REM) sleep. This is an epoch (120 sec.) from an overnight polysomnogram showing a mixed (obstructive and central) apnea during phasic REM sleep. The event begins with a central apnea and turns into an obstructive pattern, as can be seen by the absence of effort in chest and abdominal sensors initially, followed by the beginning of respiratory effort in both sensors. Significant oxygen desaturation is present. Snoring is terminated during the event. There is recurrence of airflow before complete opening of the airway, as indicated by small nasal pressure deflections and snoring. The arousal begins with the partial reopening of the airway as indicated by chin electroymyogram augmentation and an increased electroencephalogram frequency. Abdomen—abdominal respiratory effort; C4A1, C3A2—central electroencephalogram; Chest—chest respiratory effort; Chin EMG—chin electromyogram; ECG—electrocardiogram; LOCA2—left electro-oculogram; Micro—snore microphone; Nasal—nasal airflow; O1A2—occipital electroencephalogram; Oral—oral airflow; ROCA1—right electro-oculogram; SaO$_2$—oxygen saturation.

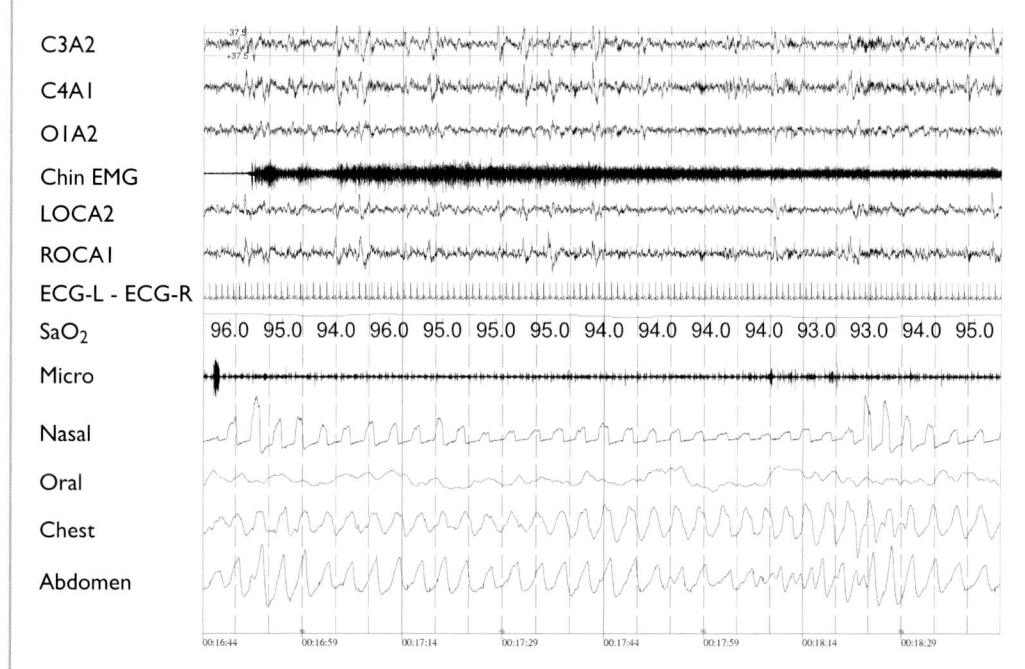

Figure 6-11. Obstructive hypopnea during non–rapid eye movement (REM) sleep. This epoch (120 sec) from an overnight polysomnogram shows a long obstructive hypopneic event during stage 2 sleep, characterized by at least a 50% reduction in airflow from baseline (baseline breaths can be seen on the left and right side of the epoch). The event begins about 20 seconds into the epoch and lasts for approximately 80 seconds. There is a change in the nasal flow contour that includes not only a reduction in amplitude but also a flattening of the wave contour during inspiration. The chest channel indicates a progressive increase in deflection that is interpreted as an indication of increased thoracoabdominal effort. The event ends with a clear change in electroencephalogram frequency indicative of a short arousal. Abdomen—abdominal respiratory effort; C4A1, C3A2—central electroencephalogram; Chest—chest respiratory effort; Chin EMG—chin electromyogram; ECG—electrocardiogram; LOCA2—left electro-oculogram; Micro—snore microphone; Nasal—nasal airflow; O1A2—occipital electroencephalogram; Oral—oral airflow; ROCA1—right electro-oculogram; SaO$_2$—oxygen saturation.

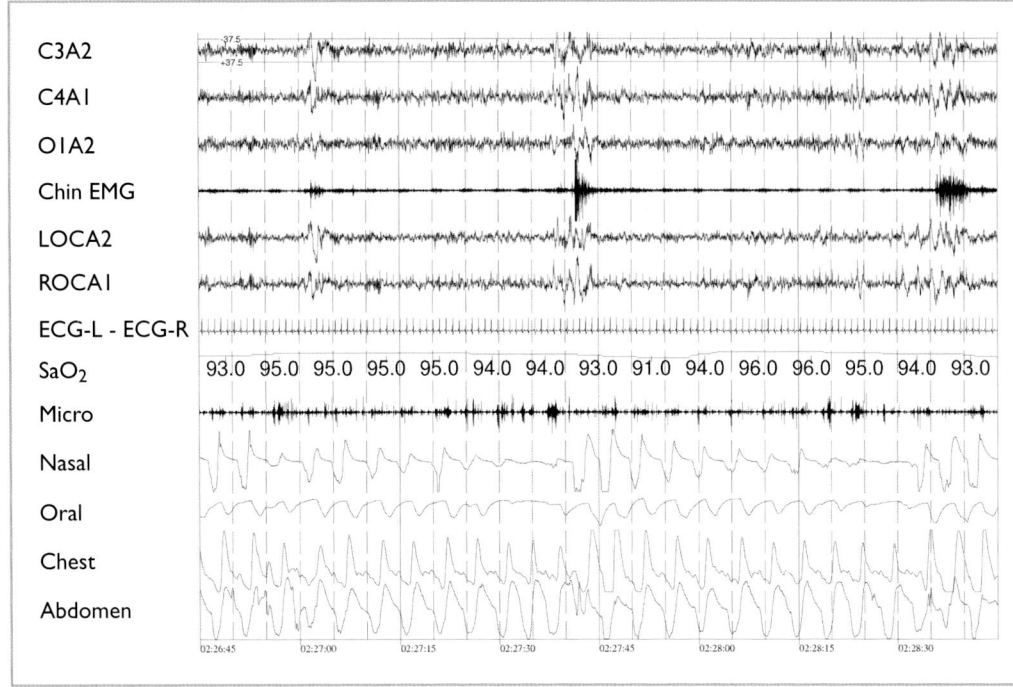

Figure 6-12. Obstructive hypopneas during non–rapid eye movement (REM) sleep. This epoch (120 sec) shows several obstructive hypopneic events during stage 2 sleep. The first event begins at 40 seconds into the epoch, and the second event begins at 80 seconds into the epoch. Both are characterized by at least 50% reduction in airflow, and both are followed by a 3% reduction in oxygen saturation. There is a progressive decrease in airflow after the arousal—particularly on the right event—which leads to a complete short obstructive apnea. Both events are terminated by an arousal seen in central and occipital leads. Abdomen—abdominal respiratory effort; C4A1, C3A2—central electroencephalogram; Chest—chest respiratory effort; Chin EMG—chin electromyogram; ECG—electrocardiogram; LOCA2—left electro-oculogram; Micro—snore microphone; Nasal—nasal airflow; O1A2—occipital electroencephalogram; Oral—oral airflow; ROCA1—right electro-oculogram; SaO_2—oxygen saturation.

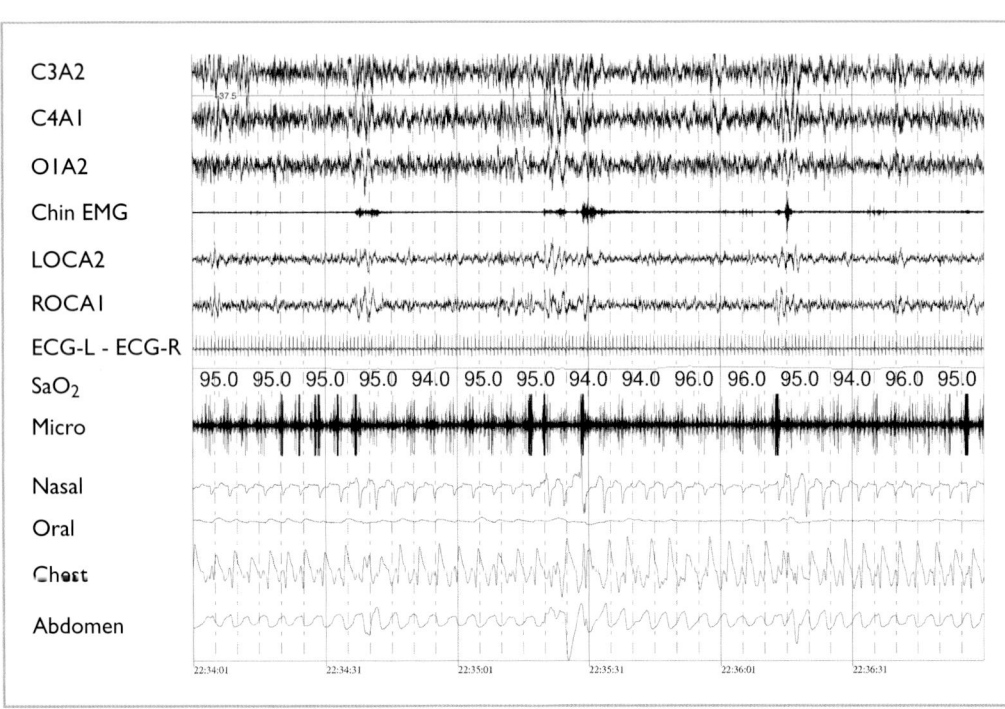

Figure 6-13. Repetitive obstructive hypopneas. This epoch (120 sec) is showing a pattern of repetitive obstructive hypopneic events as indicated by an at least 50% reduction in airflow during non–rapid eye movement (REM) sleep. The repetitive hypopneas are associated with electroencephalogram arousals, and snoring varies in intensity during each hypopneic event. Chest and abdominal efforts are sustained during the events. The EEG leads present bursts of high amplitude slow waves followed by return to background EEG. These combinations have been defined as a cyclic alternating pattern (CAP). The high-amplitude bursts have been defined as phase A of CAP and the return to background EEG as phase B. An abnormal amount of CAP is an indicator of non-REM sleep instability and even in the absence of repetitive EEG arousal has been correlated with complaints of daytime fatigue and daytime sleepiness. Abdomen—abdominal respiratory effort; C4A1, C3A2—central electroencephalogram; Chest—chest respiratory effort; Chin EMG—chin electromyogram; ECG—electrocardiogram; LOCA2—left electro-oculogram; Micro—snore microphone; Nasal—nasal airflow; O1A2—occipital electroencephalogram; Oral—oral airflow; ROCA1—right electro-oculogram; SaO_2—oxygen saturation.

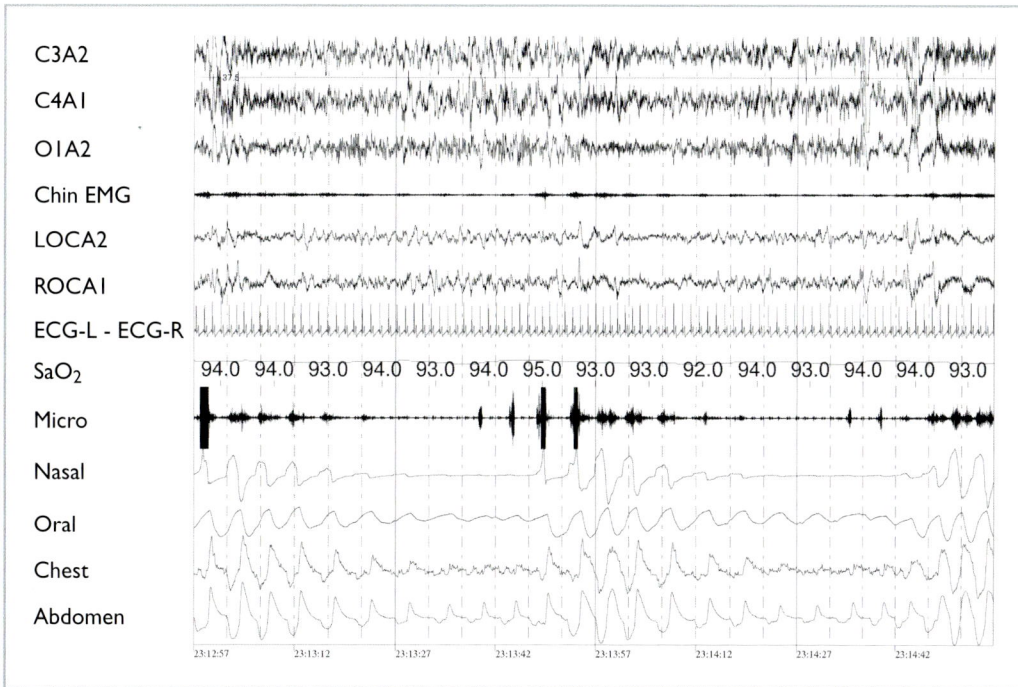

Figure 6-14. Hypopneas with decreased respiratory effort in non–rapid eye movement (REM) sleep. This epoch (120 sec) contains several hypopneic events during non-REM sleep. There is absence of airflow at the nasal cannula. Oral breathing is present. Decreased efforts are seen in chest and abdominal sensors. There is a small drop in oxygen saturation—from 95% to 92%. Arousals are seen at the end of each hypopneic event. Snoring is terminated at the beginning of the events and resumes with improvement in airflow. Abdomen—abdominal respiratory effort; C4A1, C3A2—central electroencephalogram; Chest—chest respiratory effort; Chin EMG—chin electromyogram; ECG—electrocardiogram; LOCA2—left electro-oculogram; Micro—snore microphone; Nasal—nasal airflow; O1A2—occipital electroencephalogram; Oral—oral airflow; ROCA1—right electro-oculogram; SaO_2—oxygen saturation.

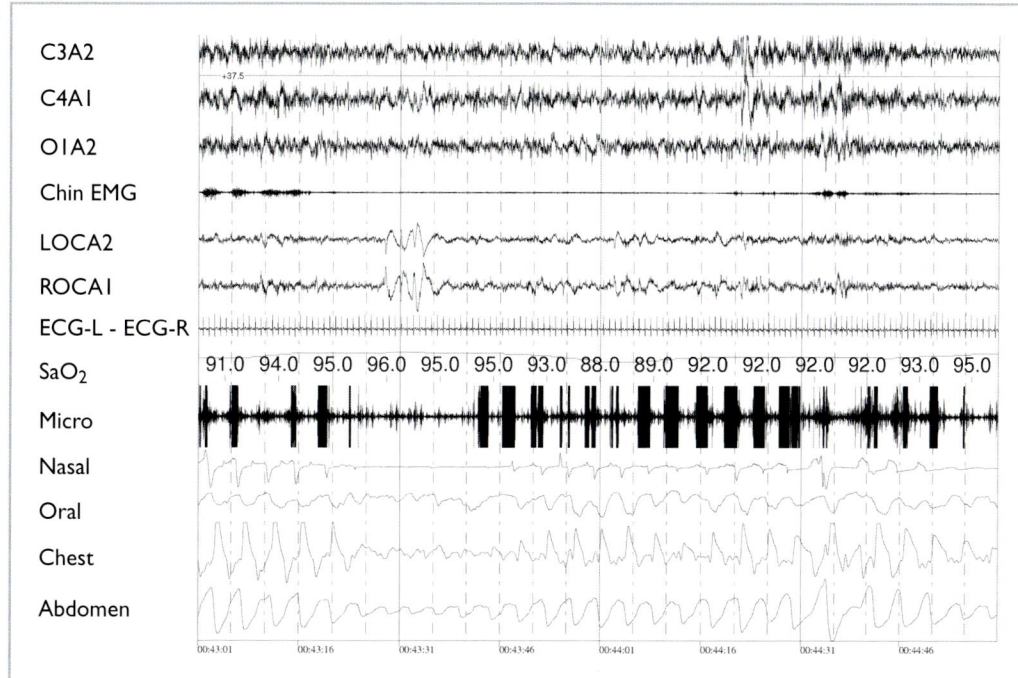

Figure 6-15. Hypopnea in association with phasic event of rapid eye movement (REM) sleep. This epoch (120 sec) contains a hypopneic event during phasic event of REM sleep as characterized by rapid eye movements. There is much more limited mouth breathing. Respiratory effort as shown by thoracic and abdominal sensors is significantly reduced. Significant oxygen desaturation is present following the event. Snoring is terminated at the start of the event and resumes with improvement in airflow. Abdomen—abdominal respiratory effort; C4A1, C3A2—central electroencephalogram; Chest—chest respiratory effort; Chin EMG—chin electromyogram; ECG—electrocardiogram; LOCA2—left electro-oculogram; Micro—snore microphone; Nasal—nasal airflow; O1A2—occipital electroencephalogram; Oral—oral airflow; ROCA1—right electro-oculogram; SaO_2—oxygen saturation.

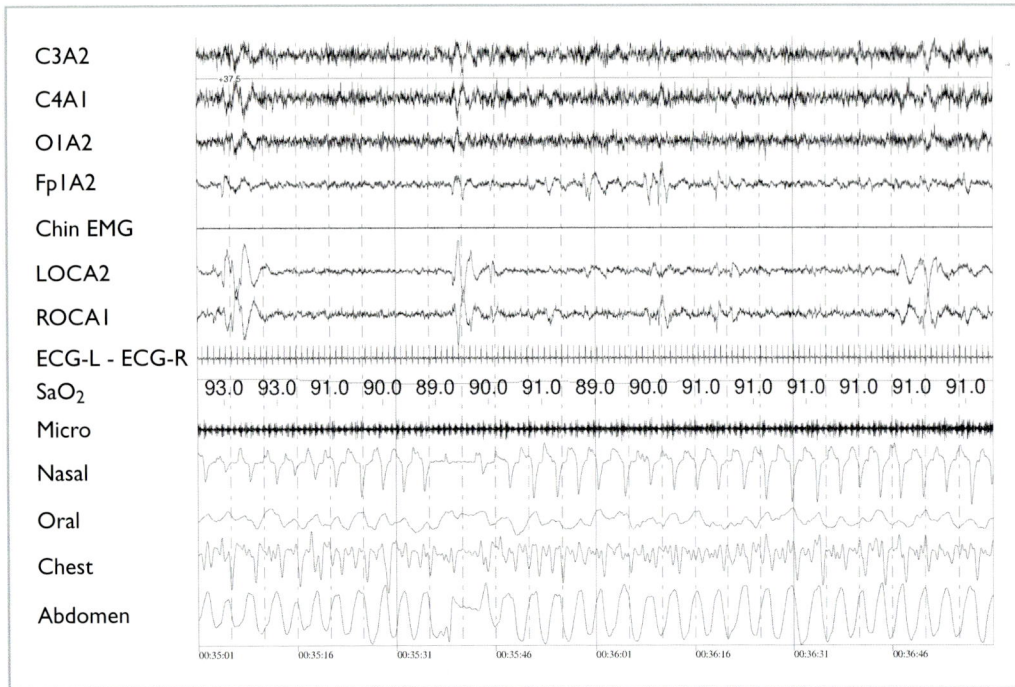

Figure 6-16. Hypoventilation during rapid eye movement (REM) sleep. This epoch (120 sec) from an overnight polysomnogram shows persistent hypoventilation as seen by persistently low oxygen saturation during a REM sleep phasic event. There is persistence of thoracic and abdominal movements and airflow at the nose. Despite respiratory movements, oxygen saturation remains low—indicative of a low tidal volume. Abdomen—abdominal respiratory effort; C4A1, C3A2—central electroencephalogram; Chest—chest respiratory effort; Chin EMG—chin electromyogram; ECG—electrocardiogram; Fp1A2—frontal electroencephalogram; LOCA2—left electro-oculogram; Micro—snore microphone; Nasal—nasal airflow; O1A2—occipital electroencephalogram; Oral—oral airflow; ROCA1—right electro-oculogram; SaO_2—oxygen saturation.

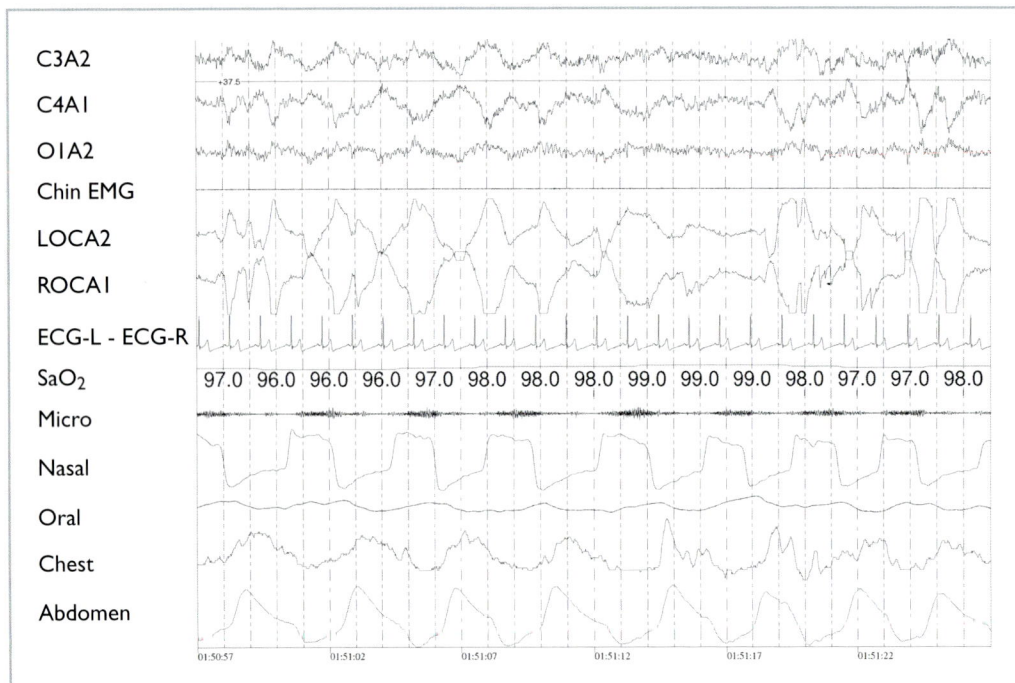

Figure 6-17. Flow limitation during rapid eye movement (REM) sleep. This epoch (60 sec) shows an example of airflow limitation during REM sleep. The nasal pressure wave contour is abnormal as characterized by a flattened wave contour. The drop in amplitude of each breath is limited and is much less than 30% of a normal breath. There is association with snoring. This pattern is significant for increased upper airway resistance causing airflow limitation. Oxygen saturation is maintained. Abdomen—abdominal respiratory effort; C4A1, C3A2—central electroencephalogram; Chest—chest respiratory effort; Chin EMG—chin electromyogram; ECG—electrocardiogram; LOCA2—left electro-oculogram; Micro—snore microphone; Nasal—nasal airflow; O1A2—occipital electroencephalogram; Oral—oral airflow; ROCA1—right electro-oculogram; SaO_2—oxygen saturation.

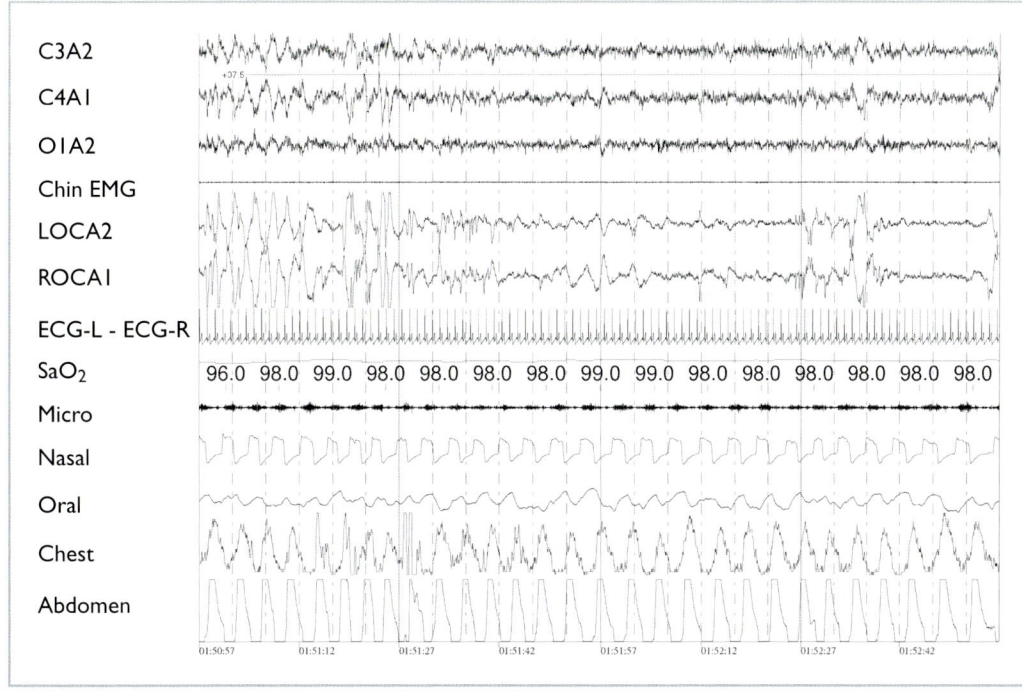

Figure 6-18. Flow limitation during rapid eye movement (REM) sleep. This epoch (120 sec) from an overnight polysomnogram shows an example of airflow limitation during REM sleep seen at 120-second intervals. The flow limitation may last for several minutes and is terminated by an electroencephalogram arousal. Note the persistently flattened wave contour from the nasal transducer tracing throughout the entire epoch. This pattern does not fit the definition of hypopnea or apnea, but it does lead to sleep fragmentation, and it is associated with daytime complaints of fatigue and sleepiness. Abdomen—abdominal respiratory effort; C4A1, C3A2—central electroencephalogram; Chest—chest respiratory effort; Chin EMG—chin electromyogram; ECG—electrocardiogram; LOCA2—left electro-oculogram; Micro—snore microphone; Nasal—nasal airflow; O1A2—occipital electroencephalogram; Oral—oral airflow; ROCA1—right electro-oculogram; SaO_2—oxygen saturation.

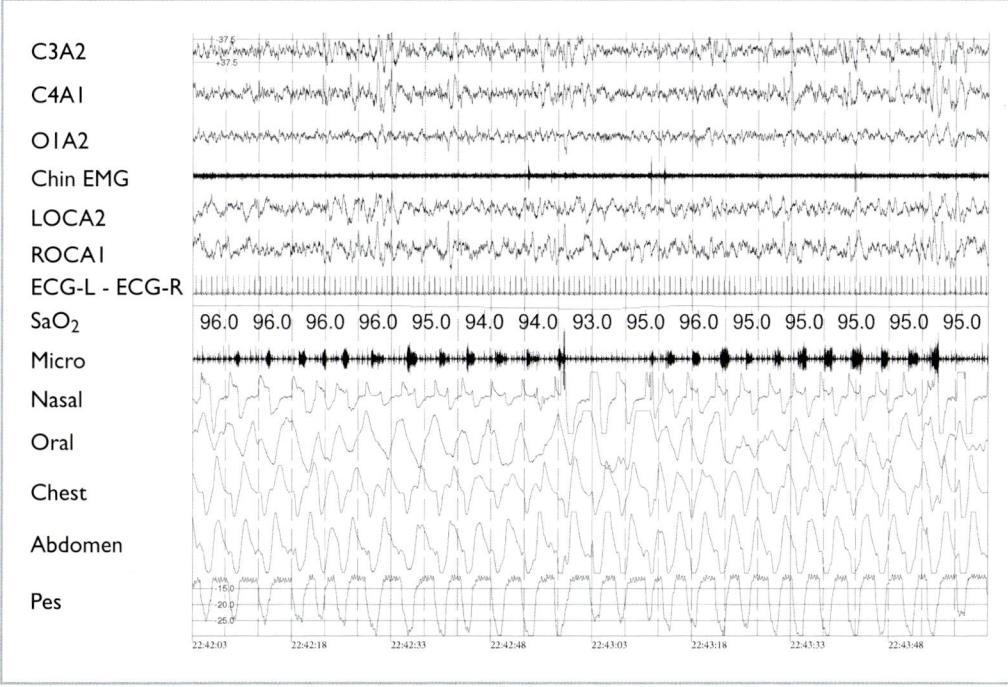

Figure 6-19. Airflow limitation with esophageal pressure (Pes) crescendo and reversal during non–rapid eye movement (REM) sleep. This epoch (120 sec) from an overnight polysomnogram shows airflow limitation complemented by a Pes monitor during non-REM sleep. The nasal cannula shows abnormal wave contour with a progressive decrease in flow and clear evidence of flow limitation. The Pes indicates variation in respiratory efforts with presence of Pes crescendo and Pes reversal. The pattern repeats itself again. Improvement in nasal airflow is seen during Pes reversal. Snoring is associated with the event, but there is no oxygen desaturation. Cyclic alternating pattern (CAP) is seen on electroencephalogram with bursts of slow wave and return to background EEG, a pattern that indicates instability of non-REM sleep and which is associated with daytime complaints of sleepiness and fatigue. Abdomen—abdominal respiratory effort; C4A1, C3A2—central electroencephalogram; Chest—chest respiratory effort; Chin EMG—chin electromyogram; ECG—electrocardiogram; LOCA2—left electro-oculogram; Micro—snore microphone; Nasal—nasal airflow; O1A2—occipital electroencephalogram; Oral—oral airflow; ROCA1—right electro-oculogram; SaO_2—oxygen saturation.

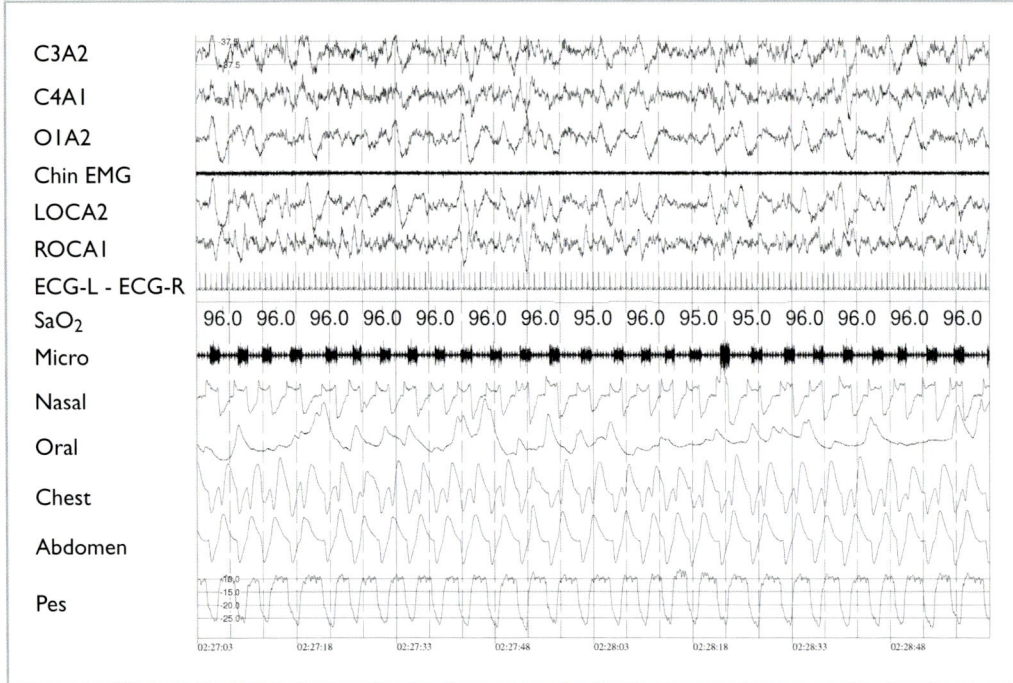

Figure 6-20. Persistent respiratory effort by esophageal pressure (Pes). This epoch (120 sec) shows continuous snoring, an abnormal nasal cannula wave pattern, and an abnormal continuous increase in respiratory effort demonstrated by Pes monitor recording. The nasal cannula shows absence of normal contour with flattening during each inspiratory breath. There is an increase in inspiratory effort indicated by Pes monitoring (Pes deflection is normally a maximum of 7 cm H_2O during nonobstructive and nonsnoring breathing in non–rapid eye movement sleep in this patient). In this epoch, Pes deflection is significantly increased (20 cm H_2O). This abnormal pattern is sustained for several minutes and terminates with an EEG arousal. This patient has no apnea or hypopneas but complains of excessive daytime sleepiness, and the patient's bed partner reports chronic continuous snoring during sleep. Abdomen—abdominal respiratory effort; C4A1, C3A2—central electroencephalogram; Chest—chest respiratory effort; Chin EMG—chin electromyogram; ECG—electrocardiogram; LOCA2—left electro-oculogram; Micro—snore microphone; Nasal—nasal airflow; O1A2—occipital electroencephalogram; Oral—oral airflow; ROCA1—right electro-oculogram; SaO_2—oxygen saturation.

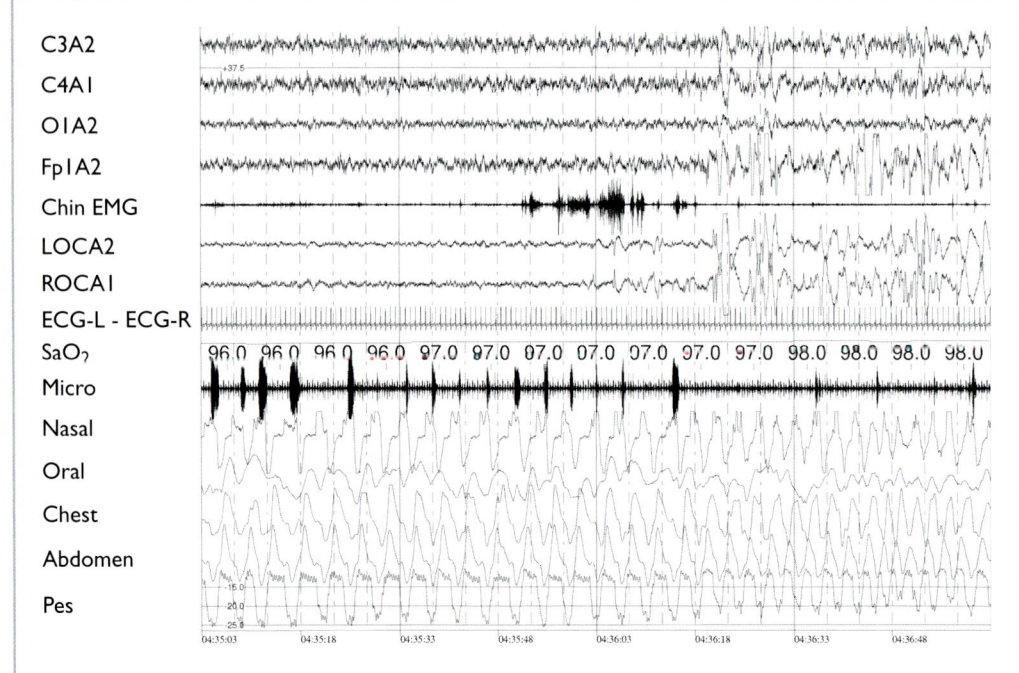

Figure 6-21. Tonic and phasic rapid eye movement (REM) sleep and abnormal respiration. The left part of this epoch shows tonic REM sleep without rapid eye movement, and the right part shows phasic REM sleep with bursts of rapid eye movement. The patient presents with snoring. The nasal cannula wave contour is abnormal because of its shape, but the drop in nasal flow is not present. Mouth breathing is present. Respiratory effort is also present, as shown by esophageal pressure (Pes) monitoring. The respiratory rate is slower during tonic REM sleep and increases during the REM sleep phasic event. There is no drop in oxygen saturation. This pattern ends with an electroencephalogram rousal associated with a decrease in respiratory effort. This patient complains of sleep maintenance insomnia with nocturnal sleep awakenings and "too much dreaming." Abdomen—abdominal respiratory effort; C4A1, C3A2—central electroencephalogram; Chest—chest respiratory effort; Chin EMG—chin electromyogram; ECG—electrocardiogram; Fp1A2—frontal electroencephalogram; LOCA2—left electro-oculogram; Micro—snore microphone; Nasal—nasal airflow; O1A2—occipital electroencephalogram; Oral—oral airflow; ROCA1—right electro-oculogram; SaO_2—oxygen saturation.

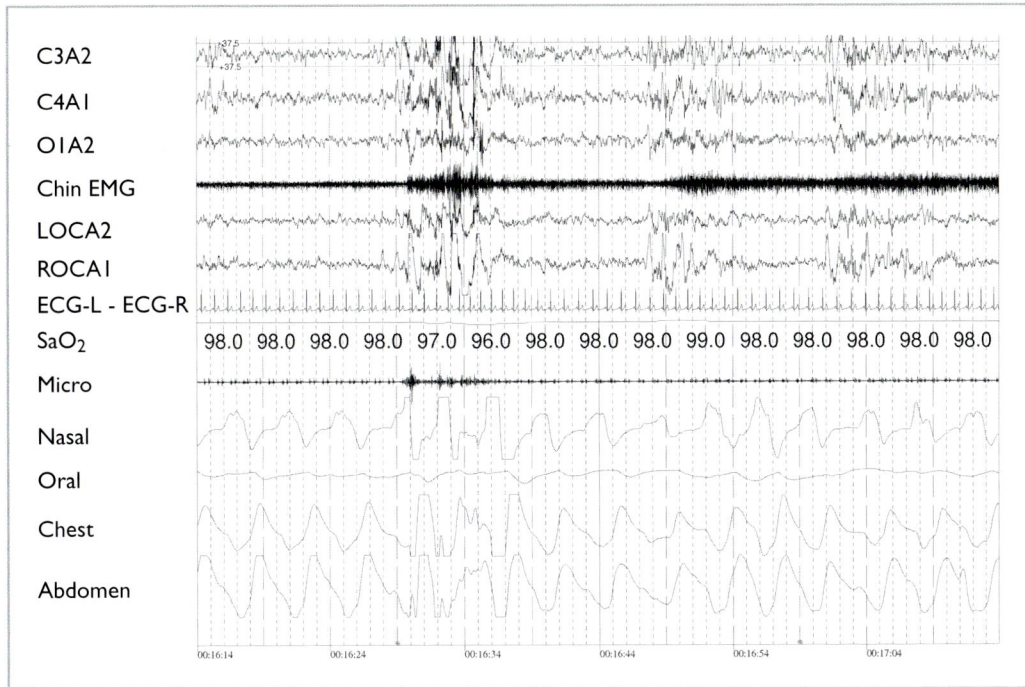

Figure 6-22. Hypopnea during non–rapid eye movement (REM) sleep. This patient presents with three short hypopneic events. During the second hypopnea, there is a lengthening of inspiration with a clear change in the wave contour of the nasal cannula. This important lengthening translates to an increase in inspiratory effort, leading to an electroencephalogram change and an electromyogram burst. The EEG arousal associated with this second hypopnea does not respond to the short EEG arousal as defined by the American Sleep Disorders Association, but the pattern responds to a cyclic alternating pattern definition (phase A2 followed by phase B). This pattern indicates instability of non-REM sleep associated with daytime clinical complaints. Abdomen—abdominal respiratory effort; C4A1, C3A2—central electroencephalogram; Chest—chest respiratory effort; Chin EMG—chin electromyogram; ECG—electrocardiogram; LOCA2—left electro-oculogram; Micro—snore microphone; Nasal—nasal airflow; O1A2—occipital electroencephalogram; Oral—oral airflow; ROCA1—right electro-oculogram; SaO_2—oxygen saturation.

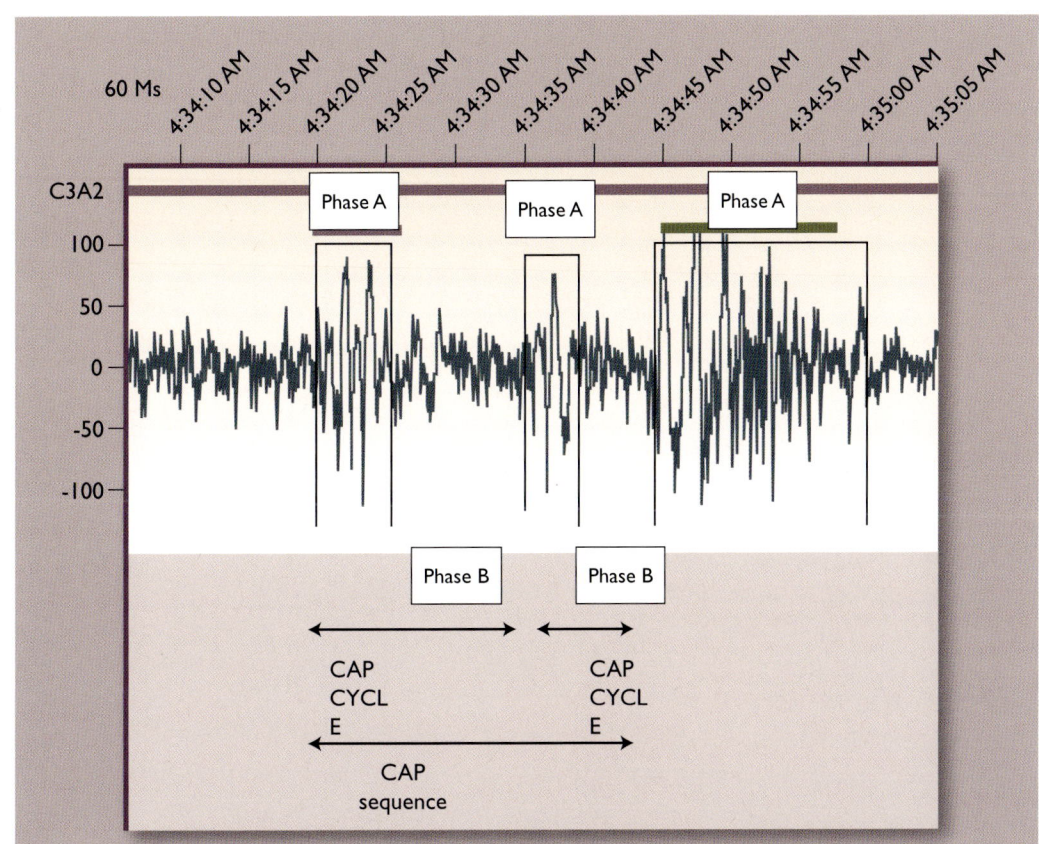

Figure 6-23. Cycling alternating pattern (CAP) scoring.

| Sleep Disordered Breathing |

RECOMMENDED READING

Aittokallio T, Saaresranta T, Polo-Kantola P, et al.: Analysis of inspiratory flow shapes in patients with partial upper-airway obstruction during sleep. *Chest* 2001, 119:37–44.

Bao G, Guilleminault C: Upper airway resistance syndrome—one decade later. *Curr Opin Pulm Med* 2004, 10:461–467.

EEG arousals: scoring rules and examples: a preliminary report from the Sleep Disorders Atlas Task Force of the American Sleep Disorders Association. *Sleep* 1992, 15:173–184.

Guilleminault C, Poyares D, Palombini L, et al.: Variability of respiratory effort in relation to sleep stages in normal controls and upper airway resistance syndrome patients. *Sleep Med* 2001, 2:397–405.

Hosselet JJ, Norman RG, Ayappa I, Rapoport DM: Detection of flow limitation with a nasal cannula/pressure transducer system. *Am J Respir Crit Care Med* 1998, 157:1461–1467.

Montserrat JM, Farre R, Ballester E, et al.: Evaluation of nasal prongs for estimating nasal flow. *Am J Respir Crit Care Med* 1997, 155:211–215.

Norman RG, Ahmed MM, Walsleben JA, Rapoport DM: Detection of respiratory events during NPSG: nasal cannula/pressure sensor versus thermistor. *Sleep* 1997, 20:1175–1184.

Sleep-related breathing disorders in adults: recommendations for syndrome definition and measurement techniques in clinical research. The Report of an American Academy of Sleep Medicine Task Force. *Sleep* 1999, 22:667–689.

Terzano MG, Parrino L, Boselli M, et al.: Polysomnographic analysis of arousal responses in obstructive sleep apnea syndrome by means of the cyclic alternating pattern. *J Clin Neurophysiol* 1996, 13:145–155.

Terzano MG, Parrino L, Smerieri A, et al.: Atlas, rules, and recording techniques for the scoring of cyclic alternating pattern (CAP) in human sleep. *Sleep Med* 2002, 3:187–199.

LOWER RESPIRATORY TRACT INFECTIONS: ACUTE EXACERBATION OF CHRONIC BRONCHITIS

Antonio Anzueto and G. Douglas Campbell Jr

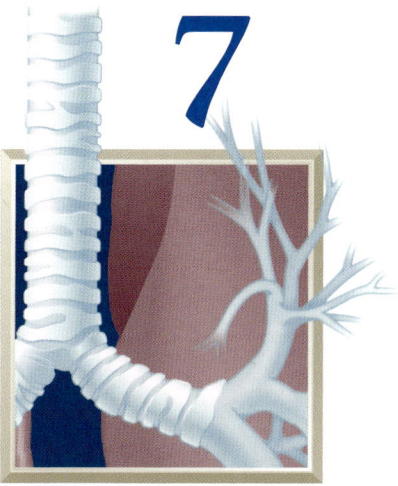

Chronic obstructive pulmonary disease (COPD) affects a large number of patients and is associated with significant morbidity, disability, and mortality [1,2]. COPD is complicated by frequent and recurrent acute exacerbations, which are associated with enormous health care expenditures and high morbidity. An exacerbation of COPD is defined as an event in the natural course of the disease characterized by a change in the patient's baseline dyspnea, cough, and/or sputum, beyond normal day-to-day variations, that is acute in onset and may warrant a change in regular medication [3,4]. Exacerbations are categorized in terms of either clinical presentation (number of symptoms) or health care resource utilization [3,4].

Exacerbations of COPD result in over 110,000 deaths and over 500,000 hospitalizations per year, with over $18 billion spent in direct costs annually [1,2,4,5]. In addition to the financial burden required to care for patients with COPD, other costs such as days missed from work and severe limitations in quality of life (QOL) are important features of this condition [6,7].

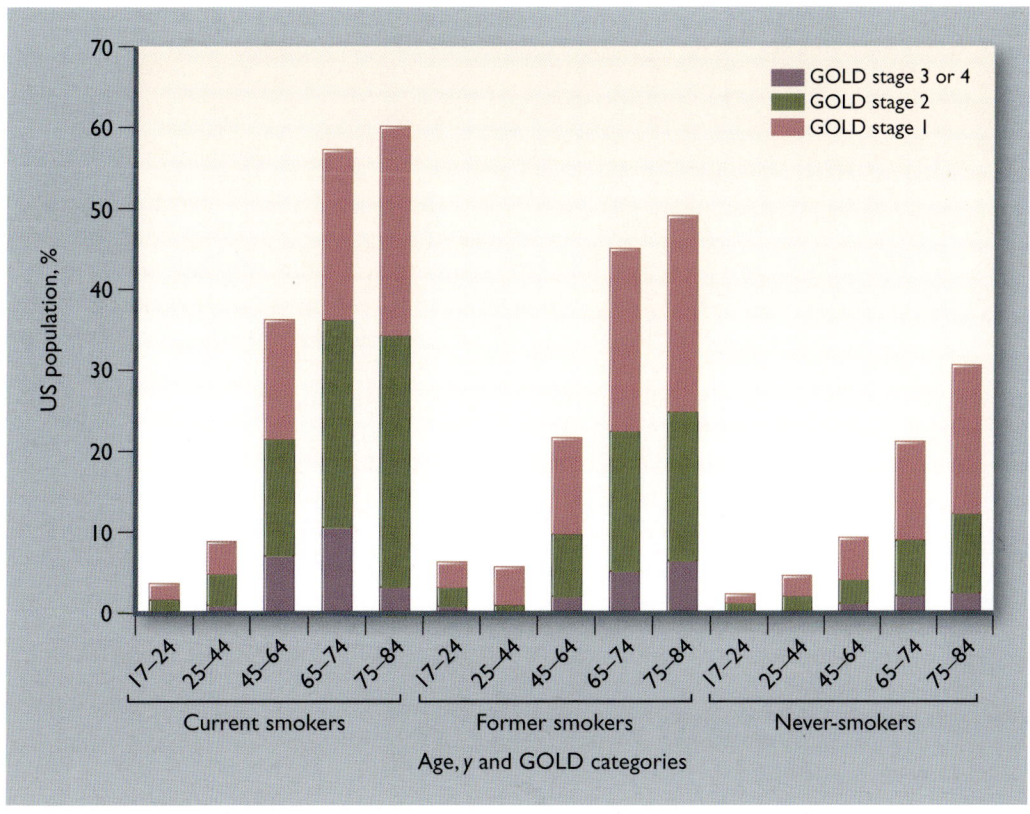

Figure 7-1. Prevalence of chronic obstructive pulmonary disease is influenced predominantly by smoking and age. This figure shows age-specific Global Initiative for Chronic Obstructive Lung Disease (GOLD) categories of chronic obstructive pulmonary disease (COPD) stratified by smoking status. The data shows that a high proportion of people aged 65 years or older have evidence of COPD [8]. Analysis of participants in the National Health and Nutrition Examination Survey demonstrated that current and former smokers with GOLD stage 3 or 4 COPD had a significantly increased mortality risk compared with participants without lung disease. However, never-smokers with GOLD stage 3 or 4 did not have an increased mortality risk [9].

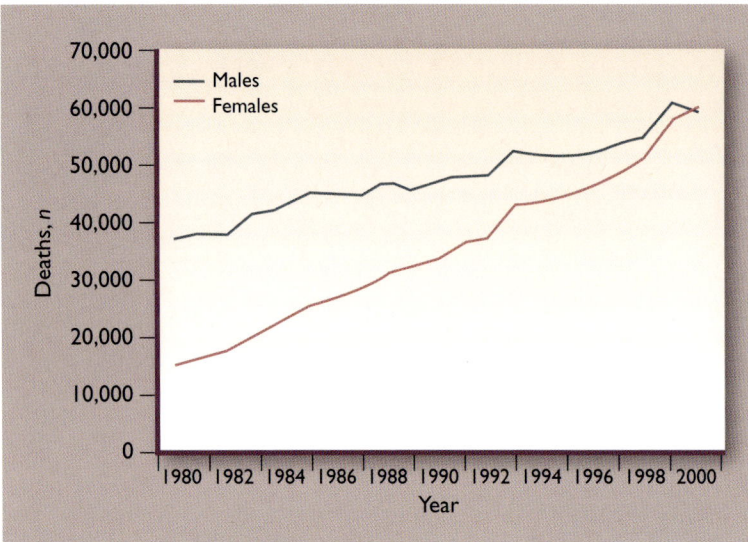

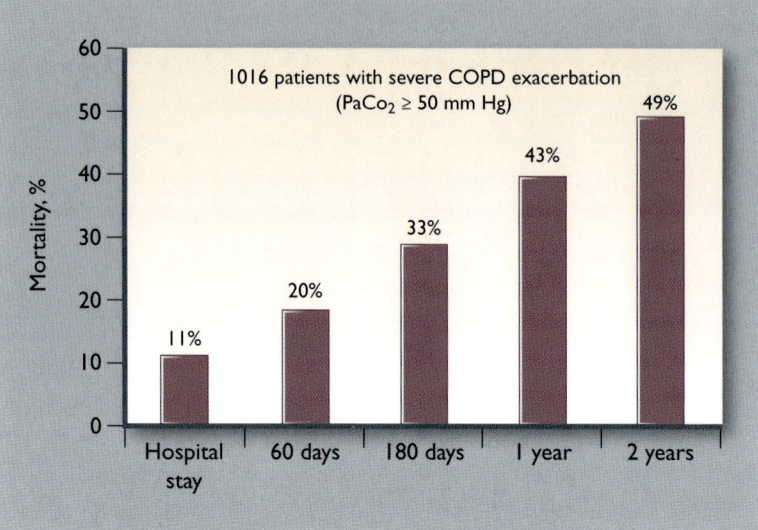

Figure 7-2. Recently reported data from the Centers for Disease Control on chronic obstructive pulmonary disease (COPD) mortality in the United States from 1980 to 2000 [2]. This information was obtained from the National Vital Statistics System. During 2000, an estimated 10 million U.S. adults reported physician-diagnosed COPD. From 1980 to 2000, the overall death rate from COPD increased 67%. The most significant change during the period analyzed was the increase in the COPD death rate for women, from 20.1 in 100,000 in 1980 to 82.6 in 100,000 in 2000. In 2000, for the first time, the number of women who died from COPD surpassed the number of men who died from the disease (59,936 vs 59,118). The COPD death rate among men increased 13%; however, death rates among men have remained steady since 1985. Other changes include an increase in the death rate of more than 87% in African Americans (*Adapted from* Mannino *et al.* [2].)

Figure 7-3. Clinical studies have reported a high mortality rate in patients admitted to the hospital with an acute exacerbation of chronic obstructive pulmonary disease (COPD) [10–14]. The Study to Understand Prognosis and Preferences for Outcomes and Rates of Treatment [10], which enrolled patients with severe acute exacerbations of COPD, reported an in-hospital mortality rate of 11% in patients with acute hypercapnic respiratory failure. The 180-day mortality rate was 33%, and the 2-year mortality rate was 49%. Significant predictors of mortality include acute physiology and chronic health evaluation score, body mass index, age, functional status 2 weeks prior to admission, ratio of partial pressure (tension) of oxygen to fraction of inspired oxygen (PO_2 to FiO_2), occurrence of congestive heart failure, serum albumen level, cor-pulmonale, activities of daily living score, and scores on the Duke Activity Status Index. The study also reported that only 25% of patients were alive and able to report a good, very good, or excellent quality of life 6 months after discharge [10]. The reported in-hospital mortality rate varies between 11% and 24 % [10] and 22% and 35.6% after 1 and 2 years, respectively [11–13].

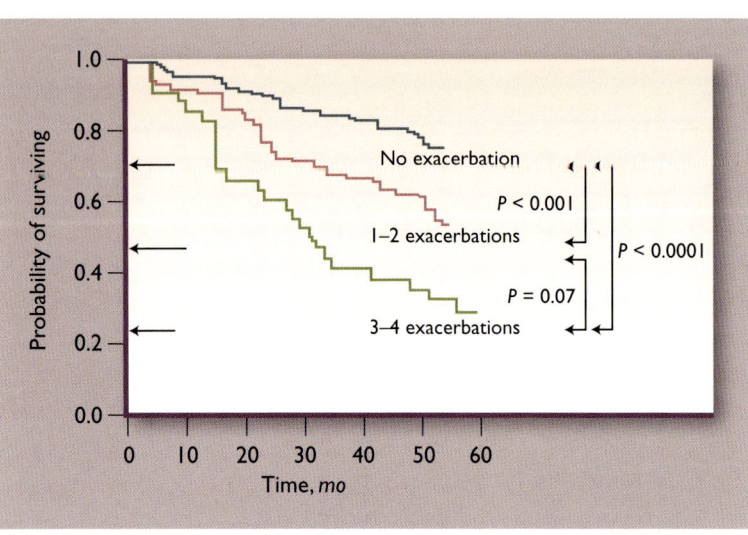

Figure 7-4. Survival probability of patients with chronic obstructive pulmonary disease (COPD). No studies have specifically examined the prognostic influence of acute exacerbation by itself. Soler-Cataluna *et al.* [14] were the first to report that severe exacerbations of COPD have an independent negative prognostic impact, with mortality increasing with the frequency of severe exacerbations and with the need for hospitalization. Patients with frequent exacerbations had the highest mortality rate ($P < 0.001$) with a risk of death 4.3 times greater (95% confidence interval [CI] 2.62 to 7.02) than that of patients requiring no hospital management.

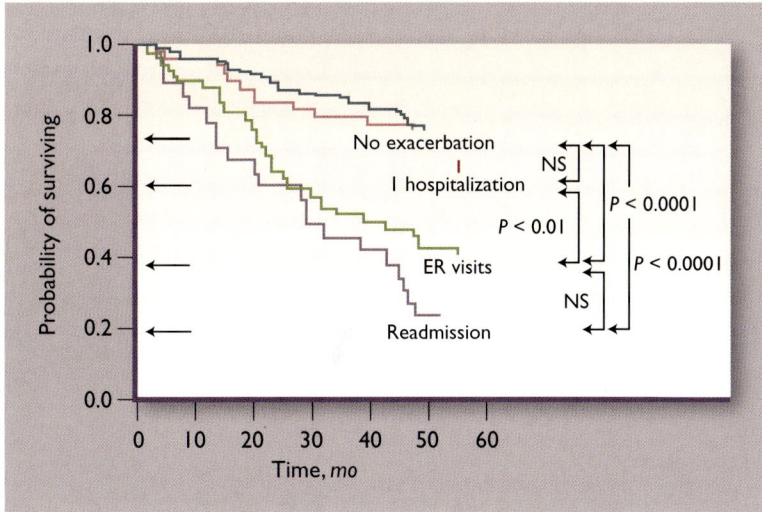

Figure 7-5. Survival probability and health care utilization in patients with chronic obstructive pulmonary disease (COPD). Soler-Cataluna et al. [14] were also able to demonstrate the relationship between health care utilization due to COPD exacerbation, emergency room (ER) utilization, and hospitalization with poor outcomes. Therefore, exacerbations themselves are a significant factor associated with increased mortality from COPD.

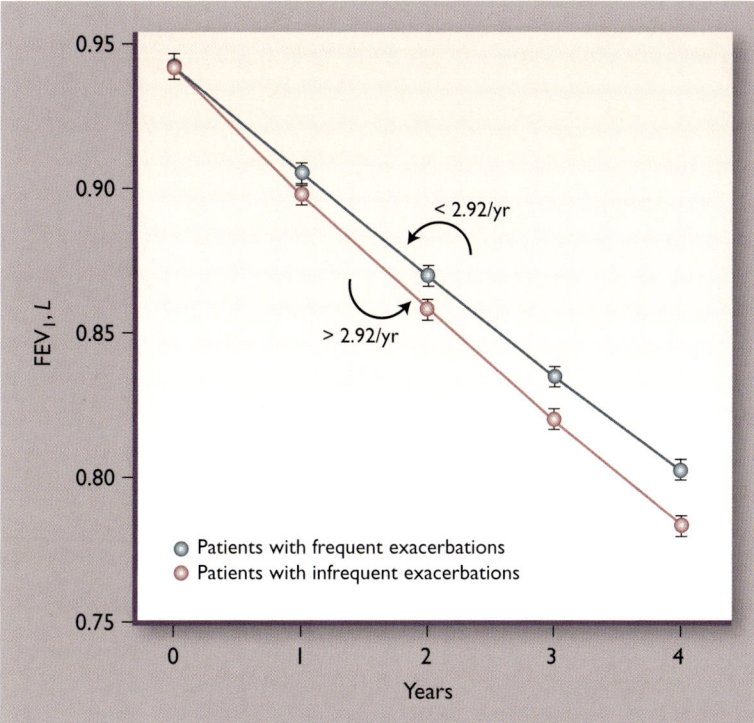

Figure 7-6. Chronic obstructive pulmonary disease (COPD) is characterized by both an accelerated decline in lung function and by periods of acute exacerbation. Donaldson et al. [15] studied the potential relationship between these factors by considering a large cohort of 109 COPD patients (81 men, median [IQR] age 68 [63–74] years; forced expiratory volume in 1 second [FEV_1] 1.00 [0.7–1.3 L], forced vital capacity 2.51 [1.9–3.0 L]). Exacerbations were identified based on symptoms, and the effect of frequent (> 2.92 per year) or infrequent (< 2.92 per year) exacerbations on lung function was examined using cross-sectional, random effect models. The 109 patients experienced 757 exacerbations. Patients with frequent exacerbations had a significantly faster decline in FEV_1 (-40.1 mL/year [n = 16]) and in peak expiratory flow [PEF] (-2.9 L/min/year [n = 46]) than those with infrequent exacerbations, in whom FEV_1 changed by -32.1 mL/year (n = 16) and PEF by -0.7 L/min/year (n = 63). Those with frequent exacerbations also had a greater decline in FEV_1 when allowance was made for smoking status. This figure shows the percentage change in FEV_1 with standard errors over 4 years. The FEV_1 decline in those with frequent exacerbations was 4.22% per year, which is greater than the 3.59% decline in those with infrequent exacerbations. Similar results were found if the patients were stratified by annual rate of reported exacerbations into two groups: those with fewer than 1.5 exacerbations per year and those with more than 1.5 per year. Donaldson et al.'s [15] study thus shows that exacerbation frequency is an important determinant of decline in lung function in patients with COPD. Strategies for prevention of COPD exacerbations may have an important impact on the natural course of this disease and on the morbidity and mortality rates of patients.

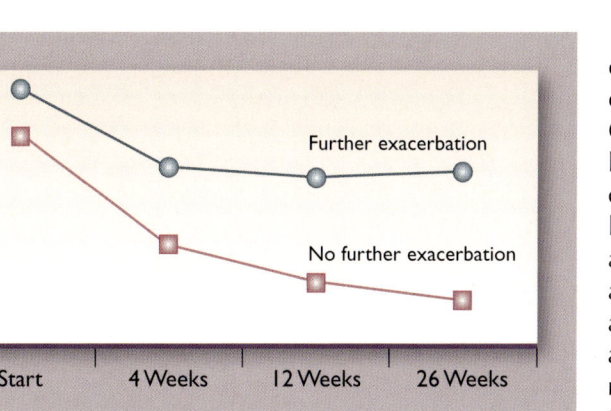

Figure 7-7. Chronic obstructive pulmonary disease (COPD) exacerbations have been shown to dramatically impact patients' feelings of wellbeing. Differences between scores on heath-related quality of life (HRQL) questionnaires completed during the stable phase of COPD and during exacerbations are great in magnitude. Connors et al. [10] reported on quality-of-life outcomes for patients hospitalized with acute exacerbations of COPD. At 6 months, 54% of patients required assistance with at least one activity of daily living, and 49% considered their health status to be fair or poor. No analysis was conducted on the relationship between readmissions and perceived quality of life. The recovery of HRQL parameters after an acute COPD exacerbation may be affected by several factors. In a study by Spencer et al. [16] patients with exacerbations who did not relapse during follow-up showed significant improvement on the St. George's Respiratory Questionnaire (SGRQ), when compared with patients with additional exacerbations. Seemungal et al. [17] showed that only 75% of patients return to their baseline peak flow values 35 days after the episode.

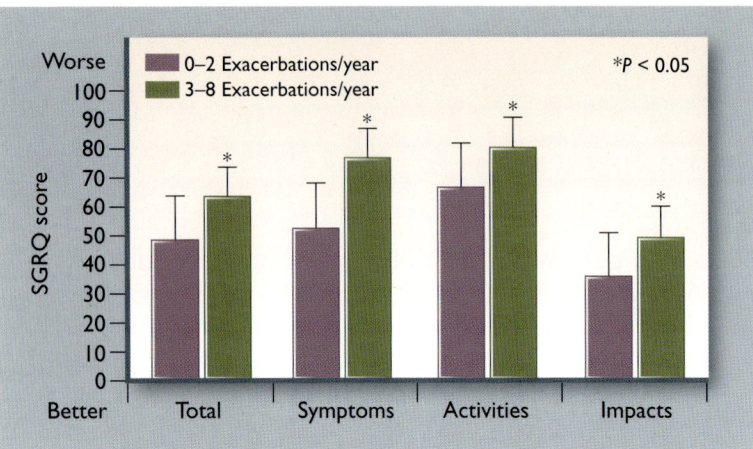

Figure 7-8. Results of St. George's Respiratory Questionnaires (SGRQs). SGRQs were completed by patients at the end of the study [16]. Exacerbations were more frequent in patients with frequent previous exacerbations (odds ratio = 5.5, $P = 0.001$). Using the median number of exacerbations, patients were classified as infrequent exacerbators (0–2) or frequent exacerbators (3–8). SGRQ total score was significantly worse in frequent exacerbators (mean difference 14.8, $P < 0.001$).

Signs and Symptoms of Acute Exacerbation of Chronic Bronchitis

	Patients, %	
Symptoms	Anthonisen et al. [18] (n = 173)	Ball et al. [20] (n = 471)
Increased dyspnea	90	45
Increased sputum production	69	77
Purulent sputum	60	66
Increased cough	82	Not Reported
Fever	29	12
Average number of exacerbations	2.56/y	3/y

Figure 7-9. The clinical presentation of acute exacerbation of chronic bronchitis is variable. Anthonisen et al. [18] classified the severity of exacerbation based on three major signs: increase in dyspnea, increase in sputum production, and presence of purulent sputum. Three levels of exacerbation were recognized. Type I is the most severe and involves worsening dyspnea with increased sputum volume and purulence. Type II is less severe and involves any two of the three previously mentioned symptoms. Type III is the least severe and involves only one of the symptoms associated with fever or upper respiratory tract infections. There is a wide variability in the presence of these symptoms in clinical trials. In a publication by Stockley et al. [19], the presence of purulent sputum is said to suggest an infectious process and is associated with positive Gram stain, positive culture, and many microorganisms isolated in the culture of sputum samples. (Adapted from Anthonisen et al. [18] and Ball et al. [20,21].)

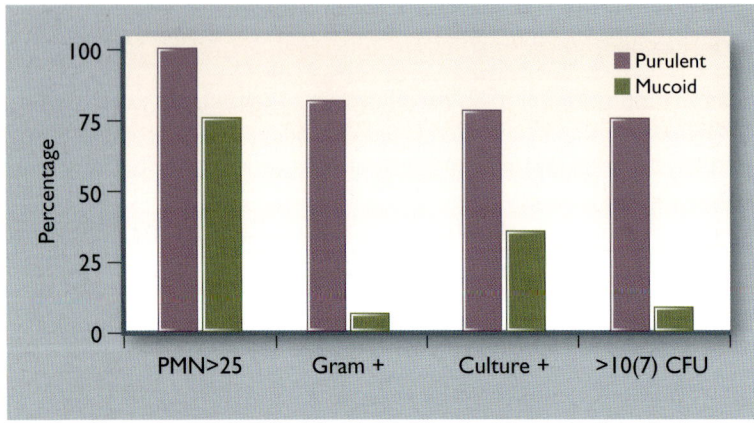

Figure 7-10. Sputum in acute exacerbation of chronic obstructive pulmonary disease (AECOPD). The relationship between sputum color and isolation of bacteria remains controversial in AECOPD. Stockley et al. [19] conducted a longitudinal study of patients presenting with AECOPD on the basis of sputum color and related this to the isolation and number of viable bacteria recovered by culture. Sputum samples from 121 patients with AECOPD were assessed on the day of presentation (89 of the patients produced a satisfactory sputum sample for analysis). Two months later, when they had returned to a stable clinical state, 109 patients were assessed. The expectoration of green, purulent sputum was taken as the primary indication of a need for antibiotic therapy, and white or clear sputum was considered irrepresentative of a bacterial episode and therefore not an indication of a need for antibiotic therapy. The bacterial culture of the sputum was positive in 84% of patients with purulent sputum on presentation, compared to only 38% of patients with mucoid sputum ($P < 0.0001$). When restudied in the stable clinical state, the incidence of a positive bacterial culture was similar for both groups (38% and 41%, respectively). In the stable clinical state, sputum color improved significantly in the group presenting with purulent sputum, from a median color number of 4.0 (interquartile range [IQR], 4.0–5.0) to 3.0 (IQR, 2.0–4.0; $P < 0.0001$). The figure shows the number of samples with more than 25 polymorphonuclear neutrophils (PMN), positive Gram stain and culture, and more than 10^7 pathogens isolated. The investigators showed that the presence of green (purulent) sputum was 94.4% sensitive and 77.0% specific for the yield of a high bacterial load, and identified a subset of patients who would likely benefit most from antibiotic therapy. All patients who produced white (mucoid) sputum during the acute exacerbation improved without antibiotic therapy, and sputum characteristics remained the same, even when the patients had returned to a stable clinical state. CFU—colony-forming units. (Adapted from Stockley et al. [19].)

Causes of Chronic Obstructive Pulmonary Disease Exacerbations			
Bacteria	**Viruses**	**Atypical organisms**	**Pollutants**
Haemophilus influenzae	Rhinovirus (common cold)	Mycoplasma pneumoniae	Nitrogen dioxide
Streptococcus pneumoniae	Influenza	Chlamydia pneumoniae	Particulates (PM$_{10}$)
Moraxella catarrhalis	Parainfluenza		Sulphur dioxide
Staphylococcus aureus	Coronavirus		Ozone
Psuedomonas aeruginosa	Adenovirus		
	Respiratory syncytial virus		
	Picornavirus		
	Metapneumovirus		

Figure 7-11. Causes of chronic obstructive pulmonary disease exacerbations. Although respiratory infections are frequent causes of exacerbations, other conditions exist, such as seasonal allergies, or exposure to toxic products or air pollutants [22–25]. During bacterial infection in acute exacerbation of chronic obstructive pulmonary disease, a variety of micro-organisms have been shown to be associated with these exacerbations, including *Haemophilus influenzae*, *Haemophilus parainfluenzae*, *Moraxella catarrhalis*, and *Streptococcus pneumoniae*. Several investigators report that a minority of patients may have atypical pathogens such as *Mycoplasma pneumoniae* and *Chlamydia pneumoniae*, but because of limitations in diagnosis, the true prevalence of these organisms is not known. Clinical studies have demonstrated that the patients with the most severe obstructive lung disease have a significantly higher prevalence of Gram-negative organisms such as *Enterobacteriaceae* and *Pseudomonas* species.

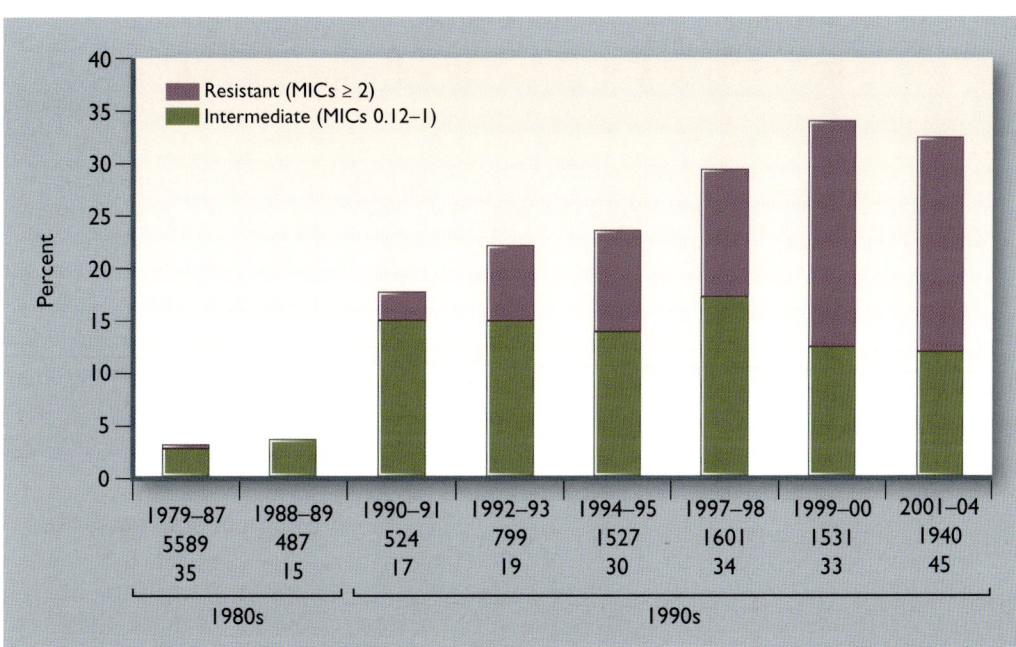

Figure 7-12. There was an increasing prevalence of penicillin resistance to *Streptococcus pneumoniae* in the United States from 1979 to 1999—from less than 5% to 34%. Since 2000, the resistant strain has remained about 35%. The plateau in this resistance is believed to be due to the introduction of the 7 serotype vaccine in children. Several publications have reported a significant decrease in invasive *Streptococcus pneumoniae* in adults [26–28]. MICs—minimal inhibitory concentrations.

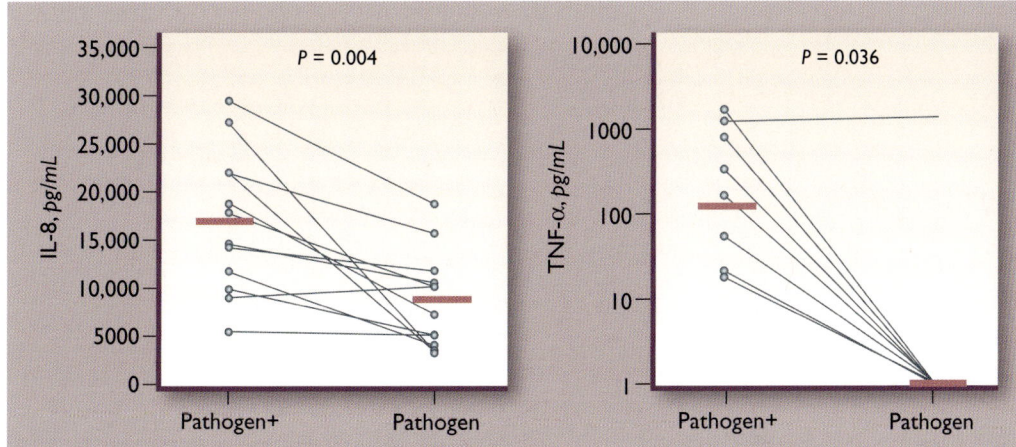

Figure 7-13. Interleukin-8 and tumor necrosis factor-α in acute exacerbation of chronic bronchitis–paired samples. The role of infection has been controversial in patients with acute exacerbation of chronic bronchitis. Recent work by Manso et al. [29] and other investigators using fiberoptic bronchoscopy to sample the lower airways of patients with chronic obstructive pulmonary disease has demonstrated that potential respiratory bacterial pathogens are present in the airways of these patients in up to 50% of the exacerbations. Several investigators have demonstrated that the presence of pathogens in the airways is associated with a significant inflammatory response. Sethi et al. [24] demonstrated that neutrophil airway infiltration is greater during exacerbations associated with the isolation of bacteria than during exacerbations with negative sputum. These investigators have demonstrated an increase of inflammatory cytokines, primary tumor necrosis factor (TNF)-α, and interleukin (IL)-8, as well as improvement when the pathogens are eradicated.

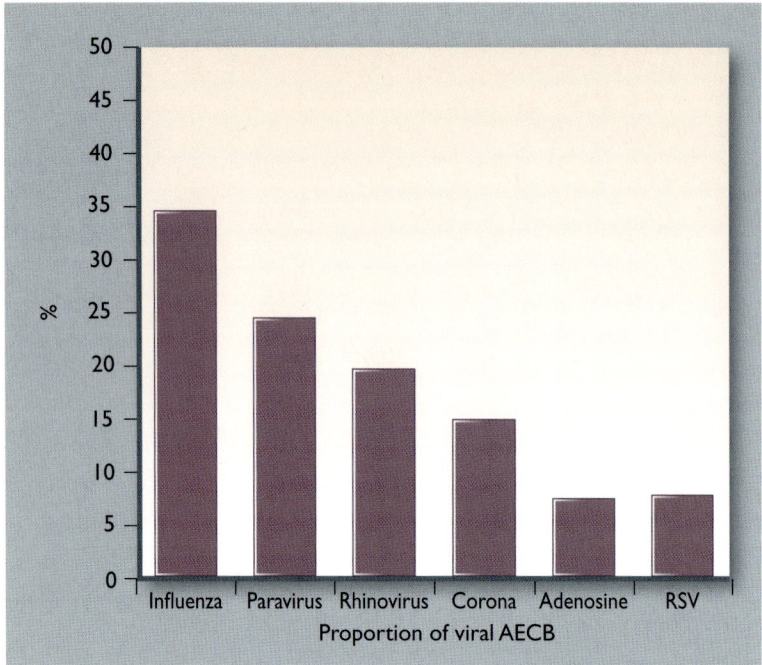

Figure 7-14. Viral etiology of acute exacerbation of chronic bronchitis (AECB). The role of viral infection in AECB is controversial. Several investigators have reported a viral infection associated with AECB; this has been manifested mainly by an increase in antibody titers or culture of respiratory secretions [30]. Furthermore, patients infected with the influenza virus have a threefold increase in the bacteria infection later. Secondary bacterial infections have been reported after other viral infections, including herpesvirus and rhinovirus [30]. The relationship between the viral infection and the bacterial infection requires further investigation, but it is clear that in some patients a viral process will precede the presence of a bacterial infection. Viral infection is associated with 30% of AECB cases, as is a fourfold increase in antibody titer. RSV—respiratory syncytial virus.

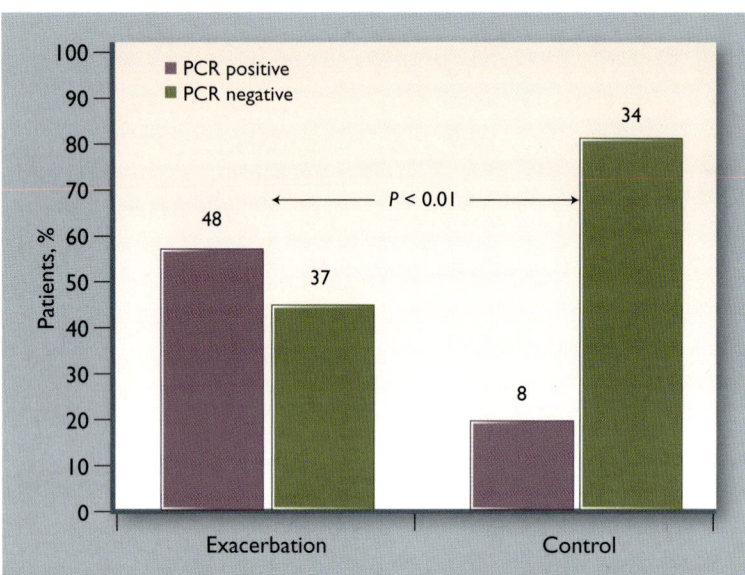

Figure 7-15. Role of respiratory tract infections in acute exacerbation of chronic bronchitis (AECB). Many AECBs are believed to be caused by upper and/or lower respiratory tract viral infections, but the incidence of these infections is undetermined. Rhode et al. [31] performed a prospective case-control study of two groups of patients with chronic obstructive pulmonary disease (COPD): one group with acute exacerbation and the other (a control group) with stable disease. This study was a 2:1 case–control setup: it involved 85 hospitalized patients with AECB and 42 patients with stable COPD admitted for other medical reasons. Respiratory syncytial virus (RSV), influenza A and B, parainfluenza 3, and picornaviruses were detected by nested reverse transcription polymerase chain reaction (PCR) in upper (nasal lavage) and lower (induced sputum) respiratory tract specimens. The two study groups had comparable demographic characteristics. In patients with AECB, forced expiratory volume in 1 second (FEV_1) on admission showed increased airflow limitation compared with controls ($P < 0.01$), as well as clinically more frequent wheezing and rhonchi ($P < 0.01$). Respiratory viruses were detected in sputum and nasal lavage in 48 of the 85 patients (56%) with AECB and in eight of the 42 controls (19%) ($P < 0.001$). Multiple viruses were more frequently detected in AECB patients. The most common viruses were picornaviruses (36%), influenza A (25%), and RSV (22%). When specimens were analyzed separately, this difference was seen in induced sputum (AECB 47% vs stable 10%; $P < 0.01$) but was not significant in nasal lavage (AECB 31% vs stable 17%, $P = 0.14$). The investigators concluded that viral respiratory pathogens are found more often in respiratory specimens of hospitalized patients with AECB than in control patients. Induced sputum detects respiratory viruses more frequently than nasal lavage in these patients.

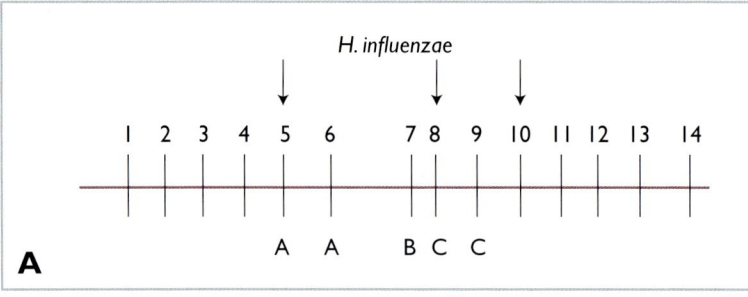

Figure 7-16. Pathogen characteristics and acute exacerbation of chronic bronchitis (AECB). The role of bacterial pathogens in AECB is controversial. In some studies, the rates of isolation of bacterial pathogens from sputum were the same during acute exacerbations and stable disease. However, these studies did not differentiate among strains within a bacterial species and therefore could not detect changes in strains over time. Sethi et al. [32] hypothesized that the acquisition of a new strain of a pathogenic bacterial species is associated with AECB. They conducted a prospective study in which clinical information and sputum samples for culture were collected monthly and during exacerbations from 81 outpatients with chronic obstructive pulmonary disease (COPD). Molecular typing was performed on sputum isolates of nonencapsulated *Haemophilus influenzae*, *Moraxella catarrhalis*, *Streptococcus pneumoniae*, and *Pseudomonas aeruginosa*.

Continued on the next page

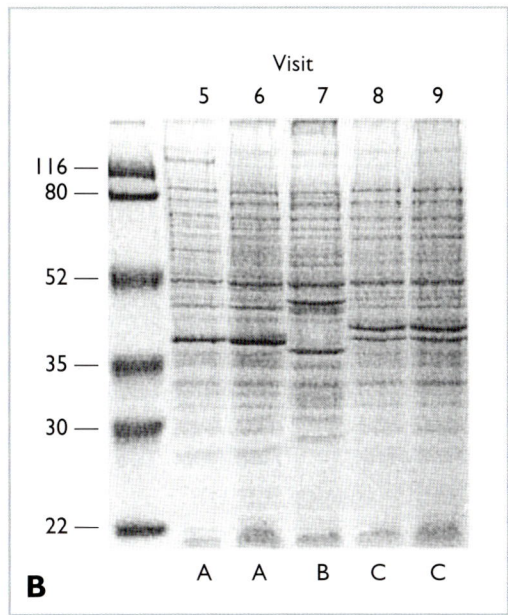

Figure 7-16. *(Continued)* Over a period of 56 months, the 81 patients made a total of 1975 clinic visits, 374 of which were during exacerbations (a mean of 2.1 per patient per year). On the basis of molecular typing, an exacerbation was diagnosed at 33.0% of the clinic visits that involved the isolation of a new strain of a bacterial pathogen, as compared with 15.4% of visits during which no new strain was isolated ($P < 0.001$; relative risk of an exacerbation: 2.15; 95% confidence interval [CI]: 1.83–2.53). Isolation of a new strain of *H. influenzae*, *M. catarrhalis*, or *S. pneumoniae* was associated with a significantly increased risk of exacerbation. Thus the association between an exacerbation and the isolation of a new strain of a bacterial pathogen supports the causative role of bacteria in AECB. **A** and **B,** Timelines and molecular typing for one patient. The *horizontal lines* are timelines, with each *number* indicating a clinic visit. **A,** The *arrows* indicate exacerbations. Isolates of each bacterial species were assigned types on the basis of banding patterns on gel electrophoresis. The first isolate was assigned the letter A, as were all subsequent isolates with identical banding patterns. Subsequent isolates with different banding patterns were assigned consecutive letters (B, C, D, and so forth). Each letter under the timeline represents a positive sputum culture for *H. influenzae* in one patient. Molecular typing was performed with sodium dodecyl sulfate–polyacrylamide-gel electrophoresis and staining with Coomassie blue. **B,** Whole bacterial-cell lysates of isolates recovered at visits 5 through 9 are shown. Three molecular types were identified. (*Adapted from* Sethi *et al.* [32].)

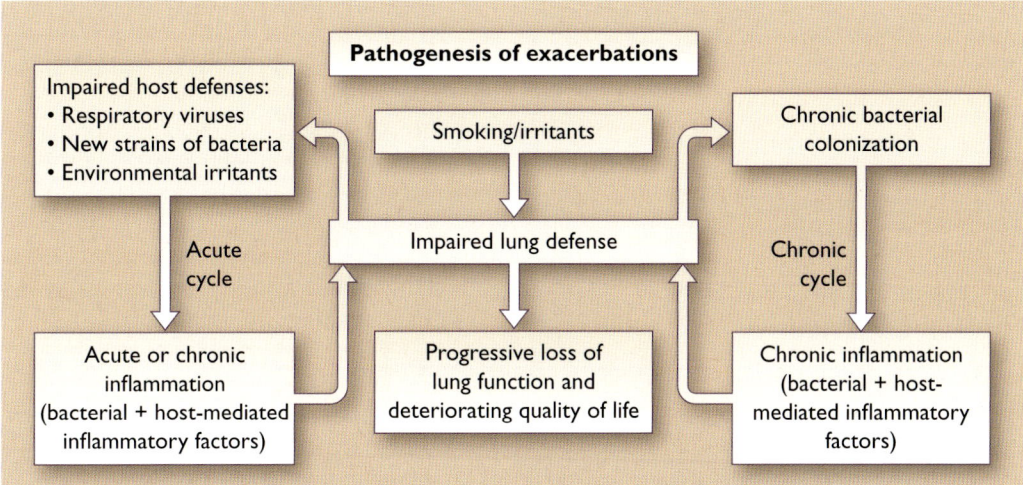

Figure 7-17. Pathogenesis of exacerbations. Sethi *et al.* [33] recently proposed a new interaction between pathogens and hosts in chronic obstructive pulmonary disease exacerbation. The balance between host defense and pathogen virulence determines the level of proliferation of the pathogen (the bacterial load), which in turn determines the increase in airway inflammation. Large increases in airway inflammation result in greater changes, which lead to symptoms so intense that the patient seeks health care and is often diagnosed as experiencing an exacerbation. On the other hand, limited increases in airway inflammation may not cause symptoms to increase to such an intensity that an exacerbation is diagnosed. Over time, development of adaptive immune response may limit the proliferation of the pathogen, or regulatory mechanisms could dampen the inflammation, although the bacterial strain may still persist. In these situations, the bacterial infection would be addressed as colonization.

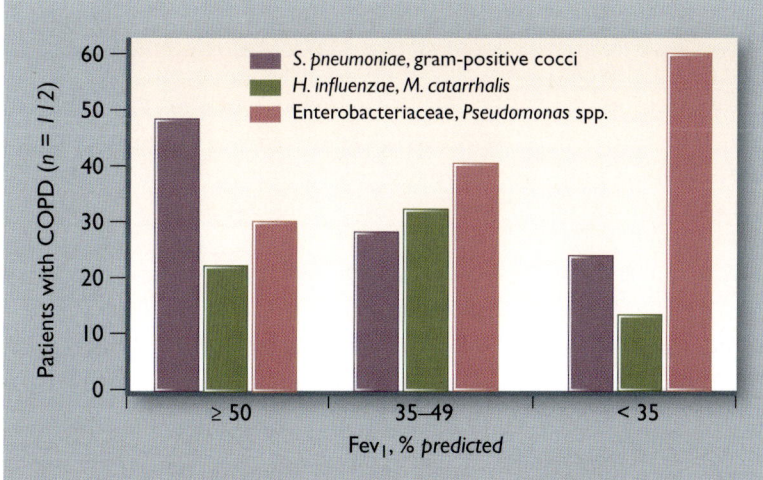

Figure 7-18. Relationship between disease severity and respiratory pathogens. There have been several studies showing that patients with more severe obstructive lung disease have a significantly higher prevalence of gram-negative organisms during an acute exacerbation [34,35]. Eller *et al.* [34] evaluated sputum cultures from 112 inpatients with acute exacerbation of chronic bronchitis (AECB). Sixty-four percent of patients with an forced expiratory volume in 1 second (FEV_1) of 35% or less of that predicted, versus only 30% of those with an FEV_1 of 50% or more ($P = 0.16$), had evidence of gram-negative organisms in their sputum. The most commonly isolated organisms included Enterobacteriaceae and *Pseudomonas*, *Proteus vulgaris*, *Serratia marcescens*, *Stenotrophomonas maltophilia*, and *Escherichia coli*. Miravitlles *et al.* [35] recently published a study with similar results that supports these findings, evaluating the relationship between FEV_1 and the isolation of diverse pathogens from 91 patients with chronic obstructive pulmonary disease (COPD) who had type I (severe) or type II (moderate) symptoms of AECB. Patients were separated into groups by FEV_1 (> 50% or < 50% of predicted). There was significantly more *Haemophilus influenzae* and *Pseudomonas aeruginosa* in the group with FEV_1s of less than 50% of that predicted ($P = 0.05$). In contrast, there were significantly more potentially nonpathogenic microorganisms in the group with FEV_1s of 50% or greater ($P < 0.5$). These investigators also performed a multivaried logistic analysis and found that *H. influenzae* was cultured significantly more commonly in patients who were actively smoking (odds ratio [OR] 8.2; confidence interval [CI] 1.9–43) and whose FEV_1 was less than 50% of that predicted (OR 6.85; CI 1.6–52). *P. aeruginosa* was also cultured significantly more frequently in those with poor lung function, FEV_1 less than 50% (OR 6.6; CI 1.2–124).

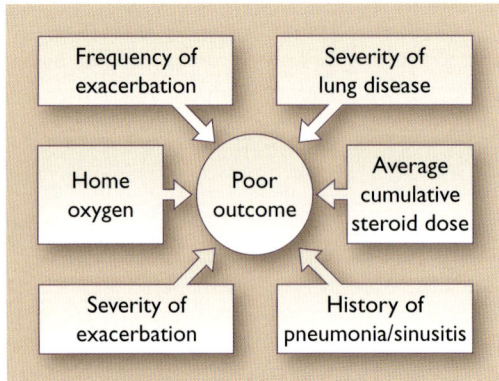

Figure 7-19. Acute exacerbation of chronic bronchitis (AECB) factors associated with poor treatment outcomes. Because the morbidity and mortality for AECB are high, many investigators have attempted to describe clinical characteristics that could be used to stratify patients with AECB. The clinical parameters that are implicated as possible risk factors for treatment failure in AECB are as follows: (1) older age (> 65 years), (2) severe underlying chronic obstructive pulmonary disease (COPD) (forced expiratory volume in 1 second [FEV_1] < 35% of that predicted), (3) frequent exacerbations (> 4 yearly), (4) more severe symptoms at diagnosis (Anthonisen types I and II), (5) comorbidities (especially in cardiopulmonary disease, but also in congestive heart failure, diabetes mellitus, chronic renal failure, and chronic liver disease), and (6) prolonged history of COPD (> 10 y) [36,37]. Recently, Dewan et al. [38] reported a study of 107 patients with 232 exacerbations over 2 years. The treatment failure rate of these exacerbations was 15%. The investigators noted that the patients who had more than four exacerbations during the 2-year period had a 100% failure rate. They also noted that the use of home oxygen and maintenance systemic corticosteroid therapy was associated with a significant relapse rate. (*Adapted from* Dewan et al. [38].)

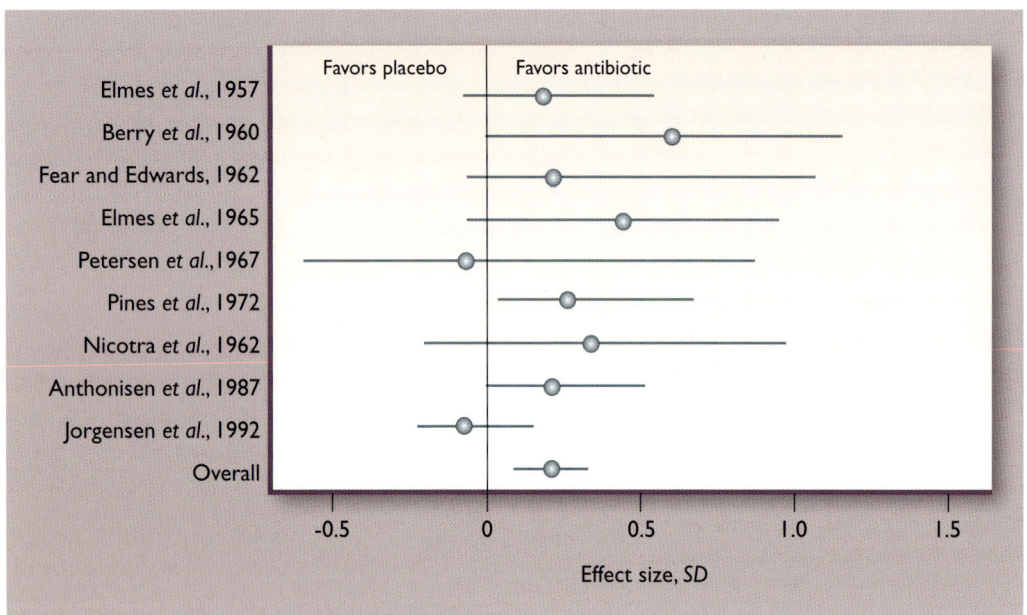

Figure 7-20. Clinical improvement with antibiotics: meta-analysis of placebo-controlled clinical trials. One way to assess the efficacy of antibiotic therapy in the treatment of acute exacerbation of chronic bronchitis (AECB) is to evaluate clinical outcomes. Saint et al. [39] reported the result of a meta-analysis of the role of antibiotics in the treatment of AECB. These investigators analyzed nine placebo-controlled, randomized studies published between 1957 and 1992 that were conducted in outpatient settings. The study showed a statistically significant overall benefit for antibiotic-treated patients. Analysis of the studies that provided data on expiratory flow noted an improvement of 10.75 L/min in the antibiotic-treated group. The authors concluded that these antibiotic-associated improvements may be clinically significant, particularly in patients with low baseline peak flow rates and limited respiratory reserves. The classic study that has addressed the use of antibiotics in AECB was reported by Anthonisen et al. [18]. These investigators conducted a large-scale, placebo-controlled trial designed to determine the effectiveness of antibiotics in the treatment of AECB. In this study, 173 patients with chronic bronchitis were followed for 3.5 years, during which time they had 362 episodes of exacerbation. The patients were randomized and given antibiotics or placebos in a double-blind, crossover fashion. Three oral antibiotics were used for 10 days (amoxicillin, trimethoprim sulfamethoxazole, and doxycycline). Approximately 40% of exacerbations were type I (severe), 40% were type II (moderate), and 20% were type III (mild). Patients with the most severe exacerbations (type I) received a significant benefit from antibiotics, whereas no significant difference was noted between antibiotics and placebos in patients who had only one of the defined symptoms (type III). Overall, the patients treated with antibiotics showed a more rapid improvement in peak flow, a greater percentage of clinical success, and a smaller percentage of clinical failure than those who received placebos. The length of illness decreased by 2 days in the antibiotic-treated group. The major criticisms of this study were that no microbiology was performed and that all antibiotics were assumed to be equivalent. Allegra and Grassi [40] found significant benefits for the use of amoxicillin–clavulanate therapy in comparison to placebos in patients with severe disease. Patients who received these antibiotics had a higher success rate (86.4% vs 50.3% in the placebo group, $P < 0.1$) and fewer recurring exacerbations.

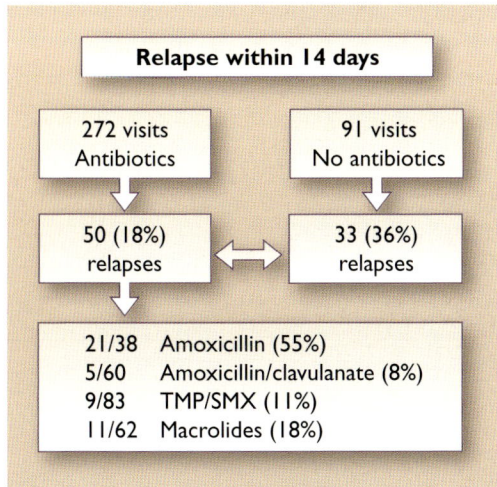

Figure 7-21. Efficacy of antibiotics for treating chronic obstructive pulmonary disease (COPD) exacerbations. If antibiotics have an effect on the outcome of acute exacerbation of chronic bronchitis, the next step is to determine if there are differences between antibiotics. Most of the recently published antibiotic clinical trials were designed to compare a new antibiotic with an established compound for the purpose of new registration and licensing. Equivalency is the desired outcome of such trials; therefore, the agent chosen for comparison is considered unimportant. In addition, these trials frequently include patients with poorly defined severity (often without any obstructive lung disease) and with acute illness of varying severity. The recent retrospective study of outpatients with documented COPD evaluated the risk factors for therapy failure at 14 days after an acute exacerbation [41]. The participating patients had a total of 362 exacerbations over an 18-month period. One group received antibiotics (270 visits), and the second group (92 visits) did not. Both groups had similar demographics and severity of underlying COPD. The patients' mean age was 67, ±10 years, 100% of patients smoked more than 50 packs of cigarettes per year, and 45% were active smokers. According to the American Thoracic Society's COPD classification, 39% had mild disease, 47% had moderate disease, and 14% had severe disease. The majority (45%) with severe symptoms at diagnosis (type I) received antibiotics, versus 40% of those with mild symptoms. The overall relapse rate (defined as a return visit within 14 days, accompanied by persistent or worsening symptoms) was 22%. In the multivariate analysis, the major risk factor for relapse was the lack of antibiotic therapy (32% vs 19%; $P < 0.01$ compared with the antibiotic-treated group). The type of antibiotic used was also an important variable associated with the 14-day treatment failure. Patients treated with amoxicillin had a 54% relapse rate with only 13% of other antibiotics ($P < 0.1$). Furthermore, treatment with amoxicillin resulted in a higher incidence of failure, even when compared with those who did not receive antibiotics ($P = 0.06$). Other variables, such as COPD severity, types of exacerbations, prior or concomitant use of corticosteroids, and use of oxygen therapy, were not significantly associated with the 14-day relapse. This study showed that the use of antibiotics was associated with a significantly lower rate of therapy failure. Furthermore, patients who received antibiotics and failed within 14 days had a significantly higher rate of hospital admission than those who did not receive antibiotics. These data emphasize the importance of giving antibiotics and providing appropriate therapy. A likely explanation of this failure could be that the pathogens were resistant to amoxicillin. TMP/SMX—trimethoprim/sulfamethoxazole. (*Adapted from* Adams et al. [41].)

Differences in Characteristics Based on Antibiotic Selection

	First-line	Second-line	Third-line
Days of therapy	8.9 ± 3.3	8.3 ± 2.3	7.5 ± 2.5*
Weeks between AECB	17.1 ± 22	22.7 ± 30	34.3 ± 35.5*
14-day failure rate (n = 36)	19%	16%	7%*
Hospitalizations (% of total failures)	53%	14%	8%*
Cost per episode, $	942 ± 2173	563 ± 2296	542 ± 1946

Data are presented in percentages (as indicated) and otherwise in mean ± standard deviation.
*$P \leq 0.05$ third line versus first line.

Figure 7-22. Differences in characteristics based on antibiotic selection. Destache et al. [42] reported the impact of antibiotic selection, antimicrobial efficacy, and related cost in acute exacerbation of chronic bronchitis (AECB). This study was a retrospective review of 60 outpatients from a pulmonary clinic at a teaching institution who were diagnosed with chronic obstructive pulmonary disease and chronic bronchitis. The participating patients had a total of 224 episodes of AECB requiring antibiotic treatment. The antibiotics were divided arbitrarily into three groups: first-line (amoxicillin, cotrimoxazole, and tetracycline), second-line (cephradine, cefuroxime, cefaclor, cefprozil), and third-line (amoxicillin–clavulanate, azithromycin, and ciprofloxacin) agents. The failure rates were significantly higher (at 14 days) for the first-line compared with the third-line agents (19% vs 7%, $P < 0.5$). When compared with the patients who received the first-line agents, those treated with third-line agents had a significantly longer time between exacerbations (34 wk vs 17 wk, $P < 0.2$), fewer days of therapy (8.9 ±3.3 d vs 17.5 ±2.5 d, $P < 0.02$), and fewer hospitalizations (3 of 26 [12%] vs 18 of 26 [69%], $P < 0.2$). The initial pharmaceutical cost was higher in the third-line agents ($8.3 ±$8.76 vs $45.4 ±$11.11, $P < 0.0001$), but the total cost of therapy was lower ($542 vs $942).

Dimipoulus et al. [43] performed a systematic review of the PubMed and Cochrane Central Register of Controlled Trials databases and identified 12 randomized controlled trials that met their inclusion criteria. Trials must have compared the use of first- and second-line antibiotics for AECB and must present data on efficacy or tolerability. First-line antibiotics were considered to include amoxicillin, ampicillin, pivampicillin, trimethroprim (TMP) plus sulfamethoxazole (SMX), and doxycycline. Second-line antibiotics included amoxicillin–clavulanic acid, macrolides (such as azithromycin), third-generation cephalosporins (such as cefaclor), and quinolones. The authors found that first-line antibiotics were associated with lower treatment success than second-line antibiotics in the clinically evaluable patients (odds ratio [OR], 0.51; 95% confidence interval [CI], 0.34 to 0.75). In microbiologically evaluable patients no difference was evident in terms of treatment success, adverse effects, or mortality. Adverse effects of antimicrobial therapy were similar for first- and second-line agents and included abdominal pain, nausea, vomiting, diarrhea, and, in some cases, dizziness and insomnia. This meta-analysis has substantial limitations that need to be considered when interpreting the data. For instance, the trials included mixed populations of patients (inpatients and outpatients), did not look at risk factors for worse outcomes (and thus the need for more aggressive antibiotic therapy), and did not allow sufficient intent-to-treat data for pooled analysis. These investigators concluded that advanced antibiotics are preferable to old antibiotics in patients with AECB. (*Adapted from* Destache et al. [42].)

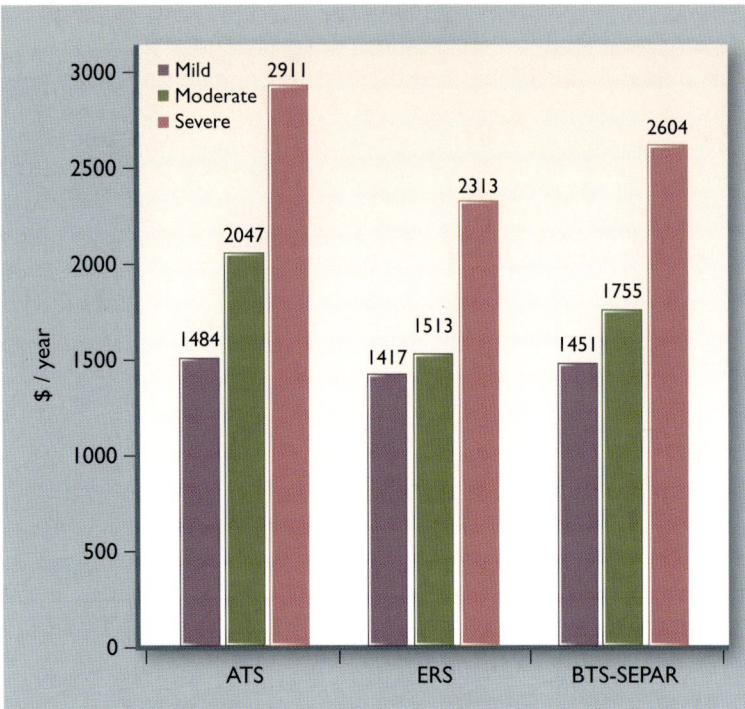

Figure 7-23. Direct medical costs of chronic obstructive pulmonary disease (COPD) by degrees of severity. COPD constitutes an important health problem associated with increased use of health care resources, with disability, and even with death, creating a great social and economic burden. The economic impact of this disease has been estimated to be billions of dollars, but no prospective studies have been aimed at qualifying the direct medical cost incurred by patients with COPD in the community. Miravitlles et al. [44] attempted to determine prospectively the total direct costs derived from the management of patients with chronic bronchitis and COPD in an ambulatory setting. These investigators assembled a cohort of 1510 patients recruited from 268 primary care practices throughout Spain. The patients' mean age was 66.5, ±11.5 years, and their mean forced expiratory volume at 1 second was 56.5%, ±16.3%. Patients were monitored for 1 year, and all direct medical costs incurred by the cohort and related to their respiratory disease were quantified. Costs were calculated for each patient according to the severity of that patient's COPD. The cohort members had a mean of 1.9 acute exacerbations during 1 year and visited their primary care physicians a mean of 5.1 times. The mean number of emergency department visits was 0.5 per patient per year, and the mean hospitalization was 0.2 per patient per year. The global mean direct yearly cost was $1876. The cost was double for patients with severe COPD in comparison with those who had mild COPD: $2911 and $1484, respectively. Hospitalization represented 43.8% of costs, drug acquisition 40.8%, and clinic visits and diagnostic tests only 15.4%. The figure shows the direct medical costs of COPD by degrees of severity, comparing the severity stratification criteria of the American Thoracic Society (ATS), European Respiratory Society (ERS), and British Thoracic Society and Spanish Society of Pneumology and Thoracic Surgery (BTS-SEPAR). Regardless of the severity stratification used, patients with more severe COPD had significantly higher medical costs. The investigators concluded that COPD represents a great health care burden that is worse in patients with more severe disease. The aging of the population, and continued smoking habits, make it seem likely that costs will only continue to increase in the future.

Cost of Treatment of Acute Exacerbation of Chronic Bronchitis

Age group	Hospital costs, millions of $	Outpatient costs, millions of $
≥ 65 years	1141	34
< 65 years	408	14
All ages	1549	48

Figure 7-24. Treatment costs of exacerbations of chronic obstructive pulmonary disease. It has been suggested that many episodes of in acute exacerbation of chronic bronchitis are noninfectious or are produced by a variety of nonpathogenic agents and will therefore resolve spontaneously without antibiotic therapy. Work by Adams et al. [41] and Destache et al. [42] has shown that the failure of therapy is associated with a very high cost. Niederman et al. [45] recently reported that an age greater than 65 years and inpatient treatment are the major determinants contributing to the overall cost of acute exacerbation of chronic bronchitis. The cost was estimated at $1.2 billion for the 27,540 inpatients 65 years of age or older versus $452 million for 5.8 million outpatients in the same group. The mean length of stay was longer and the in-hospital mortality rate was significantly higher for those older than 65 years. (Adapted from Niederman et al. [45].)

Characteristics of an Ideal Antibiotic

Activity against most likely organisms: *Streptococcus pneumoniae*, *Haemophilus influenzae*, *Moraxella catarrhalis*

Resistant to destruction by beta-lactamase

Good penetration into bronchial tissue

Well-tolerated/conveniently dosed

Cost effective

Figure 7-25. Characteristics of an ideal antibiotic. In order to determine the most important characteristics to take into consideration when selecting antimicrobial agents for the treatment of acute exacerbation of chronic bronchitis, one should ask the following questions: (1) How active is the agent against the most common pathogens isolated in acute exacerbation of chronic bronchitis (AECB), and are there significant gaps in the coverage of these organisms? (2) Does the antibiotic cover the spectrum of causative organisms based on clinical risk factors? (3) How likely are the pathogens to be resistant to the agents chosen? (4) How much of the antibiotics can penetrate the sputum, bronchial mucosa, and epithelial lining fluid? (5) How difficult is it to take the medication, and what are its major side effects? (6) How cost-effective is the agent? The ideal antibiotic should satisfy all of these criteria. However, because all antimicrobial agents possess only portions of these characteristics, the goal of a treating physician must be to weigh the importance of these factors for each patient with AECB. After all these factors are considered, it is possible to make an informed choice about the most appropriate antibiotic to administer to a patient who has AECB.

Percentage of Serum Concentrations of Antibiotic Achieved in Sputum, Epithelial Lining Fluid, and Bronchial Mucosa

	Antibiotic	Sputum, %	ELF, %	Bronchial mucosa, %
Penicillin	Amoxicillin		13	40
	Piperacillin	10–14		27–40
Cephalosporins	Cefixime			34–36
	Ceftazidime	2–15		51
	Cefuroxime	14		
	Doxycycline	18		
Macrolides	Erythromycin	5	114	
	Azithromycin		3200–5700	
	Clarithromycin		3900–10,300	
Quinolones	Ciprofloxacin	200	140–185	240
	Levofloxacin		1250	360
	Moxifloxacin		870	170
Aminoglycosides	Amikacin	10		
	Gentamicin	20		
	Tobramycin		50	

Figure 7-26. Antibiotic penetration. Good antibiotic penetration into sputum, bronchial mucosa, and epithelial lining fluid (ELF) is the ideal. The goal of antimicrobial therapy is to deliver the appropriate drug to the specific site of infection. In acute exacerbation of chronic bronchitis (AECB), the bacteria are found predominantly in the airway lumen, along the mucosa cell surfaces, and within the mucosa tissue. Various antibiotic classes showed markedly different degrees of penetration into the tissues and secretions of the respiratory tract. Although no studies show that the concentration of antibiotics at one particular intrapulmonary site is better than any at other site, the concentration of antibiotics in sputum, bronchial mucosa, and macrophages is thought to be predictive of clinical efficacy. These antibiotics exhibited a concentration–effect relationship in bacteria eradication [46,47]. (*Adapted from* Nix [46] and Fick and Stillwell [47].)

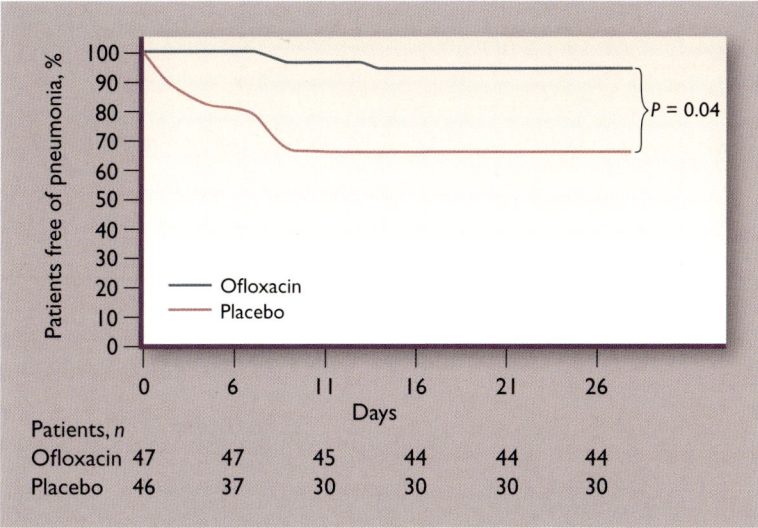

Figure 7-27. Ofloxacin efficacy. The eradication of bacteria by antibiotics is thought to break the vicious cycle of infection—lung destruction leading to progression of lung disease. Nouira *et al.* [48] reported a prospective, randomized, double-blind, placebo-controlled trial, evaluating the use of ofloxacin in 90 consecutive patients with acute exacerbation of chronic obstructive pulmonary disease who required mechanical ventilation. This study demonstrated a significant number of Gram-negative organisms (including *Escherichia coli, Proteus mirabilis,* and *Pseudomonas aeruginosa*) in their population of patients with severe chronic obstructive pulmonary disease exacerbations. In addition to supporting the findings of the previously reported studies, this trial demonstrated treatment of these pathogens to be important for improving outcomes in this high-risk population. The antibiotic-treated group had a significantly lower in-hospital mortality rate (4% vs 22%, $P = 0.01$) and a significantly reduced length of hospital stay (14.9 d vs 24.5 d, $P = 0.01$) compared with the placebo group. In addition, the patients receiving ofloxacin were less likely to develop pneumonia than those on placebos, especially during the first week of mechanical ventilation (7.2 ±2.2 days [range 4–11] vs 10.6 ±2.9 days [range 9–14], $P = 0.04$ by log-rank test).

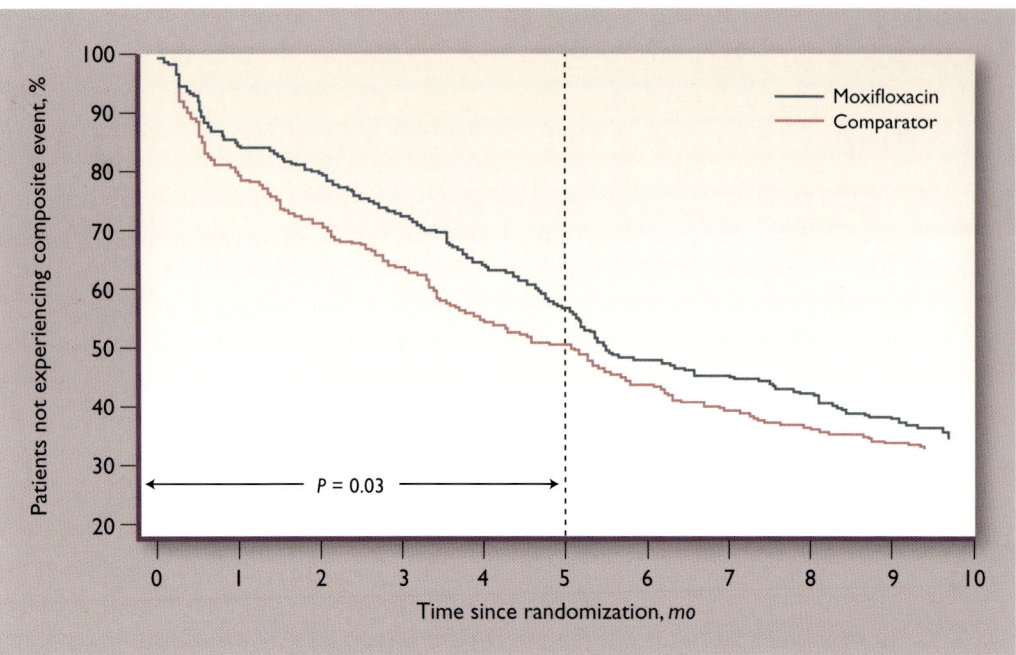

Figure 7-28. Moxifloxacin efficacy. Wilson et al. [49] reported the short- and long-term outcomes of moxifloxacin compared to standard antibiotic treatment in acute exacerbations of chronic bronchitis (AECB) (MOSAIC study). Patients were prospectively randomized (stratified based on corticosteroid use) between moxifloxacin (400 mg/d for 5 days) and standard antibiotic therapy (amoxycillin [500 mg three times daily for 7 days], clarithromycin [500 mg twice daily for 7 days], or cefuroxime-axetil (250 mg twice daily for 7 days]). Outpatients 45 years old or older, with stable chronic bronchitis, smoking more than 20 packs of cigarettes yearly, having two or more cases of acute exacerbation of chronic obstructive pulmonary disease in the previous year, and having a forced expiratory volume in 1 second (FEV_1) greater than 85% of the predicted value were studied. Patients were enrolled when stable, and those exacerbating within 12 months of enrollment were randomized; 354 patients received moxifloxacin, and 376 received standard antibiotic therapy. Clinical success was seen in 83.0% to 87.6% of patients across treatment arms and populations, with statistical equivalence in all populations except a significant difference in favor of moxifloxacin in patients not receiving steroids. Cure rates were superior with moxifloxacin. A significantly lower proportion of patients required additional antimicrobials in the moxifloxacin arm. Time to next exacerbation was longer with use of moxifloxacin: median and mean times for new AECB in patients who did not require any further antibiotic were 131.0 and 132.8 days for moxifloxacin, compared with 103.5 and 118.0 days for those without moxifloxacin ($P = 0.03$). Treatment failures, new exacerbations, and uses of further antibiotics were less frequent in the moxifloxacin group for up to 5 months ($P = 0.03$). Bacteriological eradication was superior with the use of moxifloxacin. These studies demonstrated that fluoroquinolones are superior to standard antibiotic therapy for clinically relevant measures including cure rate, the need for additional antimicrobial treatment, greater rates of bacteriologic eradication, and longer times to next exacerbation. Conventional end-points for the efficacy of antibiotics treatment in AECB include the symptoms and bacteriological resolution measured 2 to 3 weeks after the treatment was started. Most of these end-points rely solely on subjective reports of symptom improvement; although they have been used for drug registration purposes, they lack clinical relevance. It has been suggested by several reports that other parameters, such as rate of symptom resolution, interval between exacerbations, improvement in quality of life, need for hospitalization, and mortality, may be more suitable end-points in this patient population. In this study, for patients treated with oral fluoroquinolones (moxifloxacin), Wilson et al. [49] reported a significant increase in the length of time between exacerbations when compared with patients treated with commonly used antibiotics such as clarithromycin, amoxicillin, and cefuroxime. This end-point may reflect the ability of the antibiotics to achieve adequate bacteriologic eradication of the airway. This finding can be translated into cost savings, improved quality of life, and potentially slower progression of the underlying airway obstruction.

Patient Profiles from the Canadian Chronic Bronchitis Guidelines

Acute bronchitis (group 1)
  Healthy people without previous respiratory problems

"Simple" chronic bronchitis (group 2)
  Age ≤ 65 years and
  Fewer than four exacerbations per year and
  Minimal or no impairment in pulmonary function and
  No comorbid conditions

"Complicated" chronic bronchitis (group 3)
  Age > 65 years or
  Four or more exacerbations per year

"Complicated" chronic bronchitis with comorbid illness (group 4)
  Criteria for group 3 and
  Congestive heart failure or diabetes or chronic renal failure or chronic liver failure or other chronic disease

Figure 7-29. Profiles of patients with chronic bronchitis. Based on the concept of risk classification of patients by clinical parameters, a target approach for treatment of acute exacerbation of chronic bronchitis (AECB) has been proposed by the Canadian Bronchitis Symposium [50]. This group of investigators developed a classification for patients with symptoms of AECB by using the following factors: (1) number and severity of acute symptoms, (2) age, (3) severity of airflow obstruction (measured by forced expiratory volume in 1 second [FEV_1]), (4) frequency of exacerbations, and (5) history of comorbid conditions. This society suggested that patients could be profiled adequately into different categories. Acute bronchitis (group 1) includes healthy people without previous respiratory problems. Simple AECB (group 2) includes patients younger than 65 years, those who have had four or fewer exacerbations per year, those with minimal or no impairment in lung function (as reported by pulmonary function test), and those without any comorbid conditions. Complicated AECB (group 3) includes patients older than 65 years, those with FEV_1 of 50% or less of the predicted value, or those with four or more exacerbations per year. Finally, complicated AECB with associated comorbid illness (group 4) includes patients with congestive heart failure, liver disease, diabetes, or chronic renal failure as well as all the factors associated with the other groups. (*Adapted from Balter et al.* [50].)

Antibiotic Treatment in Exacerbations of Chronic Obstructive Pulmonary Disease*†

	Oral treatment (no particular order)	Alternative oral treatment (no particular order)	Parenteral treatment (no particular order)
Group A	Patients with only one cardinal symptom should not receive antibiotics‡	β-Lactam/β-lactamase inhibitor (co-amoxiclav)	
	If indication then:	Macrolides (azithromycin, clarithromycin, roxithromycin)¶	
	β-Lactam (penicillin, ampicillin/amoxicillin)§	Cephalosporins: second or third generation	
	Tetracycline		
	Trimethoprim-sulfamethoxazole		
Group B	β-Lactam/β-lactamase inhibitor (co-amoxiclav)	Fluoroquinolones¶ (gemifloxacin, levofloxacin, moxifloxacin)	β-Lactam/β-lactamase inhibitor (co-amoxiclav, ampicillin/sulbactam)
			Cephalosporins: second or third generation
			Fluoroquinolones¶ (levofloxacin, moxifloxacin)
Group C	Fluoroquinolones (ciprofloxacin, levofloxacin—high dose)**		Fluoroquinolones (ciprofloxacin, levofloxacin—high dose**) or
			β-Lactam with *Pseudomonas aeruginosa* activity

*All patients with symptoms of a COPD exacerbation should be treated with additional bronchodilators ± glucocorticosteroids.
†Classes of antibiotics are provided (with specific agents in parentheses); in countries with high incidence of Streptococcus pneumoniae resistant to penicillin, high doses of amoxicillin or co-amoxiclav are recommended.
‡Cardinal symptoms include increased dyspnea, sputum volume, sputum purulence.
§This antibiotic is not appropriate in areas where there is increased prevalence of β-lactamase producing Haemophilus influenzae and Moraxella catarrhalis and/or of S. pneumoniae resistant to penicillin.
¶Not available in all areas of the world.
**Dose 750 mgs effective against P. aeruginosa.

Figure 7-30. Recommendations for antibiotic therapy [4,51]. Based on antibiotics' characteristics and patient profiles, the Global Initiative for Chronic Obstructive Lung Disease (GOLD) recommendations for antibiotics are summarized in this figure. Patients with acute bronchitis but without underlying chronic obstructive pulmonary disease (COPD) are very likely to have viruses and thus to not require antibiotics. Patients with COPD and mild symptoms are likely to have *Haemophilus influenzae*, *Moraxella catarrhalis*, or *Streptococcus pneumoniae*. For these patients, GOLD recommends that initial therapy be with ampicillin, and alternative therapy be with co-amoxiclav, oral cephalosporins, macrolides, or respiratory fluoroquinolones. For patients with more complicated exacerbations, it is very likely that pathogens will be resistant to standard antibiotics; therefore, respiratory fluoroquinolones or co-amoxiclav should be used first. Patients with severe COPD at risk for *Pseudomonas aeruginosa* should be treated with fluoroquinolones or beta-lactams with antipseudomonas.

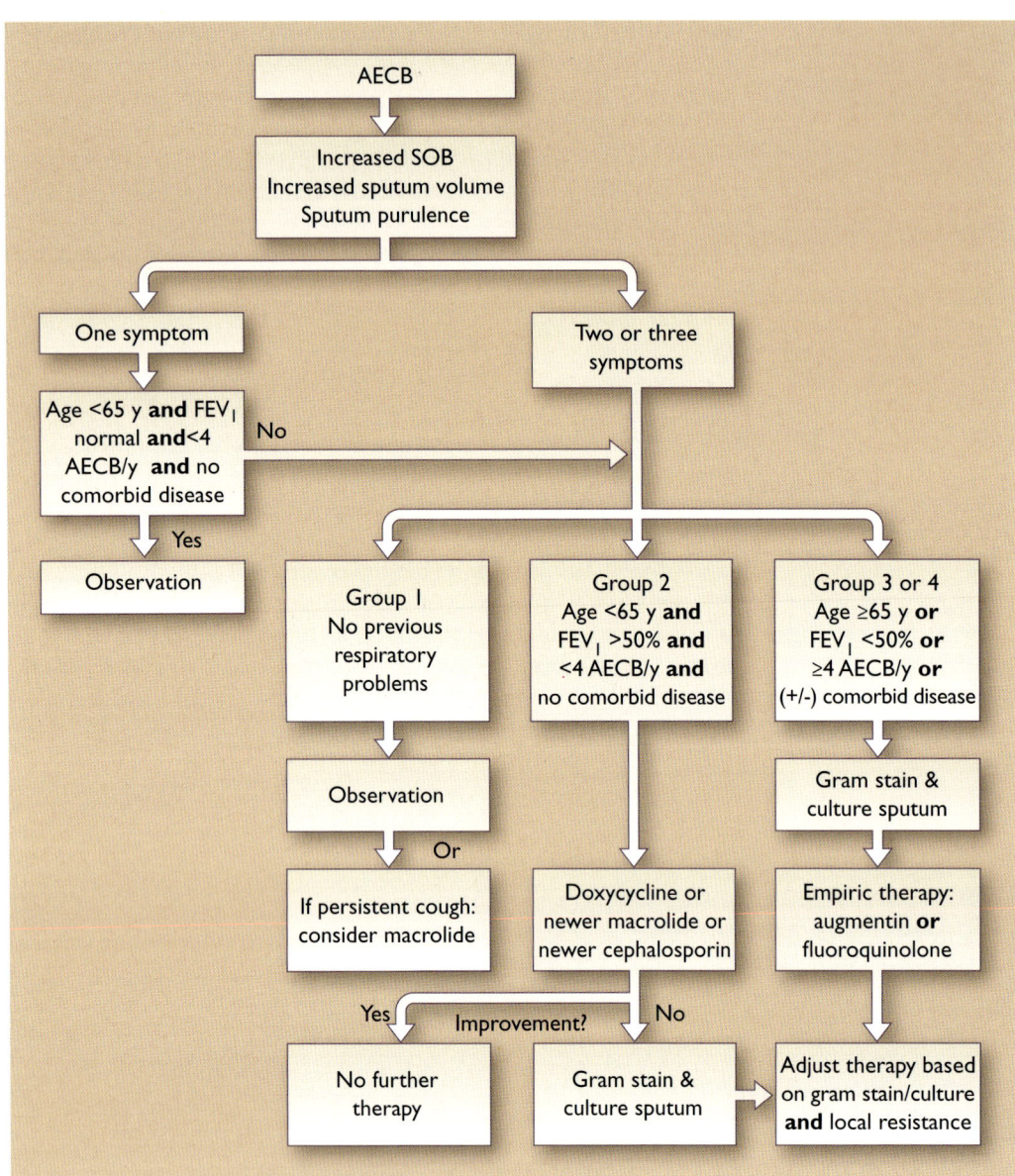

Figure 7-31. Acute exacerbation of chronic bronchitis treatment algorithm. The proposed algorithm for the treatment of patients with acute exacerbation of chronic bronchitis (AECB) takes into consideration the risk factors, microbiologic assessment, and prudent use of antimicrobial therapy. There will be many patients who do not require antibiotic therapy, but some who have significant risk factors will need to receive appropriate therapy upon initial presentation. Cx—culture; dz—disease; FEV_1—forced expiratory volume in 1 second; SOB—shortness of breath.

Therapeutic Strategies for Acute Exacerbation of Chronic Bronchitis

Agents	Comments
Corticosteroids	Improves flow rates
Ipratropium	Bronchodilator effects
β-agonists	Effects may be additive to ipratropium
Albuterol	Decreased bacterial burden
Salmeterol	
Antibiotics	May improve flow rates
	Decreases length of hospital stay
	Prolongs time between exacerbations

Figure 7-32. Therapeutic strategies for acute exacerbation of chronic bronchitis (AECB). Antibiotic therapy is one of the different treatment modalities for patients with AECB. The use of parenteral corticosteroids is not defined clearly. A randomized, double-blind, placebo-controlled trial with the use of systemic corticosteroids during acute exacerbation [52] suggested that if corticosteroids are going to be administered, they should be given for a short period of time. Short-acting $β_2$-agonists are another important therapy in this patient population. Recent reports have raised the possibility that the overuse of short-acting $β_2$-agonists may be associated with significant morbidity and cardiovascular-related mortality rates. If $β_2$-agonists will be used, our recommendation is that they be used by metered-dose inhaler with a spacer every 2 to 4 hours, not as a continuing nebulization. (*Adapted from* the American Thoracic Society [53].)

| Atlas of Pulmonary Medicine |

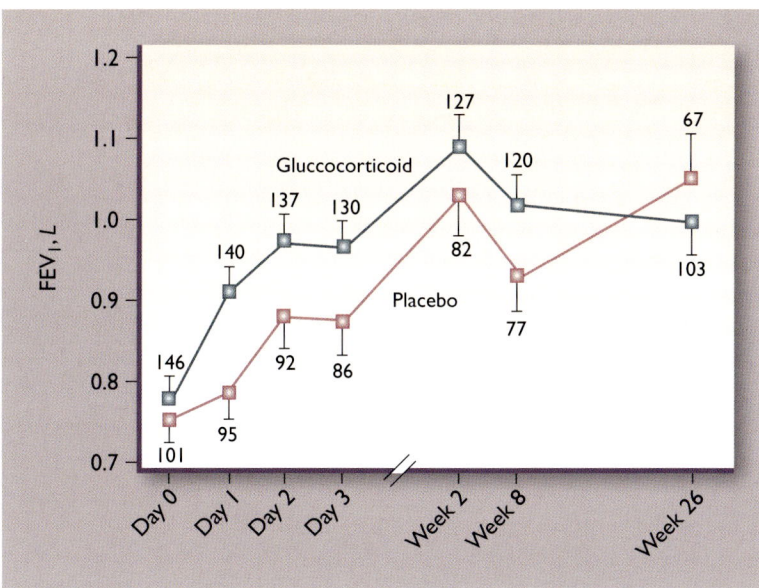

Figure 7-33. Corticosteroids in acute exacerbation of chronic obstructive pulmonary disease (AECOPD). Corticosteroids are recommended in most cases of AECOPD. There is a consensus that patients with significant bronchodilator response are more likely to benefit from this therapy, but the drug's precise role is not well understood. Corticosteroids may be administered intravenously, orally, or by inhalation. The use of inhaled corticosteroids during acute exacerbations has not been studied. In the largest study published to date, Systemic Corticosteroids in Chronic Obstructive Pulmonary Disease Exacerbations (SCCOPE) [52], 271 patients with AECOPD were enrolled. Patients received placebos or a two-dose regimen of corticosteroids for 2 or 8 weeks. This was a double-blind, randomized trial of systemic glucocorticoids or placebos, in addition to other therapies. Most other care was standardized over the 6-month follow-up period. The primary end point was treatment failure, defined as death from any cause or the need for intubation and mechanical ventilation, readmission to the hospital for chronic obstructive pulmonary disease, or intensification of drug therapy. For the combined glucocorticoid group, the risk of treatment failure compared to the placebo group was reduced by 10% (33% vs 23%, respectively) and forced expiratory volume in 1 second (FEV_1) improved statistically significantly during the first 3 days of therapy. No difference in FEV_1 existed after 2 weeks. The SCCOPE trial demonstrated equivalent outcomes between 2-week and 8-week corticosteroid regimens. The figure shows the Kaplan-Meier estimates of the rate of first treatment failure at 6 months by treatment group. The patients who received glucocorticoid therapy were more likely to have hyperglycemia requiring therapy than were those who received placebos (15% vs 4%; $P = 0.002$). Because all the published studies excluded patients who had received systemic corticosteroids within the preceding month, it is not known if corticosteroid treatment is also efficacious in these patients. (*Adapted from* Niewoehner *et al.* [52].)

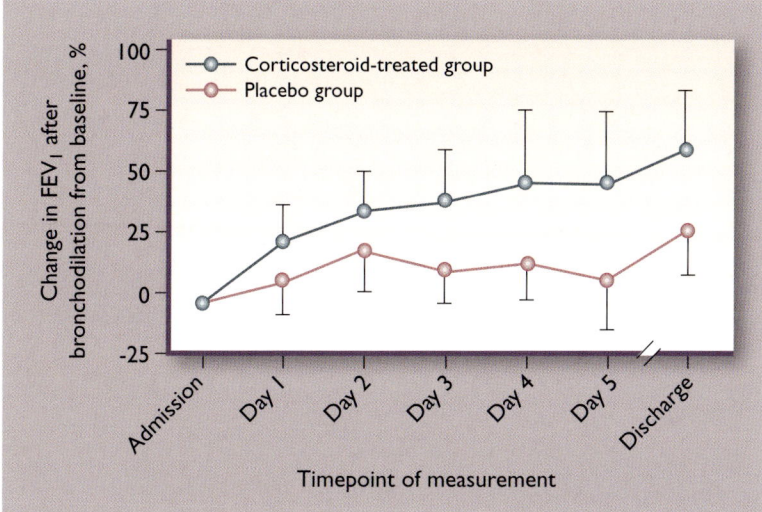

Figure 7-34. Role of corticosteroids in acute exacerbation of chronic obstructive pulmonary disease (AECOPD). The role of oral corticosteroids to treat AECOPD is controversial. Davies *et al.* [54] assessed in a prospective, randomized, double-blind, placebo-controlled trial the effect of oral corticosteroid therapy on patients with AECOPD. Patients were randomly assigned to oral prednisone, 30 mg daily ($n = 29$), or to identical placebos ($n = 27$), for 14 days, in addition to standard treatments. These investigators found that forced expiratory volume in 1 second (FEV_1) after bronchodilators increased more rapidly and to a greater extent in the corticosteroid-treated group: the percentage of predicted FEV_1 after bronchodilator use rose from 25.7% (95% confidence interval [CI], 21.0–30.4) to 32.2% (CI, 27.3–27.1) in the placebo group ($P < 0.0001$) compared with 28.2% (CI, 23.5–32.9) to 41.5% (CI, 35.8–47.2) in the corticosteroid-treated group ($P < 0.0001$). Up to the 5th day of hospital stays, FEV_1 after bronchodilator use increased by 90 mL per day (range, 50.8–129.2 mL); FEV_1 increased by 30 mL per day (range, 10.4–49.6 mL) in the placebo group ($P = 0.039$). Hospital stays were shorter in the corticosteroid-treated group. The groups did not differ at 6-week follow-up. These data suggest that oral corticosteroids may be effective in patients with AECOPD. (*Adapted from* Davies *et al.* [54].)

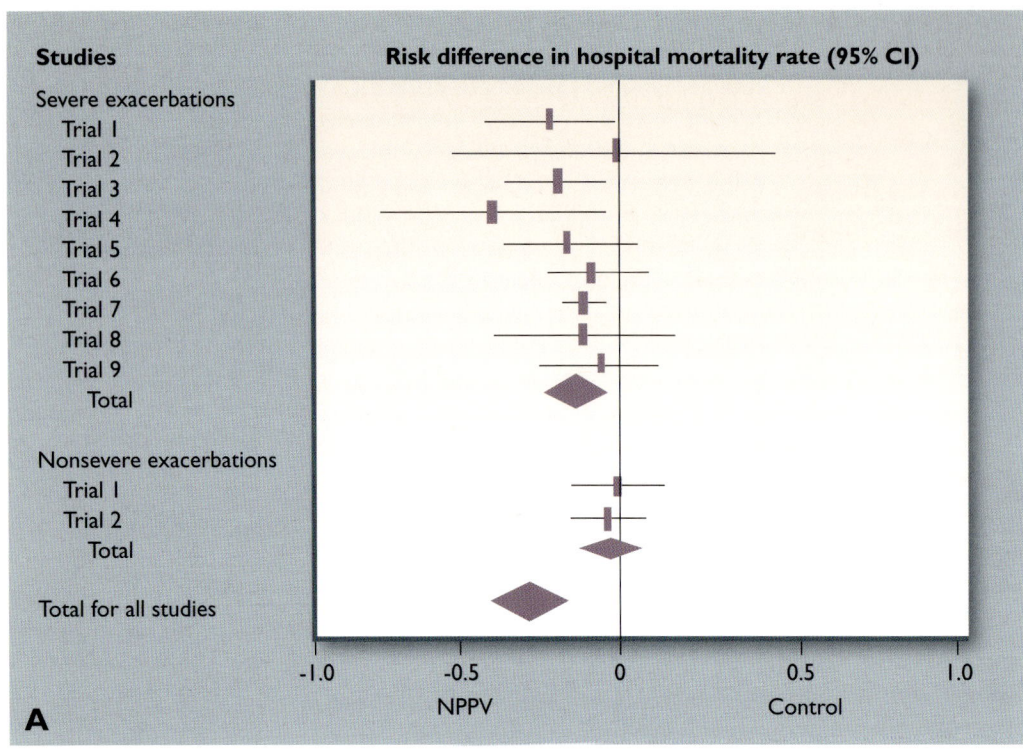

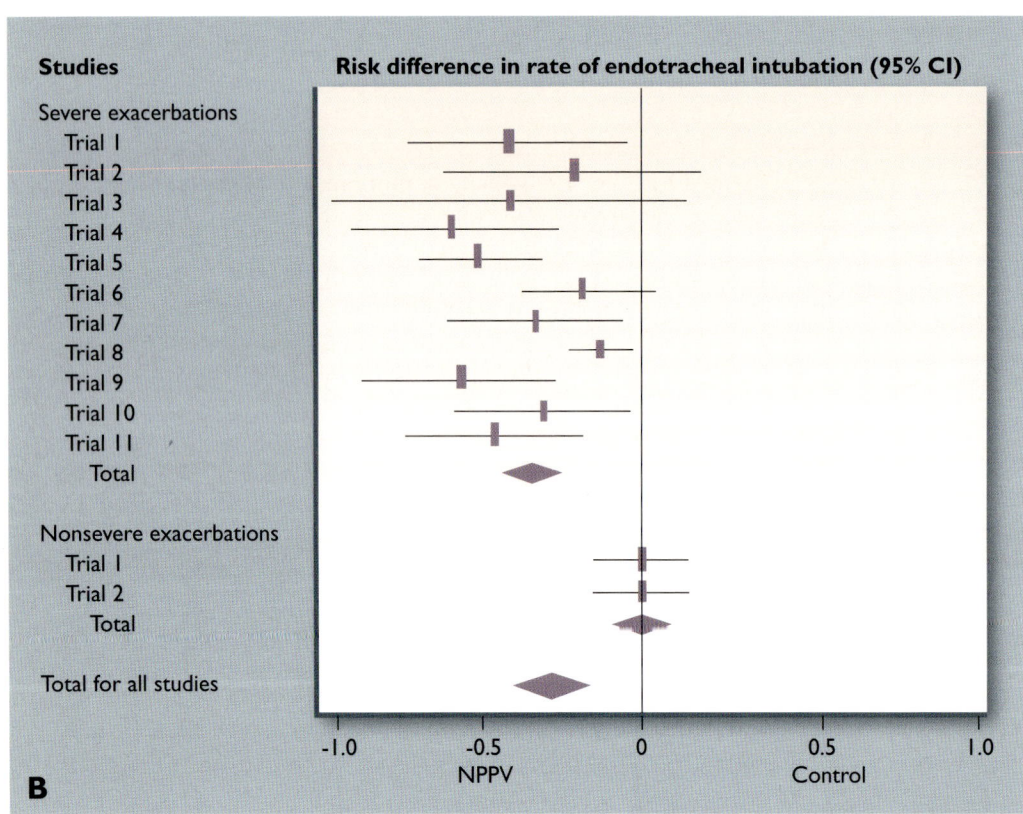

Figure 7-35. Noninvasive positive-pressure ventilation. Noninvasive positive-pressure ventilation (NPPV) is frequently used in the setting of acute exacerbation of chronic obstructive pulmonary disease (AECOPD). In order to assess the effect of NPPV on the rate of endotracheal intubation, length of hospital stay, and in-hospital mortality in patients with AECOPD, and to determine the effect of exacerbation severity on these outcomes, Keenan et al. [55] reported the results of a systematic review of the literature. The addition of NPPV to standard care decreased the rate of endotracheal intubation (RR: 28%; 95% confidence interval [CI]: 15–40), length of hospital stay (absolute reduction: 4.57 d; CI: 2.30–6.83) and in-hospital mortality rate (RR: 10%; CI: 5–15). Subgroup analysis showed that these beneficial effects occurred only in patients with severe exacerbations, not in those with milder disease. Severe exacerbations were defined as those in patients having a baseline pH less than 7.3 or an in-hospital mortality rate greater than 10% in the control group. A, Forest plot summarizing the hospital mortality as expressed by risk difference (absolute risk reduction) for individual trials and pooled results for nine trials of patients having severe exacerbations and two trials of patients having nonsevere exacerbations. B, A similar analysis of the rate of endotracheal intubation. The investigators concluded that NPPV should be added to the standard medical therapy of patients with severe AECOPD.

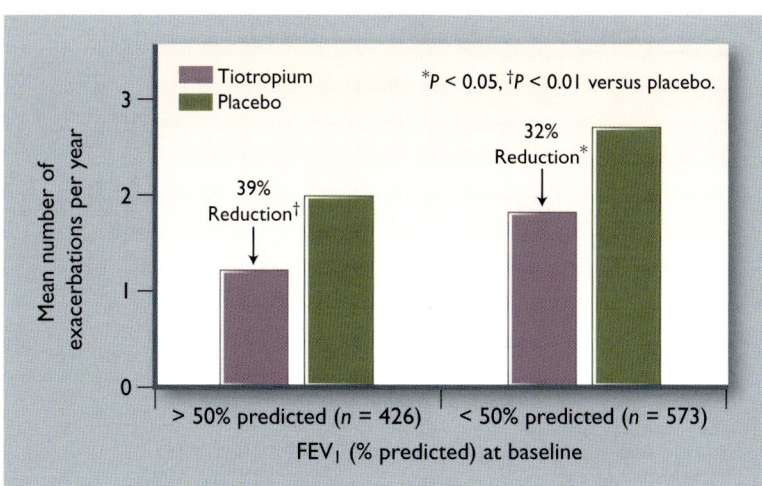

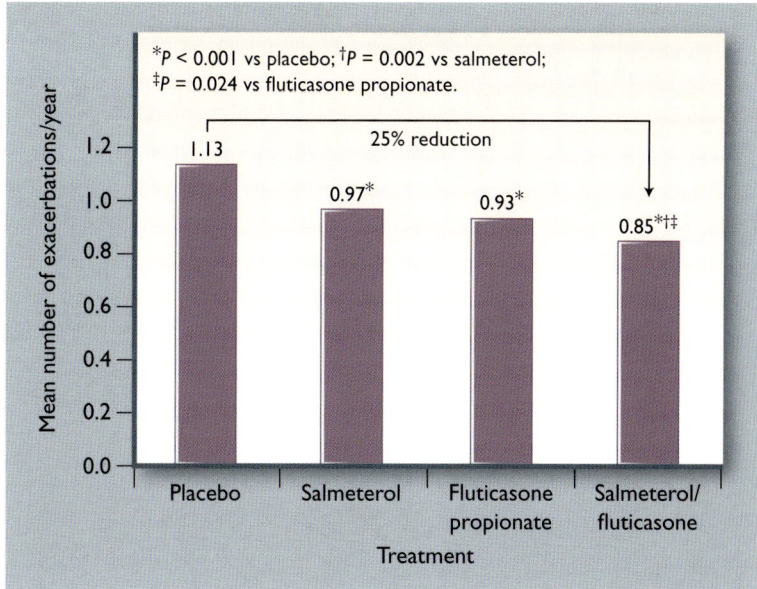

Figure 7-36. Recent clinical studies have demonstrated that chronic maintenance therapy in patients with chronic obstructive pulmonary disease can significantly decrease the frequency of exacerbations. These studies show that long-acting bronchodilators, including long-acting beta-agonists (salmeterol, formoterol) [56] and long-acting anticholinergics (tiotropium) reduce the mean rate of chronic obstructive pulmonary disease exacerbation [57,58]. FEV_1—forced expiratory volume in 1 second.

Figure 7-37. The effects of long-acting bronchodilators have also been reported in therapy combining inhaled corticosteroids and long-acting beta-agonists [59,60]. These studies have demonstrated that the reduction in exacerbations results in a significant decrease in hospitalizations and health care use [57,59].

REFERENCES

1. National Institutes of Health. National Heart, Lung, and Blood Institute: Morbidity & mortality: 2002 chart book on cardiovascular, lung and blood diseases. Accessible at http://www.nhlbi.nih.gov/resources/docs/02_chtbk.pdf. Accessed September 19, 2002.

2. Mannino DM, Homa DM, Akinbami LJ, et al.: Chronic obstructive pulmonary disease surveillance—United States, 1971-2000. *MMWR Surveill Summ* 2002, 51:1–16.

3. Fabbri L, Pauwels RA, Hurd S, GOLD Scientific Committee: Global strategy for the diagnosis, management and prevention of chronic obstructive pulmonary disease: GOLD Executive Summary, updated 2003. *COPD* 2004, 1:105–141.

4. Rabe KF, Hurd S, Anzueto A, et al.: Global strategy for the diagnosis, management and prevention of chronic obstructive pulmonary disease: Gold Executive Summary. *Am J Respir Crit Care* 2007, 176:532–555.

5. Celli BR, MacNee W: Standards for the diagnosis and treatment of patients with COPD: a summary of the ATS/ERS position paper. *Eur Respir J* 2004, 23:932–946.

6. Miravitlles M, Murio C, Guerrero T, Gisbert R, DAFNE Study Group: Decisiones sobre Antibioticoterapia y Farmacoeconomia en la EPOC. Pharmacoeconomic evaluation of acute exacerbations of chronic bronchitis and COPD. *Chest* 2002, 121:1449–1455.

7. Miravitlles M, Ferrer M, Pont A, et al., IMPAC Study Group: Effect of exacerbations on quality of life in patients with chronic obstructive pulmonary disease: a 2 year follow up study. *Thorax* 2004, 59:387–395.

8. Mannino DM, Watt G, Hole D, et al.: The natural history of chronic obstructive pulmonary disease. *Eur Respir J* 2006, 27:627–643.

9. Mannino DM, Buist AS, Petty TL, et al.: Lung function and mortality in the United States: data from the First National Health and Nutrition Examination Survey follow up study. *Thorax* 2003, 58:388–393.

10. Connors AF Jr, Dawson NV, Thomas C, et al.: Outcomes following acute exacerbation of severe chronic obstructive lung disease: the SUPPORT investigators (Study to Understand Prognoses and Preferences for Outcomes and Risks of Treatments). *Am J Respir Crit Care Med* 1996, 154:959–967.

11. Almagro P, Calbo E, Ochoa de Echaguen A, et al.: Mortality after hospitalization for COPD *Chest* 2002, 121:1441–1448.

12. Groenewegen KH, Schols AM, Wouters EF: Mortality and mortality-related factors after hospitalization for acute exacerbation of COPD. *Chest* 2003, 124:459–467.

13. Fuso L, Incalzi RA, Pistelli R, et al.: Predicting mortality of patients hospitalized for acute exacerbated chronic obstructive pulmonary disease. *Am J Med* 1995, 98:272–277.

14. Soler-Cataluna JJ, Martinez-Garcia MA, Roman Sanchez P, et al.: Severe acute exacerbations and mortality in patients with chronic obstructive pulmonary disease. *Thorax* 2005, 60:925–931.

15. Donaldson GC, Seemugal TAR, Bhowmik A, Wedzicha JA: Relationship between exacerbation frequency and lung function decline in chronic obstructive pulmonary disease. *Thorax* 2002, 57:847–852.

16. Spencer S, Jones PW, GLOBE Study Group: Time course of recovery of health status following an infective exacerbation of chronic bronchitis. *Thorax* 2003, 58:589–593.

17. Seemungal TA, Donaldson GC, Bhowmik A, et al.: Time course and recovery of exacerbations in patients with chronic obstructive pulmonary disease. *Am J Respir Crit Care Med* 2000, 161:1608–1613.

18. Anthonisen NR, Manfreda J, Warren CP, et al.: Antibiotic therapy in acute exacerbation of chronic obstructive pulmonary disease. *Ann Intern Med* 1987, 106:196–204.

19. Stockley R, O'Brien C, Pye A, Hill S: Relationship of sputum color to nature and outpatient management of acute exacerbations of COPD. *Chest* 2000, 117:1638–1645.

20. Ball P, Tillotson G, Wilson R: Chemotherapy for chronic bronchitis controversies. *Presse Med* 1995, 24:189–194.

21. Ball P: Epidemiology and treatment of chronic bronchitis and its exacerbations. *Chest* 1995, 108(Suppl 2):43S–52S.

22. Sapey E, Stockley RA: COPD exacerbations—2: Etiology. *Thorax* 2006, 61:250–258.

23. Sethi S, Wrona C, Grant BJ, Murphy TF: Strain-specific immune response to *Haemophilus influenzae* in chronic obstructive pulmonary disease. *Am J Respir Crit Care Med* 2004, 169(4):448–453.

24. Sethi S, Muscarella K, Evans N, et al.: Airway inflammation and etiology of acute exacerbations of chronic bronchitis. *Chest* 2000, 118(6):1557–1565.

25. Blasi F, Damato S, Cosentini R, et al.: *Chlamydia pneumoniae* and chronic bronchitis: association with severity and bacterial clearance following treatment. *Thorax* 2002, 57(8):672–676.

26. Doern GV, Richter SS, Miller A, et al.: Antimicrobial resistance among *Streptococcus pneumonia* in the United States: Have we begun to turn the corner on resistance to certain antimicrobial classes. *Clin Inf Dis* 2005, 41:139–148.

27. Whitney CG, Farley MM, Hadler J, et al.: Decline in invasive pneumococcal disease after the introduction of protein-polysaccharide conjugated vaccine. *N Eng J Med* 2003, 348:1737–1746.

28. Kyaw MH, Lynfield R, Schaffner W, et al.: Effect of introduction of the pneumococcal conjugated vaccine on drug-resistant *Streptococcus pneumonia*. *N Eng J Med* 2006, 354:1455–1463.

29. Manso JR, Rosell A, Manterola J, et al.: Bacterial infection in chronic obstructive pulmonary disease: study of stable and exacerbated outpatients using the protected specimen brush. *Am J Respir Crit Care Med* 1995, 152:1316–1320.

30. Hogg JC: Chronic bronchitis: the role of viruses. *Semin Respir Infect* 2000, 15:32–40.

31. Rhode G, Wiethege A, Borg I, et al.: Respiratory viruses in exacerbations of chronic obstructive pulmonary disease requiring hospitalization: a case control study. *Thorax* 2003, 58:37–42.

32. Sethi S, Evans N, Grant BJB, Murphy TF: New strains of bacteria and exacerbations of chronic obstructive pulmonary disease. *N Engl J Med* 2002, 347:465–471.

33. Sethi S: New developments in the pathogenesis of acute exacerbations of chronic obstructive pulmonary disease. *Curr Opin Infect Dis* 2004, 17:113–119.

34. Eller J, Ede A, Schaberg T, et al.: Infective exacerbations of chronic bronchitis: relation between bacteriologic etiology and lung function. *Chest* 1998, 13:1542–1548.

35. Miravitlles M, Espinosa C, Fernandez-Laso E, et al.: Relationship between bacterial flora in sputum and functional impairment in patients with acute exacerbations of COPD. *Chest* 1999, 116:40–46.

36. Murata GH, Gorby MS, Kapsner CO, et al.: A multivariate model for the prediction of relapse after outpatient treatment of decompensated chronic obstructive pulmonary disease. *Arch Intern Med* 1992, 152:73–77.

37. Ball P, Harris JM, Lowson D, et al.: Acute infective exacerbations of chronic bronchitis. *Q J Med* 1995, 88:61–68.

38. Dewan NA, Rafique S, Kanwar B, et al.: Acute exacerbation of COPD: factors associated with poor treatment outcome. *Chest* 2000, 117:662–671.

39. Saint S, Bent S, Vittinghoff E, et al.: Antibiotics in chronic obstructive pulmonary disease exacerbations: a meta-analysis. *JAMA* 1995, 273:957–960.

40. Allegra L, Grassi C: Ruolo degli antibiotici nel trattamento delle riacutizza della bronchite cronica. *Ital J Chest Dis* 1991, 45:138–148.

41. Adams S, Melo J, Anzueto A: Effect of antibiotics on the recurrence rates on chronic obstructive pulmonary disease exacerbations. *Chest* 2000, 117:1345–1352.

42. Destache CJ, Dewan N, O'Donohue WJ, et al.: Clinical and economic considerations in the treatment of acute exacerbations of chronic bronchitis. *J Antimicrob Chemother* 1999, 43:107–113.

43. Dimipoulos G, Siempos II, Korbila IP, et al.: Comparison of first-line with second-line antibiotics for acute exacerbations of chronic bronchitis: a metaanalysis of randomized controlled trials. *Chest* 2007, 132:4447–4455.

44. Miravitlles M, Murio C, Guerrero T, Gisbert R, DAFNE Study Group: Cost of chronic bronchitis and COPD: a 1-year follow-up study. *Chest* 2003, 123:784–791.

45. Niederman MS, McCombs JS, Unger AN, et al.: Treatment cost of acute exacerbations of chronic bronchitis. *Clin Ther* 1999, 21:576–592.

46. Nix DE: Intrapulmonary concentrations of antimicrobial agents. *Infect Dis Clin North Am* 1998, 12:631–646.

47. Fick RB, Stillwell PC: Controversies in the management of pulmonary disease due to cystic fibrosis. *Chest* 1989, 95:1319–1327.

48. Nouira S, Marghli S, Belghith M, et al.: Once daily oral ofloxacin in chronic obstructive pulmonary disease exacerbation requiring mechanical ventilation: a randomized placebo-controlled trial. *Lancet* 2001, 358:2020–2025.

49. Wilson R, Allegra L, Huchon G et al.: Short-term and long-term outcomes of moxifloxacin compared to standard antibiotic treatment in acute exacerbations of chronic bronchitis. *Chest* 2004, 125:953–964.

50. Balter MS, Hyland RH, Low DE, et al.: Recommendations on the management of chronic bronchitis: a practical guide for Canadian physicians. *Can Med Assoc J* 1994, 151:5–23.

51. Global strategy for the diagnosis, management and prevention of chronic obstructive pulmonary disease: GOLD Executive Summary updated 2006.

52. Niewoehner DE, Erbland ML, Deupree RH et al., for the Department of Veterans Affairs Cooperative Study Group: Effect of systemic glucocorticoids on exacerbations of chronic obstructive pulmonary disease. *N Engl J Med* 1999, 340:1941–1947.

53. American Thoracic Society: Standards for the diagnosis and care of patients with chronic obstructive pulmonary disease. *Am J Respir Crit Care Med* 1995, 152:S77–S121.

54. Davies L, Angus RM, Calverey PM: Oral corticosteroids in patients admitted to hospital with exacerbations of chronic obstructive pulmonary disease: a prospective randomized controlled trial. *Lancet* 1999, 354:456–460.

55. Keenan SP, Sinuff T, Cook DJ, Hill NS: Which patients with acute exacerbation of chronic obstructive pulmonary disease benefit from noninvasive positive-pressure ventilation? A systematic review of the literature. *Ann Intern Med* 2003, 138:861–870.

56. Mahler DA, Donohue JF, Barbee RA, et al.: Efficacy of salmeterol xinafoate in the treatment of COPD. *Chest* 1999, 15:957–965.

57. Niewoehner DE, Rice K, Cote C, et al.: Prevention of exacerbations of chronic obstructive pulmonary disease with tiotropium, a once-daily inhaled anticholinergics bronchodilator. *Ann Internal Med* 2005, 143:319–326.

58. Dusser D, Bravo ML, Iacono P: The effect of tiotropium on exacerbations and airflow in patients with COPD. *Eur Resp J* 2006, 27:547–555.

59. Hanania NA, Darken P, Horstman D, et al.: The efficacy and safety of fluticasone propionate (250 microg)/salmeterol (50 microg) combined in the Diskus inhaler for the treatment of COPD. *Chest* 2003, 124:834–843.

60. Calverley P, Celli B, Anderson JA, et al.: The TORCH (TOwards a Revolution in COPD Health). *New Engl J of Med* 2007, 356:775–789.

NOSOCOMIAL INFECTIONS INCLUDING PNEUMONIA

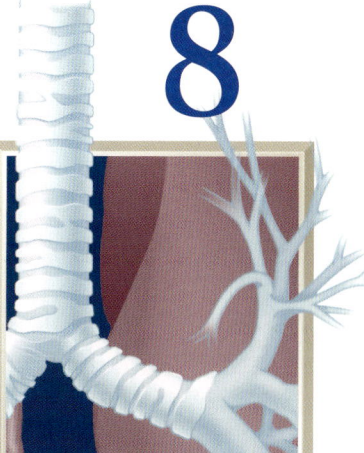

Mark J. Rumbak

Nosocomial infections are an important cause of morbidity and mortality in hospitalized patients. Pneumonia is the second most common infection in hospitals and is associated with the greatest attributable mortality, morbidity, and cost of care [1]. Hospitalized patients may develop pneumonia, but the prevalence is increased in patients requiring mechanical ventilation: the so-called ventilator-associated pneumonia (VAP). As the latter is very important, it will form the basis of this chapter.

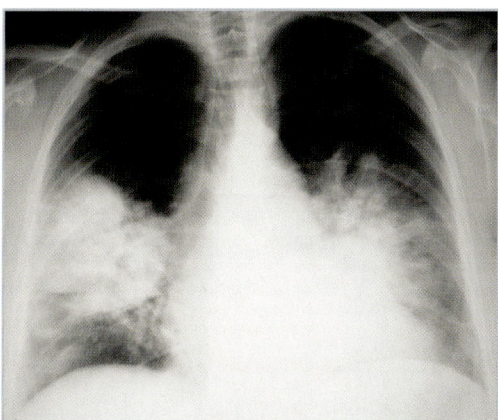

Figure 8-1. Chest radiograph of a patient with hospital-acquired pneumonia. This patient developed bilateral infiltrates after aspirating postoperatively. The leukocyte count and temperature were raised. *Pseudomonas* spp were isolated from the sputum. He was diagnosed with hospital-acquired pneumonia.

Nosocomial Infections

- Urinary tract infection
- VAP
- Hospital-acquired pneumonia (excluding VAP)
- Line sepsis
- Sinusitis
- Pseudomembranous colitis
- Bedsores
- Peritonitis
- Surgical wound infections

Figure 8-2. The most common infections occurring in hospitals. Although urinary tract infection is the most common infection, pneumonia—especially ventilator-associated pneumonia (VAP)—is the most serious. These infections are the major causes of high fever and leukocyte count in hospitalized patients.

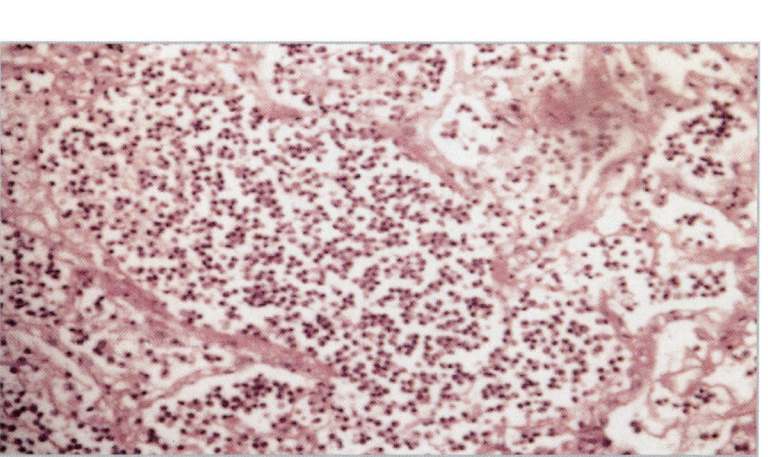

Figure 8-3. Polymorphonucleocyte infiltration in pneumonia. Typical histologic features of pneumonia include polymorphonucleocyte infiltration of the alveolar space. (Hematoxylin-eosin preparation.)

ETIOLOGY

INHALATION

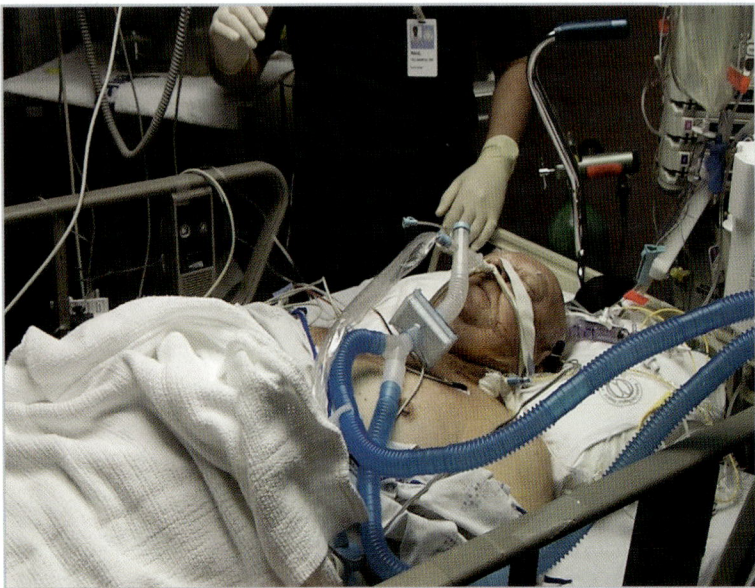

Figure 8-4. Mechanical ventilation in an intensive care unit. Appreciation of etiology is important to prevent pneumonia. Twenty-eight percent of patients who require mechanical ventilation will develop ventilator-associated pneumonia (VAP), and up to 70% may die.

There are only four routes through which microorganisms can enter the lower respiratory tract to develop into pneumonia: inhalation, aspiration, hematogenous and contiguous spread [1]. The aspiration, inhalation, and hematogenous routes are the most important. Ventilator tubing is the most common cause of aspiration VAP. Oxygen is warmed and humidified on its way from the ventilator to the patient. The tubing is cold and dry, and the water vapor precipitates in the dependent parts of the tubing and becomes infected. Microorganisms in the infected water are not nebulized very well. If the tubes are handled too frequently, the water can be aspirated into the lungs, causing VAP. Rarely, infected respiratory equipment may cause VAP [2,3].

The photograph shows a typical patient on mechanical ventilation in an intensive care unit. Notice that he is ventilated through the nose and is lying flat. The respiratory therapist is wearing gloves but did not wash his hands after attending to the previous patient. The patient is connected to the ventilator by the tubing, which is cold and dry. The air used to carry the oxygen is heated and humidified, leading to precipitation of water in the dependent part of the tubing, which becomes infected. The bacteria are not nebulized but may be aspirated into the lung by multiple manipulations of the tubing [3]. The Centers for Disease Control recommends changing the tubing weekly instead of daily, to reduce manipulation and aspiration of infected contents [1]. (*Courtesy of* David Weber, MD.)

ASPIRATION

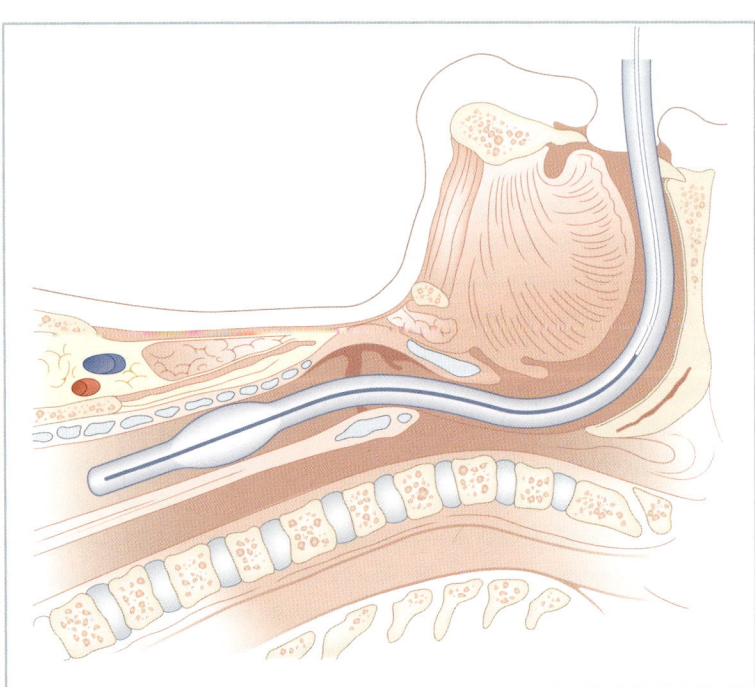

Figure 8-5. Intubation with an endotracheal tube. Pathogenic gram-negative microorganisms colonize the oropharynx in 6% of normal people, 35% of hospitalized patients, and 75% of critically ill patients. In general, patients who are colonized early have community-acquired microorganisms and those colonized late have nosocomial ones. The prevalence of ventilator-associated pneumonia (VAP) increases when microorganisms attach to the mucosa. Generally, colonization of the oropharynx is the primary jump-off point for the invasion of the lower respiratory tract. Reduction of this colonization decreases VAP dramatically [1,4,5]. How do microorganisms get to the oropharynx? The term *transcolonization* means that organisms colonizing the oropharynx come from contiguous structures [1]. These include the sinuses, teeth, plaque, and stomach. The original microorganisms come from other patients via the hands of health care workers. The role of the stomach in the etiology of VAP is very controversial [1]. It just may be that the aspiration of stomach contents physically washes the contents of the oropharynx through the open vocal cords and finally into the lungs. Sinusitis is thought to predispose the patient to VAP, and its prevention or early treatment may prevent VAP [6].

Aspiration is the main invasion route of microorganisms causing pneumonia. Intubated patients have an endotracheal tube forcibly holding the vocal cords open. Most patients are sedated and cannot cough efficiently or maintain their upper airways. Aspirated infected oropharyngeal contents pool above the inflated endotracheal tube cuff. Mechanical ventilation causes the pressure in the cuff to change, and the pooled secretions move around the cuff by capillary action and are aspirated into the distal airways. The infected secretions are then refluxed and infect the biofilm on the inner surface of the endotracheal tube. Continuous ventilation and suctioning shower infected secretions into the lungs, causing VAP [1,5].

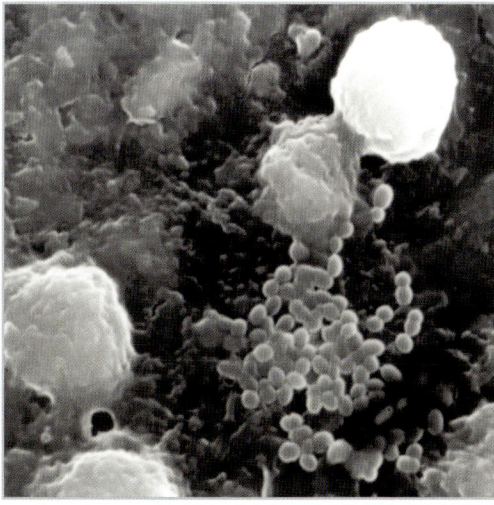

Figure 8-6. Biofilm formation. This electron microscope reveals a biofilm forming on the inner surface of the endotracheal tube [7]. (*Courtesy of* Marin Kollef, MD.)

Hematogenous Spread

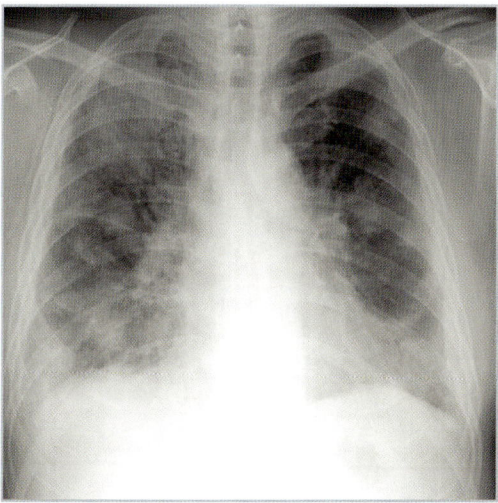

Figure 8-7. Chest radiograph showing hematogenous spread from infective endocarditis. Hematogenous spread was considered to be the most common way to develop ventilator-associated pneumonia (VAP). Bacteria were said to translocate from the gastrointestinal (GI) tract into the bloodstream and then travel to the lungs. This does not occur often because the bacteria that grow in the GI tract are different from those that cause VAP. Also, if the bacteria are spread hematogenously, the pneumonia will be diffuse and not in the dependent areas of the lungs [1]. This radiograph shows a pneumonia that spread to the lungs from the heart. The patient developed infective endocarditis, and the image shows multiple irregular ball-like lesions of different sizes. These are the so-called septic emboli.

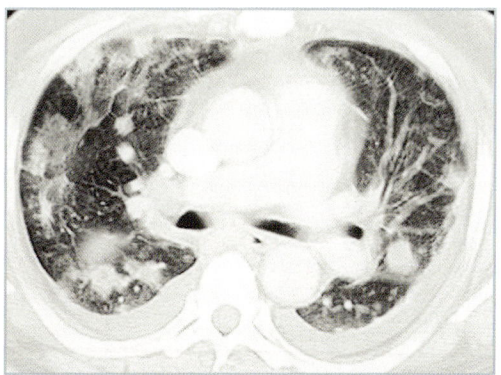

Figure 8-8. CT image of septic emboli to the lungs showing hematogenous spread from infective endocarditis. The scan was performed on the chest of the patient in Figure 8-7. The CT image further delineates the ball-like lesions of different sizes.

PREVENTION OF PNEUMONIA

Acceptable Methods of Pneumonia Prevention

- Prevention of transmission of bacteria
- Hand washing and disinfection
- Changing ventilator circuit no more than once per week
- Orotracheal tube cuff blown up
- Orotracheal rather than nasotracheal intubation
- Semireclining position
- Avoidance of paralysis
- Avoidance of reintubation
- Noninvasive ventilation
- Avoidance of patient transport
- Suctioning above the cuff
- Early tracheotomy

Figure 8-9. Acceptable methods to prevent ventilator-associated and other types of hospital-acquired pneumonia. Prevention of pneumonia is possible, and as the saying goes: An ounce of prevention is better than a pound of cure. All the methods listed in the table have been proven to prevent pneumonia [8].

Controversial Methods of Pneumonia Prevention

- Selective digestive decontamination
- Antibiotics post intubation
- Early enteral feeding
- Heat and moist-air exchanges on ventilators
- Avoidance of in-line nebulizers
- Antibiotic crop rotation
- Lateral rotational beds

Figure 8-10. Probable and controversial methods used to prevent hospital-acquired pneumonia.

Treatments Shown to Prevent Pneumonia

- Chlorhexidine and mupirocin in long-term ventilator patients
- Sulfamethoxazole/trimethoprim in burn patients
- Nasal treatment of *Staphylococcus* spp in trauma patients

Figure 8-11. Cases that prove prevention works. The three special cases listed in the table have been shown to decrease ventilator-associated pneumonia (VAP) due to *Staphylococcus* spp. Cohorting patients and decreasing the *Staphylococcus* load by twice-weekly total body wash with chlorhexidine and nasal application of mupirocin decreases VAP in patients requiring prolonged mechanical ventilation. Similar treatment of nasal carriage of *Staphylococcus* prevents *Staphylococcus* VAP in burn and trauma patients [8].

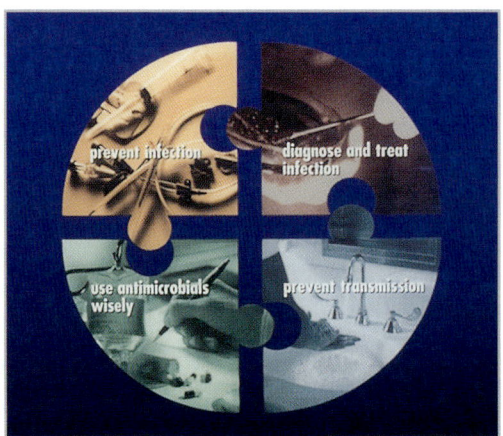

Figure 8-12. Centers for Disease Control (CDC) guidelines for preventing pneumonia. The CDC believes that prevention is paramount. The figure was redrawn from the CDC website, www.cdc.gov/drugresistance/healthcare, accessed December 2001.

Atlas of Pulmonary Medicine

DIAGNOSIS OF VENTILATOR-ASSOCIATED PNEUMONIA

CDC Criteria for the Diagnosis of Hospital-acquired Pneumonia

Chest radiograph revealing a new or progressive infiltrate plus one of the following:
Viral, bacterial, or fungal isolation or detection in respiratory secretions
Pathologic evidence of pneumonia
Elevated IgM or fourfold rise in IgG antibody for pathogen or clinical signs of pneumonia plus one of the following:
New-onset purulent sputum
Change in sputum character
Positive blood culture
Isolation of pathogen from lower respiratory tract secretions

Figure 8-13. Centers for Disease Control and Prevention (CDC) criteria for diagnosing hospital-acquired pneumonia. The diagnosis of ventilator-associated pneumonia is very controversial, with advocates of clinical versus invasive diagnostic methods often squaring off. Some investigators use the clinical criteria of high leukocyte count, a new infiltrate on the chest radiograph, and fever as enough proof for the diagnosis of pneumonia. Others advocate invasive diagnosis using protected specimen brush, bronchoalveolar lavage (BAL), or even mini-BAL [9]. Many clinicians use the clinical criteria as the sole method of diagnosing pneumonia [10].

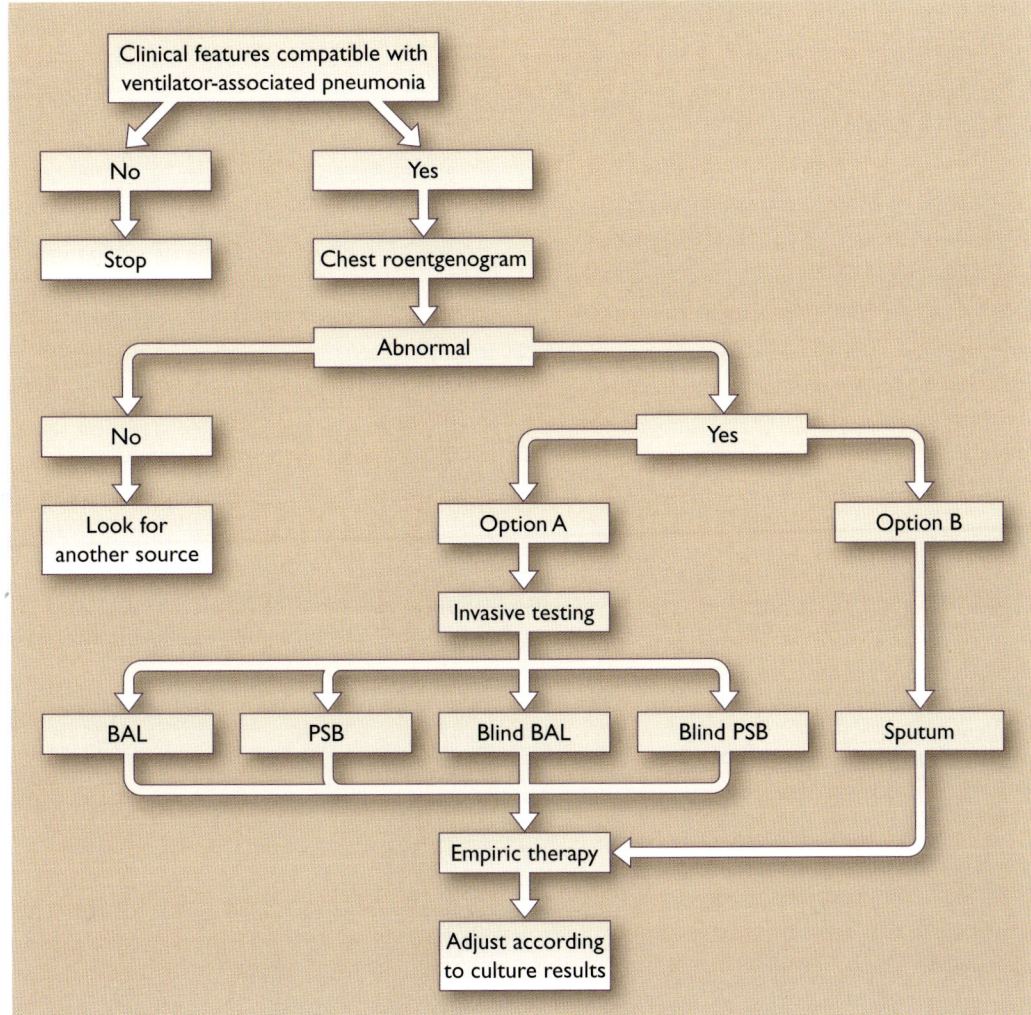

Figure 8-14. The diagnosis of ventilator-associated pneumonia is controversial, and the American College of Chest Physicians has suggested a compromise scheme. This guide may be used by clinicians who believe in the clinical diagnosis as well as by those who believe in the invasive diagnosis. BAL—bronchoalveolar lavage; PSB—protected specimen brush. (*Adapted from* Grossman and Fein [9].)

| Nosocomial Infections Including Pneumonia |

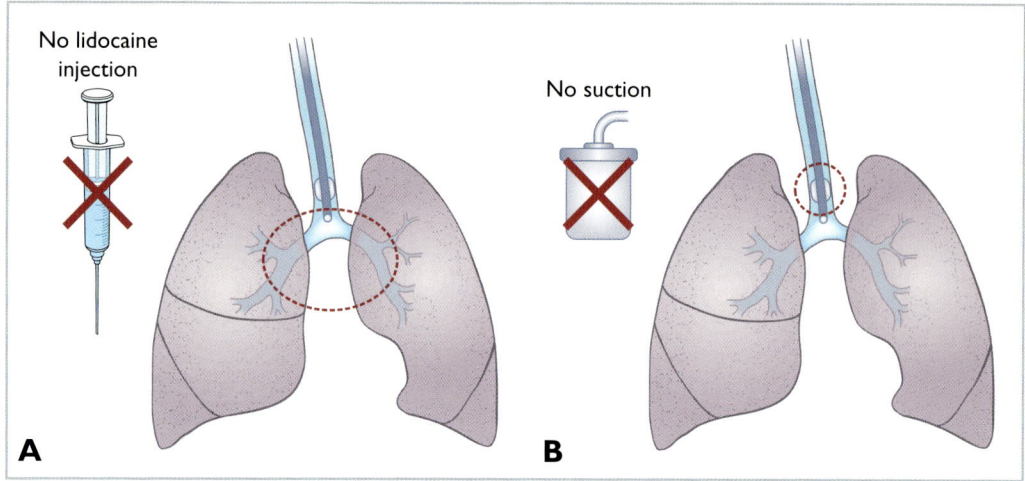

Figure 8-15. Bronchoalveolar lavage (BAL). BAL must be performed the correct way, and the figure shows the best way to obtain credible results. **A**, The method used without lidocaine prevents contamination of the airway (circled area). **B**, Prevention of suctioning prevents contamination of the bronchoscope. (*Courtesy of* GU Meduri, MD.)

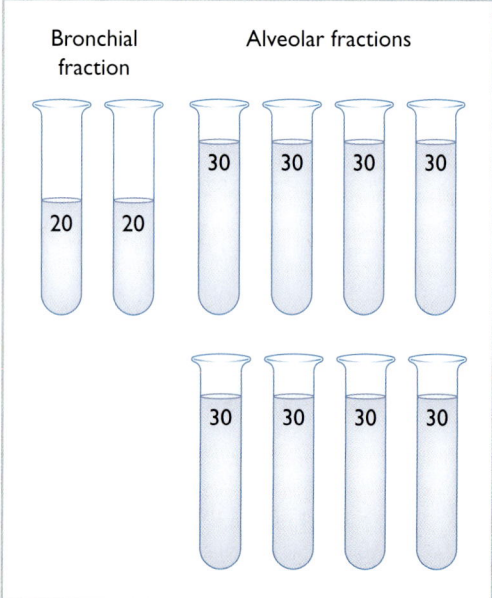

Figure 8-16. The correct way to perform bronchoalveolar lavage (BAL). Twenty milliliters of lavage fluid (normal saline, water, or similar fluid) is injected into the bronchus. The aspirate is kept separately and sent to a laboratory for tuberculosis, cancer, fungal, or viral investigation; this is the bronchial fraction. The next four aliquots of 30 mL are mixed and sent for all investigations needed; this is the alveolar fraction of the BAL. (*Adapted from* International Consensus Conference [11].)

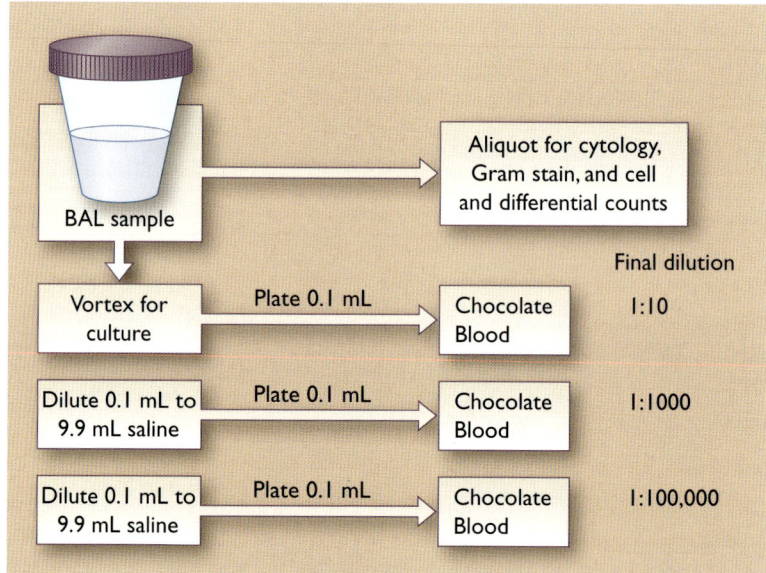

Figure 8-17. The bronchoalveolar lavage (BAL) sample. When BAL or mini-BAL is used to make an invasive diagnosis, this scheme is followed to obtain semiquantitative cultures. (*Courtesy of* Robert Baughmann, MD.)

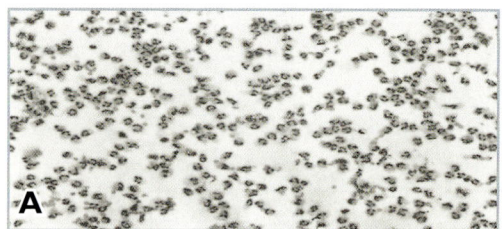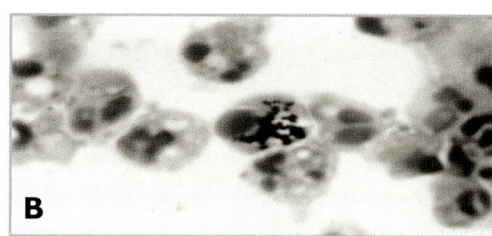

Figure 8-18. Microscopy of bronchoalveolar lavage (BAL). **A**, Inflammatory cells in the BAL sample. **B**, Macrophages phagocytosing bacteria. The panels present two features compatible with the diagnosis of ventilator-associated pneumonia.

Atlas of Pulmonary Medicine

TREATMENT OF VENTILATOR-ASSOCIATED PNEUMONIA

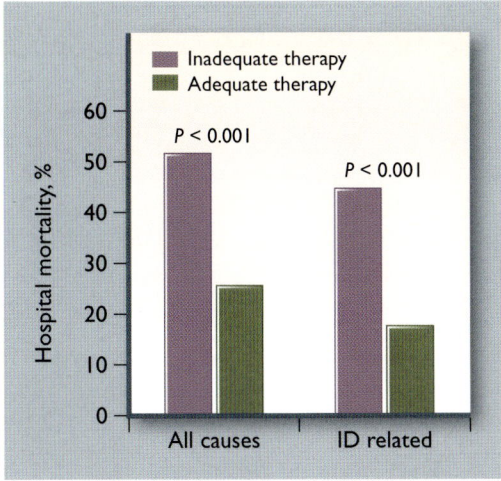

Figure 8-19. Hospital mortality. Patients who have severe sepsis must be treated with the correct antibiotics up front, as quickly as possible. Once the cultures are received, the antibiotics are tailored to them, a method called de-escalation therapy. Many clinicians advocate continued antibiotic treatment only until the clinical signs resolve, which is usually approximately 8–10 days. *Pseudomonas* spp is usually treated for 14–15 days [1]. Kollef *et al.* [12] studied the mortality in patients who were treated with adequate versus inadequate therapy. Those treated with adequate therapy had better all cause, as well as infection-related, survival. ID—infectious disease.

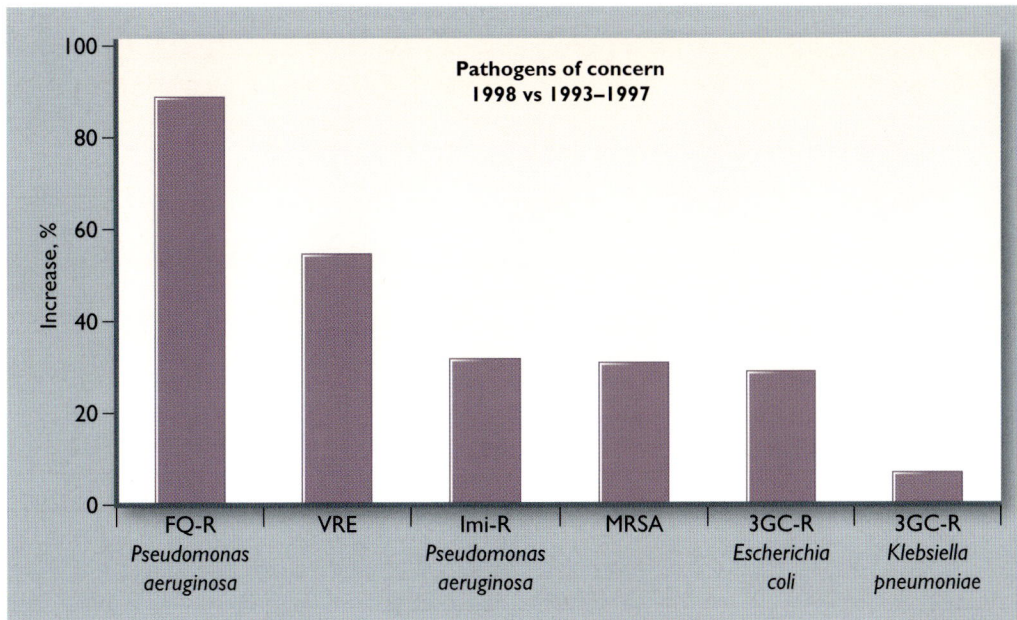

Figure 8-20. The remarkable increase in drug-resistant pathogens. Care must be taken to cover all the pathogenic bacteria in each unit. FQ-R—fluoroquinolone resistant; VRE—vancomycin-resistant Enterococcus; Imi-R—imipenem resistant; MRSA—methicillin-resistant Staphylococcus aureus; 3GC-R—third-generation cephalosporin resistant [13].

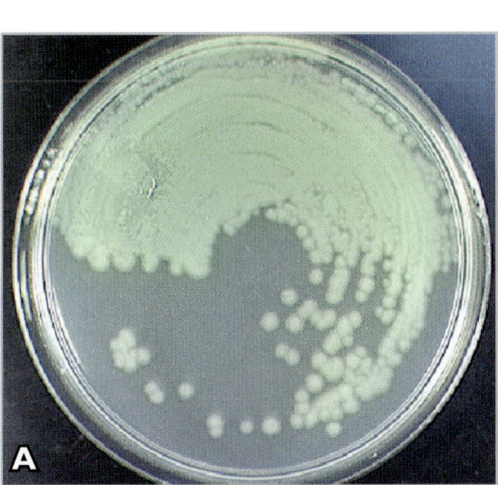
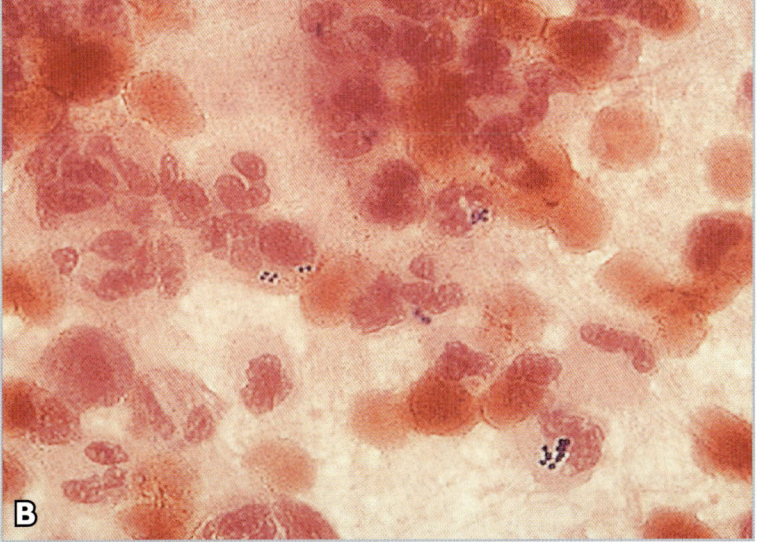

Figure 8-21. Bacteria that most commonly cause ventilator-associated pneumonia (VAP). These three bacteria, as well as bacteria producing extended-spectrum β-lactamases, must be covered. **A**, *Pseudomonas* spp are the most common gram-negative bacteria in VAP. **B**, *Acinetobacter* are not as common but are usually multidrug resistant.

Continued on the next page

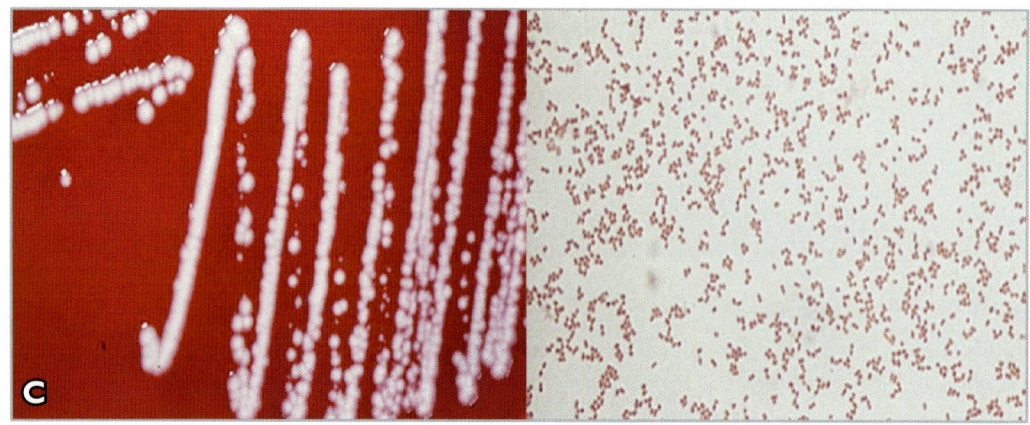

Figure 8-21. *(Continued)* **C,** *Staphylococcus* spp are the most common gram-positive bacteria and are also usually resistant.

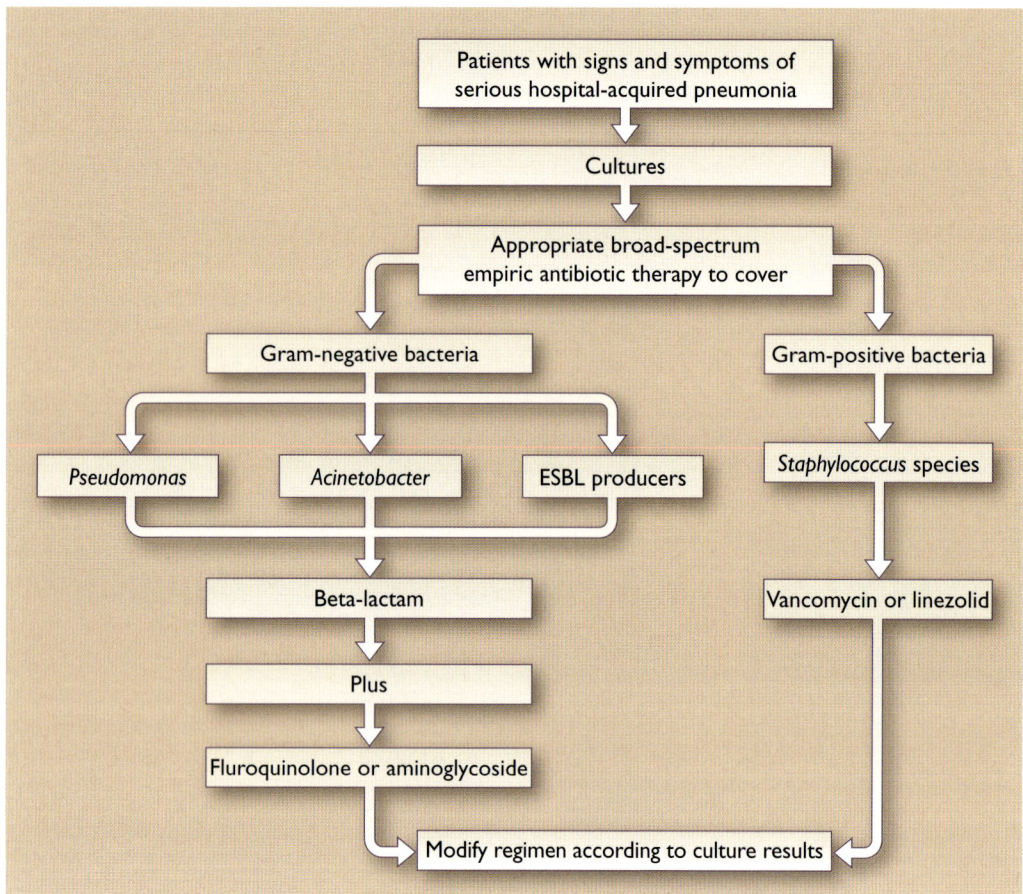

Figure 8-22. Treatment of patients with ventilator-associated pneumonia (VAP). This algorithm suggests initial broad-spectrum antibiotics to cover gram-negative and gram-positive bacteria. Once the cultures are back from the laboratory, the antibiotics are tailored to the bacteria. "β-Lactams" here include carbapenems and monolactams. Extended-spectrum β-lactams (ESBLs) and *Acinetobacter* may respond best to carbapenems [14].

REFERENCES

1. Rumbak MJ: The pathogenesis of ventilator-associated pneumonia. *Semin Respir Crit Care Med*, 23:427–434.

2. Craven DE, Goularte TA, Make BJ: Contaminated condensate in mechanical-ventilator circuits: a risk factor for nosocomial pneumonia? *Am Rev Respir Dis* 1984, 129:625–628.

3. Craven DE, Connolly MG Jr, Lichtenberg DA, *et al.*: Contamination of mechanical ventilators with tubing changes every 24 or 48 hours. *N Engl J Med* 1982, 306:1505–1509.

4. Macrae W, Wallace P: Aspiration around high-volume, low pressure endotracheal cuff. *Brit Med J (Clin Res Ed)* 1981, 283:1220.

5. Torres A, Aznar R, Gatell JM, *et al.*: Incidence, risk factors and prognostic factors of nosocomial pneumonia in mechanical ventilated patients. *Am Rev Respir Dis* 1990, 142:523–528.

6. Caplan ES, Hoyt NJ: Nosocomial sinusitis. *JAMA* 1982, 247:639–641.

7. Feldman C, Kassel M, Cantrell J, *et al.*: The presence of endotracheal tube colonization in patients undergoing mechanical ventilation. *Eur Respir J* 1999, 13:546–551.

8. Rumbak MJ: Ventilator-associated pneumonia. *J Respir Dis* 2000, 21:321–327.

9. Grossman RF, Fein A: Evidence-based assessment of diagnostic tests for ventilator-associated pneumonia. Executive summary. *Chest* 2000, 117:177S–181S.

10. Garner JS, Jarvis WR, Emori TG, *et al.*: CDC definitions for nosocomial infections, 1988. *Am J Infect Control* 1988, 16:128–140.

11. International Consensus Conference. *Chest* 1992, 102:557S.

12. Kollef MH, Sherman G, Ward S, Fraser VJ: Inadequate antimicrobial treatment of infections: a risk factor for hospital mortality among critically ill patients. *Chest* 1999, 115:462–474.

13. National Nosocomial Infection Surveillance/Centers for Disease Control: Surveillance report. February 2000.

14. Kollef MH: Hospital-acquired pneumonia and de-escalation of antimicrobial treatment. *Crit Care Med* 2001, 29:1473–1475.

TUBERCULOSIS AND NONTUBERCULOUS MYCOBACTERIAL INFECTIONS

Michael Lauzardo, Joanne Julien, and David Ashkin

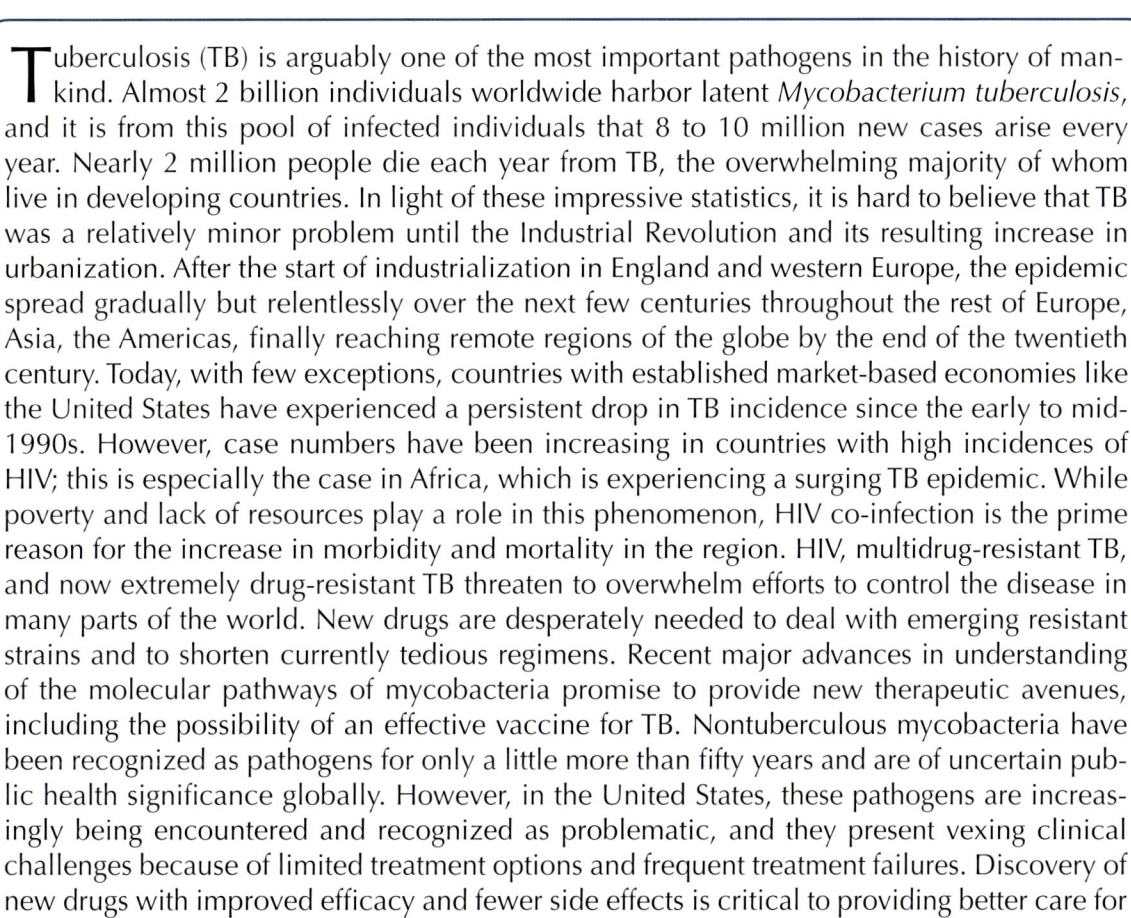

Tuberculosis (TB) is arguably one of the most important pathogens in the history of mankind. Almost 2 billion individuals worldwide harbor latent *Mycobacterium tuberculosis*, and it is from this pool of infected individuals that 8 to 10 million new cases arise every year. Nearly 2 million people die each year from TB, the overwhelming majority of whom live in developing countries. In light of these impressive statistics, it is hard to believe that TB was a relatively minor problem until the Industrial Revolution and its resulting increase in urbanization. After the start of industrialization in England and western Europe, the epidemic spread gradually but relentlessly over the next few centuries throughout the rest of Europe, Asia, the Americas, finally reaching remote regions of the globe by the end of the twentieth century. Today, with few exceptions, countries with established market-based economies like the United States have experienced a persistent drop in TB incidence since the early to mid-1990s. However, case numbers have been increasing in countries with high incidences of HIV; this is especially the case in Africa, which is experiencing a surging TB epidemic. While poverty and lack of resources play a role in this phenomenon, HIV co-infection is the prime reason for the increase in morbidity and mortality in the region. HIV, multidrug-resistant TB, and now extremely drug-resistant TB threaten to overwhelm efforts to control the disease in many parts of the world. New drugs are desperately needed to deal with emerging resistant strains and to shorten currently tedious regimens. Recent major advances in understanding of the molecular pathways of mycobacteria promise to provide new therapeutic avenues, including the possibility of an effective vaccine for TB. Nontuberculous mycobacteria have been recognized as pathogens for only a little more than fifty years and are of uncertain public health significance globally. However, in the United States, these pathogens are increasingly being encountered and recognized as problematic, and they present vexing clinical challenges because of limited treatment options and frequent treatment failures. Discovery of new drugs with improved efficacy and fewer side effects is critical to providing better care for patients with nontuberculous mycobacterial lung disease.

EPIDEMIOLOGY

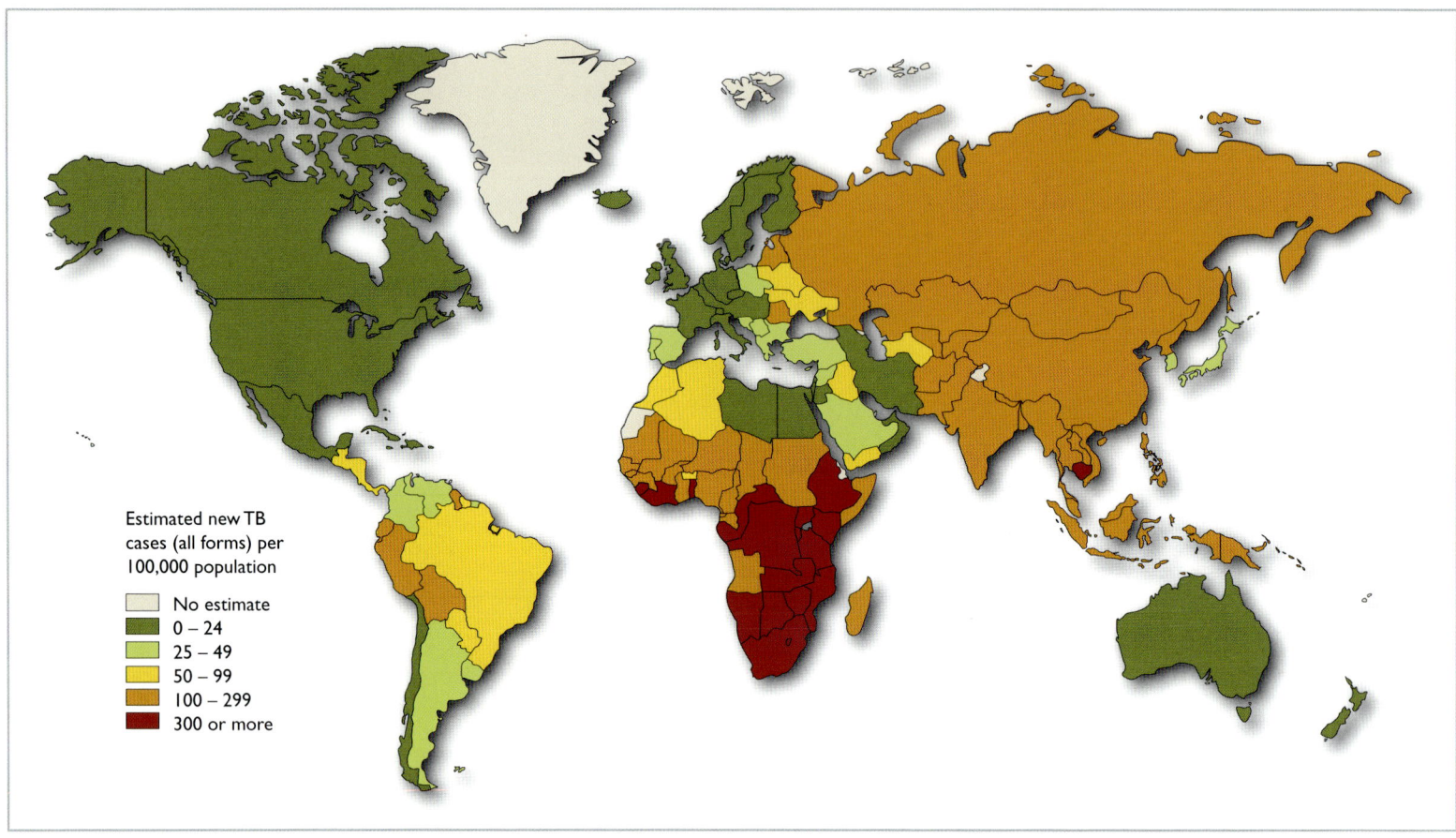

Figure 9-1. Estimated worldwide tuberculosis incidence rate. There were nearly 9 million new cases of tuberculosis (TB) worldwide in 2005, with 80% occurring in Asia and in sub-Saharan Africa. Approximately 1.6 million people died of TB, including 195,000 who were co-infected with HIV. Despite these daunting numbers, the incidence of TB has remained level since 2002. Unfortunately, while the incidence of TB is stable or declining in most areas of the world, the number of cases continues to increase in Africa, particularly in those areas already hard hit by the HIV pandemic. Multidrug-resistant TB (MDR-TB) is defined as TB that is resistant to isoniazid and rifampin, and is found in all regions of the world. It is estimated that there are approximately 455,000 new cases of MDR-TB each year. Extensively drug-resistant TB (XDR-TB) is defined as MDR-TB plus resistance to two of the most important second-line drugs for treating TB, the quinolones and injectable agents such as capreomycin, kanamycin, or amikacin. Data now suggest that XDR-TB, too, has a global distribution. In the United States, the majority of new cases of TB now occur among those born outside of the United States, usually those who hail from high–TB incidence countries. In total, 13,779 TB cases (a rate of 4.6 cases per 100,000 persons) were reported in the United States in 2006. This represents a 2.1% decline in the rate from 2005. The 2006 TB rate was the lowest recorded since national reporting began in 1953. In 2006, the TB rate in foreign-born persons in the United States (22.0 cases per 100,000 persons) was 9.5 times greater than that of US-born persons (2.3 cases per 100,000 persons). Elimination of TB in the United States will require interventions that address the global aspects of the disease [1–3].

Commonly Used Genotyping Methods

Method	Genomic Target	Uses	Comment
IS6110 RFLP	IS6110 insertion sequence	Current gold standard Determining clusters	Technically difficult Expensive Requires cultures be done first Weeks to get results
SPOLIGOTYPING	DR locus	Screening large numbers of isolates Determining strain family	Less discrimination than RFLP Technically easier of techniques Low cost Cultures not necessary
VNTR-MIRU	MIRU	Determining clusters	Can be automated so a large number of isolates can be evaluated simultaneously Faster than RFLP Cultures not necessary Results available in days

Figure 9-2. The ability to determine the molecular "fingerprint" or genotype of various strains of tuberculosis (TB) has revolutionized our understanding of its epidemiology. For example, conventional teaching held that only about 10% of new TB cases were the result of recent transmission; however, genotyping has since shown that between 20% and 50% of cases in urban areas are the result of recent transmission. Genotyping studies considering Mycobacterial laboratories have shown that approximately 3% of all positive TB cultures are the result of lab contamination.

Continued on the next page

| Atlas of Pulmonary Medicine |

Figure 9-2. *(Continued)* Other valuable insights into the transmission of TB include the identification of strain families such as the Beijing strain, which is common in Asia, but is increasingly becoming more common around the world and has been shown by some studies to be more virulent than other strains. Determinations in the future regarding what molecular features exist in common strains will conceivably shed more light on the molecular determinants of virulence. TB control programs are increasingly using molecular data on TB strains to identify groups at risk for TB, to improve contact investigations, and to evaluate program performance. The three most commonly used techniques for genotyping TB are RFLP, Spoligotyping, and VNTR-MIRU. Because of the ability to be automate, VNTR-MIRU is likely to become the gold standard for genotyping [4–7].

DIAGNOSIS

Use of the Laboratory in the Diagnosis of Active Tuberculosis

Staining and Microscopic Examination

The detection of acid-fast bacilli in stained smears is the easiest and most rapid test that can be performed. Approximately 50%–60% of patients with pulmonary tuberculosis will have positive sputum smears. The sensitivity of this test is limited in paucibacillary disease, as there must be a minimum of 5000–10,000 bacilli/mL present in the specimen for bacteria to be detected in the stained smears.

Nucleic Acid Amplification

RNA and DNA amplification kits are commercially available and allow for direct detection of *Mycobacterium tuberculosis* from a specimen within 8 hours. Target sequences of nucleic acid are amplified and detected though the use of nucleic acid probes. The presence of as few as 10 bacilli is required for a positive result, making this test a more sensitive test than smears. The sensitivity in smear-positive cases approaches 98% and is 70%–80% in smear-negative cases. The specificity is 98% in smear-positive cases.

Culture

All suspected mycobacterial specimens should be cultured in order to confirm speciation and to eventually perform antimicrobial susceptibility testing. Cultures are still considered to be the gold-standard in diagnosing tuberculosis, with a sensitivity of 80%–85% and a specificity of 95%. Of note, approximately 20% of patients with active tuberculosis disease will have culture-negative tuberculosis (negative cultures with signs or symptoms compatible with tuberculosis, a chest radiograph compatible with tuberculosis, a positive PPD, and clinical improvement when the patient is started on antituberculosis medications). Liquid media systems allow for rapid growth (within 1–3 weeks) when compared with solid media, where growth takes 3–8 weeks.

Drug Susceptibility Testing and Rapid Molecular Susceptibility Tests

Drug susceptibility tests should be performed on initial isolates to identify resistance patterns. Repeat testing is done on patients who continue to produce positive sputum cultures after 3 months of treatment. Recently, DNA-based tests that use PCR and reverse hybridization have been developed to rapidly detect genetic mutations associated with tuberculosis drug resistance. The assays are currently being studied to determine clinical utility in select patient populations in which drug resistance is suspected. At the present time, their widespread use is limited by expense and by dependence on sophisticated laboratory infrastructure.

Figure 9-3. Use of the laboratory in the diagnosis of active tuberculosis. *Mycobacterium tuberculosis* is a slow-growing microbe that proliferates best under aerobic conditions. After inhalation, the droplet nucleus bypasses the upper airway and is deposited in a respiratory bronchiole or alveolus. The bacillus then divides every 25 to 32 hours within the macrophage. Over the subsequent 2 to 12 weeks, when the baciili are 10^3 to 10^4 in number, they become abundant enough to elicit a cellular immune response that can be detected by the tuberculin skin test. Approximately 10% of individuals who acquire the infection will go on to develop active tuberculosis. The organism's thick, waxy coat is the basis for the acid-fast staining technique that has been in use for over 100 years. Smears are less sensitive and specific than culture techniques. Cultures are essential for species identification, drug susceptibility testing, and monitoring response to therapy [8,9]. PCR—polymerase chain reaction; PPD—purified protein derivative (skin test).

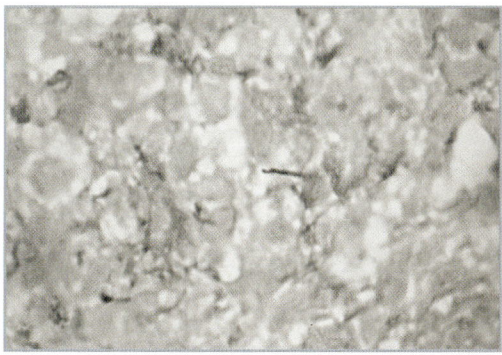

Figure 9-4. Acid-fast stain (Ziehl-Neelsen) showing *Mycobacterium tuberculosis*. Stained smears of sputum become positive when the microbial count equals or exceeds 10,000 organisms/mL. When one organism is seen per oil emersion field, the microbial concentration is approximately 100,000/mL. DNA amplification techniques may be used to detect *M. tuberculosis* in smear-positive sputum. When the smear is negative for bacilli, DNA amplification gives about 30% false-negative results. These methods are also available for histologic specimens that have been fixed in formalin and are applied to other body fluids, such as urine and pleural and cerebrospinal fluids. New methods using DNA microarray technology are now under development for identification of *M. tuberculosis* [10,11].

A. Presentation of Mycobacterium Tuberculosis Infection Versus Acute Disease

Criteria	Infection	Disease
PPD+	Yes	Yes/no (up to 33% of active cases are PPD-)
Symptoms	No	Yes
Chest radiograph	Normal (patients may have an abnormal chest radiograph unrelated to tuberculosis)	Abnormal
Communicable	No	Yes

B. Clinical Conditions That Lead to Active Tuberculosis After Infection

- HIV
- Silicosis
- Diabetes mellitus
- Chronic renal failure/hemodialysis
- Malnutrition associated with gastrectomy or jejunoileal bypass
- Solid organ transplantation (renal/cardiac)
- Carcinoma of head or neck
- Prolonged corticosteroids (> 15 mg/d) and other immunosuppressive agents
- Treatment with TNF-α blockers such as infliximab or adalimumab

Figure 9-5. A, Presentation of *Mycobacterium tuberculosis* infection versus active disease. After exposure to *M. tuberculosis* and the development of an immune response (positive tuberculin skin test), patients have a 5% chance of developing active disease in the next 2 years. Over the rest of the lifetime, there is an additional 5% risk of disease. **B,** In the presence of any of the risk factors listed in this figure, the odds of developing active disease are much higher. A person infected with HIV and exposed to *M. tuberculosis* has a 10% chance per year of developing active disease, unless adequate prophylactic measures are taken [12]. PPD+/- —positive/negative purified protein derivative (skin test for tuberculosis). TNF—tumor necrosis factor.

Criteria for Tuberculin Positivity by Risk Group

Reaction ≥ 5 mm of Induration	Reaction ≥10 mm of Induration	Reaction ≥15 mm of Induration
HIV-positive persons	Recent immigrants (ie, within the last 5 y) from high-prevalence countries	Persons with no risk factors for TB
Recent contacts of tuberculosis (TB) case patients	Injection drug users	
Fibrotic changes on chest radiograph consistent with prior TB	Residents and employees[†] of the following high-risk congregate settings: prisons and jails, nursing homes and other long-term facilities for the elderly, hospitals and other health care facilities, residential facilities for patients with AIDS, and homeless shelters	
Patients with organ transplants and other immunosuppressed patients (receiving the equivalent of ≥15 mg/d of prednisone for 1 mo or more)[*]	Mycobacteriology laboratory personnel	
	Persons with the following clinical conditions that place them at high risk: silicosis, diabetes mellitus, chronic renal failure, some hematologic disorders (eg, leukemias and lymphomas), other specific malignancies (eg, carcinoma of the head or neck and lung), weight loss of > 10% of ideal body weight, gastrectomy, and jejunoileal bypass	
	Children younger than 4 y or infants, children, and adolescents exposed to adults at high risk	

*Risk of TB in patients treated with corticosteroids increases with higher dose and longer duration.
†For persons who are otherwise at low risk and are tested at the start of employment, a reaction of ≥ 15 mm induration is considered positive.

Figure 9-6. The tuberculin skin test. Approximately 75% of newly diagnosed cases of tuberculosis are tuberculin skin test (TST)–positive when first diagnosed, although almost all cases become TST–positive after approximately 2 months of successful chemotherapy. Vaccination with bacille Calmette-Guérin produces a positive TST in most subjects, but this reaction tends to wane over time. After 10 years, most subjects are TST–negative, unless they have inhaled viable *Mycobacterium tuberculosis* in the interim. For those at high risk of becoming infected with *M. tuberculosis*, such as some health care workers, prison employees, and workers in homeless shelters, annual TSTs are advised. For these groups, a "two-step" baseline test is recommended. The initial skin test should be repeated in 2 to 4 weeks if the first reading shows less than 10 mm of induration. The second TST may elicit a "booster reaction," giving a larger degree of induration on the second test; the second test reading should be recorded as the baseline measure of the skin test [12].

CLINICAL PRESENTATION

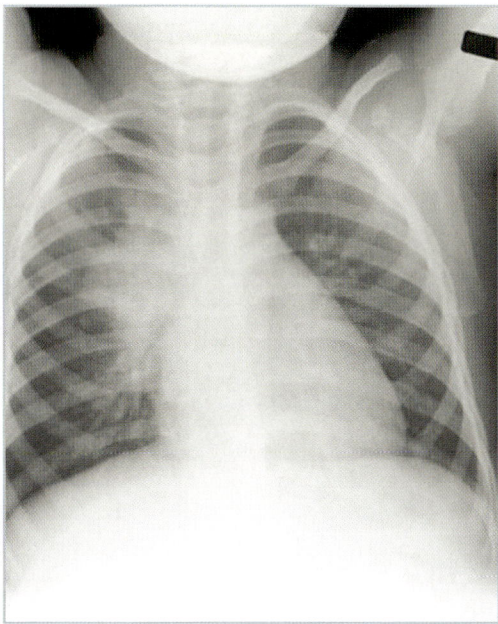

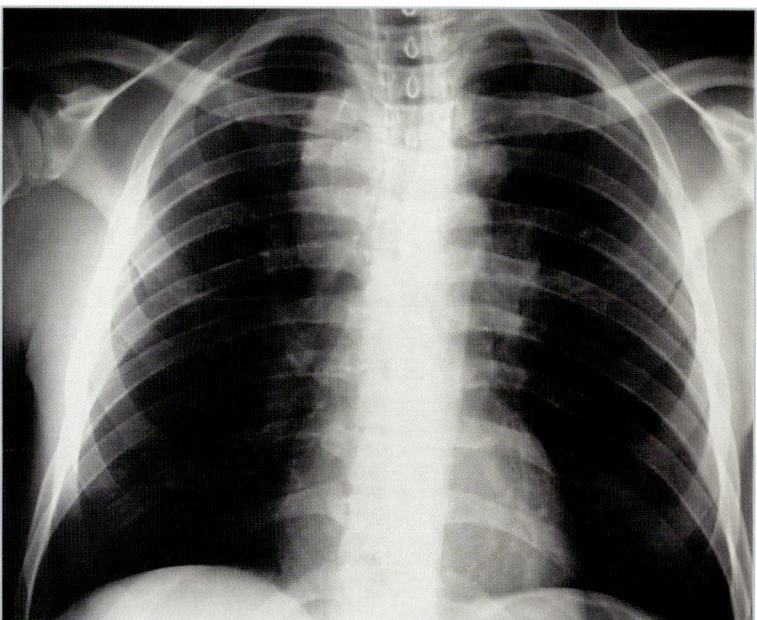

Figure 9-7. Progressive primary tuberculosis in a 6-year-old child after exposure to a case of smear-positive pulmonary disease. Children, especially those under the age of 5, develop tuberculosis as a complication of exposure to an active infectious case and are more likely to progress directly to active disease with a short or even absent period of latency. Radiographically, disease in children is manifested by intrathoracic adenopathy and associated atelectasis. Cavitation is very rare in this patient population. Because young children progress quickly to disease after exposure, children who are in contact with individuals with potentially infectious cases should be identified quickly and should receive isoniazid, even if their skin test is negative, until another skin test 8 to 10 weeks after the last exposure to the potentially infectious case can be performed. If that skin test is 5 mm or greater, isoniazid should be continued for a total of 9 months. Therapy for active disease is similar to that for adults, but ethambutol is used with caution because of the difficulty in assessing for ocular toxicity.

Figure 9-8. Paratracheal adenopathy in an immunosuppressed patient with smear-positive disease. Patients with immunosuppression—be it from HIV, chemotherapy, or advanced age—can have atypical chest radiograph manifestations of tuberculosis disease. This is particularly true for patients with advanced HIV. This patient had a CD4 count of 10 and was smear- and culture-positive for tuberculosis despite a lack of obvious parenchymal infiltrates. Remember, as much as 20% of patients with HIV and pulmonary tuberculosis will have normal chest radiographs. Always maintain a high index of suspicion for tuberculosis in the appropriate clinical and epidemiological context.

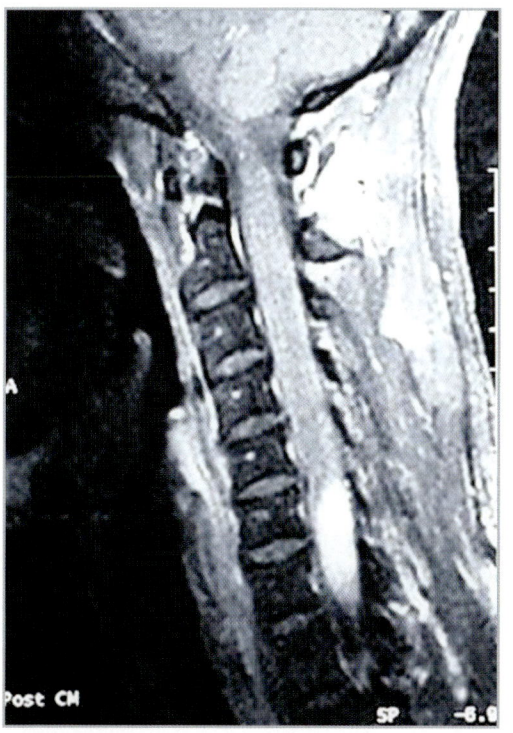

Figure 9-9. Immune reconstitution syndrome (paradoxical reactions). This is the sagittal view of the spinal cord in a 42-year-old man with immune reconstitution syndrome. This patient was diagnosed with tuberculosis (TB) after a biopsy of an enlarged cervical lymph node. He was found to be HIV positive at the time of the TB diagnosis with an initial CD4 count of 20 and a viral load of 250,000 copies/mL. He was started on four-drug anti-TB therapy, and after 6 weeks, he was started on highly active antiretroviral therapy. Within one month of dual therapy he had an excellent clinical response and an improved CD4 and viral load but developed a sudden onset of quadraparesis. Note the hyperlucent lesion within the spinal cord. This patient eventually regained strength in his extremities, and the lesion largely resolved with steroid therapy. Paradoxical reactions are most often reported in patients co-infected with HIV and usually occur within 2 to 10 weeks of initiating anti-TB or anti-HIV therapy. Patients present with transient worsening of tuberculosis signs and symptoms such as increased lymphadenopathy, fevers, malaise, and worsening pulmonary infiltrates. In addition, previously unidentified sites of infection may be unmasked, such as in the above case where central nervous sytem disease was not previously suspected. The reaction is attributed to an inflammatory response produced by rapid strengthening of the immune system; therefore, initiation of antiretroviral therapy should be delayed 6 to 8 weeks if possible after starting anti-TB medications [13].

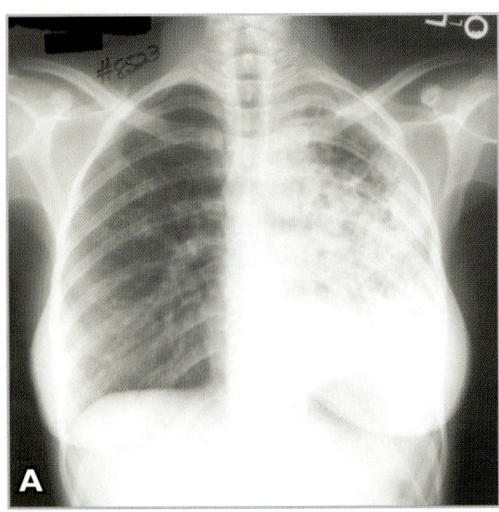
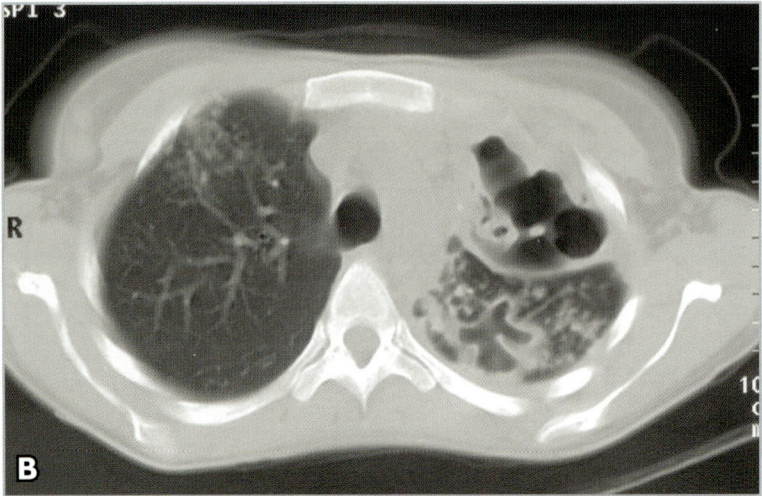

Figure 9-10. Cavitary pulmonary disease from tuberculosis. These images are from a 15-year-old woman who was a recent arrival from a high-incidence country in the Caribbean. (**A**) One can appreciate the dense consolidation with concomitant areas of increased lucency, suggesting cavitation of the left upper lobe. (**B**) This figure is a CT from the same patient that shows no normal appearing lung parenchyma on the left and minimal fibronodular changes in the right lung, most likely representing endobronchial spread of the disease to the contralateral lung. This patient eventually had a left pneumonectomy, once she was culture-negative. Complete destruction of the lung from tuberculosis is fairly uncommon in the United States, but when it does occur, it usually occurs in the left lung, possibly as a result of the more acute take-off of the left mainstem bronchus.

TREATMENT

A — First-line Antituberculosis Agents

Drug	Dosage Form	Daily Dose	Once-weekly Dosage	Twice or Three Times Weekly Dose
Isoniazid	Oral, intravenous, intramuscular	5 mg/kg (300 mg)	15 mg/kg (900 mg)	15 mg/kg (900 mg)
Rifampin	Oral, intravenous	10 mg/kg (600 mg)	—	10 mg/kg (600 mg)
Ethambutol	Oral	See below	—	
Pyrazinamide	Oral	See below	—	
Rifapentine	Oral	—	10 mg/kg (continuation phase) (600 mg)	—
Rifabutin	Oral	5 mg/kg (300 mg)	—	5 mg/kg (300 mg)

Suggested Ethambutol and Pyrazinamide Dosing, mg

	Weight, kg*		
	40–55	56–75	76–90
Ethambutol			
Daily	800	1200	1600
Three times weekly	1200	2000	2400
Twice weekly	2000	2800	4000
Pyrazinamide			
Daily	1000	1500	2000
Three times weekly	1500	2500	3000
Twice weekly	2000	3000	4000

*Based on estimated lean body weight.

Figure 9-11. A, Treatment guidelines for tuberculosis in the United States were revised in 2003. Active cases should be treated with four drugs: isoniazid, rifampin, ethambutol, and pyrazinamide. All isolates must have drug-susceptibility testing performed, and if drug resistance is identified, the treatment regimen must be modified accordingly. Treatment strategies should always emphasize an adherence plan including directly observed therapy [14].

Continued on the next page

B. Adverse Reactions/Drug Interactions of Antituberculosis Agents

Drug	Adverse Reactions	Drug Interactions
Isoniazid	Elevated transaminases, hepatitis, peripheral neuropathy, lupuslike syndrome, fever, rash	Phenytoin, disulfiram, corticosteroids
Rifampin	Pruritus, rash, fever, myalgias, hepatitis, orange discoloration of urine	Oral contraceptives, methadone, warfarin, antiretroviral agents, corticosteroids, β-blockers, digoxin, hormone replacements, tamoxifen, cyclosporine
Ethambutol	Retrobulbar (optic) neuritis, peripheral neuritis, rash	Aluminum salts
Pyrazinamide	Hepatitis, nausea, vomiting, nongouty/gouty polyarthralgia, hyperuricemia	Allopurinol

C. Second-line Antituberculosis Agents

Drug	Dosage Form	Daily Dose	Adverse Reactions	Drug Interactions
Ethionamide	Oral	250–750 mg daily	Nausea, vomiting, hepatitis, pituitary-adrenal dysfunction	H2-blockers, antacids
P-aminosalicylic	Oral	4–6 g twice daily	Abdominal bloating, diarrhea, hepatitis	H2-blockers, antacids
Fluoroquinolones				
Levofloxacin*	Oral, intravenous	500–1000 mg	Bone marrow suppression, arthralgias, CNS effects, nausea, vaginitis	Antacids, multivitamins, iron supplements, calcium
Moxifloxacin*		400–800 mg		
Gatifloxacin*		400–800 mg		
Streptomycin	Oral, intravenous	15 mg/kg/d (1 g) and 10 mg/kg in persons > 59 y (750 mg) for the first 2–4 months of treatment	Eighth nerve toxicity (hearing loss, tinnitus, vestibular changes), nephrotoxicity	NSAIDs, other aminoglycosides, vancomycin, amphotericin B
Capreomycin		15–30 mg/kg, up to 1 g	Renal, auditory, vestibular	Furosemide, ethacrynic acid, amphotericin B, vancomycin, cisplatin, other aminoglycosides, mannitol
Amikacin*		15–30 mg/kg	Renal, auditory, vestibular	See above
Kanamycin*		15–30 mg/kg	Renal, auditory, vestibular	See above

*Not approved by the US Food and Drug Administration for use in the treatment of tuberculosis. Gatifloxacin taken off US market in 2006 but still used in other countries.

Figure 9-11. *(Continued)* **B,** Adverse reactions and drug interactions of tuberculosis agents. **C,** Second-line antituberculosis agents are used when there is multidrug resistance involving all or almost all first-line drugs. Second-line drugs are generally more toxic, are less effective, and require careful monitoring by specialists fully familiar with their use. CNS—central nervous system; H2—histamine; NSAIDs—nonsteroidal anti-inflammatory drugs.

Drug Regimens for Culture-Positive Pulmonary Tuberculosis Caused by Drug-Susceptible Organisms

	Initial phase			Continuation Phase			Rating[‡] (Evidence)[§]	
Regimen	Drugs	Interval and Doses* (Minimal Duration)	Regimen	Drugs	Interval and Doses*[†] (Minimal Duration)	Range of Total Doses (Minimal Duration)	HIV−	HIV+
1	INH	7 d/wk for 56 doses (8 wk) or 5 d/wk for 40 doses (8 wk)[¶]	1a	INH/RIF	7 d/wk for 126 doses (18 wk) or 5 d/wk for 90 doses (18 wk)[¶]	182–130 (26 wk)	A (I)	A (II)
	RIF		1b	INH/RIF	Twice weekly for 36 doses (18 wk)	92–76 (26 wk)	A (I)	A (II)**
	PZA		1c[††]	INH/RIF	Once weekly for 18 doses (18 wk)	74–58 (26 wk)	B (I)	E (I)
	EMB							
2	INH	7 d/wk for 14 doses (2 wk), then twice weekly for 12 doses (6 wk) or 5 d/wk for 10 doses (2 wk),[¶] then twice weekly for 12 doses (6 wk)	2a	INH/RIF	Twice weekly for 36 doses (18 wk)	62–58 (26 wk)	A (II)	B (II)**
	RIF		2b[††]	INH/RPT	Once weekly for 18 doses (18 wk)	44–40 (26 wk)	B (I)	E (I)
	PZA							
	EMB							
3	INH	Three times weekly for 24 doses (8 wk)	3a	INH/RIF	Three times weekly for 54 doses (18 wk)	78 (26 wk)	B (I)	B (II)
	RIF							
	PZA							
	EMB				7 d/wk for 217 doses			
4	INH	7 d/wk for 56 doses (8 wk) or 5 d/wk for 40 doses (8 wk)	4a	INH/RIF	7 d/wk for 217 doses (31 wk) or 5 d/k for 155 doses (31 wk)[¶]	273–195 (39 wk)	C (I)	C (II)
	RIF		4b	INH/RIF	Twice weekly for 62 doses (31 wk)	118–102 (39 wk)	C (I)	C (II)
	EMB							

*When directly observed therapy is used, drugs may be given 5 d/wk and the necessary number of doses adjusted accordingly; although there are no studies that compare five with seven daily doses, extensive experience indicates this would be an effective practice.
[†]Patients with cavitation on initial chest radiograph and positive cultures at completion of 2 months of therapy should receive a 7-month (31-week; either 217 doses [daily] or 62 doses [twice weekly]) continuation phase.
[‡]Evidence ratings: A—preferred; B—acceptable alternative; C—offer when A and B cannot be given; E—should never be given.
[§]Evidence ratings: I—randomized clinical trial; II—data from clinical trials that were not randomized or were conducted in other populations; III—expert opinion.
[¶]Five-day-a-week administration is always given by directly observed therapy; rating for 5 d/wk regimens is AIII.
**Not recommended for HIV-infected patients with CD4+ cell counts less than 100 cells/mL.
[††]Options 1c and 2b should be used only in HIV-negative patients who have negative sputum smears at the time of completion of 2 months of therapy and who do not have cavitation on the initial chest radiograph (see text); for patients started on this regimen and found to have a positive culture from the 2-month specimen, treatment should be extended an extra 3 months.

Figure 9-12. Therapeutic regimens for active tuberculosis. Treatment regimens have recently been modified based on evidence from clinical trials and have been rated according to the strength of the recommendation and to the quality of evidence supporting the regimen. These regimens are designated A through C and I through III, accordingly. There are four recommended regimens for treating patients with tuberculosis (TB) caused by drug-susceptible organisms. Each regimen has an initial 2-month phase followed by a choice of several options for the continuation phase of either 4 or 7 months. The number of doses ingested, as well as the duration of treatment administration, defines treatment completion. Directly observed therapy is recommended for all cases of active TB. Because of the increasing incidence of isoniazid resistance, four drugs are necessary in the initial phase for the 6-month regimen. Treatment of multidrug-resistant tuberculosis should be based on susceptibility data and should include at least three drugs to which the isolate is susceptible. These cases present a significant clinical challenge and should be supervised by an expert. EMB—ethambutol; INH—isoniazid; PZA—pyrazinamide; RIF—rifampin; RPT—rifapentine.

Treatment of Tuberculosis in Special Cases

Pregnancy and Breastfeeding

- Untreated TB represents a far greater hazard to a pregnant woman and her fetus than does the treatment of the disease
- The initial regimen should consist of isoniazid, rifampin, and ethambutol, and if pyrazinamide is not used, the duration of teatment is nine months
- Although pyrazinamide is not routinely recommended because of insufficient data to determine safety, it should be considered in cases of drug-resistant or drug-intolerant cases
- Streptomycin is the only TB drug documented to have teratogenic effects
- Breastfeeding should not be discouraged in women being treated with first-line agents

Renal Insufficiency and End-stage Renal Disease

- Some medications used to treat TB are cleared by the kidney and require dose modification based on creatinine clearance
- Decreasing the dose of the TB medications is not the best option because of lower peak levels; therefore, increasing the dosing interval is preferred
- Isoniazid and rifampin are metabolized by the liver, so conventional dosing is used, but pyrazinamide and ethambutol require dose modification
- Administer medications after dialysis by directly observed therapy and consider therapeutic drug monitoring in all patients with TB and renal insufficiency

Hepatic Disease

- Poses special challenges because of the hepatotoxicity associated with TB medications
- Consider using a regimen with fewer potentially liver-toxic drugs such as rifampin or rifabutin plus ethambutol for a year, or rifampin or rifabutin, ethambutol, and pyrazinamide for 6 months
- Consultation is advised in these cases

Figure 9-13. Treatment suggestions for special cases of tuberculosis. Because of the myriad comorbid conditions found in tuberculosis (TB) patients, therapy can be quite challenging. The figure above lists some suggested strategies. In addition to the suggestions above, it should be remembered that not all TB medications are available parenterally, but the following drugs are available: isoniazid, rifampin, streptomycin, capreomycin, kanamycin, amikacin, and the quinolones [15].

Candidates for Treatment of Latent Tuberculosis Infection

Isoniazid treatment should be offered to adult tuberculin skin test–positive reactors with the following risk factors:
- HIV-positive
- Recent tuberculin skin test conversion (within 2 years)
- Close contact with an infectious patient
- Therapy with immunosuppressive drugs
- Immunosuppressed state such as diabetes, renal failure, and profound malnutrition
- Chest radiograph abnormalities and clinical evaluation suggesting old tuberculosis fibrotic lesions
- Silicosis
- Immigrants who are recent arrivals from countries with high prevalence

Figure 9-14. Candidates for treatment of latent tuberculosis infection. Isoniazid administered for 12 months reduces the risk of tuberculosis developing by more than 90% over the lifetime of the subject. Treatment for 6 months provides protection at a level of approximately 70%. Treatment for 9 months provides greater protection than does 6 months of treatment; 9 months of treatment is advised as a minimum for most patients. The dosage in adults is 300 mg once daily. A 4-month regimen of daily rifampin may be used for patients who cannot tolerate isoniazid. For HIV-positive adults, a 9-month course of isoniazid is recommended; however, if necessary, rifabutin may be used in some circumstances. Rifabutin may be used safely with indinavir, nelfinavir, amprenavir, ritonavir, and efavirenz, but not with hard-gel saquinavir or delavirdine [12,16].

Diagnosis of Latent Tuberculosis Infection

Test	QuantiFERON-Gold	Tuberculin Skin Test (TST)
Type of test	In vitro	In vivo
Antigens	Specific *Mycobacterium tuberculosis* antigens	Antigens cross react with other mycobacterial species
Result interpretation	No inter-reader variability	Inter-reader variability
Results	Available in one day	Available in 2–3 days

Figure 9-15. The tuberculin skin test produces a delayed hypersensitivity reaction to antigenic components of the organisms contained in the culture filtrate. Some antigens in the test are shared with other mycobacteria, which explains why up to 20% of patients may have false-positive reactions after bacillus Calmette-Guérin vaccinations or infection with nontuberculous mycobacteria. In addition, a false-negative rate of 25% is reported in patients with active tuberculosis disease. Newly developed blood tests such as QuantiFERON-Gold (QFT-G) (Cellestis, Valencia, CA) measure interferon-gamma release from the lymphocytes of sensitized persons when their blood is incubated with peptide mixtures of specific *Mycobacterium tuberculosis* proteins. This confers the advantage of increased specificity when compared to the tuberculin skin test (TST). The Center for Disease Control currently recommends that QFT-G can be used in all circumstances in which the TST is currently used [17].

Multidrug-Resistant Tuberculosis

Description

Resistance to both isoniazid and rifampin
1%–2% of TB patients in the US are resistant to isoniazid and rifampin

Contributing Factors

HIV
Close contact with patients with MDR TB
Noncompliance with TB therapy and inadequate follow-up
Increased immigration from areas of high prevalence (Asia, Africa, Latin America, the former Soviet Union)
Increased numbers of the homeless, intravenous drug users, and institutionalized patients
Cutbacks in public funding of TB control programs

MDR—multidrug-resistant; TB—tuberculosis.

Figure 9-16. Multidrug-resistant tuberculosis. Transmission of strains doubly resistant to isoniazid and rifampin was recognized in the late 1980s and increased in the 1990s. Such strains take their origin from patients who do not respond to treatment because of a large bacillary population of organisms (cavitary disease), inadequate ingestion of a prescribed regimen, or physician error in prescribing. Probable treatment failure should be considered when a positive culture from a patient does not convert to a negative culture within 3 months of therapy initiation. Repeat drug-sensitivity studies should be obtained at this point, and at least three new drugs to which the infecting organism is sensitive should be added. If the patient is not on directly observed therapy, such supervised therapy should begin at this point. Never add only one new drug to a failing regimen. Intermittent therapy should not be used except for injectable agents. Patients with multidrug-resistant tuberculosis or strains resistant to rifampin alone are at increased risk for failure and should be referred to a specialist for management.

Extensively Drug-Resistant Tuberculosis

Definition

Resistance to izoniazid and rifampin + any fluoroquinolone + one of the three following injectable drugs (capreomycin, kanamycin, or amikacin)

Contributing factors

Same as MDR-TB

Figure 9-17. Extensively drug-resistant tuberculosis (XDR-TB). Initially reported in 2005 in a group of predominantly HIV-positive South African patients, XDR-TB is presently found around the world, including the United States, China, and Russia. Like multidrug-resistant tuberculosis, the most common causes are related to nonadherence; however, transmission from person to person has been widely reported. The strain is considered highly lethal, particularly in HIV-positive patients, with mortality rates up to 98% reported in some studies. Clinical consultation is strongly recommended [3,18].

Recommendations For Co-Administering Antiretroviral Therapy and Rifamycin Agents

Protease Inhibitor	Antiretroviral Dose Change	Rifabutin Dose Change	Comments
Amprenavir	None	Decrease to 150 mg/day or 300 mg 3x/week	Rifabutin AUC ↑ by 193%, no change in aprenavir
Fos-aprenavir	None	Decrease to 150 mg/day or 300 mg 3x/week	
Atazanavir	None	Decrease to 150 mg every other day or 150 mg 3x/week	Rifabutin AUC ↑ by 250%
Indinavir	↑1000 mg q8h	Decrease to 150 mg/day or 300 mg 3 x/week	Rifabutin AUC ↑ by 204%; indinivir AUC ↓ by 32%
Nelfinavir	↑1000 mg q8h	Decrease to 150 mg/day or 300 mg 3 x/week	Rifabutin AUC ↑ by 207%; nelfinavir ↓ AUC by 32%
Ritonavir	None	Decrease to 150 every other day or 150 mg 3 x/week	Rifabutin AUC ↑ by 430%; no change in ritonavir
Duel Protease Inhibitor	**Antiretroviral Dose Change**	**Rifabutin Dose Change**	**Comments**
Kaletra	None	Decrease to 150 every other day or 150 mg 3x/week	Rifabutin AUC ↑ by 303%
Ritonavir with saquinavir, indinavir, amprenavir, fos-amprenavir or atazanavir amprenavir	None	Decrease to 150 every other day or 150 mg 3 x/week	
NNRTI	**Antiretroviral Dose Change**	**Rifabutin Dose Change**	**Comments**
Efavirenz	None	Increase to 450 mg/day or 600 mg 3x/week	Rifabutin ↓ by 38%. Effect of efavirenze and protease inhibitor on rifabutin concentration has not been studied
Nevirapine	None	300 mg/day or 300 mg 3x/week	Rifabutin and nevirapine AUC not significantly changed
Delavirdine	Rifabutin and delavirdine should not be used together		

Figure 9-18. Co-administering antiretroviral agents and rifamycins. Understanding the drug reactions between protease inhibitors (PI) and some non-nucleoside reverse transcriptase inhibitors (NNRTIs) with rifamycin agents is essential when prescribing an antituberculosis regimen. Rifamcyins induce hepatic P450 and CYP3A4 enzymes that accelerate the metabolism of many antiretroviral agents.

Continued on the next page

Figure 9-18. *(Continued)* Rifampin is a more potent inducer than rifabutin. In addition, it has been shown that certain antiretroviral agents can decrease the concentration of rifamycins. In general, rifampin should not be used in patients on antiretroviral therapy, and most experts will use rifabutin. All patients on rifabutin should be closely monitored for toxicity such as hepatitis, leucopenia, and arthralgia. (*Adapted from* http://www.cdc.gov/nchstp/tb/TB_HIV_Drugs/Rifabutin.htm.)

Preventing Transmission of Tuberculosis in Health Care Facilities

Administrative Controls

The first and most important level of TB control is the use of administrative measures to reduce the risk for exposure to persons who might have TB disease; this will include conducting a TB risk assessment of the setting

Developing and instituting a written TB infection control plan to ensure prompt detection, airborne precautions, and treatment of persons who have suspected or confirmed TB disease

Implementing effective work practices for the management of patients with suspected or confirmed TB disease

Ensuring proper cleaning and sterilization or disinfection of potentially contaminated equipment (usually endoscopes)

Screening and evaluating HCWs who are at risk for TB disease or who might be exposed to *Mycobacterium tuberculosis* (ie, TB screening program)

Coordinating efforts with the local or state health department

Environmental Controls

The second level of the hierarchy is the use of environmental controls to prevent the spread and reduce the concentration of infectious droplet nuclei in ambient air

Primary environmental controls consist of controlling the source of infection by using local exhaust ventilation to remove contaminated air

Secondary environmental controls consist of controlling the airflow to prevent contamination of air in areas adjacent to the source and cleaning the air by using high efficiency particulate air (HEPA) filtration, or UVGI

Respiratory-Protection Controls

The third level of the hierarchy is the use of respiratory protective equipment

Implementing a respiratory protection program

Training HCWs on respiratory protection,

Training patients on respiratory hygiene and cough etiquette procedures

Figure 9-19. Transmission of *Mycobacterium tuberculosis* is a risk in health care settings, and pulmonologists are frequently consulted with regard to risks after exposures. Although the risk of tuberculosis (TB) in the United States and other economically advanced countries is gradually decreasing, the risk to health care workers (HCWs) persists. The magnitude of the risk varies by setting, occupational group, prevalence of TB in the community, patient population, and effectiveness of TB infection-control measures. Regarding health care settings, associated transmission of *M. tuberculosis* has been linked to close contact with persons with TB disease during various procedures, including bronchoscopy, intubation, and autopsy, to name a few. The most recent guidelines from the Centers for Disease Control and Prevention recommend decreased frequency of tuberculosis screening based on the risk level of the setting and also give recommendations concerning personal respirator fit testing, ultraviolet germicidal irradiation (UVGI), and the use of blood assays for *M. tuberculosis*, such as the recently US Food and Drug Administration-approved QuantiFERON (Cellestis, Valencia, CA) test. For more detailed and updated information please visit the Centers for Disease Control website at http://www.cdc.gov/tb//TB_HIV_Drugs/default.htm [19].

NONTUBERCULOUS MYCOBACTERIAL LUNG DISEASE

Diagnostic Criteria for Pulmonary Nontuberculous Mycobacterial Infection

Clinical

Symptoms compatible with the disease including but not limited to cough, weight loss, fatigue, and hemoptysis

Nodules and/or cavitations noted on chest radiographs. High resolution CT scan of the chest with multi-focal bronchiectasis with nodules. Characteristic "tree-in-bud" appearance

Microbiologic

Positive cultures from at least two sputum specimens or

Positive culture result from one bronchial wash or

A histopathological specimen with AFB or granulomatous inflammation and a positive culture from either tissue, bronchial washing, or sputum

Figure 9-20. Nontuberculous mycobacteria. The diagnosis of nontuberculous mycobacteria (NTM) is challenging for a variety of reasons, including the fact that the disease may mimic tuberculosis (TB), and the fact that its organisms are found in the environment, especially in water and soil. Despite similarities to TB in clinical presentation, an important epidemiological distinction between TB and NTM is that, in the case of the latter, human-to-human transmission is not known to occur. When mycobacteria in clinical specimens are encountered, consultation with experts is recommended. If patients meet only some of the diagnostic criteria, and the clinical index of suspicion is high, patients should be followed until the diagnosis is confirmed or excluded. Once the diagnosis is established, the risks and potential benefits of treatment need to be assessed, and a decision to treat may be deferred if the patient is likely to be intolerant of therapy [20].

Treatment of Common Pulmonary NTM Pathogens

Treatment	Mycobacterium avium complex nodular disease	Mycobacterium avium complex cavitary disease	Mycobacterium abcessus	Mycobacterium kansasii
Macrolide	Clarithromycin 1000 mg TIW or 500–600 mg TIW azithromycin 500–600 mg TIW	Clarithromycin 500–1000 mg daily or azithromycin 250–300 mg daily	May use in combination with aminoglycosides and other injectables to suppress the disease; not curative	Use in rifampin-resistant cases as part of three-drug regimen
Rifamycin	Rifampin 600 mg TIW	Rifampin 450–600 mg daily	None	Rifampin 10 mg/kg max 600 mg daily
Ethambutol	Ethambutol 25 mg/kg TIW	Ethambutol 15 mg/kg daily	None	Ethambutol 15 mg/kg daily
Aminoglycoside	None	Consider streptomycin or amikacin	May use in combination with macrolides and other injectables to suppress the disease. Not curative.	None
Isoniazid	No role for isoniazid	No role for isoniazid	No role for isoniazid	Isoniazid 5my/kg max 300 mg daily
Surgery	Consider in treatment failures with localized disease	Consider in treatment failures with localized disease	Surgery for localized disease is the only predictable curative therapy	No clear role

Figure 9-21. Treatment regimens. Treatment regimens for the most common nontuberculous mycobacteria (NTM) causing pulmonary disease are listed in Figure 9-21. Although the macrolides have proven to be a very important addition to the care of patients with pulmonary disease caused by NTM, therapy remains very challenging for most patients. Drug intolerance and relapses are common, and therapeutic options remain few. In general, patients with disease due to either *Mycobacterium avium* complex or *Mycobacterium kansasii* should receive therapy for 1 year after culture conversion to negative. Close clinical monitoring for response to therapy and monitoring for drug toxicity is important because of the high rate of toxicity and failed therapy. The regimens listed in the figure are for the pathogens listed. Caution should be used in extrapolating these recommendations to other less common pulmonary NTM pathogens. Unlike with tuberculosis, in-vitro susceptibility data is not closely correlated with clinical response. Clinicians encountering these patients are strongly encouraged to seek expert consultation [20].

REFERENCES

1. World Health Organization: Tuberculosis. http://www.who.int/tb/en/.
2. World Health Organization: Tuberculosis challenges. http://www.who.int/tb/challenges/en/.
3. Centers for Disease Controls and Prevention: trends in tuberculosis incidence—United States, 2006. *MMWR* 2006, 56(11).
4. Barnes PF, Cave MD: Molecular epidemiology of tuberculosis. *N Engl J Med* 2003, 349:1149–1156.
5. Burman WJ, Reves RR: Review of false positive cultures for *Mycobacterium tuberculosis* and recommendations for avoiding unnecessary treatment. *Clin Infect Dis* 2000, 31:1390–1395.
6. Jou R, Chiang C, Huang W: Distribution of the Beijing family genotypes of *Mycobacterium tuberculosis* in Taiwan. *J Clin Microbiol* 2005, 43(1):95–100.
7. Bifani PJ, Mathema B, Kurepina NE, Kreiswirth BN: Global dissemination of the *Mycobacterium tuberculosis* W-Beijing family strains. *Trends Microbiol* 2002, 10(1):45–52.
8. Pai M, Kalantri S, Dheda K: New tools and emerging technologies for the diagnosis of tuberculosis, part II: active tuberculosis and drug resistance. *Expert Rev Mol Diagn* 2006, 6(3):423–432.
9. American Thoracic Society and the Centers for Disease Control and Prevention: diagnostic standards and classification of tuberculosis in adults and children. *Am J Respir Crit Care Med* 2000, 161:1376–1395.
10. Salian NV, Rish JA, Eisenach KD, et al.: Polymerase chain reaction to detect *Mycobacterium tuberculosis* in histological specimens. *Am J Respir Crit Care Med* 1998, 158:1150–1155.
11. Soini H, Musser JM: Molecular diagnosis of mycobacteria. *Clin Chem* 2001, 47:809–814.
12. American Thoracic Society: targeted tuberculin testing and treatment of latent tuberculosis infection. *MMWR Recomm Rep* 2000, 49(RR-6):1–43.
13. Narita M, Ashkin D, Hollender ES, Pichenik AE: Paradoxical worsening of tuberculosis following antiretroviral therapy in patients with AIDS. *Am J Respir Crit Care Med* 1998, 158(1):157–161.
14. American Thoracic Society, CDC, and Infectious Diseases Society of America: treatment of tuberculosis. *MMWR Recomm Rep* 2003, 52(RR11):1–77.
15. Centers for Disease Control and Prevention: treatment of tuberculosis. *MMWR* 2003, 52 (11):1–77.
16. Centers for Disease Control and Prevention and the American Thoracic Society: update: adverse event data and revised American Thoracic Society/CDC recommendations against the use of rifampin and pyrazinamide for treatment of latent tuberculosis infection—United States, 2003. *MMWR Morb Mortal Wkly Rep* 2003, 52:735–739.
17. Centers for Disease Control and Prevention: guidelines for the investigation of contacts of persons with infectious tuberculosis. *MMWR* 2005, 54.
18. Ghandi NR, Moll A, Sturm AW, et al.: Extensively drug resistant tuberculosis as a cause of death in patients co-infected with tuberculosis and HIV in a rural area of South Africa. *Lancet* 2006, 386:1575–1580.
19. Centers for Disease Control and Prevention: guidelines for preventing transmission of *Mycobacterium tuberculosis* in health care settings—2005. *MMWR* 2005, 54(RR-17): 1–141.
20. Griffith DE, Aksamit T, Brown-Elliott BA, et al.: An official ATS/IDSA statement: diagnosis, treatment, and prevention of nontuberculous mycobacterial diseases. *Am J Respir Crit Care Med* 2007, 175(4):367–416.

HIV/AIDS AND IMMUNOCOMPROMISED HOSTS

Laurence Huang, Matthew Fei, and Michael B. Gotway

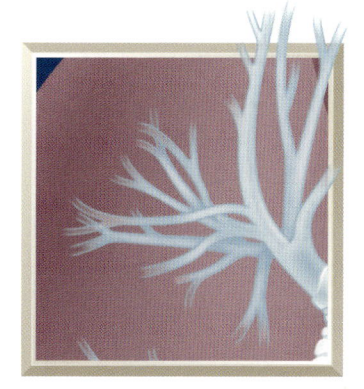
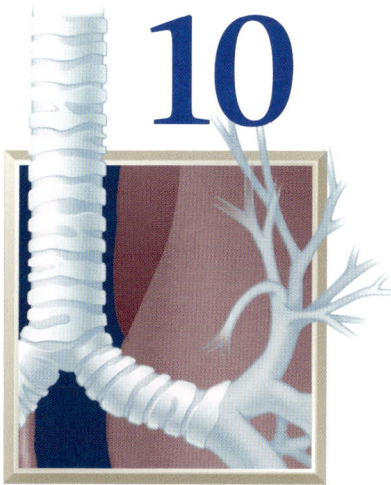
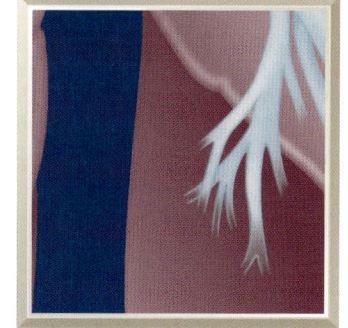

Over the past 25 to 30 years, the number of people with compromised immune systems has grown and will continue to do so. Immune compromise that leads to pulmonary infections is caused by 1) humoral, or B cell, deficiency; 2) cellular, or T cell, deficiency; and 3) neutrophil deficiency (neutropenia). Patients are at risk for developing infections from different pathogens depending on the deficiency present and the arm(s) of the immune system compromised.

The human immunodeficiency virus (HIV) is the cause of AIDS. While the disease predominantly leads to destruction of T-cell–mediated immunity, B-cell dysfunction often coexists. This places individuals at risk for a variety of usual as well as opportunistic processes. Prior to the HIV/AIDS epidemic, Pneumocystis pneumonia (PCP) was rare. In 1981, cases of PCP heralded the onset of the HIV/AIDS epidemic, and PCP became the leading AIDS-defining opportunistic infection. Currently, bacterial pneumonia is the leading HIV-associated opportunistic pneumonia in the United States, while worldwide, tuberculosis is the most common opportunistic pneumonia.

Several other major patient groups comprise the growing population of immunocompromised individuals. These include people with cancer who are receiving chemotherapy, people with either bone marrow or solid organ transplantation, and people who are receiving immunosuppressive medications. The type of chemotherapy used, the degree of immunosuppression required after transplantation, and the length of time one is immunosuppressed after transplantation plays a key role in defining specific pathogen risk. Advances in cancer chemotherapeutics, transplant technology, and antirejection agents have led to more patients being at risk for opportunistic pneumonias.

HIV/AIDS

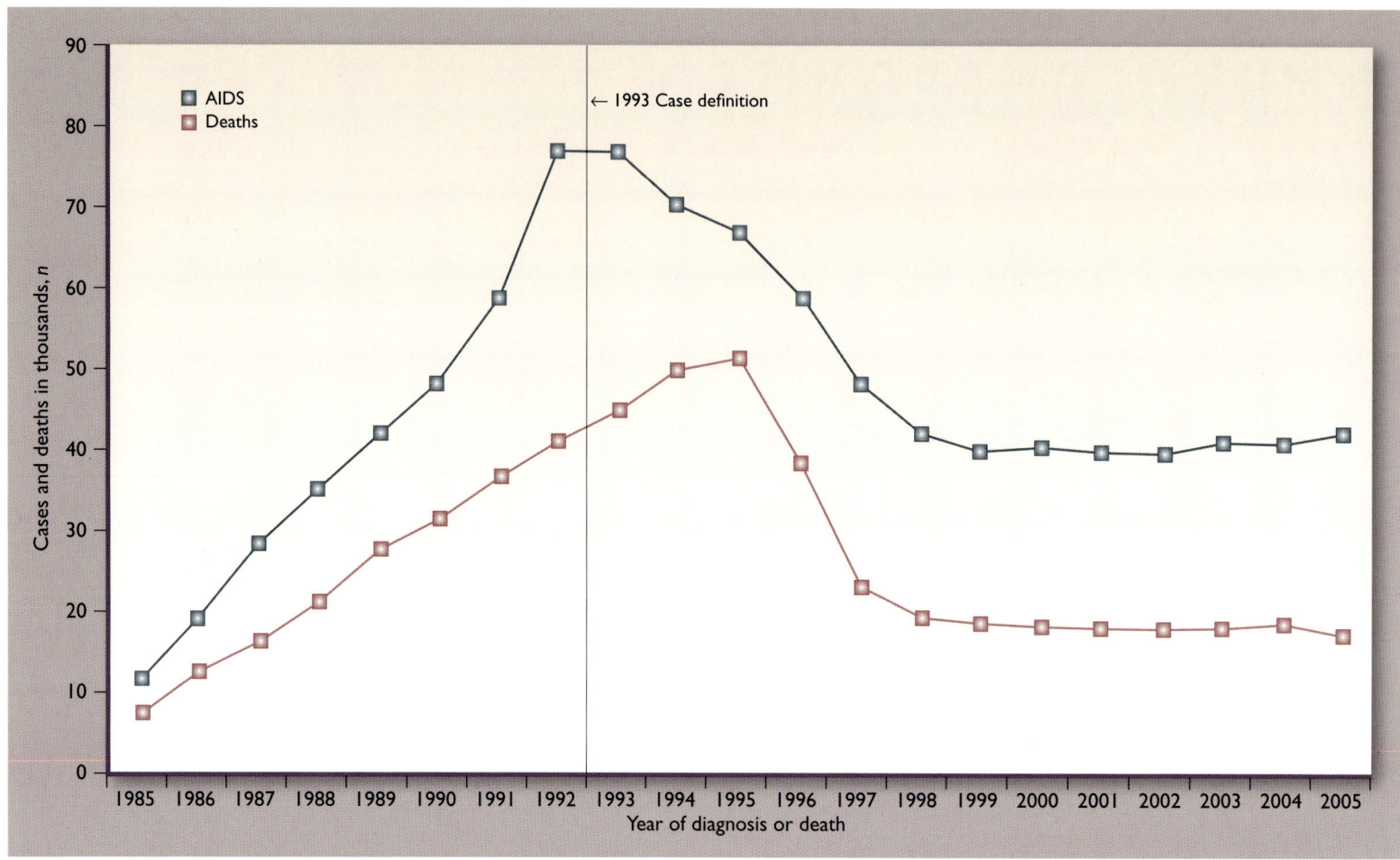

Figure 10-1. Estimated number of new AIDS cases and deaths among adults and adolescents with AIDS, 1985–2005: United States and dependent areas. The upper curve represents the estimated number of new AIDS cases (AIDS incidence); the lower curve represents the estimated number of deaths among adults and adolescents with AIDS. The peak in 1993 was associated with the expansion of the AIDS surveillance case definition implemented that year. Overall, AIDS incidence and deaths of persons with AIDS have declined. The declines are due in part to the success of combination antiretroviral therapy, which was introduced in 1996. (*Adapted from* the Centers for Disease Control and Prevention [1].)

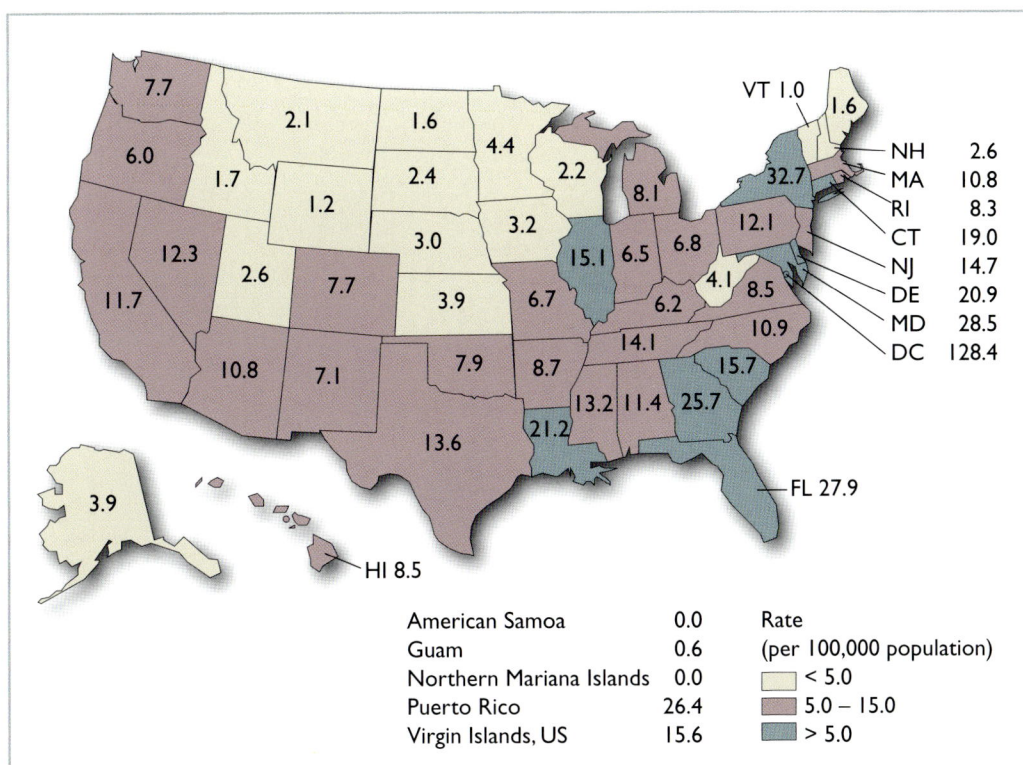

Figure 10-2. AIDS rates, 2005: United States and dependent areas. AIDS rates (cases per 100,000 population) for the year 2005 are shown for each state, the District of Columbia, American Samoa, Guam, the Northern Mariana Islands, Puerto Rico, and the US Virgin Islands. Areas with the highest rates in 2005 were the District of Columbia, New York, Maryland, and Florida. (*Adapted from* the Centers for Disease Control and Prevention [1].)

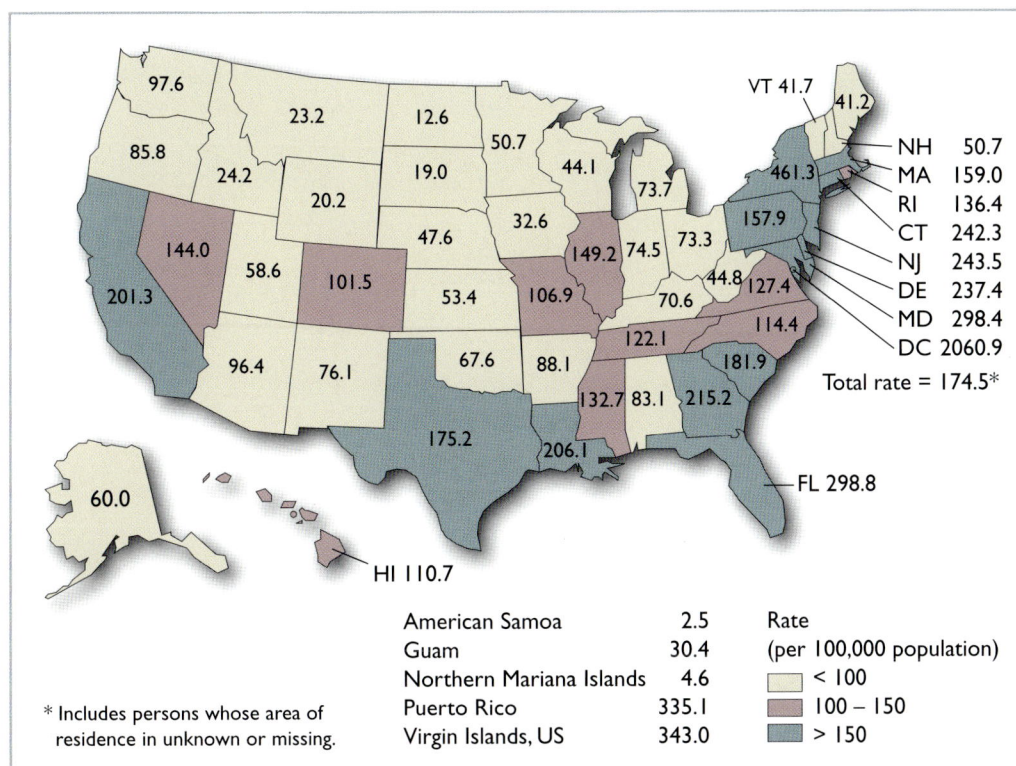

Figure 10-3. Estimated prevalence rates for adults and adolescents living with AIDS (per 100,000 population), 2005: United States and dependent areas. In the United States and dependent areas, the prevalence rate of AIDS among adults and adolescents was estimated at 174.5 per 100,000 at the end of 2005. The rate for adults and adolescents living with AIDS ranged from an estimated 2.5 per 100,000 in American Samoa to an estimated 2,060.9 per 100,000 in the District of Columbia. (*Adapted from* the Centers for Disease Control and Prevention [1].)

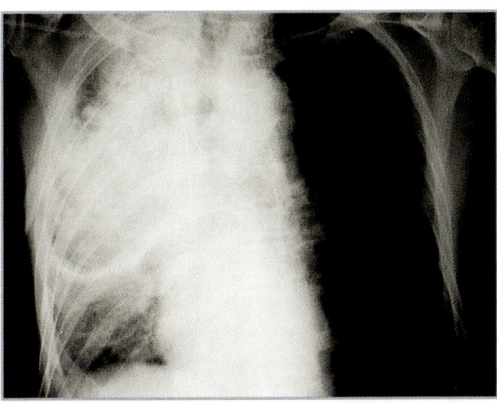

Figure 10-4. Chest radiograph of an HIV-infected patient, CD4+ cell count less than 200 cells/µL, with right lung consolidation. Blood and sputum cultures revealed *Streptococcus pneumoniae*. Bacterial pneumonia is the most common HIV-associated opportunistic pneumonia, and *S. pneumoniae* is the most frequently identified bacterial pathogen reported. In HIV-infected patients, pneumococcal pneumonia is often accompanied by bacteremia, especially when the CD4+ cell count is less than 200 cells/µL. (*Courtesy of* Laurence Huang, MD.)

| HIV/AIDS and Immunocompromised Hosts |

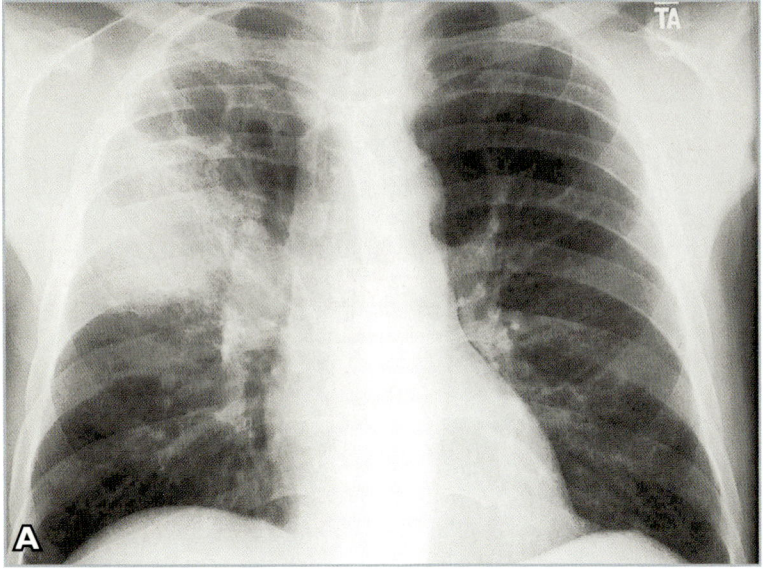
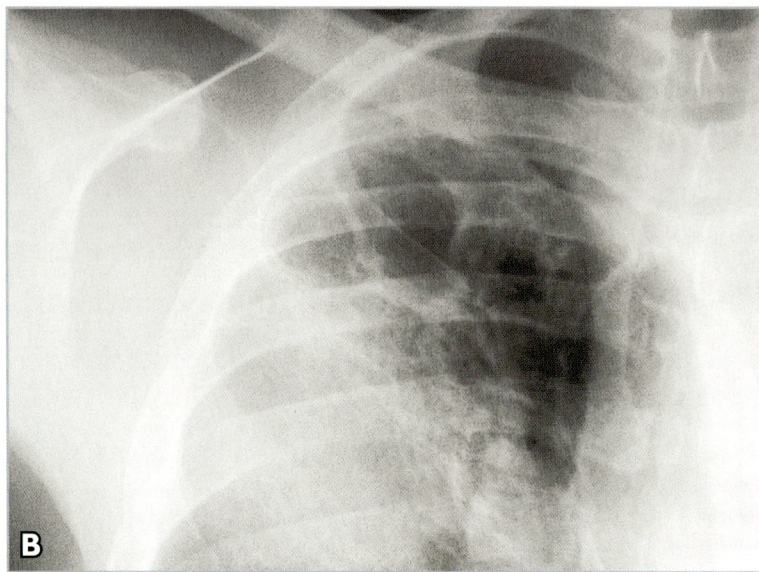

Figure 10-5. Chest radiograph of an HIV-infected patient, CD4+ cell count greater than 200 cells/μL, with right upper lobe infiltrate (**A**) and areas of cavitation (**B**). Multiple sputum acid-fast bacillus (AFB) stains were positive and AFB cultures grew *Mycobacterium tuberculosis*. Worldwide, tuberculosis is the most common opportunistic pneumonia found in HIV-infected patients. Typically, tuberculosis presents with upper lung zone opacities and areas of cavitation when the CD4+ cell count is greater than 200 cells/μL. The diagnosis and treatment of tuberculosis in HIV-infected persons is similar to that of individuals without HIV. (*Courtesy of* Laurence Huang, MD.)

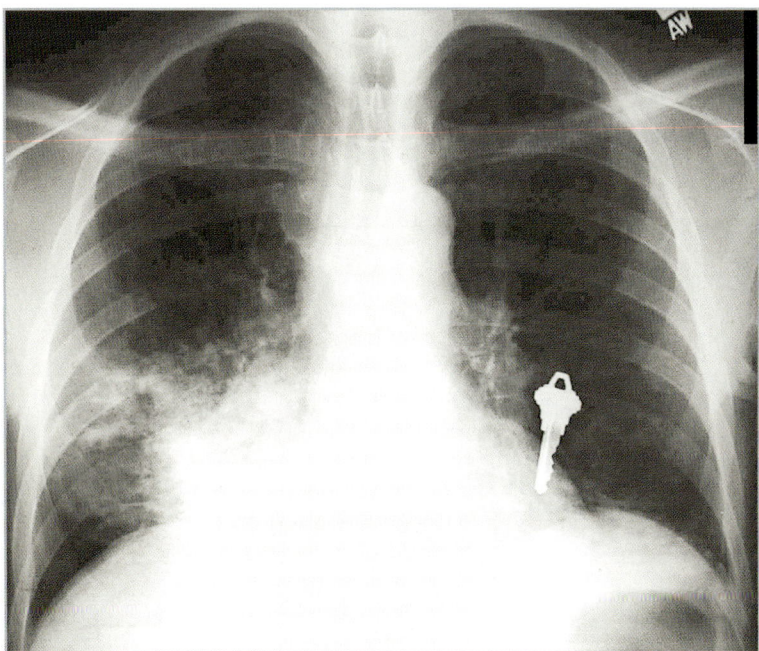
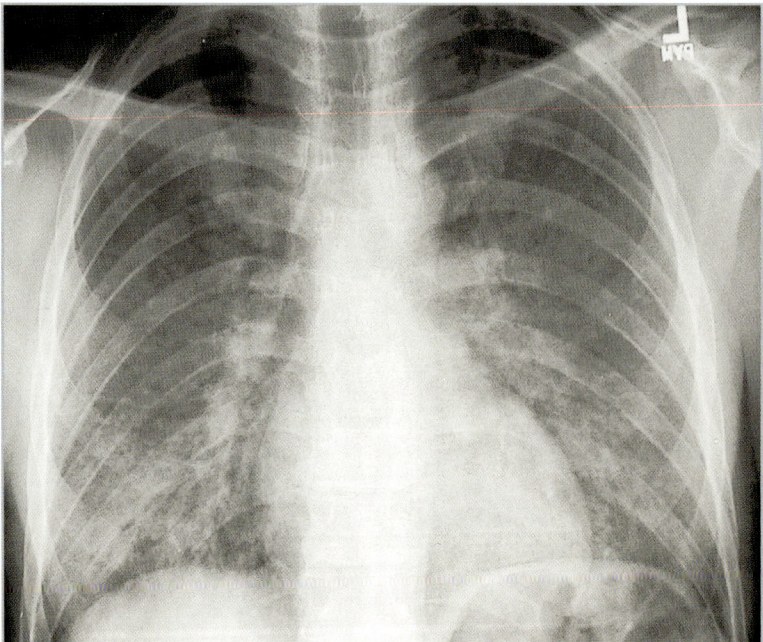

Figure 10-6. Chest radiograph of an HIV-infected patient, CD4+ cell count less than 200 cells/μL, demonstrating right lower lung zone consolidation with air bronchograms. Several sputum acid-fast bacillus cultures grew *Mycobacterium tuberculosis* that was resistant to rifampin. In this case, the key to the diagnosis of tuberculosis was knowledge of the patient's CD4+ cell count and an understanding that tuberculosis frequently presents with middle and/or lower lung opacities in such individuals (*key*). Prompt recognition of this presentation is essential for proper clinical management and for prevention of transmission. (*Courtesy of* Laurence Huang, MD.)

Figure 10-7. Chest radiograph of an HIV-infected patient, CD4+ cell count less than 200 cells/μL, revealing bilateral, diffuse granular opacities characteristic of *Pneumocystis* pneumonia. Bronchoscopy with bronchoalveolar lavage fluid examination revealed *Pneumocystis* organisms. Although its incidence has decreased, *Pneumocystis* pneumonia remains a significant cause of morbidity and mortality among HIV-infected and other immunocompromised persons. Bronchoscopy with bronchoalveolar lavage remains the gold standard procedure for diagnosing *Pneumocystis*. Trimethoprim-sulfamethoxazole is the recommended first-line treatment. (*Courtesy of* Laurence Huang, MD.)

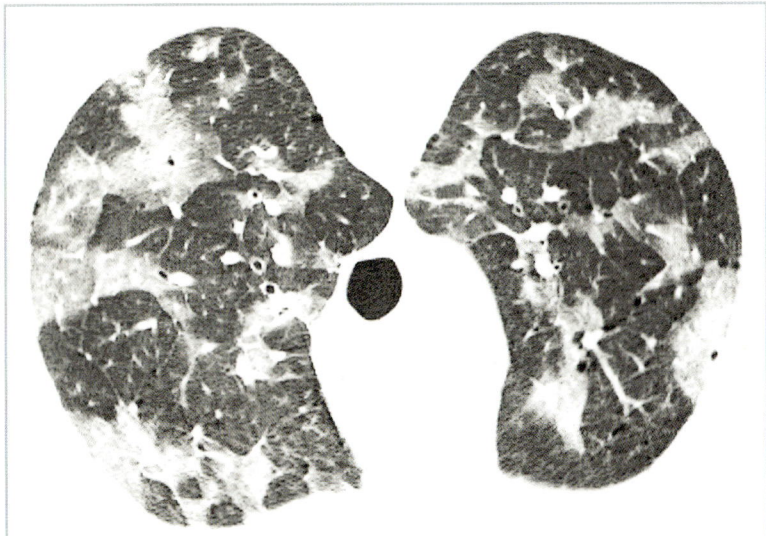

Figure 10-8. Chest high-resolution CT of an HIV-infected patient, CD4+ cell count less than 200 cells/μL, whose chest radiograph was normal, demonstrating patchy areas of ground glass opacities characteristic of *Pneumocystis* pneumonia. Induced sputum examination revealed *Pneumocystis* organisms. HIV-infected patients with *Pneumocystis* pneumonia may present with a normal or minimally abnormal chest radiograph. In these cases, high-resolution CT may be a useful test. Patients with ground glass opacities should undergo procedures to diagnose *Pneumocystis*, whereas those without ground glass opacities are unlikely to have *Pneumocystis* pneumonia, so close observation or procedures to diagnose non-*Pneumocystis* pathogens should be considered. (*Courtesy of* Laurence Huang, MD.)

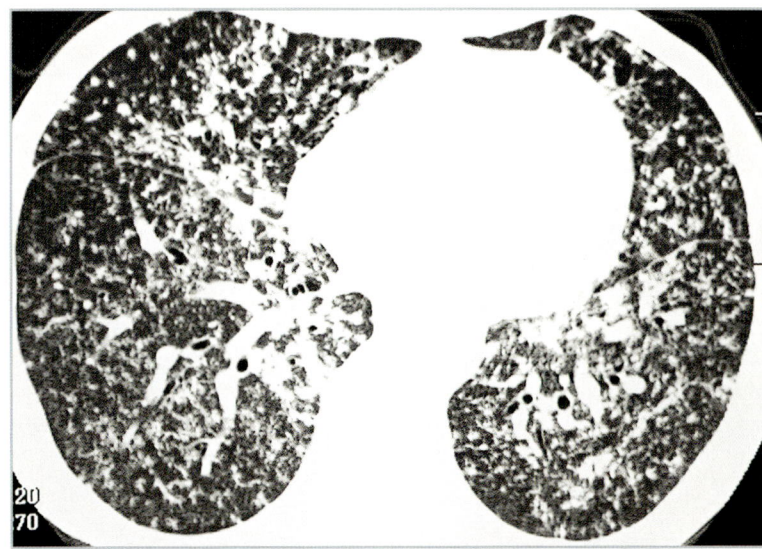

Figure 10-9. Chest CT of an HIV-infected patient, CD4+ cell count less than 50 cells/μL, revealing a miliary or micronodular pattern. The diagnosis of coccidioidomycosis was established by sputum, blood, and bronchoalveolar lavage fluid cultures. In HIV-infected persons, coccidioidomycosis often presents with disseminated extrapulmonary disease. The diagnosis was first suggested by the patient's history of extensive time spent in an area endemic for *Coccidioides immitis*. (*Courtesy of* Laurence Huang, MD.)

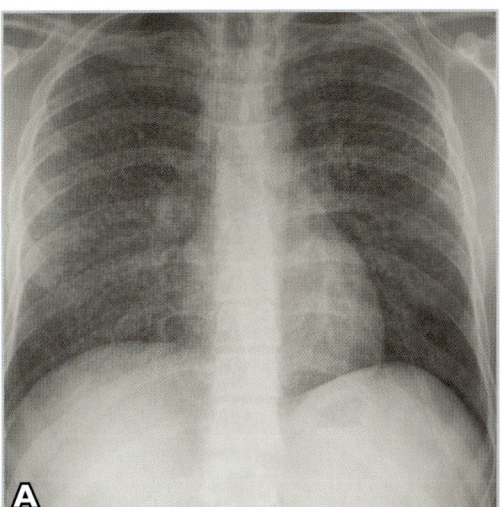
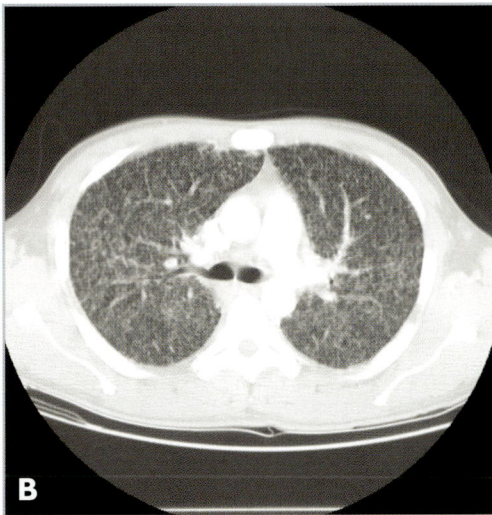

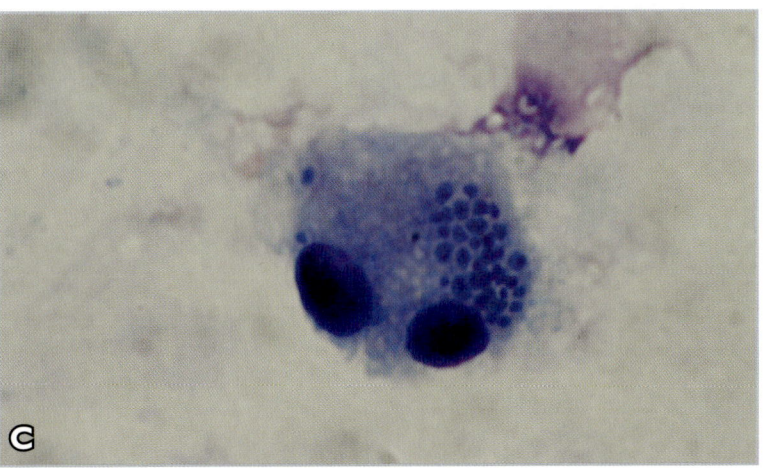

Figure 10-10. Chest radiograph (**A**) and chest CT (**B**) of an HIV-infected patient, CD4+ cell count less than 50 cells/μL, demonstrating a diffuse miliary pattern. The patient was started on empiric antituberculous therapy without improvement. Bronchoscopy with bronchoalveolar lavage and transbronchial biopsies revealed *Histoplasma capsulatum* (**C**). The urine *Histoplasma* antigen was also positive. A miliary pattern is nonspecific in HIV-infected persons, and *Mycobacterium tuberculosis* and endemic fungal pneumonias due to *Coccidioides immitis* and *H. capsulatum* are chief considerations. (*Courtesy of* Matthew Fei, MD.)

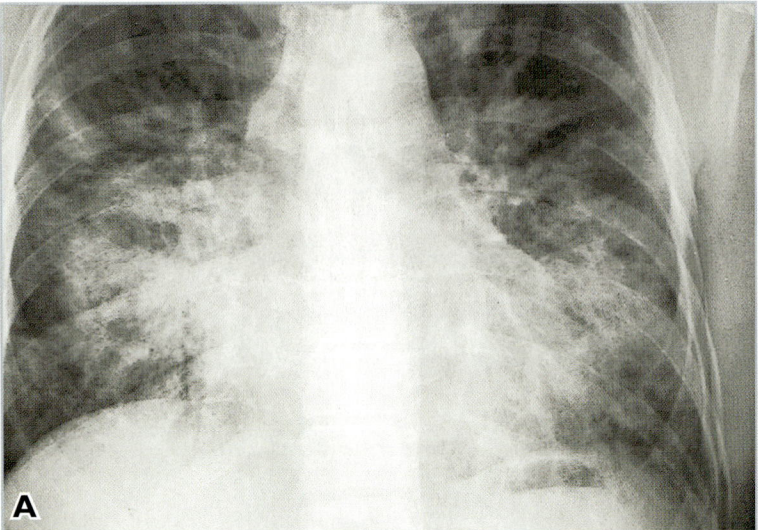
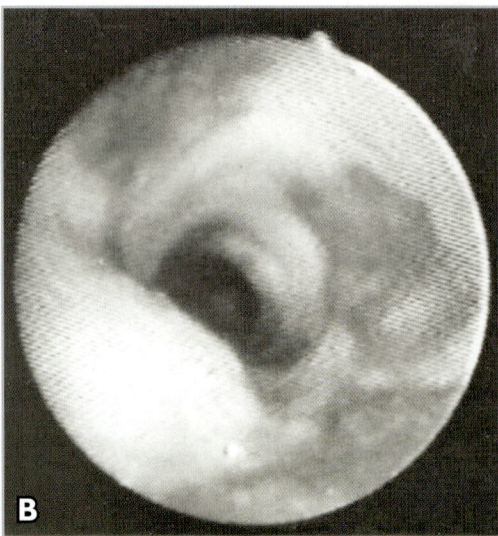

Figure 10-11. Chest radiograph of an HIV-infected patient, CD4+ cell count less than 100 cells/μL, demonstrating the characteristic bilateral, middle-lower lung zone, perihilar appearance of pulmonary Kaposi's sarcoma (**A**). Although the patient had no evidence of mucocutaneous Kaposi's sarcoma lesions, bronchoscopy revealed multiple Kaposi's lesions within the tracheobronchial tree (**B**). Kaposi's sarcoma is an AIDS-defining condition and is associated with human herpesvirus 8 infection. (*Courtesy of* Laurence Huang, MD.)

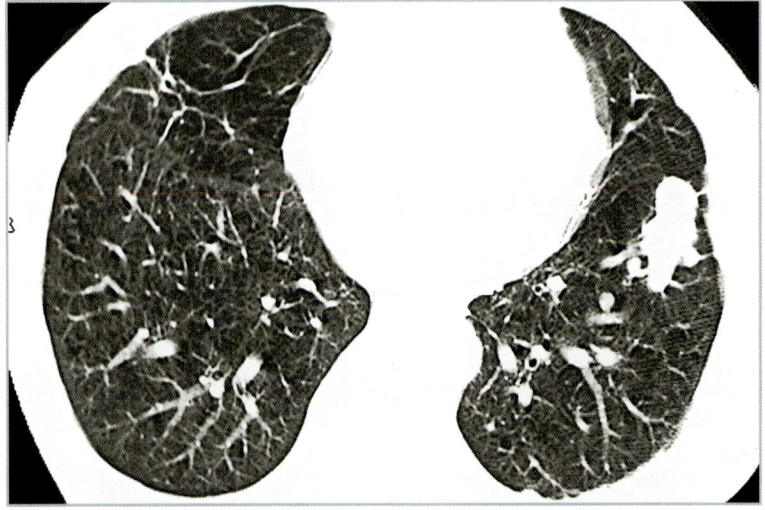

Figure 10-12. Chest CT of an HIV-infected patient, CD4+ cell count less than 100 cells/μL, demonstrating a lobulated left lung mass. CT-guided fine needle aspiration diagnosed non-Hodgkin's lymphoma. Non-Hodgkin's lymphoma is a common HIV-associated neoplasm. (*Courtesy of* Laurence Huang, MD.)

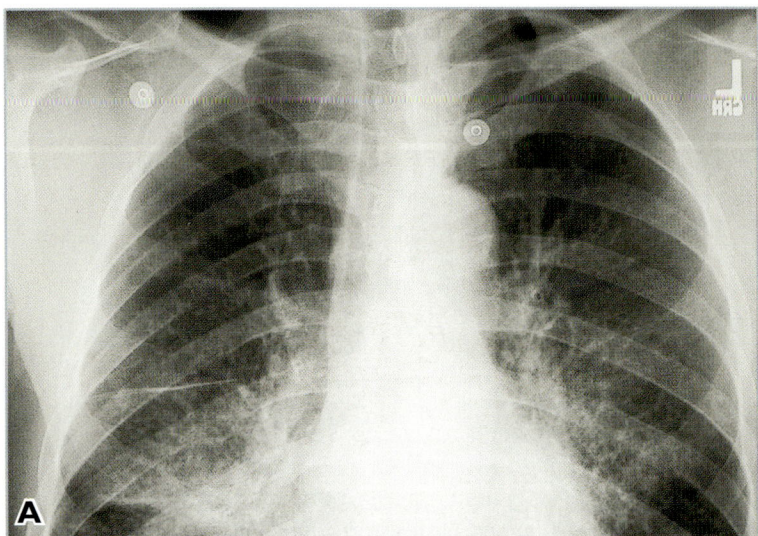
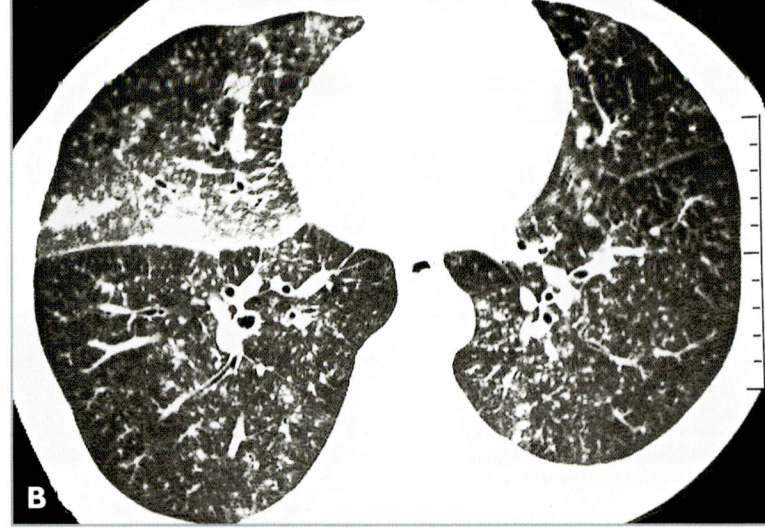

Figure 10-13. Chest radiograph (**A**) and chest high resolution CT (**B**) of an HIV-infected patient, CD4+ cell count less than 200 cells/μL, revealing bilateral, diffuse micronodules and right lower lobe consolidation. Although the presentation was most suspicious for mycobacterial or fungal pneumonia, the patient was diagnosed with lymphocytic interstitial pneumonitis by lung biopsy.

Continued on the next page

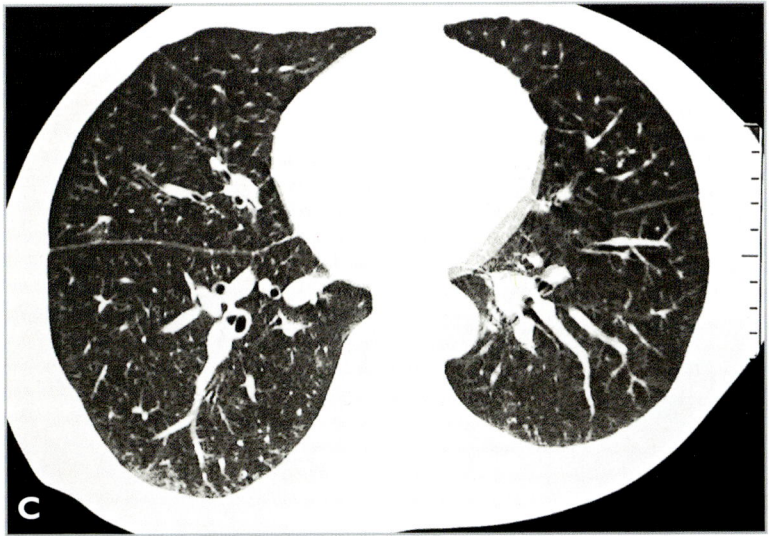

Figure 10-13. *(Continued)* The patient was treated with combination antiretroviral therapy alone, and there was subsequent improvement in his radiographic findings (**C**). Lymphocytic interstitial pneumonitis is an uncommon pulmonary disorder in HIV-infected adults but is more common in HIV-infected children [2]. (*Courtesy of* Laurence Huang, MD.)

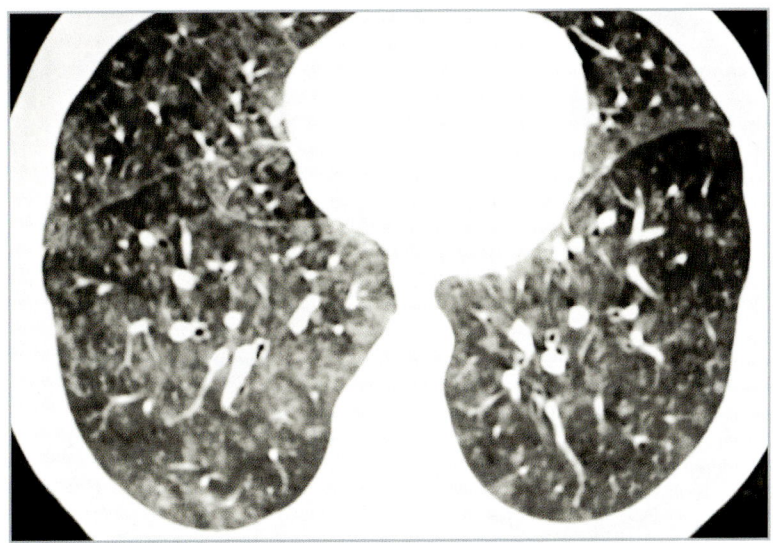

Figure 10-14. Chest high-resolution CT of an HIV-infected patient, with a nadir CD4+ cell count less than 100 cells/μL, which subsequently increased to 300 cells/μL with combination antiretroviral therapy. The patient developed progressive dyspnea and cough during the course of her immune reconstitution. The chest high-resolution CT reveals bilateral ground glass opacities, which were initially most concerning for *Pneumocystis* pneumonia. Of note, the patient reported owning two lovebirds, one button quail, and a diamond dove, which shifted the diagnostic evaluation toward interstitial lung disease. Subsequently, she was diagnosed with hypersensitivity pneumonitis by video-assisted thoracoscopic lung biopsy. Her symptoms and radiographic findings completely resolved after removal of the birds [3]. (*Courtesy of* Laurence Huang, MD.)

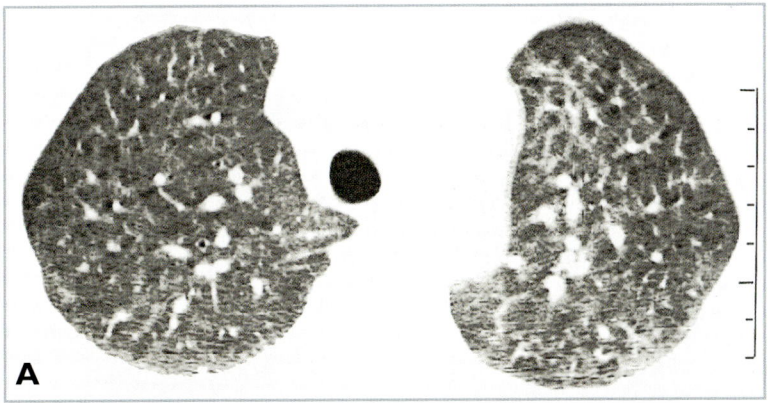
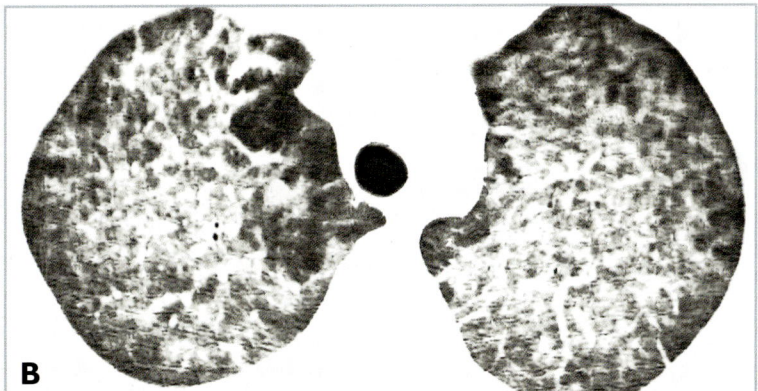

Figure 10-15. Chest high-resolution CTs of an HIV-infected patient, CD4+ cell count less than 100 cells/μL, who was diagnosed with *Pneumocystis* pneumonia (**A**) and then developed immune reconstitution syndrome after the subsequent initiation of combination antiretroviral therapy (**B**). HIV-infected patients with opportunistic infections who receive concurrent treatment for both opportunistic and HIV infections may develop a paradoxical worsening due to immune reconstitution syndrome. The diagnosis of immune reconstitution syndrome, however, must be one of exclusion. (*Courtesy of* Laurence Huang, MD.)

OTHER IMMUNOCOMPROMISED HOSTS

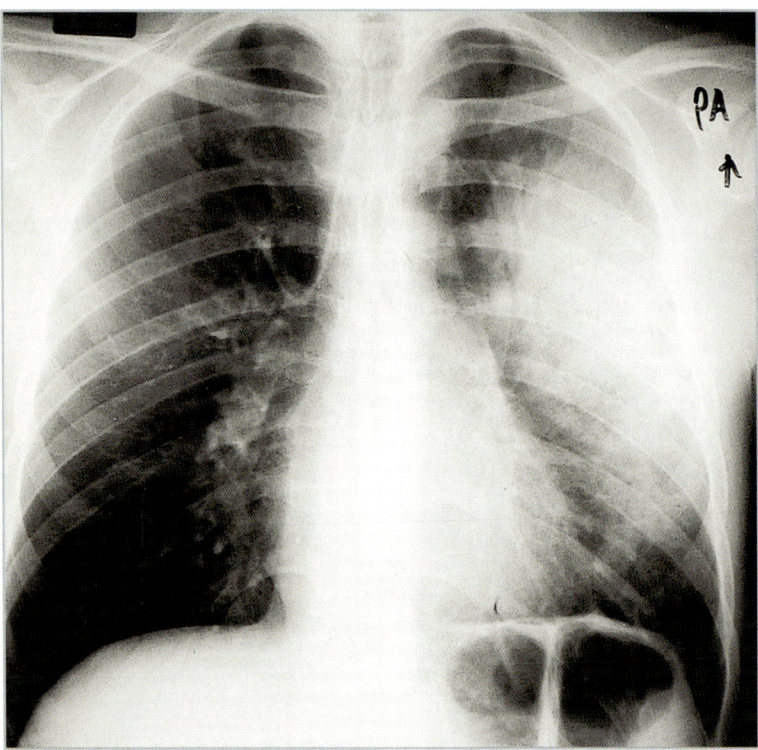

Figure 10-16. Chest radiograph of a neutropenic patient, absolute neutrophil count less than 100 cells/mm^3, with left lung consolidation. Blood and sputum cultures revealed *Escherichia coli*. Pneumonia in patients with severe neutropenia is often secondary to Enterobacteriaceae organisms. (*Courtesy of* Chin-Tang Huang, MD, and Laurence Huang, MD.)

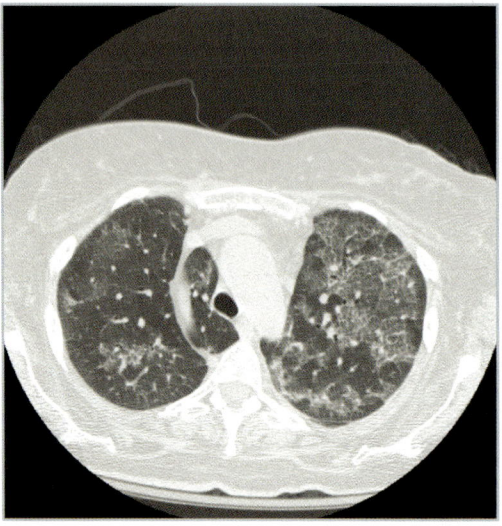

Figure 10-17. Chest CT of a patient on high-dose prednisone for polymyositis, demonstrating bilateral ground glass opacities, and interlobular and intralobular septal thickening. This radiographic pattern has been called "crazy paving" and can be seen in a variety of alveolar and interstitial diseases. This patient was HIV negative and had *Pneumocystis* organisms on bronchoscopy with bronchoalveolar lavage. Similar to HIV-infected persons, individuals receiving chronic immunosuppression with prednisone are also at risk for *Pneumocystis* pneumonia. (*Courtesy of* Matthew Fei, MD.)

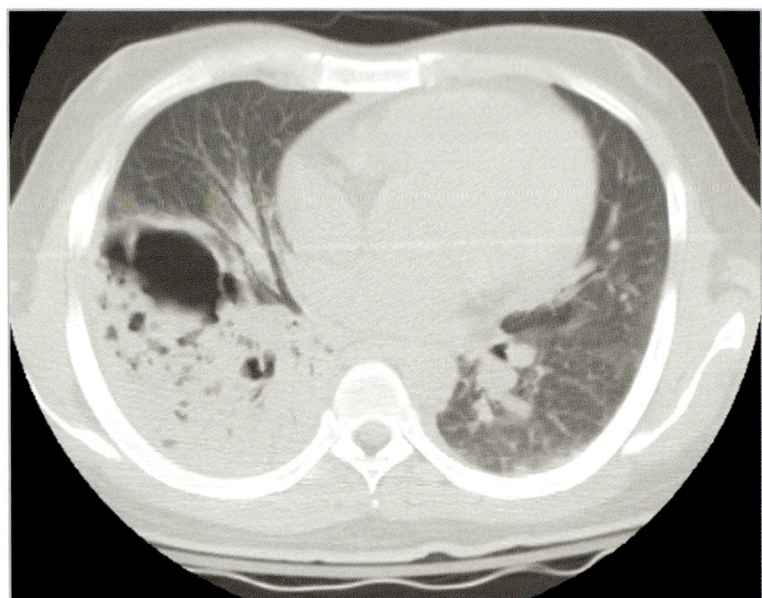

Figure 10-18. Chest CT of a patient on high-dose prednisone for autoimmune hepatitis, revealing large thick-walled cavities in the right upper and lower lobes. Multiple sputum cultures grew *Aspergillus fumigatus*. (*Courtesy of* Matthew Fei, MD.)

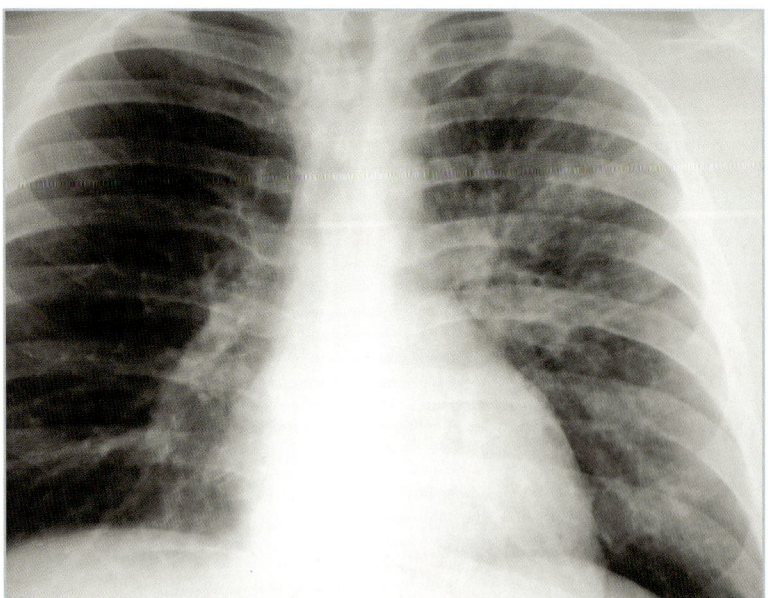

Figure 10-19. Chest radiograph of a patient after renal transplantation, revealing left lung opacities due to *Legionella pneumophila*. Transplant recipients are at an increased risk for *Legionella* species infection. The primary host defense mechanism against *Legionella* and other intracellular pathogens is cell-mediated immunity. Depression of cell-mediated immunity by medications used in transplantation predisposes the host to *Legionella* infection. (*Courtesy of* Michael B. Gotway, MD.)

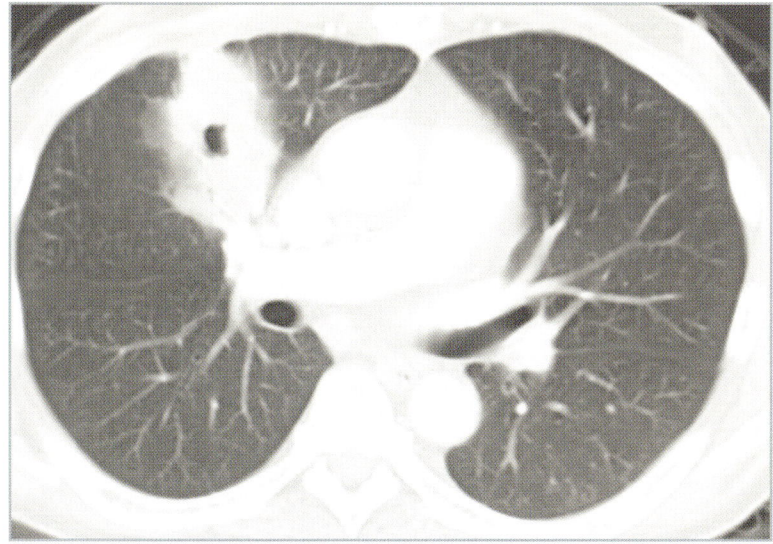

Figure 10-20. Chest CT of a patient after cardiac transplantation, demonstrating right lung cavitary pneumonia due to *Nocardia asteroides*. Transplant recipients are at an increased risk for *Nocardia* species infection. Among transplant recipients, the rate of *Nocardia* infection is highest in lung and heart transplant recipients and lowest in liver and kidney transplant recipients. (*Courtesy of* Michael B. Gotway, MD.)

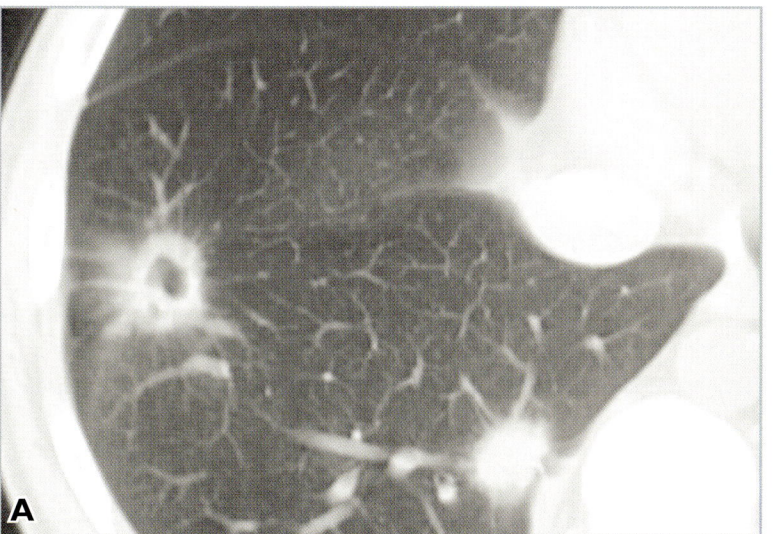
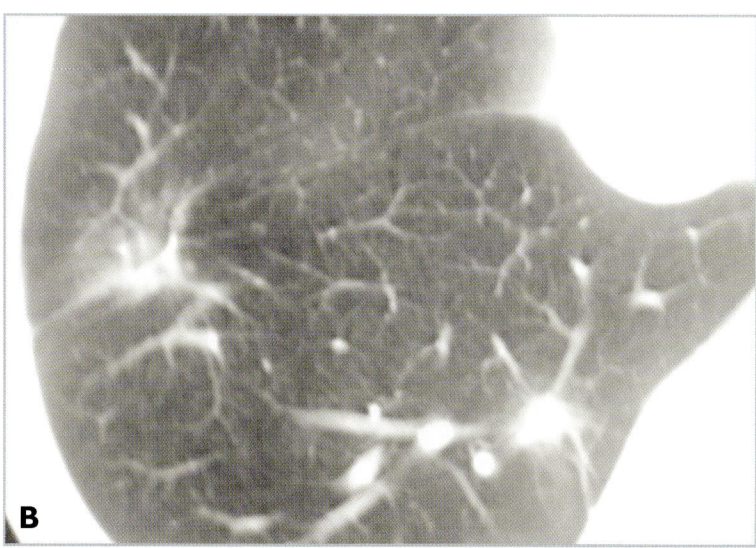

Figure 10-21. Chest CT of a patient after bone marrow transplantation, revealing right lung cavitary lesion due to *Aspergillus fumigatus* (**A**) that resolved with treatment (**B**). (*Courtesy of* Michael B. Gotway, MD.)

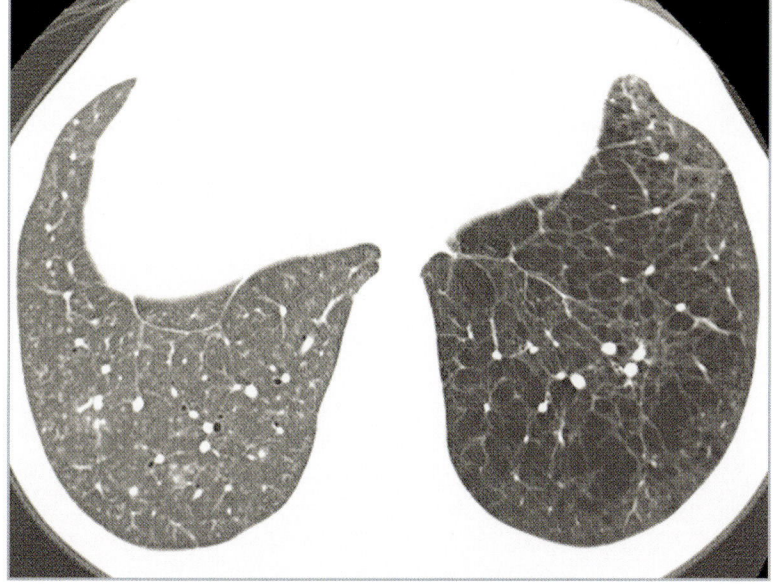

Figure 10-22. Chest CT of a patient after single-lung transplantation for severe emphysema. Right lung demonstrates pneumonia due to cytomegalovirus (CMV). CMV pneumonitis is the most common presentation of CMV disease following lung transplantation, although hepatitis, gastroenteritis, and colitis also occur. The clinical features of CMV pneumonitis may overlap with those of acute rejection. Both groups of patients may present with low-grade fever, shortness of breath, nonproductive cough, and changes in pulmonary-function testing. (*Courtesy of* Michael B. Gotway, MD.)

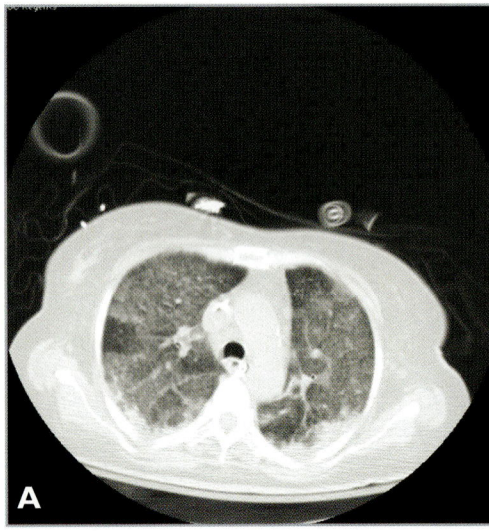
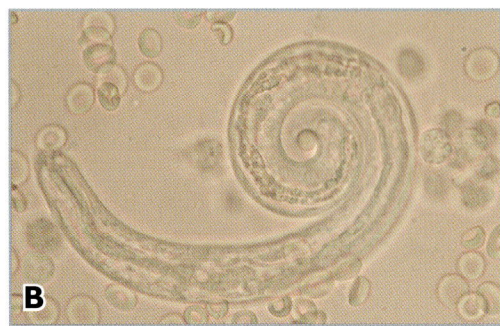

Figure 10-23. Chest CT (**A**) of a patient after renal transplantation revealing diffuse ground glass opacities. The patient was a native of Mexico and developed periumbilical purpura, suggestive of disseminated *Strongyloides stercoralis* infection. Bronchoscopy with bronchoalveolar lavage examination revealed filariform larvae (**B**) characteristic of *S. stercoralis* hyperinfection. (*Courtesy of* Matthew Fei, MD.)

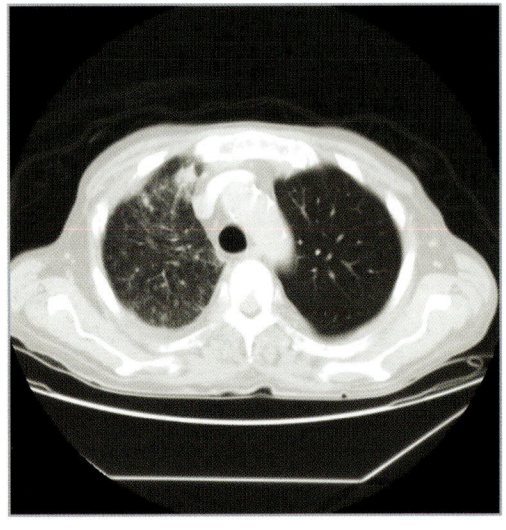

Figure 10-24. Chest CT of a patient after a recent liver transplant for autoimmune hepatitis and alcoholic cirrhosis, demonstrating right upper lobe nodules. The patient was receiving immune suppressive medications and was initially thought to have an opportunistic pneumonia. Bronchoscopy with bronchoalveolar lavage subsequently revealed cells suspicious for a metastatic carcinoma. Examination of his explanted liver revealed cholangiocarcinoma that was not diagnosed prior to transplant. It is important to remember that immunocompromised patients are at an increased risk for malignancy as well as for opportunistic infections. (*Courtesy of* Matthew Fei, MD.)

REFERENCES

1. CDC Division of HIV/AIDS Prevention: AIDS Surveillance—General Epidemiology (through 2005). Accessible at http://www.cdc.gov/hiv/topics/surveillance/resources/slides/epidemiology/index.htm. Accessed 2007.

2. Innes AL, Huang L, Nishimura SL: Resolution of lymphocytic interstitial pneumonitis in an HIV infected adult after treatment with HAART. *Sex Transm Infect* 2004, 80(5):417–418.

3. Morris AM, Nishimura SL, Huang L: Subacute hypersensitivity pneumonitis in an HIV infected patient receiving antiretroviral therapy. *Thorax* 2000, 55:625–627.

FUNGAL INFECTION

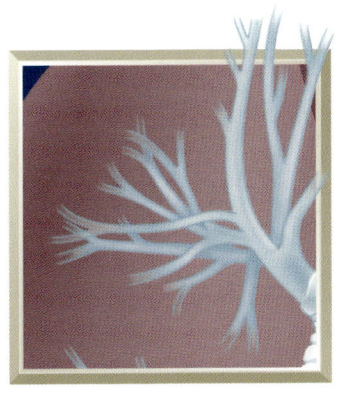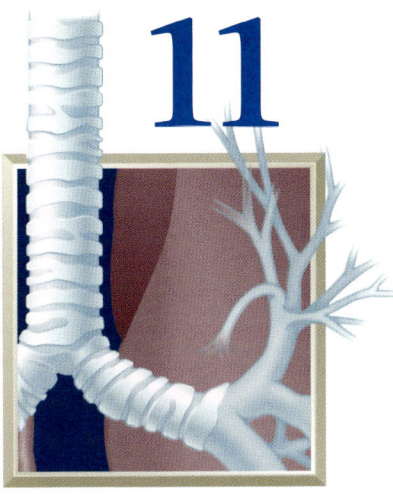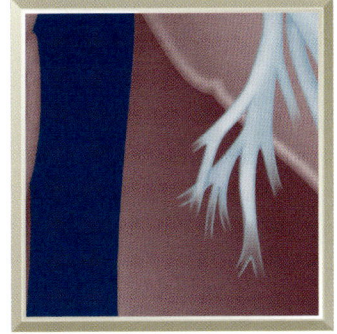

Anupama Menon and Robert W. Bradsher

There are two modes of epidemiology of fungal infections: opportunistic and endemic. The opportunistic fungi include *Aspergillus*, *Candida*, *Fusarium*, and *Rhizopus* species; some of the fungi more traditionally characterized as endemic fungi, including *Histoplasma*, *Blastomyces*, *Cryptococcus*, *Sporothrix*, and *Coccidioidomyces*, may also present as opportunistic infections in immunocompromised patients. However, the organisms considered to be opportunistic fungi do not cause endemic or geographically localized diseases. *Aspergillus*, *Candida*, *Fusarium*, and *Rhizopus* species and the like are ubiquitous in nature and are found throughout the world.

Opportunistic fungi are more likely to be nosocomial and to occur in specialized patient groups. These include those with HIV/AIDS, those having undergone transplantation and immunosuppressive chemotherapy, and those treated with corticosteroids. In addition, invasive *Candida* infections occur in patients in burn, medical, neonatal, and surgical intensive care units, as well as in other specialized patient-care areas. Resistance to antifungal chemotherapy has been increasing, particularly with *Candida* and fluconazole.

The endemic fungi, on the other hand, are more likely to present in a community-acquisition rather than a nosocomial fashion. These infections, except for sporotrichosis, originate by aerosol inhalation with primary infection occurring in the lung. This infection may never cause symptomatic disease and may resolve spontaneously, or the organism may escape host defenses and cause progressive infection in the lung or at sites of hematogenous dissemination. Therefore, disease may range from asymptomatic to life-threatening. Although there has been some evidence of development of resistance of *Histoplasma capsulatum* to fluconazole, antifungal resistance has not been a major factor in the endemic mycosis.

Risk Factors for Invasive Candidiasis	
Granulocytopenia	Hyperalimentation
Hematologic malignancy	Recent surgery
Broad-spectrum antibiotics	Prior colonization with *Candida* species
Hemodialysis or acute renal failure	Neonates: Gestational age < 32 wk; low Apgar score; intubation; length of stay; histamine-2 blockers; central venous catheters; hyperalimentation
Central vascular catheters	
Solid organ transplantation	

Figure 11-1. Risk factors for invasive candidiasis [1–4]. Invasive candidiasis is typically not seen in normal, healthy hosts. Immunocompromised hosts and patients in intensive care units are at highest risk.

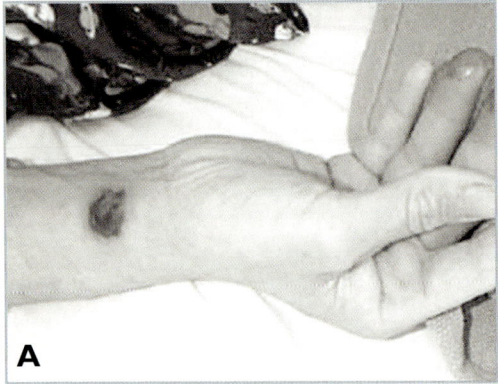
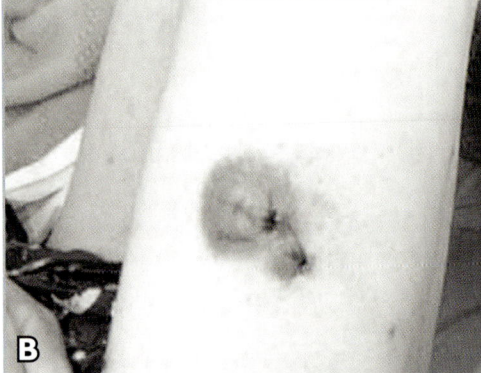

C	Forms of Invasive Candidiasis
	Catheter-related candidemia
	Acute disseminated candidiasis
	Chronic disseminated candidiasis
	Deep organ candidiasis

Figure 11-2. A–C, Forms of invasive candidiasis. In the past two decades, *Candida* species have emerged as the fourth leading cause of bloodstream infections in hospitalized patients with catheter-related candidemia. In patients with central venous catheters, primary infection occurs at the catheter or in the fibrin clot that forms around the catheter. In the acute disseminated form, candidemia is present and may have originated from an infected catheter; however, there is also evidence of dissemination to one or more organs. The most common organs involved are the eyes, kidneys, brain, skin, and myocardium. Chronic disseminated candidiasis is also known as hepatosplenic candidiasis. It almost always occurs during early recovery of neutrophils following a prolonged episode of neutropenia after treatment for hematologic malignancy. In deep organ candidiasis, blood cultures are rarely positive. Virtually any organ(s) may be involved. In each case, an episode of candidemia must have led to seeding of the affected organ(s). At the time of presentation, however, the blood is sterile. Deep organ candidiasis differs from the chronic disseminated type in that it may occur in any patient at risk for candidemia, not just in neutropenic patients.

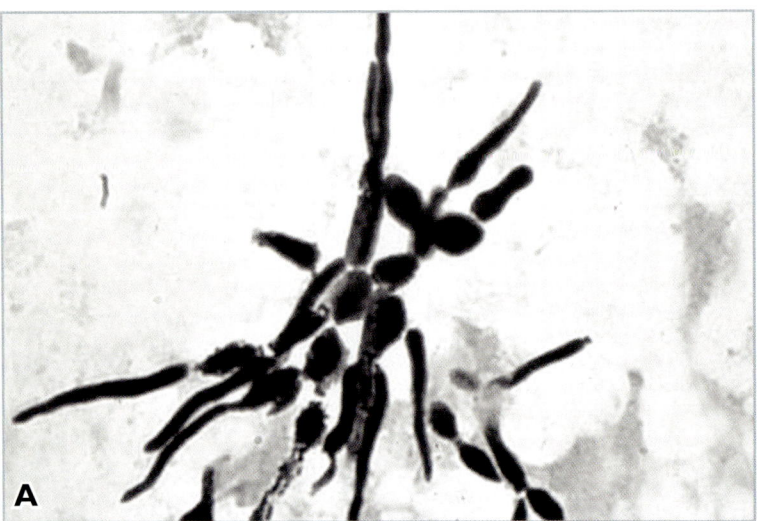

Figure 11-3. A and B, Invasive focal infections due to *Candida*. True urinary tract infection is difficult to distinguish from colonization. Funguria is very common in hospitalized patients, especially those who are older, have indwelling bladder catheters, are on antibiotics, are diabetic, or have had a prior surgical procedure. The benefit of treatment of funguria is a controversial issue that has been addressed in clinical trials. In a prospective, multicenter surveillance study of 861 patients with candiduria, clinical outcomes data were available for 530. The outcome of funguria was followed: in those who received no therapy, 76% cleared, and in those who received either fluconazole or amphotericin B bladder irrigation, 46% and 54% cleared, respectively. Only seven patients developed candidemia [5].

Continued on the next page

B. Invasive Focal Infections Caused by *Candida*

- Urinary tract infections
- Peritonitis
- Endophthalmitis
- Hepatosplenic
- Osteoarticular
- Meningitis

Figure 11-3. *(Continued) Candida pyelonephritis* most often occurs in the setting of urinary obstruction. Fungus balls may develop and require surgical or percutaneous drainage if they cause obstruction. *Candida peritonitis* occurs in the setting of intestinal perforations, postoperative wound infections, and peritoneal dialysis. Endophthalmitis may develop exogenously following trauma or surgery on the eye, or endogenously through hematogenous seeding of the retina and choroid as a complication of candidemia. This infection may be sight-threatening if it is not treated. Hepatosplenic candidiasis almost always occurs in the setting of neutrophil recovery after chemotherapy-induced neutropenia. *Candida* osteo-articular infections occur endogenously through hematogenous seeding or exogenously after trauma, intra-articular injection, or surgery. Most infections have been described in native joints. *Candida* species may cause either acute or chronic meningitis.

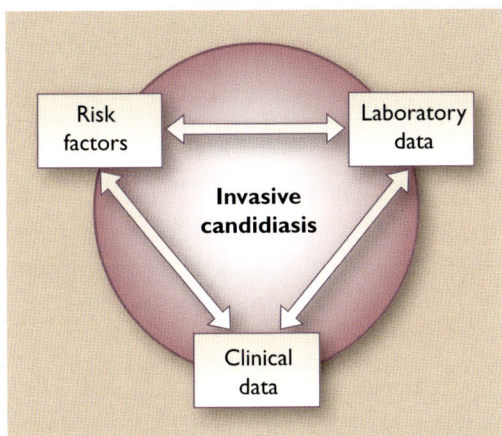

Figure 11-4. Invasive candidiasis versus colonization with *Candida*. There is no single test that reliably establishes a diagnosis of invasive candidiasis. Physicians must consider invasive candidiasis in any patient with appropriate risk factors and clinical signs and symptoms suggestive of this syndrome. Available laboratory tests are not highly sensitive, so a negative culture does not exclude infection. Retrospective studies show that blood cultures are positive in only 40% to 60% of patients with autopsy-proven invasive candidiasis [6]. Recovery of *Candida* from urine is common, particularly in hospitalized patients with urinary catheters. Neither the colony count of fungus in the urine nor the presence or absence of pyuria is uniformly reliable in determining the significance of candiduria. Because *Candida* species are part of the normal oral flora, isolation from sputum, tracheal aspirate, and even bronchoalveolar lavage fluid usually reflects contamination or colonization, particularly in critically ill patients. In this setting, radiographic findings and recovery of *Candida* from sputum or tracheal aspirate are not sufficient to make a diagnosis of *Candida* pneumonia [7]. *Candida* pneumonia is a rare entity, and some authorities recommend biopsy-proven evidence of invasion to establish this diagnosis [8].

Guidelines for Treatment of Invasive Candidiasis

Condition	Primary	Alternative	Duration
Candidemia			
Non-neutropenic adult	AmB or flu or caspo	AmB + Flu 3–7 d, then flu	14 d after last positive blood culture and resolution of signs and symptoms
Neutropenic adult	AmB or LF AmB or caspo	Flu	14 d after last positive blood culture and resolution of signs and symptoms
Chronic disseminated	AmB or LF AmB	Flu or caspo	3–6 mo and resolution of radiologic lesions
Osteomyelitis	Surgical debridement + AmB, then flu	—	AmB × 2–3 wk, then flu × 6–12 mo
Intra-abdominal infection	AmB or flu	—	2–3 wk or until resolution of signs and symptoms
Meningitis	AmB + 5-FC	—	≥ 4 wk after resolution of signs and symptoms
Endophthalmitis	AmB ± 5-FC	Flu	6–12 wk
Endocarditis	AmB or LF AmB ± 5-FC	Flu or caspo	≥ 6 wk after valve replacement

Figure 11-5. Guidelines for treatment of invasive candidiasis, 2004. Nonalbicans *Candida* species constitute up to 50% of *Candida* isolates at many centers. Of the clinically relevant species, *Candida krusei* and *Candida glabrata* may demonstrate reduced susceptibility or resistance to azole antifungal agents. *C. krusei* is uniformly resistant to fluconazole, whereas 10% to 15% of *C. glabrata* isolates were reported as being resistant to this antifungal agent in recent bloodstream infection surveys. Recent data also indicate that a significant proportion of *C. krusei* and *C. glabrata* isolates may have reduced susceptibility to amphotericin B [9]. AmB—deoxycholate amphotericin B; flu—fluconazole; caspo—caspofungin; 5-FC—5-flucytosine; LF—lipid formulation.

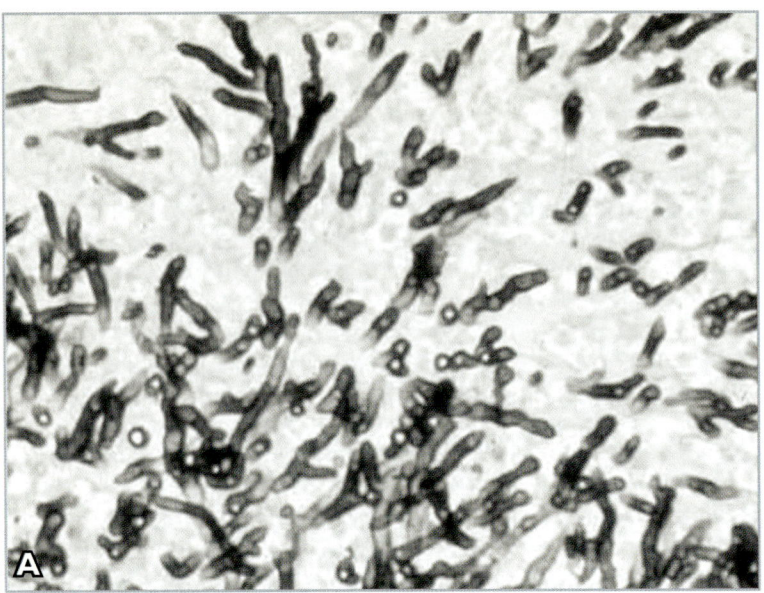
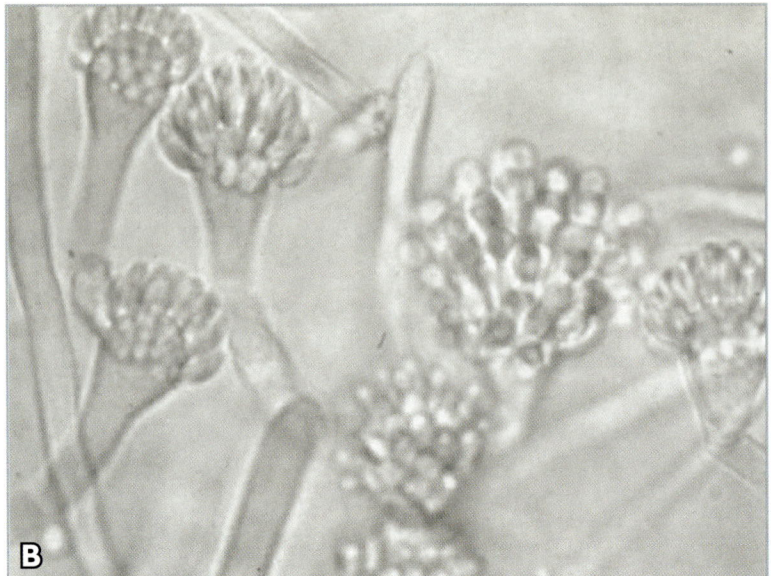

C	Manifestations of *Aspergillus* Infection
	Invasive aspergillosis
	Allergic bronchopulmonary aspergillosis
	Aspergilloma
	Semi-invasive pulmonary aspergillosis
	Disseminated aspergillosis

Figure 11-6. **A–C**, Manifestations of *Aspergillus* infection. Invasive pulmonary aspergillosis (IPA) usually presents as an acute, progressive infection characterized by invasion of the organism across tissue planes, with subsequent infarction and tissue necrosis. The most commonly involved sites include the lungs, the upper airways, and the sinuses. It is most often seen in patients with profound neutropenia or in those undergoing prolonged corticosteroid therapy. *Aspergillus* species are often secondary opportunistic pathogens in patients with bronchiectasis, carcinoma, other mycoses, sarcoidosis, and tuberculosis. Diagnosis of IPA relies on demonstration of the organism in infected tissue, combined with culture confirmation. In patients who are unable to undergo biopsy, a presumptive diagnosis of IPA may be made if bronchoalveolar lavage yields *Aspergillus* (and no other pathogen) in the presence of new pulmonary symptoms or infiltrates [10]. In May 2003, the US Food and Drug Administration (FDA) approved an enzyme immunoassay (EIA), the Platelia *Aspergillus* EIA (Bio-Rad Laboratories, Hercules, CA), for use in the diagnosis of IPA. The EIA uses a monoclonal antibody against galactomannan, a cell wall component of *Aspergillus* species, detected in serum samples. In the data evaluated by the FDA, the sensitivity and specificity were 80.7% and 89.2%, respectively. The diagnosis of IPA is strongly supported by two consecutive positive serum samples. Platelia *Aspergillus* EIA may also be used for follow-up of clinical response to antifungal therapy [11].

Allergic bronchopulmonary aspergillosis (ABPA) is a hypersensitivity reaction characterized by colonization of the airways by *Aspergillus* in patients with asthma or cystic fibrosis. Patients present with worsening asthma or pulmonary function and eosinophilic pneumonia or mucoid impaction. There is no evidence of mucosal invasion. The disease is characterized by peripheral blood eosinophilia, elevated serum IgG and IgE antibodies against *Aspergillus*, and immediate skin test reactivity to *Aspergillus* antigens. Sputum cultures may yield *Aspergillus* in up to two-thirds of patients with ABPA. Findings on chest radiography include parenchymal infiltrates, atelectasis due to mucoid impaction, and bronchiectasis. Repeated episodes of ABPA may lead to bronchiectasis, fibrosis, and respiratory compromise [12].

Aspergilloma refers to a fungus ball that develops in a cavity, usually in the lung parenchyma, brain, sinuses, or kidney. The fungus ball consists of fungal hyphae, inflammatory cells, fibrin, mucus, and amorphous debris. In the lung, an aspergilloma usually occurs within a preexisting cavity. Aspergillomas may develop in patients with tuberculosis, sarcoidosis, neoplasms, invasive aspergillosis, or any other condition associated with cavitary lung disease. Patients with aspergilloma may present with persistent productive cough, hemoptysis, wheezing, weight loss, or digital clubbing; some patients are asymptomatic. A chest radiograph or CT may show a solid mass within a cavity, surrounded by a rim of air (crescent sign, Monod's sign). If the aspergilloma is mobile, a decubitus radiograph will demonstrate that the fungus ball has moved. Sputum cultures may or may not yield *Aspergillus* [13]. Semi-invasive pulmonary aspergillosis is found following IPA after resolution of neutropenia in a patient treated with cytotoxic chemotherapy. The invasion is halted by effective polymorphonuclear neutrophil function, and cavitary disease results. Disseminated aspergillosis is the diagnosis if the organism is found with invasive disease outside the respiratory tract. Dissemination to almost any organ may occur; the most common organs affected are the central nervous system organs, the kidney, the liver, and the spleen. Very rarely, disseminated disease may develop in a normal host.

Recommendations for Treatment of *Aspergillus* Infections		
Condition	Primary	Alternative
Invasive aspergillosis	Vori or AmB or LF AmB	Itra or caspo
Allergic bronchopulmonary aspergillosis	Corticosteroids	Itra
Aspergilloma	Surgery if massive hemoptysis	—

Figure 11-7. Recommendations for the treatment of *Aspergillus* infections [14]. AmB—deoxycholate amphotericin B; caspo—caspofungin; itra—itraconazole; LF—lipid formulation; vori—voriconazole.

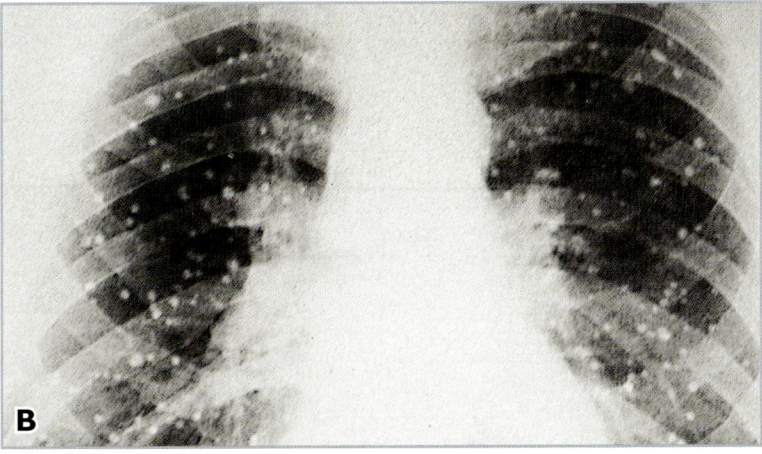

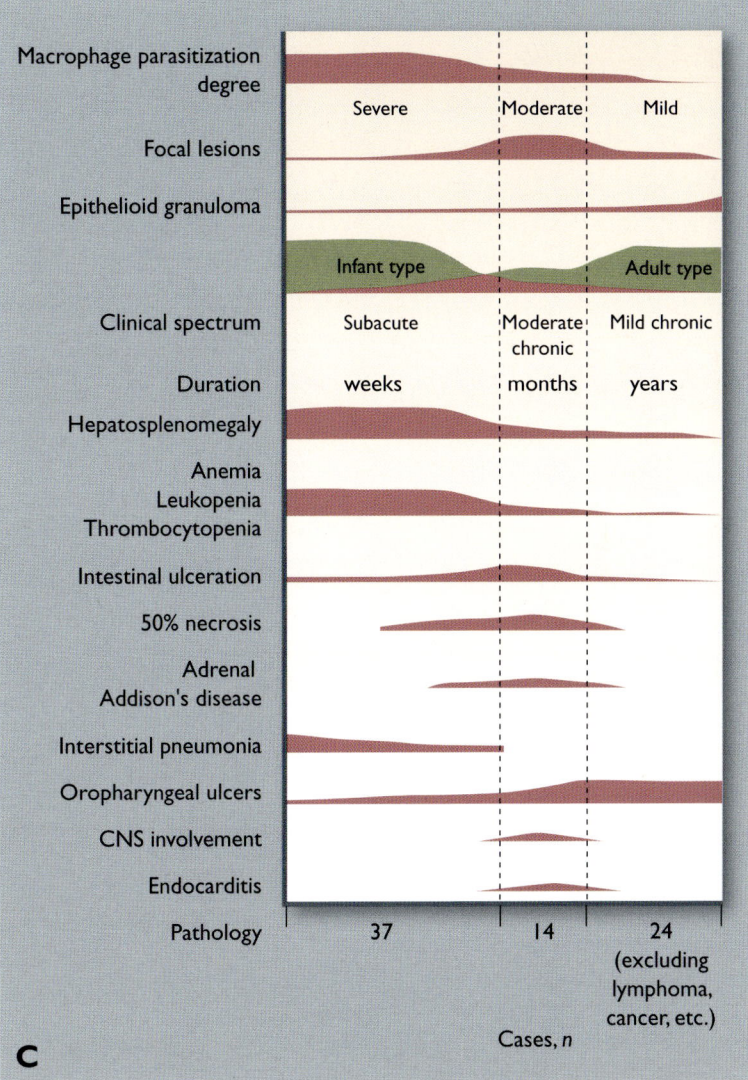

Figure 11-8. Classification of histoplasmosis. **A,** Method of Goodwin and Des Prez. **B,** Buckshot calcification as a result of prior pulmonary histoplasmosis. **C,** A schema showing correlations between degree of parasitization of the monocyte phagocytic system and pathologic and clinical manifestations of disease in disseminated histoplasmosis. The contrast between disease in infants and adults can be seen here. CNS—central nervous system. (*Adapted from* Goodwin and Des Prez [15].)

| Fungal Infection |

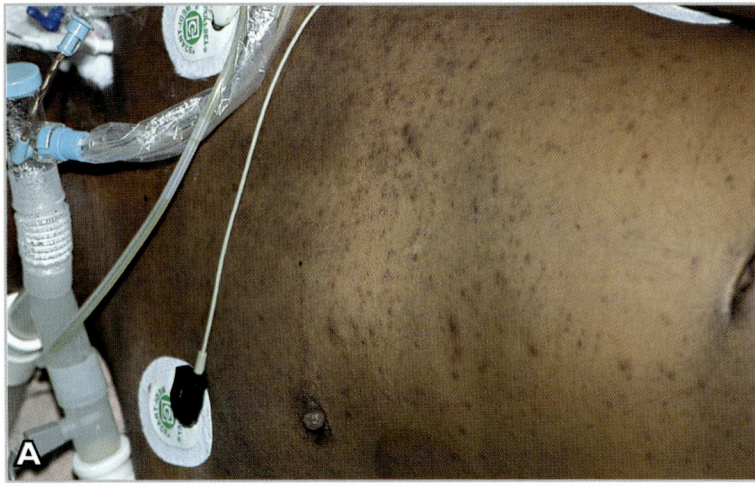
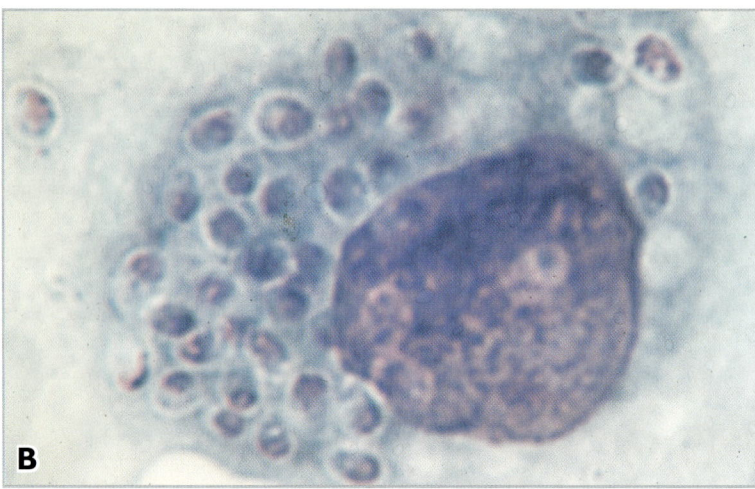

Figure 11-9. Progressive disseminated histoplasmosis [16]. In Southeast Asia, patients infected with HIV have an illness caused by *Penicillium marneffei*, which resembles histoplasmosis. Itraconazole is effective against this condition, such as it is against histoplasmosis.

A, Patient with HIV and cutaneous manifestations of progressive disseminated histoplasmosis. **B,** Organisms of *Histoplasma capsulatum* inside human macrophage.

Guidelines for Management of Patients with Histoplasmosis, 2007

Acute pulmonary	
Moderately severe or severe	Lipid AmB + methylprednisolone
Mild to moderate	None or itra if symptoms > 4 wk
Chronic cavitary pulmonary	Itra
Pericarditis	
Moderately severe or severe	Itra if prenisone used
	Prednisone in tapering doses over 2 wk
Mild	NSAID
Pulmonary nodule	None
Progressive disseminated histoplasmosis	
Moderately severe or severe	Lipid AmB
Mild to moderate	Itra
CNS histoplasmosis	Lipid AmB for 4–6 wk, followed by itra for at least 12 mo

Figure 11-10. Guidelines for management of patients with histoplasmosis, 2007. AmB—amphotericin B; CNS—central nervous system; itra—itraconazole; NSAID—nonsteroidal anti-inflammatory drug. (*Adapted from* Wheat et al. [17].)

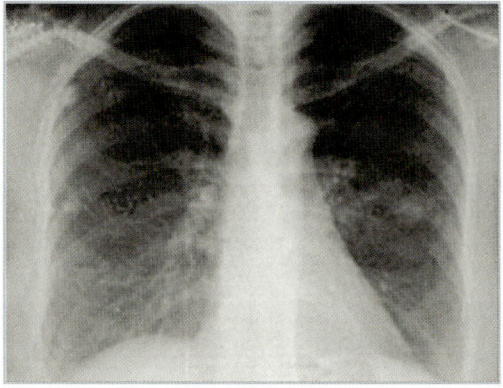

Figure 11-11. Blastomycosis. Case report of a 42-year-old patient from New Hampshire with AIDS and schizophrenia. He was on highly active antiretroviral therapy, trimethoprim/sulfamethoxazole for pneumocystis prophylaxis, and weekly azithromycin for *Mycobacterium avium-intracellulare* prophylaxis. He had 2 weeks of cough and sputum and a remote history of outdoor exposure, including eating beaver meat. The organism is *Blastomyces dermatitidis*. It is found in the south central and southeastern United States. The lung is the primary site of infection, with subsequent dissemination to skin, to soft tissue, or to other organs [18–21].

Atlas of Pulmonary Medicine

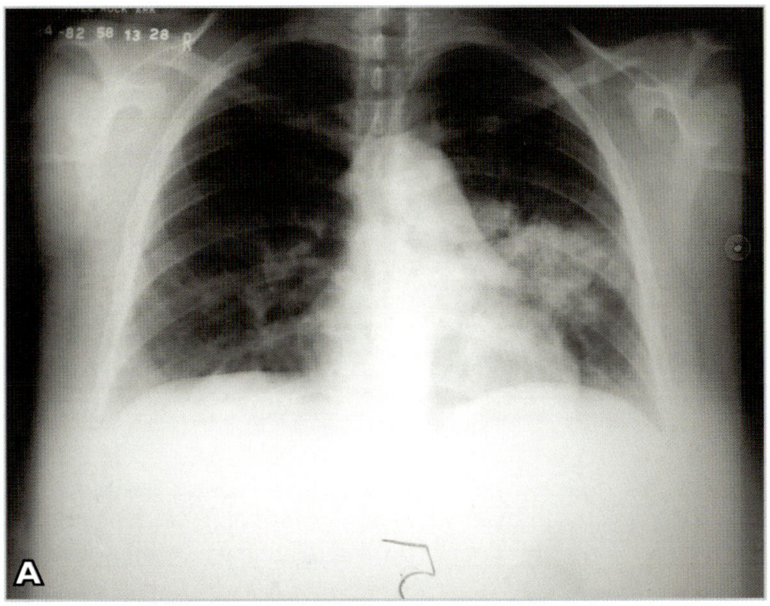

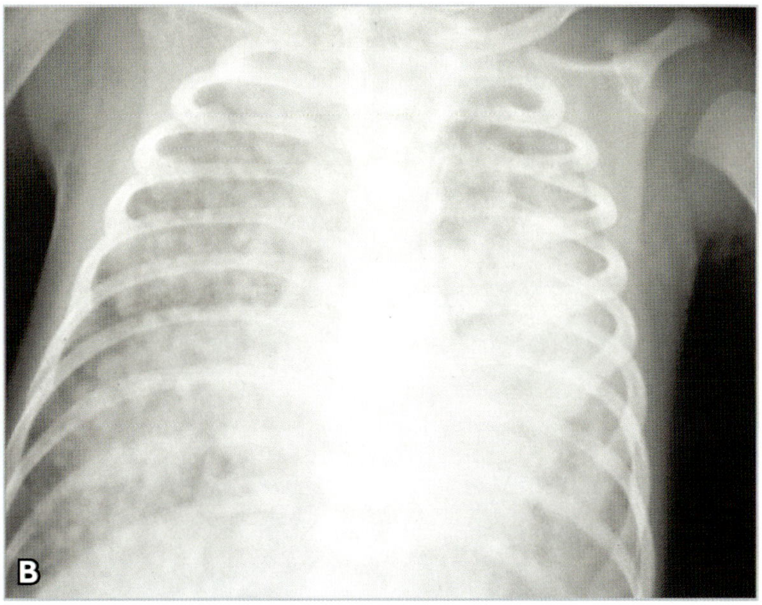

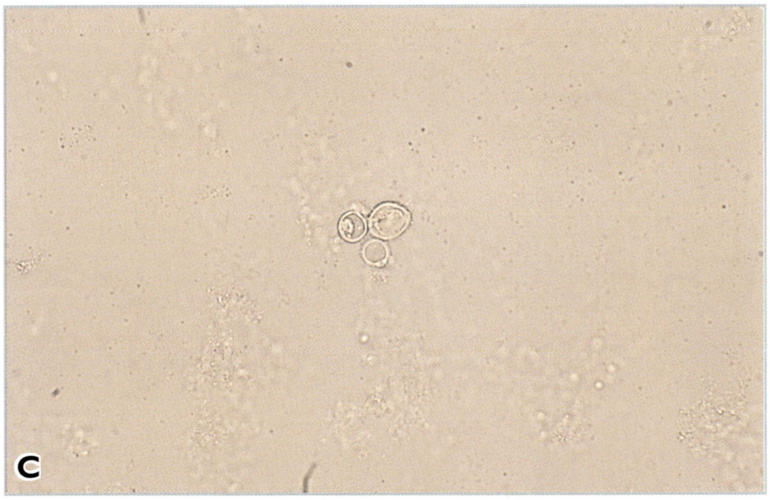

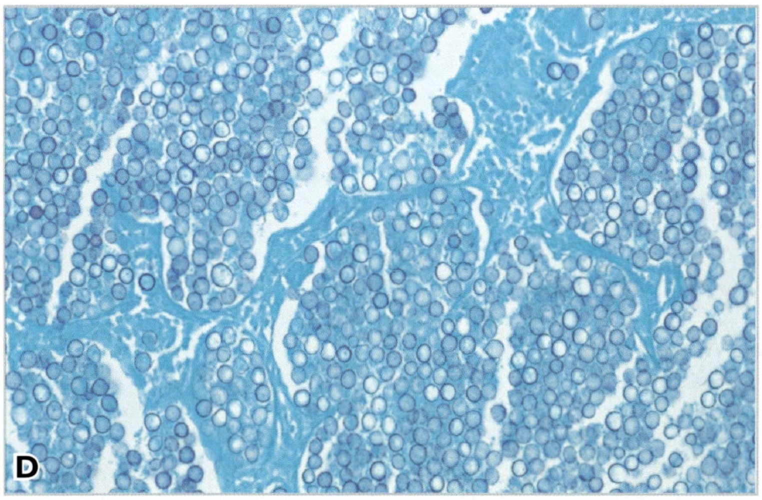

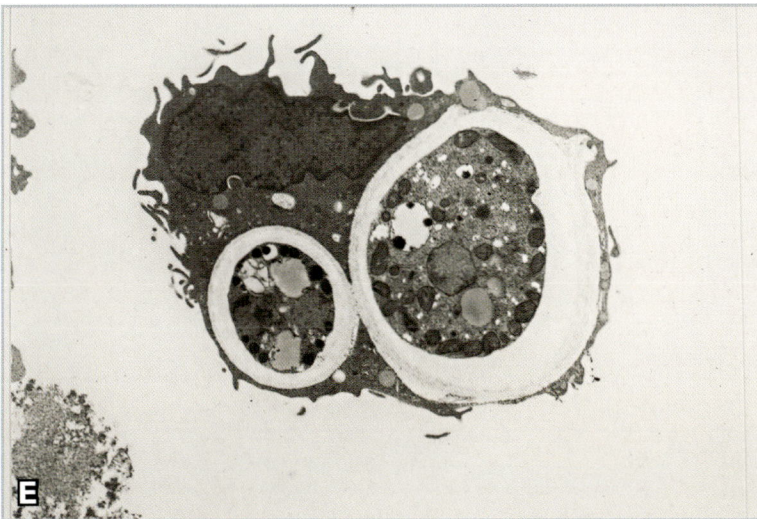

Figure 11-12. **A** and **B**, Pneumonia caused by *Blastomyces dermatitidis* may present with an acute process, like bacterial pneumonia or acute respiratory distress syndrome, as in these two examples, or with a more chronic process resembling tuberculosis or malignancy. **C**, Sputum smear positive for organism by potassium hydrozxide preparation. **D**, Lung biopsy positive for organisms by Methenamine silver stain. **E**, Organisms are phagocytized by alveolar macrophages or peripheral macrophages.

| *Fungal Infection* |

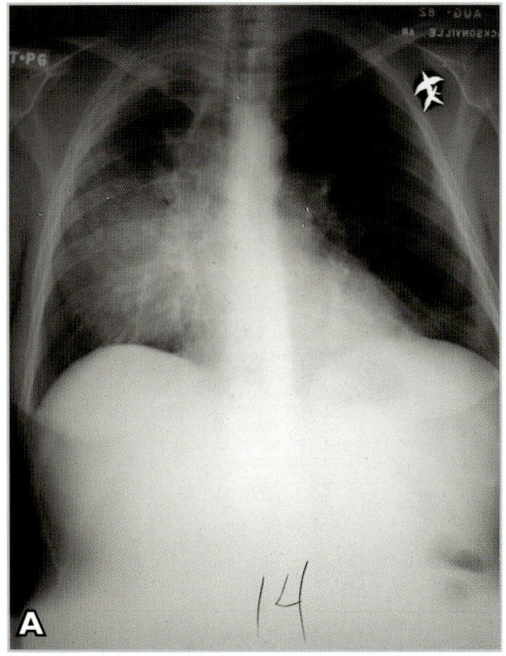
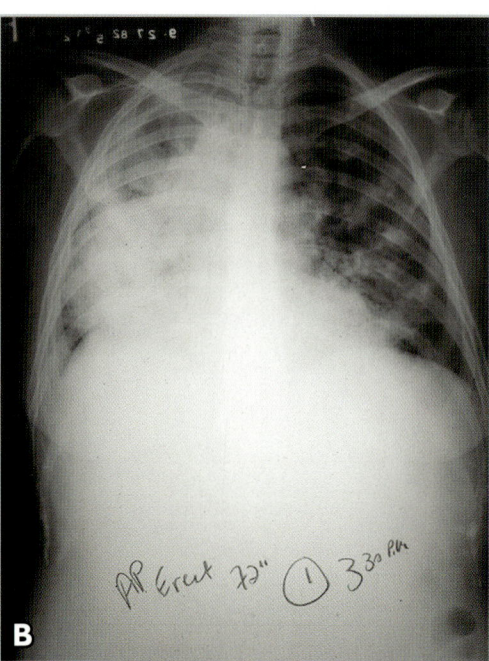

Figure 11-13. **A** and **B**, Pneumonia with blastomycosis can progress, as it did in this patient, over a 3-week period. She previously had tuberculosis and apical pleural thickening. The right lung infiltrate spread from an alveolar process to widespread and bilateral pneumonia because she was non-compliant with therapy.

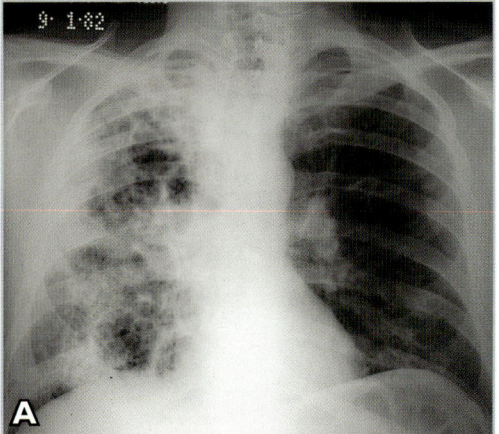
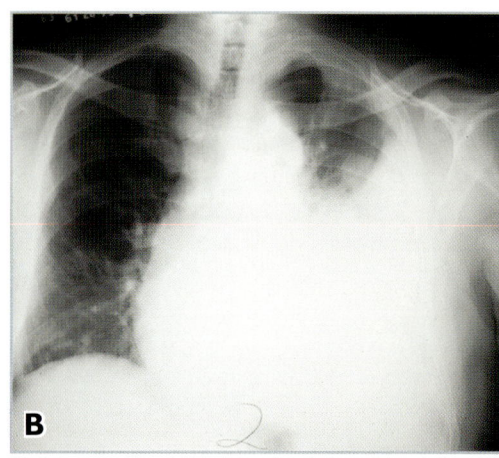

Figure 11-14. **A** and **B**, Chronic pneumonia with blastomycosis may mimic cavitary tuberculosis or lung cancer with a mass-like lesion with effusion.

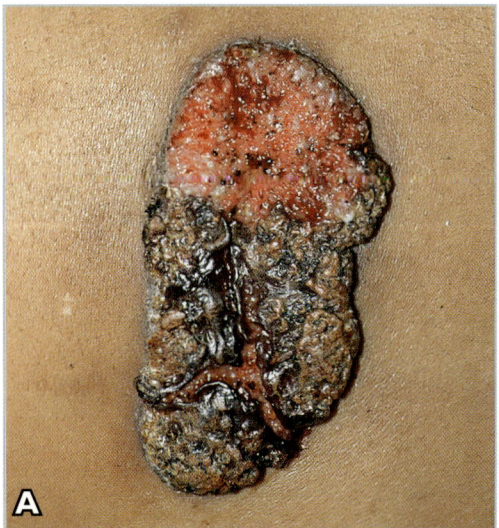
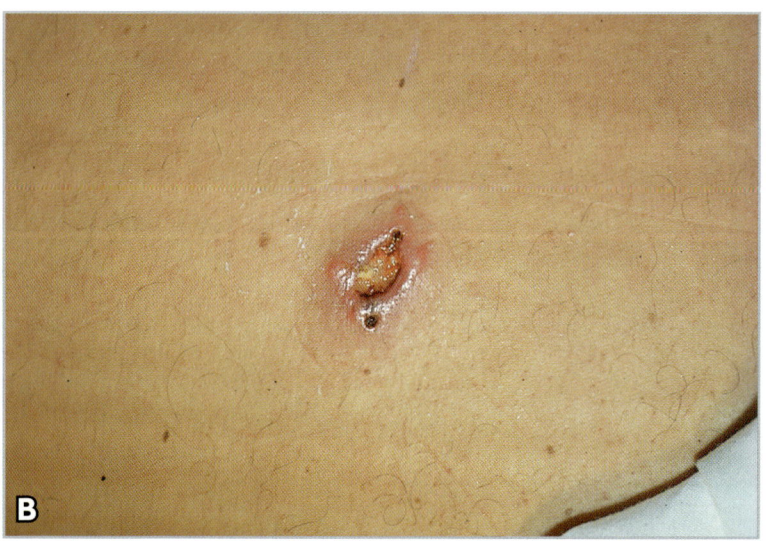

Figure 11-15. **A** and **B**, Cutaneous blastomycosis: verrucous ulcerative. The most common extrapulmonary site of blastomycosis is the skin. Lesions may have a verrucous appearance, or the roof of the lesion may slough to leave an ulcerative lesion. Microscopy of scrapings from the fungating lesion or from the base of the ulcer will show the thick-walled, budding yeast cell after destruction of human tissue with potassium hydroxide.

| Atlas of Pulmonary Medicine |

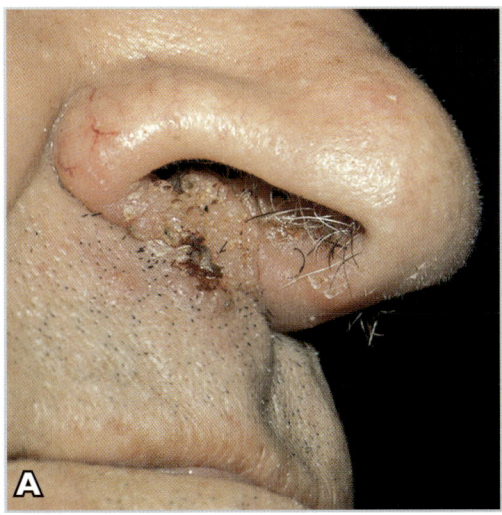 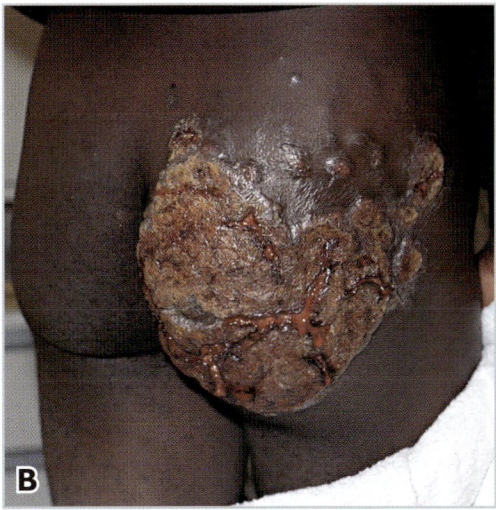 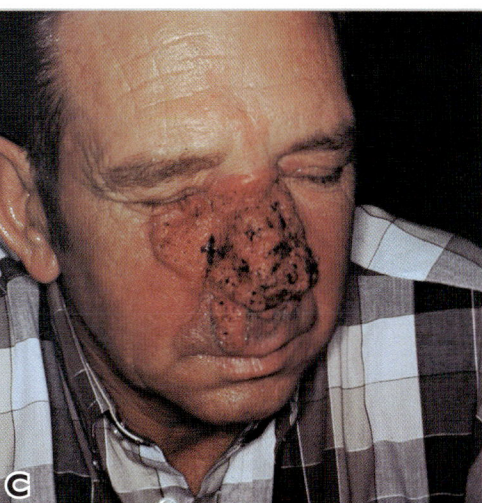

Figure 11-16. Blastomycosis may present in a range of ways: hardly noticeable lesions (**A**) to destructive and disfiguring sites of infection (**B** and **C**) may be observed.

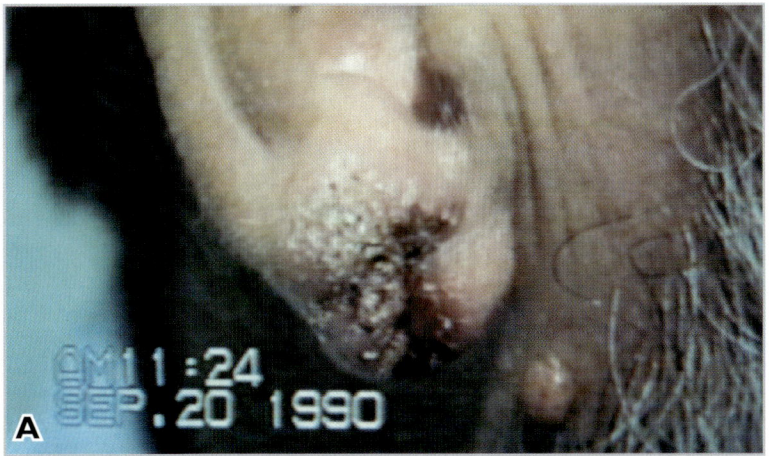 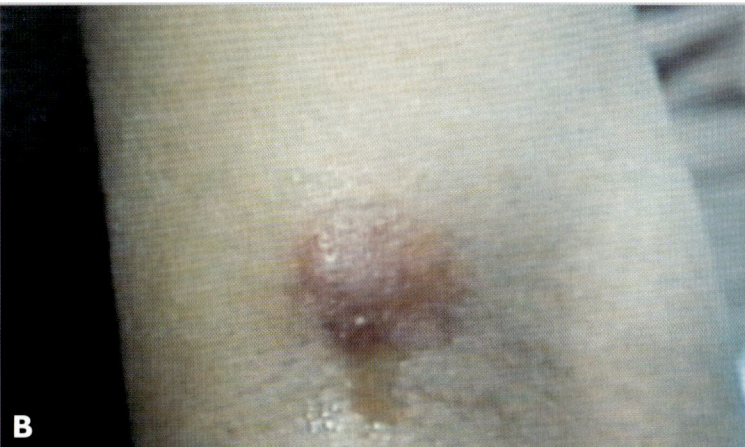

Figure 11-17. Blastomycosis (disseminated). **A**, Patient whose pulmonary blastomycosis improved with fluconazole therapy, but who developed this cutaneous lesion on his ear lobe. **B**, Patient with multiple cutaneous lesions of blastomycosis, who had developed a site of dissemination at a venipuncture site on the antecubital fossae 1 week prior.

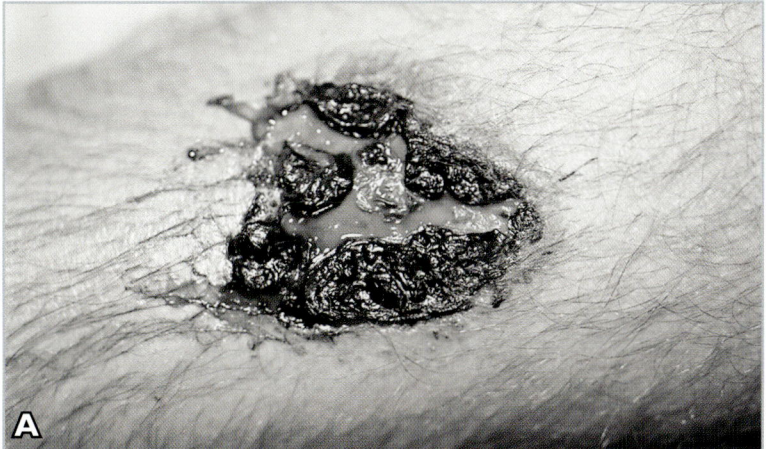 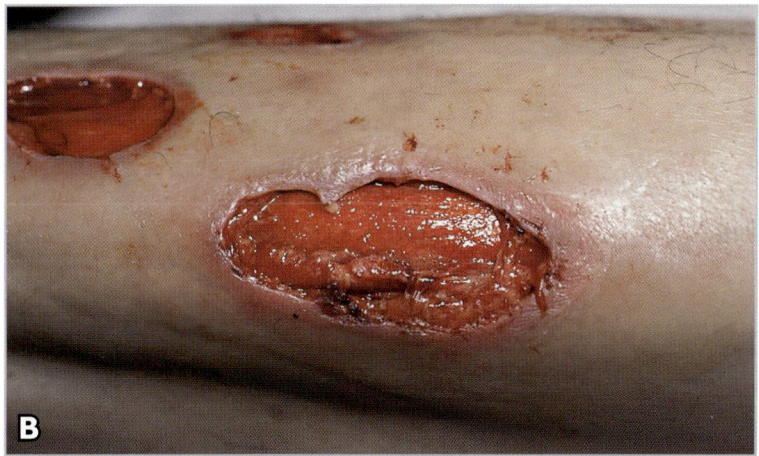

Figure 11-18. **A** and **B**, Ulcers caused by blastomycosis may have a marked degree of exudate in the base or a relative lack of inflammatory cells.

| Fungal Infection |

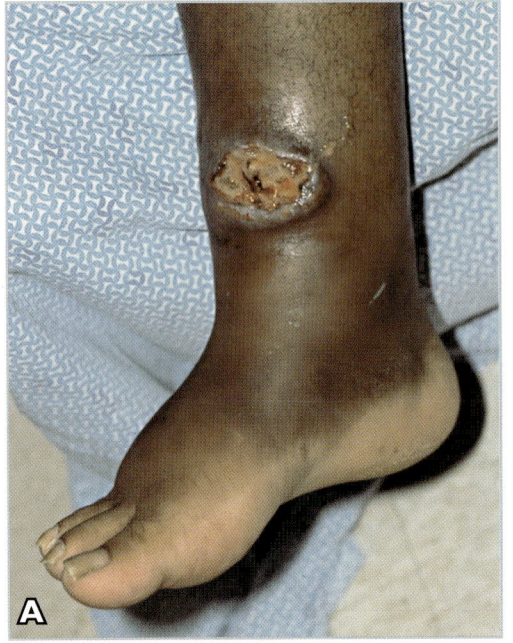
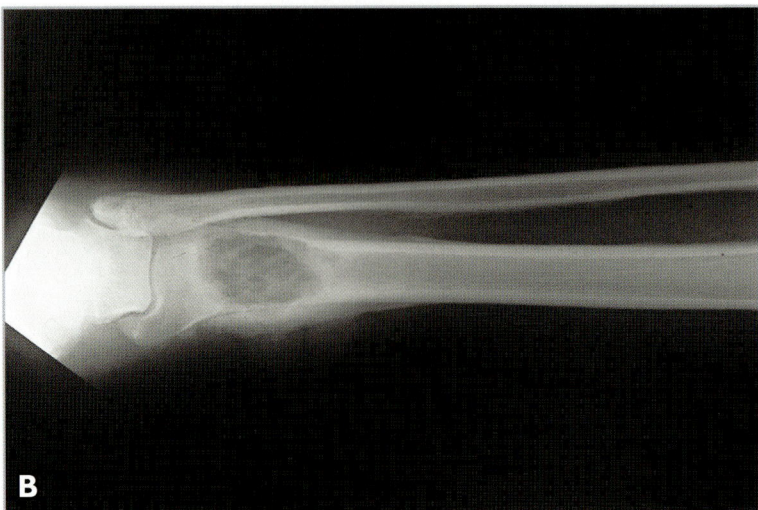

Figure 11-19. **A** and **B**, Extrapulmonary blastomycosis may present in any organ, in addition to in the skin. The next most common site of involvement is bone, followed by the genitourinary system and then the central nervous system.

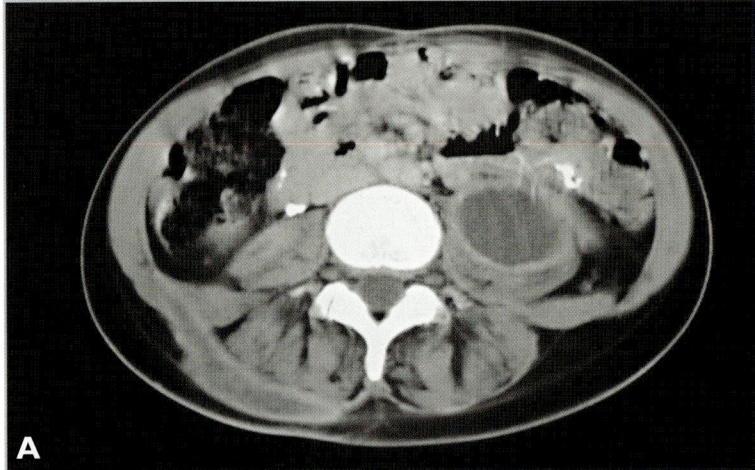
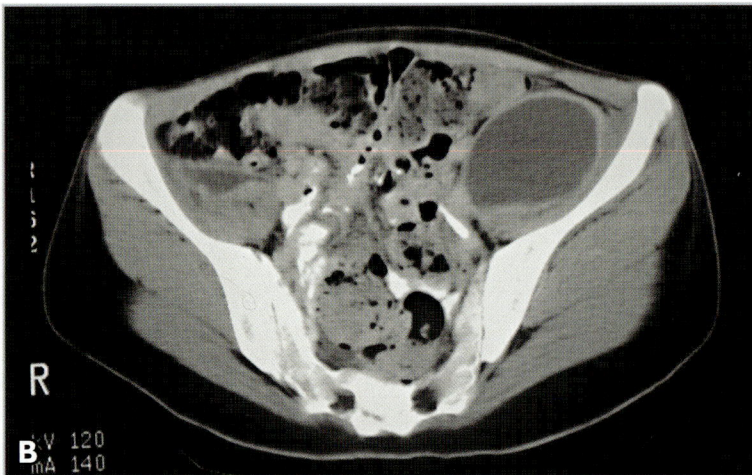
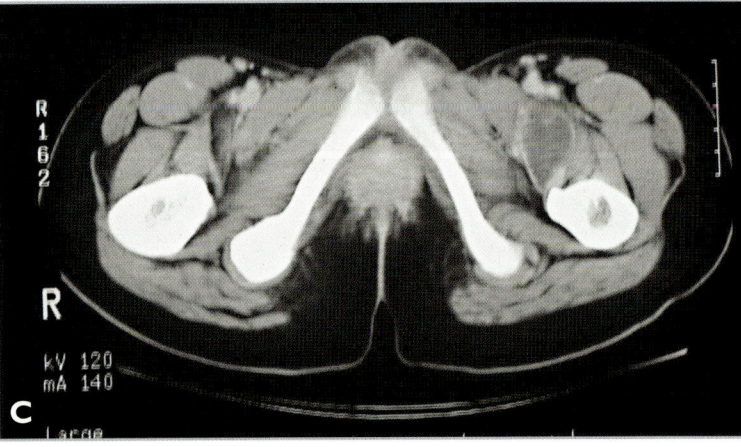

Figure 11-20. **A–C**, CT of woman with psoas abscess. This woman had a psoas abscess caused by *Blastomyces dermatitidis* that extended from her lumbar area down to her thigh. With CT-guided drainage and oral itraconazole, her infection was cured.

Atlas of Pulmonary Medicine

Guidelines for Management of Patients with Blastomycosis, 2000

Pulmonary	First-line	Alternate
Life-threatening	AmB 1.5–2.5 g	AmB; itra when stable
Mild/moderate	Itra 200–400 mg/d	Flucon/ketocon
Disseminated		
CNS	AmB > 2 g	?Flucon if intolerant
Non-CNS, severe	AmB 1.5–2.5 g	AmB; itra when stable
Non-CNS, mild/moderate	Itra 200–400 mg/d	Flucon/ketocon
Immunocompromised	AmB 1.5–2.5 g	Suppressive itra or flucon
Special circumstances		
Pregnancy	AmB	None
Pediatric	AmB or itra	?Flucon

Figure 11-21. Guidelines for management of patients with blastomycosis, 2000. AmB—amphotericin B; CNS—central nervous system; flucon—fluconazole; itra—itraconazole; ketocon—ketoconazole. (*Adapted from* Chapman *et al.* [20].)

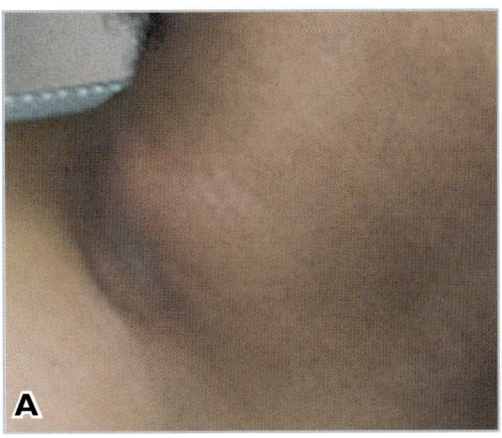 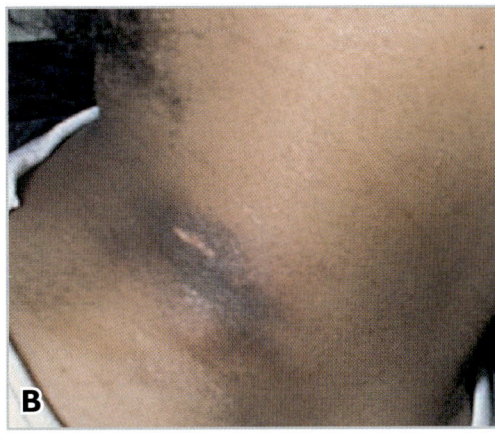 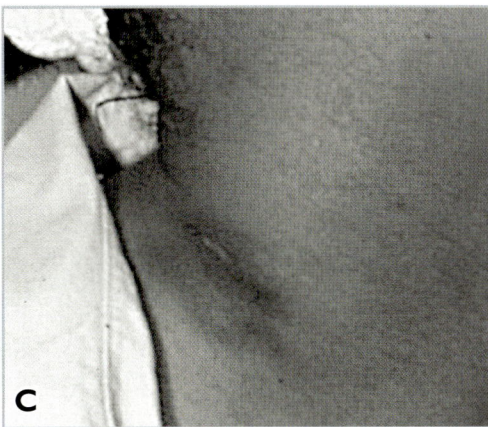

Figure 11-22. Extrapulmonary blastomycosis treated with itraconazole. This figure shows the rapid resolution of blastomycosis with oral itraconazole over 1 month. **A**, February 4, 1999. **B**, February 18, 1999. **C**, March 4, 1999.

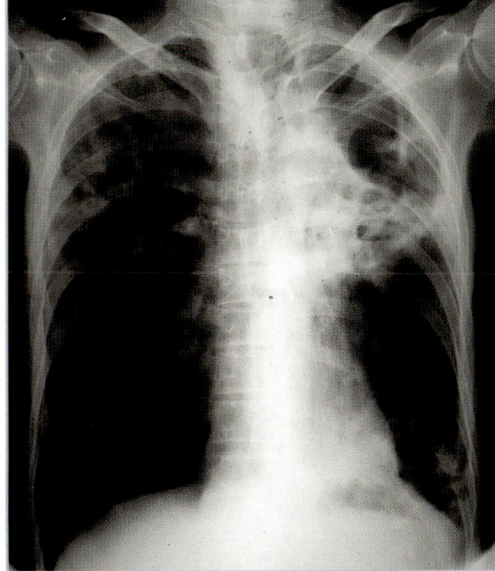 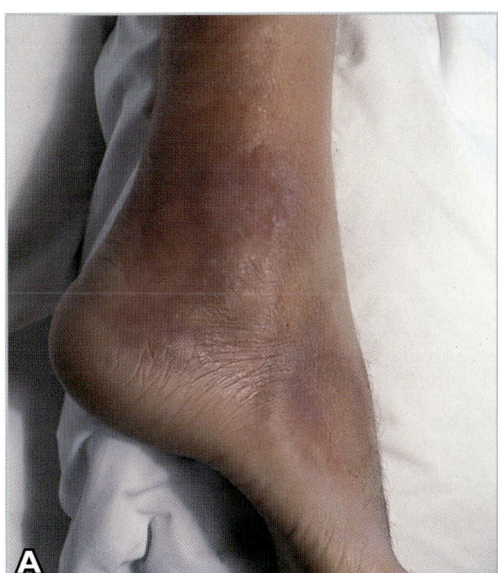 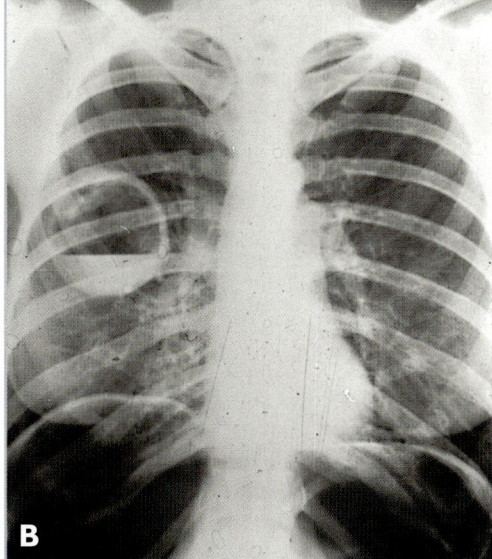

Figure 11-23. *Sporothrix schenkii* differs from other endemic fungi in that cutaneous inoculation, rather than inhalation, is the primary means of infection. Pulmonary involvement with cavitary disease may be found after dissemination, particularly in patients with chronic lung disease [26].

Figure 11-24. Cryptococcosis and sporotrichosis. **A**, *Cryptococcus neoformans* causes pneumonia but may disseminate to other sites, particularly the central nervous system, to cause meningitis. It also may disseminate to the skin, as seen in this renal transplant patient [25]. **B**, Coccidioidomycosis is an endemic fungus that occurs in the Lower Sonoran Life Zone in areas that have alkaline soil with hot summers, mild winters, and little rainfall [22–24]. Pulmonary involvement may be nodular or cavitary, typically with a thin cavitary wall, as in this radiograph from the Centers for Disease Control teaching files. Of note, this patient was from Bakersfield, CA, an area highly endemic for *Coccidioides immitis*.

Infections Caused by Fungi

Zygomycosis (Mucormycosis)	Hyalohyphomycosis	Phaeohyphomycosis
Broad, nonseptate hyphae	Nonpigmented septate hyphae	Darkly pigmented septate hyphae
Rhizopus, Mucor, Absidia, Cunninghamella	*Fusarium, Scedosporium, Pseudoallescheria*	*Curvularia, Bipolaris, Exoserhilum, Alternaria, Exophialia, Drechslera,* others
Risk factors of diabetes, neutropenia	Clinical manifestations of fusariosis	Clinical manifestations of *Curvularia* infection
Clinical manifestations	Foreign body: contact lens, CAPD catheter	Allergic: sinusitis
Sinus-rhinocerebral, necrotic, progressive	Localized: skin, nail, bone, brain	Localized: skin, nail, lung, CAPD
Lung-cavity, hemoptysis, ulcerative	Disseminated: nodular skin blood (60%)	Disseminated: heart, lung, CNS, deep abscess
Skin/wound trauma, burns, necrotic	Therapy: ?response to amphotericin B, surgery	Therapy: amphotericin B, surgery, itraconazole
Disseminated CNS, heart, kidney, gastrointestinal		
Treatment: surgery, amphotericin B		

Figure 11-25. Zygomycosis (mucormycosis), hyalohyphomycosis, and phaeohyphomycosis. CAPD—continuous ambulatory peritoneal dialysis; CNS—central nervous system.

Penicillium marneffei

- Immunosuppression: HIV, lymphoma
- Southeast and East Asia
- Clinical presentation similar to histoplasmosis
- Skin, nodes, bone, joints, liver, spleen
- Oval yeast with cross wall septation
- Dimorphic at room/body temperatures
- Therapy with amphotericin B or itraconazole

Figure 11-26. *Penicillium marneffei* [27–31].

REFERENCES

1. Blumberg HM, Jarvis WR, Soucie JM, *et al.*: Risk factors for candidal bloodstream infections in surgical intensive care unit patients: the NEMIS prospective multicenter study. The National Epidemiology of Mycosis Survery. *Clin Infect Dis* 2001, 33:177–186.

2. Saiman L, Ludington E, Pfaller M, *et al.*: Risk factors for candidemia in neonatal intensive care unit patients. The National Epidemiology of Mycosis Survey study group. *Pediatr Infect Dis J* 2000, 19:319–324.

3. Karabinis A, Hill C, Leclercq B, *et al.*: Risk factors for candidemia in cancer patients: a case-control study. *J Clin Microbiol* 1988, 26:429–432.

4. Ostrosky-Zeichner L, Pappas PG: Invasive candidiasis in the intensive care unit. *Crit Care Med* 2006, 34:857–863.

5. Kauffman CA, Vazquez JA, Sobel JD, *et al.*: Prospective multicenter surveillance study of funguria in hospitalized patients. *Clin Infect Dis* 2000, 30:14–18.

6. Pizzo PA, Walsh TJ. Fungal infections in the pediatric cancer patient. *Semin Oncol* 1990, 173(Suppl 6):6–9.

7. Barenfanger J, Arakere P, Cruz RD, *et al.*: Improved outcomes associated with limiting identification of *Candida spp.* in respiratory secretions. *J Clin Microbiol* 2003, 41:5645–5649.

8. Edwards JE: Candida species. In *Principles and Practice of Infectious Diseases*, 6th ed. Edited by Mandell GL, Bennett JE, Dolin R. Philadelphia: Elsevier Churchill Livingstone; 2005:2938–2957.

9. Pappas PG, Rex JH, Sobel JD, *et al.*: Guidelines for treatment of Candidiasis. *Clin Infect Dis* 2004, 38:161–189.

10. Sugar AM: Clinical features and diagnosis of invasive aspergillosis. Accessible at http://www.uptodate.com. Accessed September 4, 2007.

11. Doctor Fungus: U.S. Food and Drug Administration approves the marketing of Platelia's Aspergillus EIA kit in USA. Accessible at http://www.doctor-fungus.org/news/aspergillosis_June1603.pdf. Accessed September 4, 2007.

12. Weller PF: Allergic bronchopulmonary aspergillosis. Accessible at http://www.uptodate.com. Accessed September 4, 2007.

13. Sugar AM: Aspergilloma. Accessible at http://www.uptodate.com. Accessed September 4, 2007.

14. Doctor Fungus: Aspergillosis. Accessible at http://www.doctorfungus.org/mycoses/human/aspergillus/aspergillosis.htm. Accessed September 4, 2007.

15. Goodwin RA Jr, Des Prez RM: Histoplasmosis. *Am Rev Respir Dis* 1978, 117:929–956.

16. Kaufman CA: Histoplasmosis: a clinical and laboratory update. *Clin Microbiol Rev* 2007, 20:115–132.

17. Wheat LJ, Freifeld AG, Kleiman MB, *et al.*: Clinical practice guidelines for the management of patients with histoplasmosis, 2007 Update, by the Infectious Diseases Society of America. *Clin Infect Dis* 2007, 45:807–825.

18. Bradsher RW: Blastomycosis. In *Clinical Mycology*. Edited by Dismukes WE, Pappas PG, Sobel JE. New York: Oxford University Press; 2003:299–310.

19. Bradsher RW, Chapman SW, Pappas PG: Blastomycosis. *Infect Dis Clin North Am* 2003, 17:21–40.

20. Chapman SW, Bradsher RW, Campbell GD, *et al.*: Practice guidelines for the management of blastomycosis. Infectious Diseases Society of America. *Clin Infect Dis* 2000, 30:679–683.

21. Pappas PG, Pottage JC, Powderly WG, *et al.*: Blastomycosis in patients with the acquired immunodeficiency syndrome. *Ann Intern Med* 1992, 116:847–853.

22. Drutz DJ, Catanzaro A: Coccidioidomycosis. *Am Rev Respir Dis* 1978, 117:559–585,727–771.

23. Anstead GM, Graybill JR: Coccidioidomycosis. *Infect Dis Clin North Am* 2006, 20:621–643.

24. Galgiani JN: Coccidioidomycosis: a regional disease of national importance. *Ann Intern Med* 1999, 130:293–300.

25. Kwon-Chung KJ: Cryptococcosis. In *Medical Mycology*. Edited by Bennett JE. Philadelphia: Lea & Febiger; 1992:397–446.

26. Kaufman CA: Endemic mycoses: blastomycosis, histoplasmosis, and sporotrichosis. *Infect Dis Clin North Am* 2006, 20:645–662.

27. Manns BJ, Baylis BW, Urbanski SJ, *et al.*: Paracoccioidomycosis: case report and review. *Clin Infect Dis* 1996, 23:1026–1032.

28. Duong RA: Infection due to *Penicillium marneffei*, an emerging pathogen: review of 155 reported cases. *Clin Infect Dis* 1996, 23:125–130.

29. Supparatpinyo K, Khamwan C, Baosoang V, *et al.*: Disseminated *Penicillium marneffei* infection in Southeast Asia. *Lancet* 1994, 344:110–113.

30. Chariyalertsak S, Sirisanthana T, Supparatpinyo K, *et al.*: Case-control study of the risk factors for *Penicillium marneffei* infection in human immunodeficiency virus-infected patients in northern Thailand. *Clin Infect Dis* 1997, 24:1080–1086.

31. Supparatpinyo K, Perrieus J, Nelson KE, Sirisanthana T: A controlled trial of itraconazole to prevent relapse of *Penicillium marneffei* infection in patients infected with the human immunodeficiency virus. *N Engl J Med* 1998, 339:1739–1743.

SARCOIDOSIS

Danielle Antin-Ozerkis and Lynn T. Tanoue

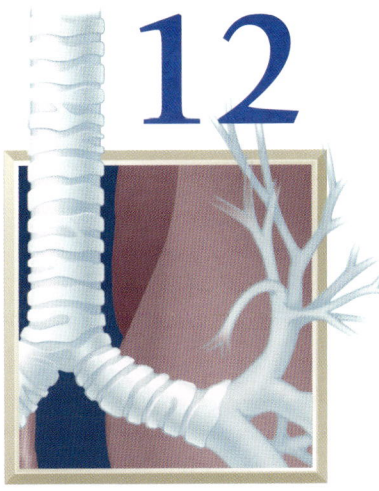
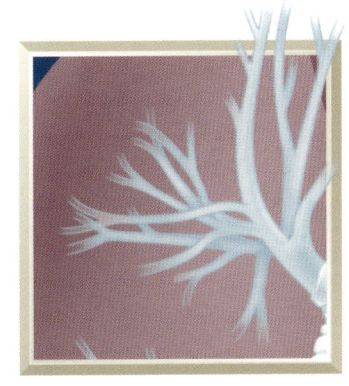
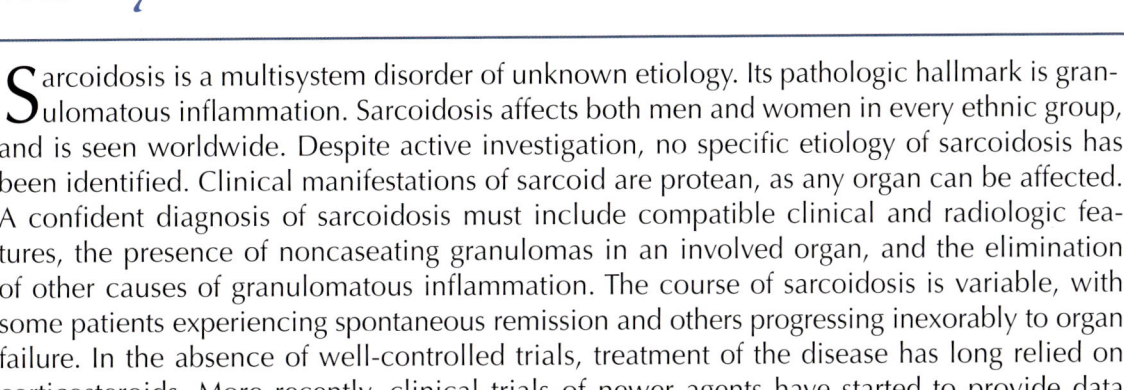
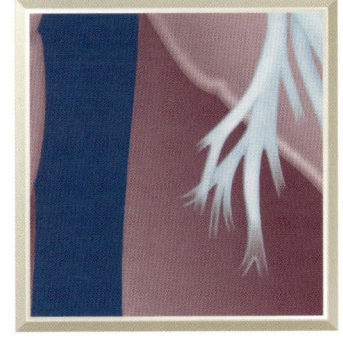

Sarcoidosis is a multisystem disorder of unknown etiology. Its pathologic hallmark is granulomatous inflammation. Sarcoidosis affects both men and women in every ethnic group, and is seen worldwide. Despite active investigation, no specific etiology of sarcoidosis has been identified. Clinical manifestations of sarcoid are protean, as any organ can be affected. A confident diagnosis of sarcoidosis must include compatible clinical and radiologic features, the presence of noncaseating granulomas in an involved organ, and the elimination of other causes of granulomatous inflammation. The course of sarcoidosis is variable, with some patients experiencing spontaneous remission and others progressing inexorably to organ failure. In the absence of well-controlled trials, treatment of the disease has long relied on corticosteroids. More recently, clinical trials of newer agents have started to provide data about alternative treatment options.

While sarcoid affects every ethnicity, African Americans and northern Europeans are disproportionately represented. It is also clear that presentation and clinical course vary by ethnicity. For example, African Americans have an increased tendency to have more progressive disease as well as an increased degree of multiorgan involvement. [1,2]. Whether this is due to a genetic effect or to socioeconomic status remains unclear [3]. Although a recent project known as A Case Control Etiologic Study of Sarcoidosis (ACCESS) did not find any specific unifying exposure, it has begun to shed light on the complex interactions between familial and environmental exposures [4,5].

One current hypothesis regarding the pathogenesis of sarcoid is that of a genetically susceptible host reacting to an environmental exposure, stimulating a granulomatous response. The nature of this stimulus could be infectious, organic or inorganic particles, or other environmental agents. It is possible that multiple exposures give rise to the entity we define as sarcoidosis. A host immune response occurs, and the clinical manifestations of the disease may depend upon another set of modifier genes. Chronic inflammation and granulomas that contain macrophages, epithelioid cells, lymphocytes, giant cells, and fibroblasts are characteristic of sarcoidosis [6]. In contrast to the peripheral blood, lung and other tissues from patients with sarcoidosis have an increased number of $CD4^+$ lymphocytes and macrophages that are activated in vivo [7]. In sarcoidosis, both $CD4^+$ and $CD8^+$ T cells have been shown to have a Th1 phenotype characterized by the increased production of interferon-γ. Tumor necrosis factor (TNF) is also produced in an exaggerated fashion and has been shown to play a critical role in granuloma formation. The alveolar macrophages in sarcoidosis tissues are similarly activated. A number of positive feedback loops are present which can contribute to sarcoidosis tissue abnormalities. An interesting feature of sarcoidosis is the frequency with which some patients undergo spontaneous remission, while others progress to fibrosis. Interleukin-10 and transforming growth factor-β1, anti-inflammatory cytokines, are upregulated in sarcoidosis, and could potentially contribute to disease remission [8].

Noncaseating epithelioid granulomas may be found in any organ. The clinical presentation of sarcoidosis is highly variable depending on which organs are symptomatically involved. Up to 60% of sarcoidosis cases are discovered incidentally in asymptomatic patients [9]. Up to 90% of patients will have pulmonary involvement at some point in their clinical course; thus, the lung is often the site of initial histologic diagnosis [10]. In the lung, typical features of sarcoidosis include varying degrees of granulomatous inflammation and tissue fibrosis. The Scadden staging system for sarcoidosis (stages 0 through IV) is based on chest radiographic findings and can offer some prognostic information [11].

Diagnosis of sarcoidosis is made after review of clinical, radiographic, and pathologic data. In patients with bilateral hilar adenopathy who are completely asymptomatic, or in those with bilateral adenopathy who present with erythema nodosum or uveitis, tissue confirmation may not be necessary [12]. In most cases, biopsy is performed both to document the presence of granulomas and to obtain tissue for culture, as infectious etiologies may be missed by histologic stains for fungi and mycobacteria [13]. Biopsy is commonly performed in the thorax because the majority of patients will have intrathoracic findings [14]. If a more accessible site is available—typically the skin or peripheral lymph nodes—it may be sampled. In many cases, a transbronchial lung biopsy performed with a flexible fiberoptic bronchoscope is the procedure of choice. Yield is higher in patients with stage II or III disease than for those with stage 0 or I disease [15]. However, with increasing numbers of biopsy specimens (up to 10), yields have been reported to be as high as 97% [16]. Endobronchial biopsy can also increase the rate of diagnosis, particularly if biopsies are taken of abnormal-appearing mucosa [17]. Additional techniques utilized during the bronchoscopic procedure, such as transbronchial needle aspiration or endobronchial ultrasound-guided biopsy of hilar and mediastinal lymph nodes can also significantly improve yield and can potentially spare the patient a more invasive procedure such as mediastinoscopy [18]. In addition to pulmonary evaluation, every patient with sarcoidosis should be thoroughly evaluated for signs and symptoms of extrapulmonary disease. In particular, manifestations of organ-threatening disease, such as sarcoidosis involving the heart, eye, or neurologic system should be sought.

Treatment for sarcoidosis has been an area of considerable controversy. Sarcoidosis is known for its predilection to wax and wane spontaneously, which renders treatment response difficult to interpret. Some have suggested that treatment with steroids may lead to more progressive and refractory disease and may prevent the host's own clearance mechanisms from occurring [19]. Many patients with sarcoidosis require no therapy. Widely accepted indications for medical treatment include organ-threatening disease, cardiac involvement, central nervous system disease, involvement of either anterior or posterior chamber of the eye, and hypercalcemia. Treatment for disease in the lung, the most common clinically involved site, is more controversial and is typically reserved for patients with progressing, higher stage disease. At present, corticosteroids remain the usual therapy—an approach based largely on nonrandomized studies conducted over the last several decades. It is generally accepted that corticosteroids provide symptomatic relief and disease improvement acutely in the majority of patients. However, long-term effects of glucocorticoids in altering disease outcomes are unclear.

The optimal medications, dosage, and duration of treatment are unknown. For patients with pulmonary sarcoidosis in whom systemic corticosteroid treatment appears warranted, treatment recommendations typically suggest beginning prednisone at a dosage of 20 to 40 mg/day and maintaining a dosage in that range for a period of 1 to 3 months [20]. At that point, an assessment regarding the benefit of treatment should be made. If there is stability or improvement, prednisone should be tapered very slowly, with an anticipated total duration of therapy of between 6 and 12 months. Relapse may occur in some patients during tapering or after treatment is discontinued, particularly in those patients who experienced remission of disease with corticosteroids [19].

Because of the known potential for corticosteroids to produce side effects and because some patients with chronic disease require maintenance treatment over years or a lifetime, there has been growing interest in the use of steroid-sparing agents. Methotrexate and azathioprine are generally used as initial steroid-sparing agents, but more recent studies of biological agents with specific activity against TNF-α, such as infliximab, have shown that these drugs may be effective for some patients with progressive disease [21,22].

For end-stage pulmonary or cardiac sarcoidosis, transplantation is an option to extend survival and to improve quality of life. No predictive models for mortality in sarcoid exist, but because mortality among sarcoid patients on the lung transplant waiting list is high, early referral should be considered for severe, fibrobullous disease that is refractory to therapy, and particularly for coexisting pulmonary hypertension and/or oxygen dependence [23]. Survival after lung transplantation for sarcoidosis is comparable to that for other lung diseases [24].

Although there have been many recent advances in our understanding of sarcoidosis, it remains a challenging disease. The clinician must maintain a high index of suspicion for sarcoidosis and be thorough in excluding other etiologies of granulomatous inflammation. Once a diagnosis is made, a comprehensive clinical assessment should be performed. Treatment decisions should be individualized. Because outcomes can vary widely, close follow-up of patients is essential.

EPIDEMIOLOGY

Sarcoidosis: Historical Timeline	
1877	"Livid papillary psoriasis" described [25]
1889	"Lupus pernio" described [26]
1899	"Multiple benign sarkoid of the skin" described [27]
1914	Multisystem nature of disease described [28]
1952	First report of beneficial effect of corticosteroids in sarcoidosis [29]
2008	Etiology remains unknown

Figure 12-1. Historical timeline of sarcoidosis. Although sarcoidosis was first described in 1877, its etiology remains unknown.

Sarcoidosis: Geographic Prevalence Rates			
	Prevalence/100,000 Persons		
Country	Men	Women	Study
United States	5.9	6.3	Henke et al. [30]
White	5.0		Gundelfinger and Britten [31]
African American	47.8		Gundelfinger and Britten [31]
United Kingdom			
British born	27.0	27.0	James and Hosoda [32]; Brett [33]
Irish born	97.0	213.0	James and Hosoda [32]; Brett [33]
Caribbean born	197.0	170.0	James and Hosoda [32]; Brett [33]
Finland	22.0	34.4	Pietinalho et al. [34]
Japan	4.9	7.0	Pietinalho et al. [34]
Sweden	16.5	21.7	Hillerdal et al. [35]

Figure 12-2. Geographic prevalence rates of sarcoidosis. Prevalence rates reported for sarcoidosis are widely varied. A sampling of prevalence rates by country and gender is outlined. Country of origin, as well as ethnicity, appears to be associated with different rates. The lack of exact case definition, the absence of specific diagnostic tests, the varied manner in which case identification is performed (eg, mass radiographic screening vs symptomatic case identification), and the absence of identifiable causative agents likely all contribute to this variation [10].

IMMUNOPATHOGENESIS

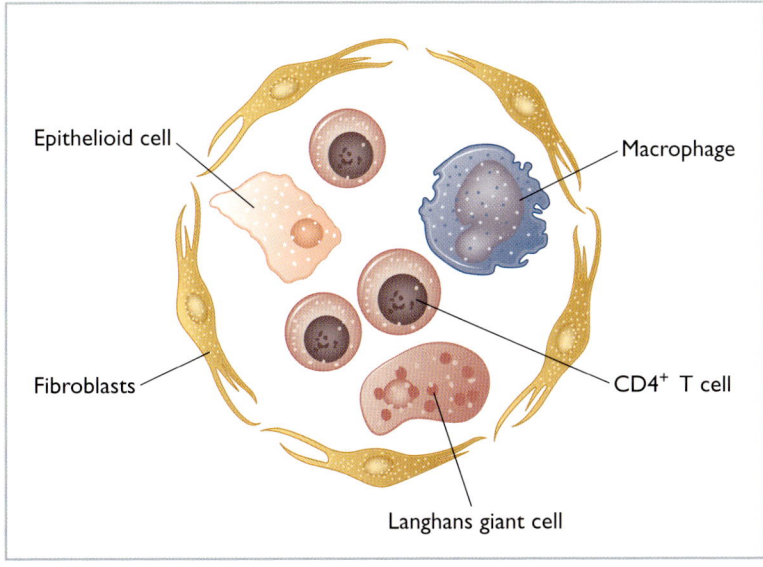

Figure 12-3. Schematic illustration of the contents of the sarcoid granuloma. The center of the granuloma frequently contains lymphocytes, macrophages, epithelioid cells, and foreign body and/or Langhans giant cells. They are frequently surrounded by a rim of fibrosis with fibroblastic cells that elaborate collagen.

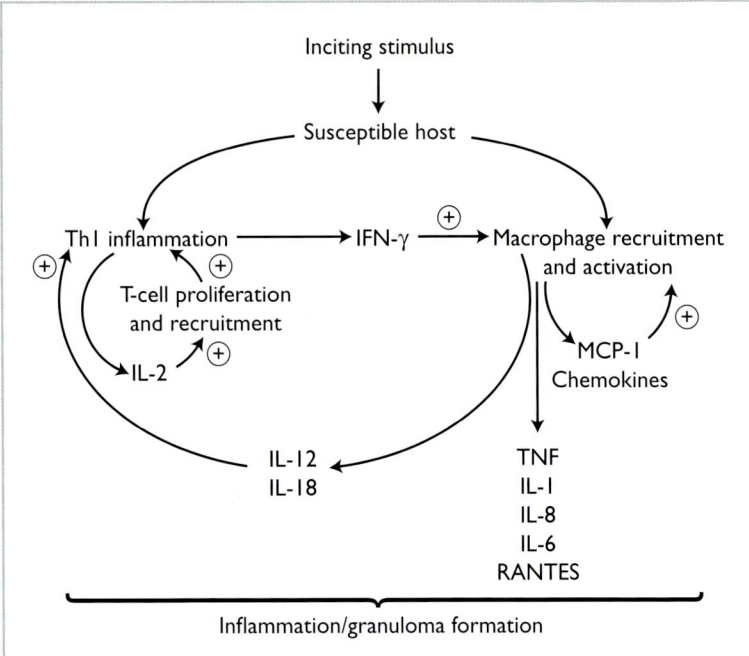

Figure 12-4. Schematic illustration of the pathogenesis of the inflammatory alterations in sarcoidosis. Sarcoidosis results from an appropriate stimulus interacting with a susceptible host. Host susceptibility may be related to altered levels of T-cell activation, increased macrophage activation, and/or altered innate immune mechanisms. Antigen exposure results in a Th1 inflammatory response characterized by the heightened production of interferon (IFN)-γ and interleukin (IL)-2. IFN-γ activates macrophages, which produce a variety of chemokines. A positive feedback loop is established, in which chemokine secretion leads to increased macrophage recruitment and activation. Activated macrophages also produce tumor necrosis factor (TNF), IL-1, IL-8, IL-6, RANTES, IL-12 and IL-18. TNF is likely an important mediator of granuloma formation. Importantly, IL-12 and IL-18 augment IFN-γ elaboration. Activated T cells also produce IL-2 and IL-16, which augment T-cell proliferation and recruitment.

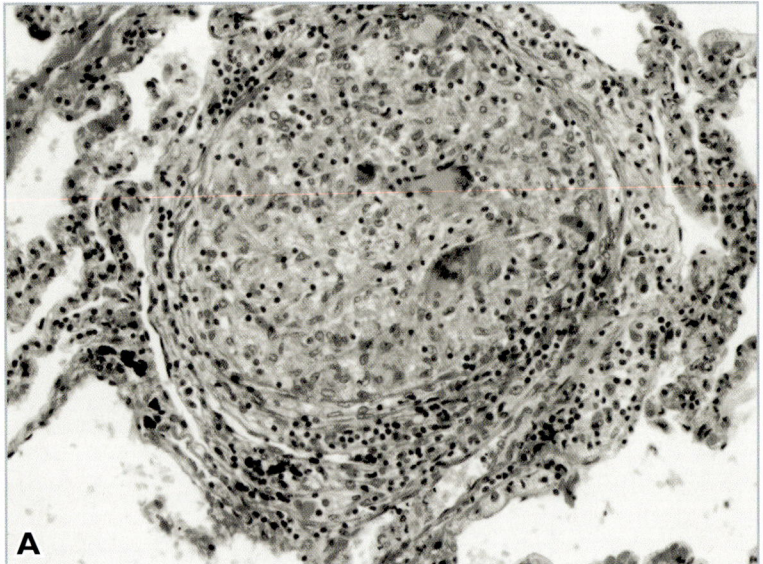

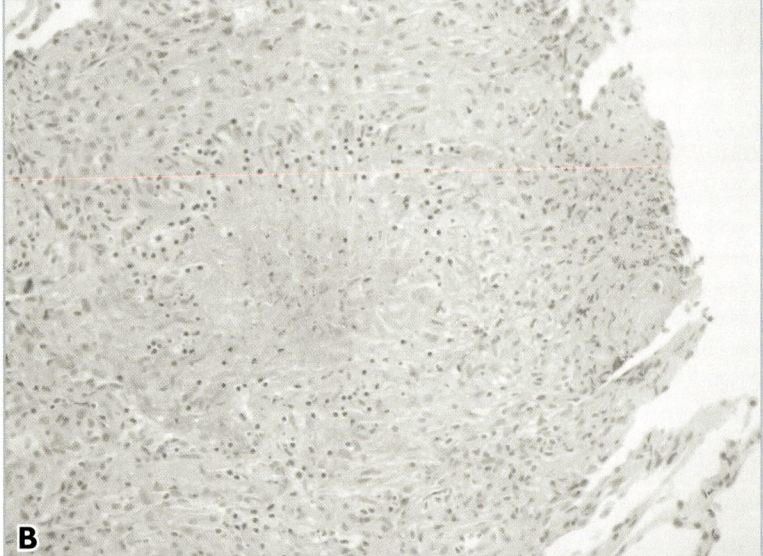

Figure 12-5. **A**, Transbronchial lung biopsy taken from a patient with pulmonary sarcoidosis. The photomicrograph demonstrates a granuloma with typical tight epithelioid histiocytes and occasional giant cells, with some surrounding concentric fibrosis. There is no local inflammation, and caseation is absent, although punctate necrosis can often be seen in sarcoidosis. The location of granuloma in peribronchial tissue is a typical feature of sarcoidosis and contributes to the high diagnostic yield of bronchoscopic biopsy. **B**, Transbronchial biopsy taken from a patient with tuberculosis. This photomicrograph demonstrates a granuloma with central caseation, which is typical of mycobacterial infection. (*Courtesy of* Dr. Robert Homer, Associate Professor of Pathology, Yale School of Medicine.)

SARCOIDOSIS CHEST RADIOGRAPHY

Staging of Sarcoidosis by Chest Radiography

Stage	Radiographic Findings	Prognosis
0	Normal	Variable, depending on extra-pulmonary organ involvement
I	Hilar, mediastinal, or paratracheal adenopathy	50%–90% spontaneously resolve
		10%–40% remain stable
		15%–30% progress to higher stage
II	Hilar, mediastinal, or paratracheal adenopathy with pulmonary parenchymal abnormalities	40%–70% spontaneously resolve
		40%–60% remain stable or have progressive disease
III	Pulmonary parenchymal abnormalities without adenopathy	10%–20% spontaneously resolve
		50%–60% remain stable
		5%–10% progress to severe lung disease
IV	Fibrobullous pulmonary parenchymal disease	Irreversible

Figure 12-6. Staging of sarcoidosis by chest radiography. The initial presentation of sarcoidosis is often in the chest, and the staging system for sarcoidosis is based on chest radiographic findings [11]. This system is useful for descriptive purposes and, to a certain degree, for defining prognosis [20,36]. However, it is lacking because it disregards involvement of organs outside the thorax. Thus, a Stage I chest radiograph, which is typically associated with good outcomes, may be seen in patients with severe extrapulmonary disease—for instance, of the heart or the neurologic system. Despite such limitations, the staging system is broadly used and remains a useful descriptive tool.

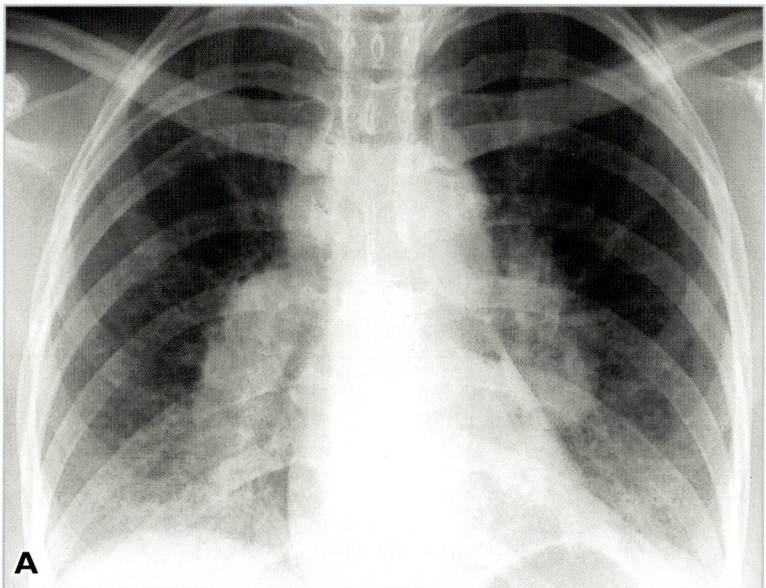

B Differential Diagnosis of Stage I Sarcoidosis

Infection
  Mycobacteria (tuberculosis, atypical mycobacteria)
  Fungal infection
  Viral infection (HIV, mononucleosis)
Malignancy
  Lymphoma
  Primary lung cancer
  Metastatic disease
Other
  Berylliosis
  Pulmonary hypertension

Figure 12-7. Sarcoidosis, stage I. **A**, Chest radiograph of a patient with stage I sarcoidosis. **B**, Differential diagnosis of stage I sarcoidosis.

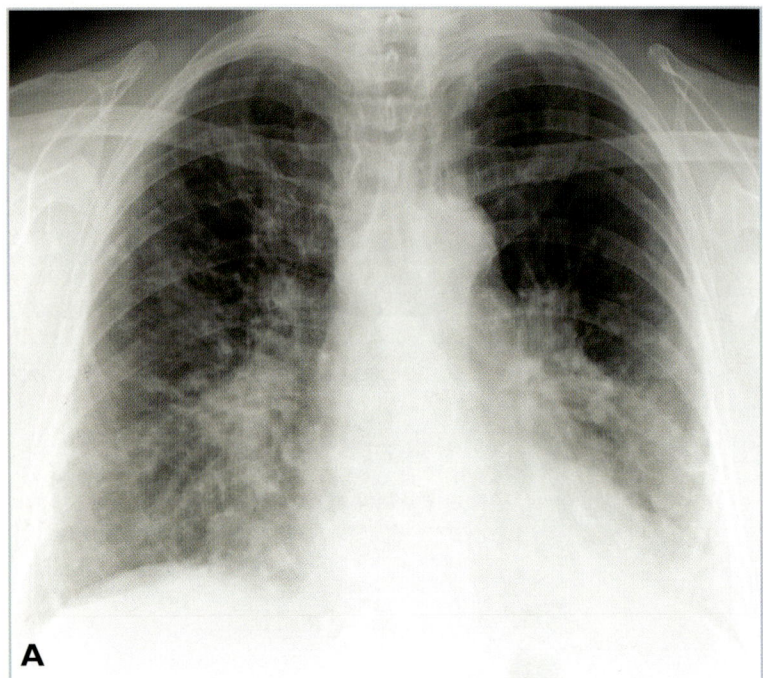

B Differential Diagnosis of Stage II Sarcoidosis

Infection
    Mycobacteria (tuberculosis, atypical mycobacteria)
    Fungal infection
    Viral infection (HIV, mononucleosis)
Malignancy
    Lymphoma
    Primary lung cancer with intrathoracic spread
    Metastatic disease
Inflammation
    Berylliosis
    Pneumoconioses
Interstitial lung diseases that may be associated with adenopathy
    Idiopathic pulmonary fibrosis
    Connective tissue disease–associated interstitial lung disease
    Allergic bronchopulmonary aspergillosis

Figure 12-8. Sarcoidosis, stage II. **A,** Chest radiograph of a patient with stage II sarcoidosis. **B,** Differential diagnosis of stage II sarcoidosis.

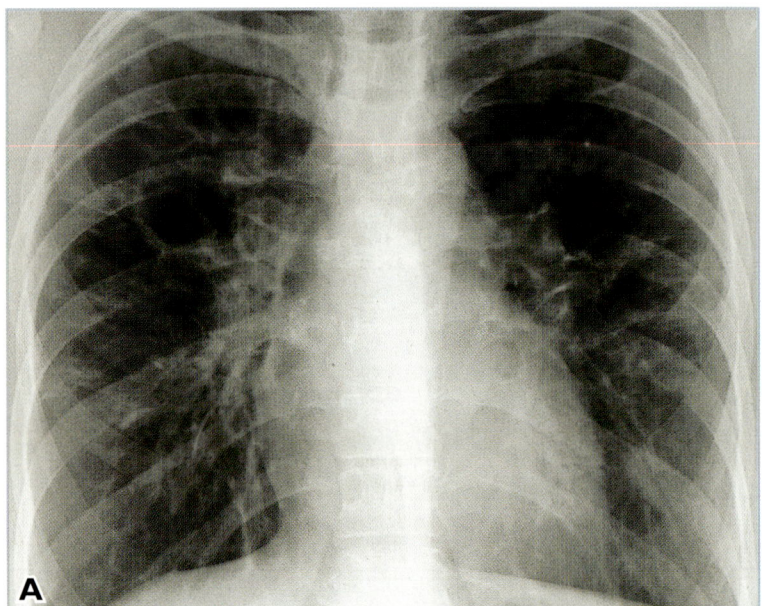

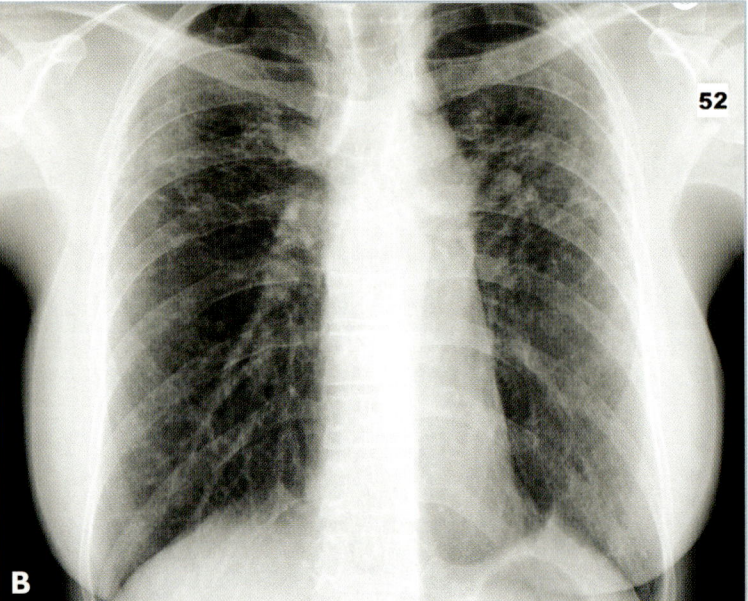

C Differential Diagnosis of Stage III Sarcoidosis

Infection
    Any diffuse pulmonary infection
    Bacterial pneumonia
    Mycobacteria (tuberculosis, atypical mycobacteria)
    Fungal infection
    Viral infection
    Pneumocystis jiroveci pneumonia
Malignancy
    Bronchoalveolar carcinoma
    Metastatic/lymphangitic spread of tumor
Inflammation/Other
    Berylliosis
    Pneumoconioses
    Interstitial lung disease
    Cystic fibrosis
    Allergic bronchopulmonary aspergillosis
    Alveolar proteinosis
    Congestive heart failure

Figure 12-9. Sarcoidosis, stage III. **A,** Chest radiograph of a 28-year-old African American woman who initially presented with a cough. Transbronchial biopsies demonstrated noncaseating granuloma, and she was believed to have pulmonary sarcoidosis, stage III. **B,** Chest radiograph of a 68-year-old Caucasian woman whose sarcoidosis was incidentally found on a routine chest radiograph. **C,** Differential diagnosis of stage III sarcoidosis.

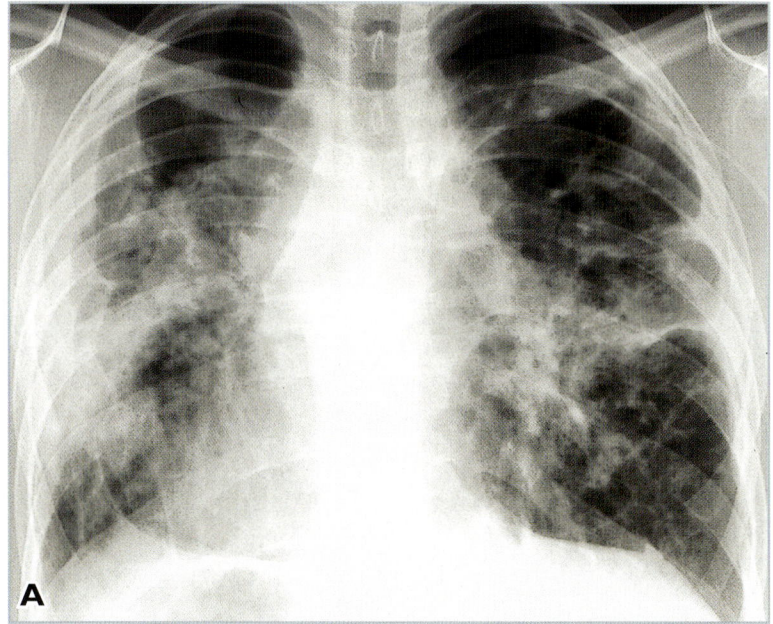

Figure 12-10. Sarcoidosis, stage IV. **A**, Chest radiograph of the same patient in Figure 12-9A, taken 10 years later. Over time, she developed progressive pulmonary disease. The radiograph shows extensive progression of pulmonary infiltrates. **B**, Differential diagnosis of stage IV sarcoidosis.

B Differential Diagnosis of Stage IV Sarcoidosis

Infection
- Mycobacteria (tuberculosis, atypical mycobacteria)
- Fungal infection
- Malignancy
- Lung cancer

Inflammation
- Silicosis
- Postradiation fibrosis

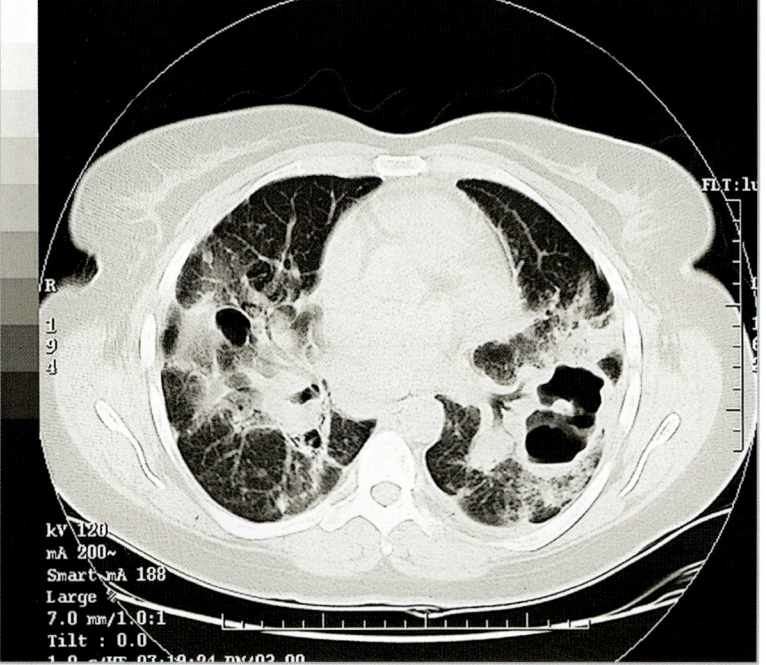

Figure 12-11. Chest CT of the same patient in Figures 12-9A and 12-10A. The patient's chest CT demonstrates extensive centrally-located infiltrates with evidence of destruction and cavitary changes in both lungs. A rounded density within the cavitary lesion in the left lung is suggestive of a mycetoma. This patient developed recurrent episodes of massive hemoptysis.

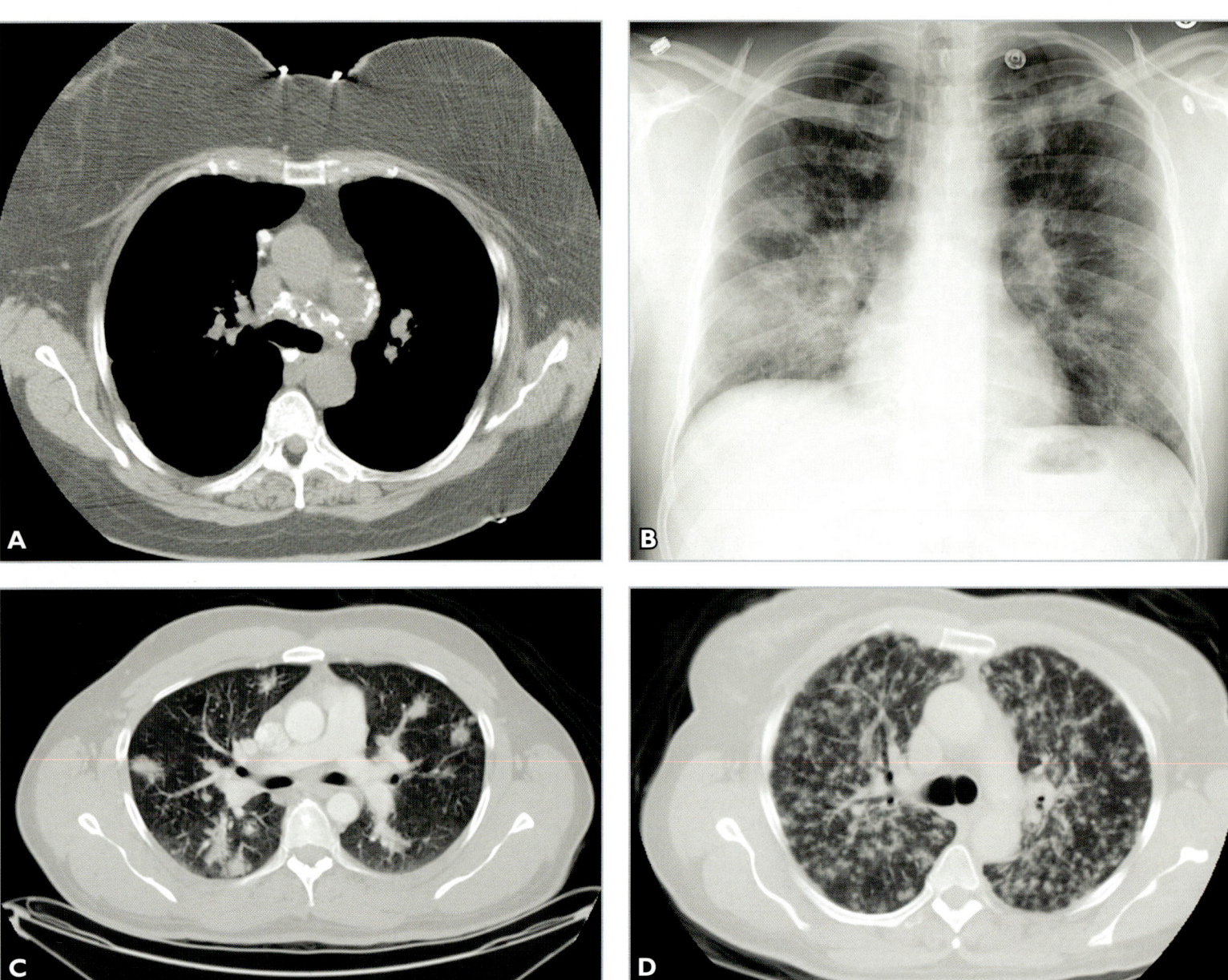

Figure 12-12. In addition to the lymphadenopathy and interstitial infiltrates routinely observed in sarcoidosis, several other radiographic findings are commonly seen. **A**, Calicified mediastinal and hilar lymph nodes. The differential diagnosis for this finding includes tuberculosis, histoplasmosis, silicosis, and Hodgkin's disease following radiation therapy to the mediastinum. **B** and **C**, Alveolar sarcoid. Sarcoidosis can have a nodular appearance with dense parenchymal opacities. The differential diagnosis for this presentation includes infection (tuberculosis, fungal, septic emboli), neoplasm (metastases, lymphoma), inflammatory diseases (Wegener's granulomatosis, cryptogenic organizing pneumonia, rheumatoid nodules), and pneumoconioses (silicosis). **D**, Multiple small nodules. The differential diagnosis for this presentation includes infection (tuberculosis and histoplasmosis), metastatic disease, and pulmonary Langerhans cell histiocytosis. The nodular infiltrates of sarcoidosis tend to have a perivascular and perilymphatic distribution.

DIAGNOSIS AND MANIFESTATIONS OF DISEASE

Characteristics of Patients Enrolled in the ACCESS Study

Specific Organ Involved		Scadding Stage at Diagnosis	
Lungs	95.0%	Stage 0	8%
Skin (not erythema nodosum)	15.9%	Stage I	40%
Lymph nodes	15.2%	Stage II	37%
Eye	11.8%	Stage III	10%
Liver	11.5%	Stage IV	5%
Erythema nodosum	8.3%		
Spleen	6.7%		
Neurologic system	4.6%		
Parotid/salivary	3.9%		
Bone marrow	3.9%		
Calcium	3.7%		
Ear, nose, and throat	3.0%		
Cardiac	2.3%		
Renal	0.7%		
Bone/joint	0.5%		
Muscle	0.4%		

Figure 12-13. Characteristics of patients enrolled in the ACCESS study. The National Heart, Lung and Blood Institute-sponsored study, A Case Control Etiologic Study of Sarcoidosis (ACCESS), enrolled over 700 newly diagnosed sarcoidosis patients. Of note, the primary investigators were pulmonologists, perhaps explaining the high rate of lung involvement. The majority of patients had stages 0 through II disease. Sarcoidosis is a systemic disease, and involvement of other organ systems was frequently observed. (*Adapted from* Baughman *et al.* [37].)

Sarcoidosis: Yield of Commonly Obtained Biopsies

Biopsy	Patients with Positive Biopsy, %	Study
Mediastinoscopy		Raghu [38], Gossot [39]
Stage I	90–95	
Stage III	50–60	
Bronchoscopy		Gilman [40], Roethe [16], Chapman and Mehta1 [5], Descombes *et al.* [41]
Stage I (7–10 specimens)	70–90	
Stage II (4–6 specimens)	85–95	
Stage III (4–6 specimens)	> 90	
Surgical lung biopsy	90–100	Raghu [38], Gossot [39]
Endomyocardial biopsy	19	Uemura [42]
Liver	40–70	Devaney [43]
Skin		
Lupus pernio*		
Erythema nodosum†		
Lymph node‡		

*The characteristic appearance of lupus pernio and the predilection for sarcoidosis to involve traumatized skin may render skin biopsy unnecessary or undesirable, particularly if tissue is available from another organ.
†The histopathology of erythema nodosum is nongranulomatous, and biopsy of these lesions will therefore be nondiagnostic for sarcoidosis.
‡The term "GLUS" (granulomatous lesions of unknown significance) is used to describe granulomatous inflammation in a lymph node or in the liver in the absence of other organ involvement.

Figure 12-14. Yields of commonly obtained biopsies in sarcoidosis.

Causes of Granulomatous Inflammation

Infection
  Mycobacteria
  Fungi
  Parasites
  Leprosy
  Cat-scratch disease
Inflammation
  Sarcoidosis
  Berylliosis
  Granulomatous vasculitidies
  Rheumatoid arthritis (necrobiotic nodules)
  Crohn's disease
  Foreign body reactions
  Hypersensitivity pneumonitis
  Biliary cirrhosis
  Eosinophilic granuloma
Malignancy
  Lymphoma

Figure 12-15. Causes of granulomatous inflammation.

Clinical Features of Extrapulmonary Organ Involvement in Sarcoidosis

Organ	Clinical Features	Organ	Clinical Features
Skin	Nodular, papular, or plaquelike lesions (especially in old scars)	Heart	Syncope, palpitations, sudden death
	Lupus pernio (specific)		Conduction system abnormalities
	Erythema nodosum (nonspecific)		Arrhythmia
Eye	Photophobia, tearing, blurred vision, conjunctival injection		Cardiomyopathy
	Lacrimal gland inflammation	Endocrine/renal	Nephrolithiasis, renal insufficiency, diabetes insipidus, hypercalcemia, hypercalciuria, pituitary insufficiency, interstitial nephritis
	Anterior chamber disease		Parotid gland swelling
	Anterior uveitis, conjunctivitis, adhesions, vision loss	Lymph nodes	Bulky adenopathy (usually asymptomatic)
	Posterior chamber disease	Spleen	Splenomegaly (usually asymptomatic)
	Posterior uveitis, chorioretinitis	Bone marrow	Cytopenias
	Optic neuritis	Musculoskeletal	Polyarthritis (acute or chronic)
Liver	Abdominal discomfort		Bone cysts
	Liver function test abnormalities		Myopathy
	Hepatomegaly		
Neurologic system	Cranial nerve palsies, headache, blurred vision, seizures, peripheral neuropathy, polyneuropathy, diabetes insipidus		
	Central nervous system		
	Aseptic basilar meningitis, cranial neuropathies, brain mass, hypothalamic and pituitary lesions, obstructing hydrocephalus		
	Peripheral nervous system		
	Polyneuropathy, peripheral neuropathy		

Figure 12-16. Clinical features of extrapulmonary organ involvement in sarcoidosis.

CUTANEOUS SARCOIDOSIS

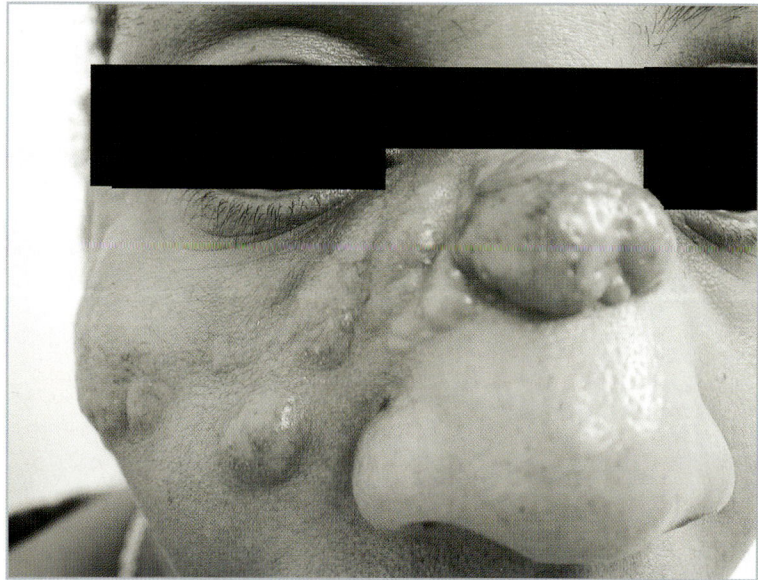

Figure 12-17. Cutaneous sarcoidosis: Lupus pernio. These granulomatous skin lesions may present as violaceous eruptions on the face, particularly around the eyes, across the bridge of the nose, on the cheeks, or on the ears. They can be papular as shown here, but they may also be macular and may be associated with scarring and deformity. Lupus pernio is more common among African Americans and generally follows a chronic course. (*Courtesy of* Dr. Peter Heald, Professor of Dermatology, Yale School of Medicine.)

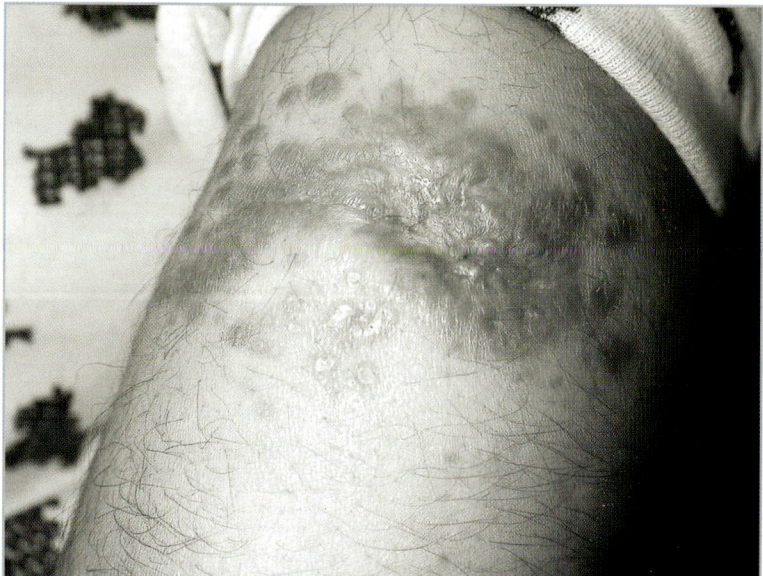

Figure 12-18. Cutaneous sarcoidosis. Granulomatous infiltration of the skin with nodular features surrounding a scar can be seen on this patient's arm. (*Courtesy of* Dr. Peter Heald, Professor of Dermatology, Yale School of Medicine.)

SARCOIDOSIS OF THE HEART

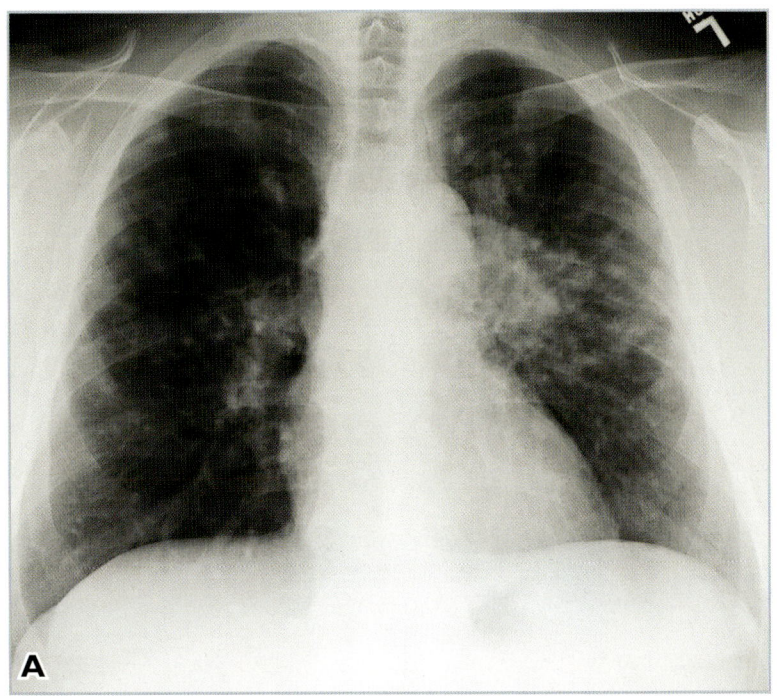
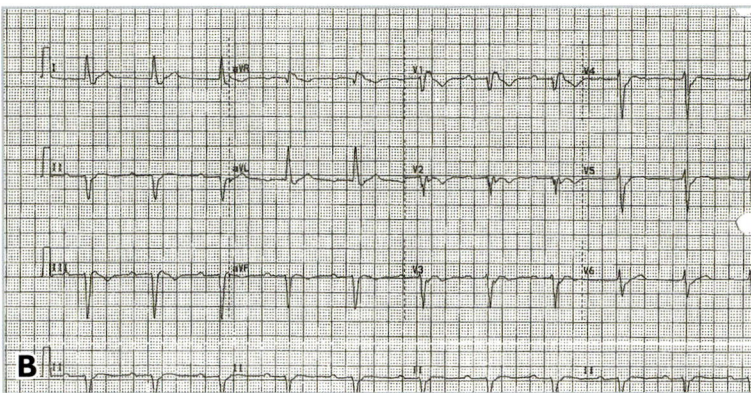
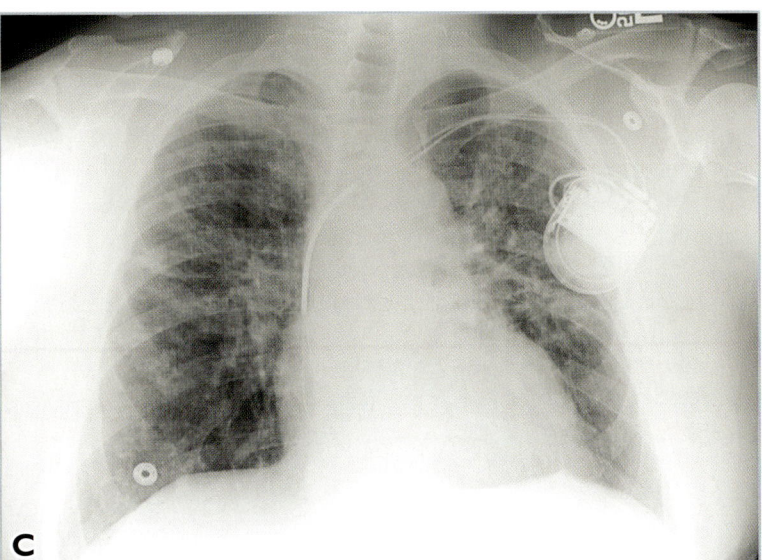
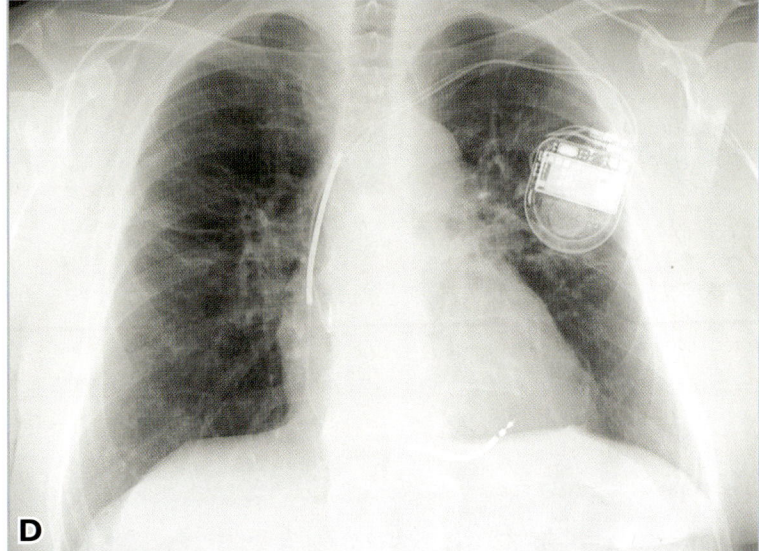

Figure 12-19. **A**, Chest radiograph of a 62-year-old white man diagnosed with sarcoidosis by transbronchial lung biopsy. The patient's baseline chest radiograph at the time of initial diagnosis demonstrates an interstitial process with bilateral hilar adenopathy, more prominent on the left than on the right. He was asymptomatic at that time and was not treated. **B**, Nine years after initial presentation, the patient presented for follow-up with complaint of exertional dyspnea. Resting electrocardiogram shows evidence of first-degree atrioventricular block, as well as a right bundle-branch block pattern. Echocardiography showed no evidence of regional wall motion abnormality and revealed an estimated left ventricular ejection fraction of 40%. The patient underwent cardiac catheterization and demonstrated no evidence of coronary artery disease. Based on the prior history of pulmonary sarcoidosis and on the presence of conduction system abnormalities and cardiomyopathy in the absence of coronary artery disease, the patient was felt to have cardiac sarcoidosis. The patient underwent electrophysiologic study, which demonstrated inducible sustained ventricular tachycardia. An implantable cardiodefibrillator device (ICD) was placed. **C**, Chest radiograph at the time of ICD placement reveals enlargement of the cardiac silhouette with worsened interstitial abnormalities, as well as the implanted defibrillator. **D**, Chest radiograph after treatment with prednisone and methotrexate. The patient's ejection fraction improved to 55% and remained stable while he was on therapy. The upper lobe interstitial and alveolar abnormalities simultaneously improved while he was on therapy for cardiac sarcoidosis.

SARCOIDOSIS OF THE NERVOUS SYSTEM

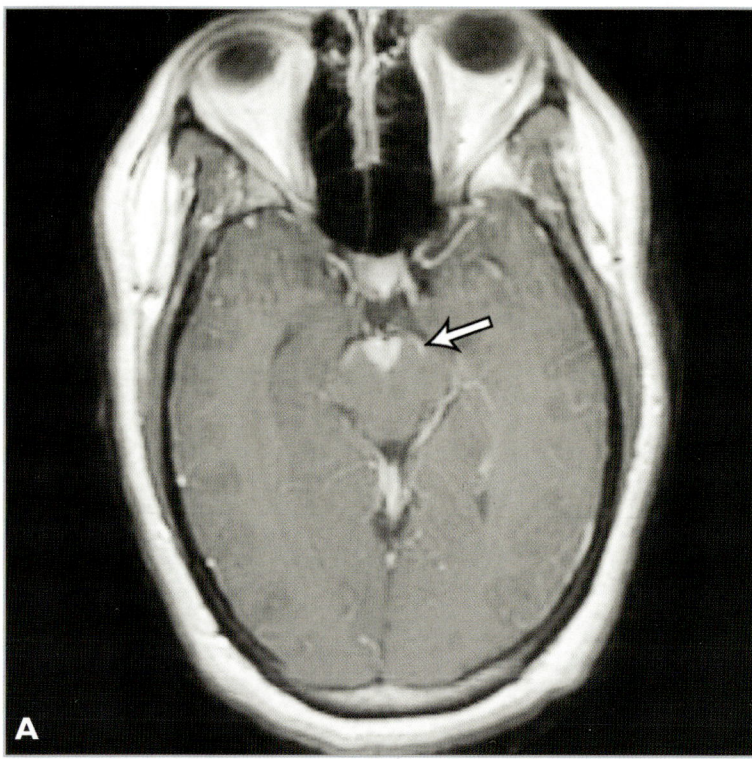 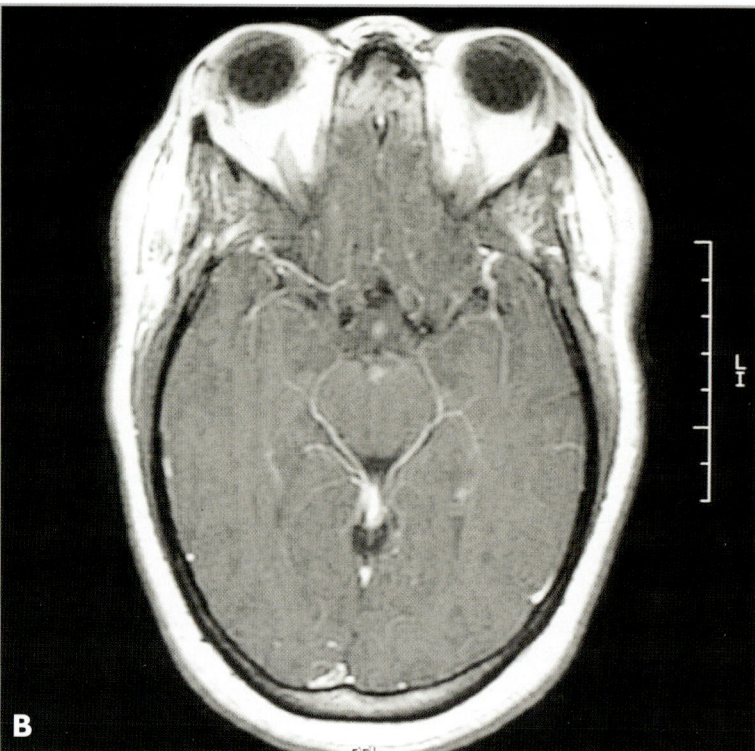

Figure 12-20. **A**, A 25-year-old African American woman presented with chief complaints of lightheadedness, visual acuity loss, and tinnitus. Neurologic evaluation at that time included MRI of the brain. The MRI demonstrates an enhancing mass in the midbrain at the base of the third ventricle (arrow), with subarachnoid enhancement in the interpeduncular cistern. Further evaluation included a chest radiograph showing bilateral hilar adenopathy without evidence of parenchymal pulmonary abnormalities. The patient underwent mediastinoscopy. Pathologic evaluation of the mediastinal lymph nodes demonstrated noncaseating granuloma. The diagnosis was felt to be sarcoidosis with neurologic involvement.

B, The patient was treated with corticosteroids, initially prednisone at 40 mg/day, for several months. She had complete resolution of her neurologic symptoms within 2 months. A follow-up MRI after 1 year of treatment demonstrates a marked decrease in the size of the mass, with some persistent enhancement in the region of the interpeduncular fossa. The patient developed severe glucose intolerance requiring insulin treatment, which necessitated a decrease in corticosteroid dosage over the first few months of treatment. Methotrexate was instituted as a steroid-sparing agent. She has subsequently remained stable on low-dosage prednisone and low-dosage methotrexate after 24 months of follow-up.

Baseline Evaluation for All Patients with Sarcoidosis

History, including occupational history

Comprehensive physical examination

Laboratory examination

  Chest radiograph

  Electrocardiogram

  CBC, BUN/Cr, calcium, liver function tests

  24-hour urinary calcium excretion analysis

  Tuberculin skin test

  Pulmonary function tests (spirometry, lung volumes, and diffusion capacity)

Slit lamp ophthalmologic examination

Other organ-specific evaluations should be directed by findings on history and physical examination

Figure 12-21. Baseline evaluation for all patients with sarcoidosis. Because the clinical presentation of sarcoidosis is highly varied, a broad-based approach to a patient with sarcoidosis should be taken. Sarcoidosis is a systemic disease. The absence of clinical symptoms does not reliably exclude the presence of clinically relevant organ involvement. Regardless of the site of initial identification of disease, every patient with sarcoidosis should have a comprehensive examination focusing on the particular organs known to be commonly affected by disease [20]. BUN/Cr—blood urea nitrogen/creatinine; CBC—complete blood count.

Proposed Access Criteria for Organ Involvement in Patients with Biopsy-Confirmed Sarcoidosis

Organ	Definite Involvement	Probable Involvement
Lung	Chest roentgenogram with one or more of the following:	Lymphocytic alveolitis by bronchoalveolar lavage
	Bilateral hilar adenopathy	Any pulmonary infiltrates
	Diffuse infiltrates	Isolated reduction in diffusing capacity for carbon monoxide
	Upper lobe fibrosis	
	Restriction on pulmonary function tests	
Skin	Lupus pernio	Macular/papular
	Annular lesion	New nodules
	Erythema nodosum	
Eye	Lacrimal gland swelling	Blindness
	Uveitis	
	Optic neuritis	
Neurologic system	Positive MRI with uptake in meninges or brainstem	Other abnormalities on MRI
	Cerebrospinal fluid with increased lymphocytes and/or protein	Unexplained neuropathy
	Diabetes insipidus	Positive electromyogram
	Bell's Palsy	
	Cranial nerve dysfunction	
	Peripheral nerve dysfunction	
Cardiac system	Treatment responsive cardiomyopathy	No other cardiac problem and either ventricular arrhythmias or cardiomyopathy
	Electrocardiogram showing intraventricular conduction defect or nodal block	
	Positive gallium scan of the heart	Abnormal thallium scan
Liver	Liver function tests greater than three times normal	Compatible CT
		Elevated alkaline phosphatase
Hypercalcemia/Hypercalciuria	Increased serum calcium with no other cause	Increased urine calcium
		Nephrolithiasis analysis showing calcium
Nonthoracic lymph node		New palpable node above waist
		Lymph node > 2 cm by CT
Parotid/salivary glands	Symmetrical parotitis with syndrome of mumps	
	Positive gallium scan ("panda sign")	

Figure 12-22. ACCESS criteria for organ involvement in patients with biopsy-confirmed sarcoidosis. The investigators from A Case Control Etiologic Study of Sarcoidosis (ACCESS), in conjunction with the National Heart, Lung, and Blood Institute, used these criteria for organ involvement in patients with a diagnosis of sarcoidosis confirmed by tissue biopsy. Organ involvement is identified as definite or probable based on clinical evidence of disease. (*Adapted from* Judson et al. [44].)

TREATMENT

Broadly Accepted Clinical Indications for Treatment of Sarcoidosis

- Progressive, symptomatic pulmonary disease
- Cardiac disease
- Disease of the central nervous system
- Severe posterior chamber eye disease
- Persistent hypercalcemia
- Debilitating constitutional symptoms
- Disfiguring skin disease
- Renal dysfunction
- Severe hepatic dysfunction
- Hypersplenism
- Pituitary disease
- Myopathy
- Painful lymphadenopathy

Figure 12-23. Broadly accepted clinical indications for treatment of sarcoidosis. The diagnosis of sarcoidosis does not mandate treatment of all patients. Widely accepted indications for initiation of treatment are listed here and in Figure 12-24.

Treatment for Pulmonary Sarcoidosis

Observe patients with
- Stage I disease, given the likelihood of stability or spontaneous remission
- Stage II or III disease who are asymptomatic and have normal pulmonary function
- Stage II or III disease with minimal symptoms and mild pulmonary function abnormalities

Consider treatment with glucocorticoids in patients with
- Stage II or III disease with symptoms and/or pulmonary function abnormalities that do not spontaneously improve after a period of observation (months)

Initiate treatment with glucocorticoids in patients with
- Stage II or III disease with symptoms and/or pulmonary function abnormalities at baseline that are progressively worsening

Figure 12-24. Treatment for pulmonary sarcoidosis. In general, glucocorticoids have been the mainstay of treatment for patients with progressive pulmonary or organ-threatening extrapulmonary disease. However, considerable controversy exists regarding the efficacy of treatment because of the lack of large randomized trials rigorously evaluating treatment benefit and because sarcoidosis can spontaneously remit.

Risk Factors for Poor Outcome in Sarcoidosis

Demographics
- African American
- Age at onset 40 or above
- Symptoms lasting longer than 6 mo
- Lower annual family income

Clinical factors
- Involvement of > 3 organ systems
- Stage III or IV pulmonary disease
- Chronic respiratory insufficiency
- Amount of supplemental oxygen used
- Pulmonary hypertension
- Right atrial pressure ≥15 mm Hg
- Progressive pulmonary disease

Signs and symptoms
- Absence of erythema nodosum
- Presence of lupus pernio
- Chronic hypercalcemia
- Nephrocalcinosis
- Chronic uveitis
- Nasal mucosal involvement

Specific organ involvement
- Neurosarcoid
- Cardiac sarcoid
- Cystic bone lesions
- Splenomegaly

Figure 12-25. Risk factors for poor outcome in sarcoidosis. It is well known that some patients with sarcoidosis will have a benign clinical course with few, if any, symptoms, and with spontaneous resolution. Others will have progressive pulmonary decline with eventual respiratory failure, whereas still others will have debilitating disease due to extrapulmonary sarcoidosis. The reasons for such variability in outcomes are still unclear, but certain clinical features have been shown to predict worse outcomes and might prompt more aggressive treatment or earlier referral for transplant evaluation [1,2,23,24,45–47].

Comparison of Studies Evaluating Oral Corticosteroids

Study	Outcome Measures	Patients, n	Duration of Therapy, mo	Outcome
James et al. [48]	Chest radiographic changes, symptoms	75	6	Treatment group had improved by the end of therapy as measured by radiographic findings and symptoms; no long term follow-up data
Israel et al. [49]	Symptoms, radiographic changes, pulmonary function	83	3	Treatment group had improved by the end of therapy as measured by radiographic findings and symptoms; no long term follow-up data
Eule et al. [50]	Chest radiographic changes and pulmonary function	280	6 or 12	Treatment group had improved by the end of therapy as measured by radiographic findings, but this benefit was not sustained at follow-up of 3 and 5 years
Selroos and Sellergren [51]	Chest radiographic changes and pulmonary function	39	7	Treatment group had improved by the end of therapy in radiographic findings, and in pulmonary function compared with placebo group, but this benefit was not sustained at follow-up of up to 48 months
Zaki et al. [52]	Chest radiographic changes and pulmonary function	159	24	No difference between treatment and placebo groups with regard to radiographic changes or pulmonary function at completion of treatment or at 4-year follow-up
Pietinalho et al. [53]	Chest radiographic changes, pulmonary function, ACE activity	154	3	Treatment group with Stage II disease had improved by the end of therapy in chest radiograph and in pulmonary function compared to placebo; beneficial effect persisted at 6 months of follow-up, but not thereafter

Figure 12-26. Comparison of studies evaluating oral corticosteroids. The role of corticosteroids in the treatment of sarcoidosis remains controversial. It is widely accepted that corticosteroids provide symptomatic relief and disease improvement acutely in the majority of patients. However, long-term effects of glucocorticoids in altering disease outcomes are unclear. Because corticosteroids are widely accepted as standard-of-care for patients with progressive or symptomatic sarcoidosis, a randomized, double-blind, placebo-controlled trial is difficult to perform. A systematic review of the medical literature by the Cochrane Library Airways Group relating to this topic included 13 randomized, double-blind, placebo-controlled trials, of which six examined the role of oral steroids (detailed in this figure) and seven examined the role of inhaled corticosteroids [54]. The findings of these studies were combined in a meta-analysis, which demonstrated a significant overall improvement in radiographic findings in the group of patients receiving oral corticosteroids. Symptoms and spirometry were also improved over 3 to 24 months. The data for inhaled corticosteroids were inadequate for meta-analysis of radiographic changes or pulmonary function. This result supports the widely held view that oral corticosteroids do result acutely in improvement in patients with stage II and III disease. However, there is no firm evidence that this benefit is sustained at long term follow-up. ACE—antiotensin converting enzyme.

Extrapulmonary Sarcoidosis: Treatment Options Other Than Glucocorticoids

Organ	Clinical Scenario	Treatment Options (Other than Oral Corticosteroids)
Skin	Lupus pernio, disfiguring skin lesions	Intralesional corticosteroid injection; topical high-potency fluorinated corticosteroids (plus occlusive dressings); antimalarials; methotrexate; other alternative agents
Eye	Anterior chamber disease	Topical corticosteroid alone may be adequate
Liver	Transaminase elevation	Patients with abnormal liver function tests, but an absence of symptoms, may not require treatment
Neurologic system	Variable presentations	Diagnosis may be made by surgical resection; anticonvulsants if indicated
Heart	Conduction system disease, arrhythmia, congestive heart failure	Pacemaker or implantable cardiodefibrillator device placement; antiarrhythmic medications; treatment for left ventricular dysfunction
Endocrine	Hypercalcemia, hypercalciuria	Reduction in calcium and vitamin D intake, hydration
Pituitary	Pituitary insufficiency, diabetes insipidus	Hormone replacement, water replacement for diabetes insipidus
Musculoskeletal system	Acute or chronic arthritis	Nonglucocorticoid anti-inflammatory agents

Figure 12-27. Oral corticosteroids are generally reserved for organ-threatening disease. For less severe extrapulmonary involvement, observation or topical treatments may suffice. For more extensive organ involvement, oral corticosteroids are used. Alternative therapies should be considered when appropriate, particularly in the setting of unacceptable steroid side effects. In the case of complicating features, such as seizures due to neurologic sarcoidosis, or cardiac arrhythmias in the case of cardiac sarcoidosis, additional medical therapies may be required.

Alternative Therapies for Sarcoidosis

Immunosuppressive agents	Antimicrobial agents
Methotrexate	Antimalarials
Azathioprine	Hydroxychloroquine
Cyclophosphamide	Chloroquine
Leflunomide	**Antibiotics**
Cyclosporin	Minocycline
Tacrolimus (topical)	Doxycycline
TNF-α inhibitors	
Infliximab	
Pentoxifylline	
Thalidomide	
Adalimumab	
Etanercept	

Figure 12-28. Alternative therapies for sarcoidosis. Often, steroid-sparing agents are required due to side effects and toxicities of corticosteroids. Methotrexate is the most commonly used alternate agent and may be efficacious in up to 60% of patients, but its full effect may not be seen for up to 6 months [22]. Additional concerns include potential hepatotoxicity and pulmonary hypersensitivity reactions. Other immunosuppressive agents have been used with varying success. Antimicrobial agents, including antimalarial drugs and antibiotics, have been useful, particularly for cutaneous sarcoidosis. The tumor necrosis factor-α (TNF-α) pathway has been found to be important in many patients with granulomatous inflammation. Agents targeting this cytokine have shown efficacy in some patients with sarcoidosis [55].

REFERENCES

1. Newman LS, Rose CS, Maier LA: Sarcoidosis. *N Engl J Med* 1997, 336(17):1224–1234.

2. Judson MA, Baughman RP, Thompson BW, *et al.*: Two year prognosis of sarcoidosis: the ACCESS experience. *Sarcoidosis Vasc Diffuse Lung Dis* 2003, 20(3):204–211.

3. Westney GE, Judson MA: Racial and ethnic disparities in sarcoidosis: from genetics to socioeconomics. *Clin Chest Med* 2006, 27(3):vi,453–462.

4. Newman LS, Rose CS, Bresnitz EA, *et al.*: A case control etiologic study of sarcoidosis: environmental and occupational risk factors. *Am J Respir Crit Care Med* 2004, 170(12):1324–1330.

5. Rossman MD, Thompson B, Frederick M, *et al.*: HLA-DRB1*1101: a significant risk factor for sarcoidosis in blacks and whites. *Am J Hum Genet* 2003, 73(4):720–735.

6. Rosen Y: Pathology of sarcoidosis. *Semin Respir Crit Care Med* 2007, 28(1):36–52.

7. Semenzato G, Bortoli M, Agostini C: Applied clinical immunolgy in sarcoidosis. *Curr Opin Pulm Med* 2002, 8:441–444.

8. Zissel G, Prasse A, Muller-Quernheim J: Sarcoidosis—immunopathogenetic concepts. *Semin Respir Crit Care Med* 2007, 28(1):3–14.

9. Lynch JP III, Kazerooni EA, Gay SE: Pulmonary sarcoidosis. *Clin Chest Med* 1997, 18(4):755–785.

10. American Thoracic Society: Statement on sarcoidosis. *Am J Respir Crit Care Med* 1999, 160(2):736–755.

11. Scadding JG: Prognosis of intrathoracic sarcoidosis in England: A review of 136 cases after five years' observation. *BMJ* 1961, 5261:1165–1172.

12. Winterbauer RH, Belic N, Moores KD: Clinical interpretation of bilateral hilar adenopathy. *Ann Intern Med* 1973, 78(1):65–71.

13. Hsu RM, Connors AF Jr, Tomashefski JF Jr: Histologic, microbiologic, and clinical correlates of the diagnosis of sarcoidosis by transbronchial biopsy. *Arch Pathol Lab Med* 1996, 120(4):364–368.

14. Teirstein AS, Judson MA, Baughman RP, *et al.*: The spectrum of biopsy sites for the diagnosis of sarcoidosis. *Sarcoidosis Vasc Diffuse Lung Dis* 2005, 22(2):139–146.

15. Chapman JT, Mehta AC: Bronchoscopy in sarcoidosis: diagnostic and therapeutic interventions. *Curr Opin Pulm Med* 2003, 9(5):402–407.

16. Roethe RA, Fuller PB, Byrd RB, Hafermann DR: Transbronchoscopic lung biopsy in sarcoidosis. Optimal number and sites for diagnosis. *Chest* 1980, 77(3):400–402.

17. Shorr AF, Torrington KG, Hnatiuk OW: Endobronchial biopsy for sarcoidosis: a prospective study. *Chest* 2001, 120(1):109–114.

18. Annema JT, Rabe KF: State of the art lecture: EUS and EBUS in pulmonary medicine. *Endoscopy* 2006, 38(Suppl 1):S118–S122.

19. Gottlieb JE, Israel HL, Steiner RM, *et al.*: Outcome in sarcoidosis: the relationship of relapse to corticosteroid therapy. *Chest* 1997, 111(3):623–631.

20. Hunninghake GW, Costabel U, Ando M, *et al.*: ATS/ERS/WASOG statement on sarcoidosis. American Thoracic Society/European Respiratory Society/World Association of Sarcoidosis and other Granulomatous Disorders. *Sarcoidosis Vasc Diffuse Lung Dis* 1999, 16(2):149–173.

21. Baughman RP, Drent M, Kavuru M, *et al.*: Infliximab therapy in patients with chronic sarcoidosis and pulmonary involvement. *Am J Respir Crit Care Med* 2006, 174(7):795–802.

22. Baughman RP, Lower EE: Novel therapies for sarcoidosis. *Semin Respir Crit Care Med* 2007, 28(1):128–133.

23. Shorr AF, Davies DB, Nathan SD: Predicting mortality in patients with sarcoidosis awaiting lung transplantation. *Chest* 2003, 124(3):922–928.

24. Shah L: Lung transplantation in sarcoidosis. *Semin Respir Crit Care Med* 2007, 28(1):134–140.

25. Hutchinson J: Case of livid papillary psoriasis. In *Illustrations of Clinical Surgery*. London: J and A Churchill; 1877:42.

26. Besnier E: Lupus pernio de la face. *Ann Dermatol Syphiligr* 1889, 10:33–36.

27. Boeck C: Multiple benign sarkoid of the skin. *J Cutan Genito-Urin Dis* 1899, 17:543–550.

28. Kuznitsky E, Bittorf A: Sarkoid mit Beteiligung innerer Organe [in German]. *Munch Med Wochenschr* 1915:1349–1353.

29. Siltzbach LE: Effects of cortisone in sarcoidosis; a study of thirteen patients. *Am J Med* 1952, 12(2):139–160.

30. Henke CE, Henke G, Elveback LR, *et al.*: The epidemiology of sarcoidosis in Rochester, Minnesota: a population-based study of incidence and survival. *Am J Epidemiol* 1986, 123(5):840–845.

31. Gundelfinger BF, Britten SA: Sarcoidosis in the United States Navy. *Am Rev Respir Dis* 1961, 84(5)Pt 2:109–115.

32. James DG, Hosoda Y: Epidemiology. In *Sarcoidosis and Other Granulomatous Disorders*. Edited by James DG. Los Angeles: Marcel Dekker; 1994:729–743.

33. Brett GZ: Prevalenceof intrathoracic sarcoidosis among ethnic groups in northern London during 1958–1967. In Proceedings of Fifth International Conference on Sarcoidosis. Edited by Levinsky L, Macholda F. Prague: University of Karlova; 1971:238–239.

34. Pietinalho A, Hiraga Y, Hosoda Y, *et al.*: The frequency of sarcoidosis in Finland and Hokkaido, Japan. A comparative epidemiological study. *Sarcoidosis* 1995, 12(1):61–67.

35. Hillerdal G, Nou E, Osterman K, Schmekel B: Sarcoidosis: epidemiology and prognosis. A 15-year European study. *Am Rev Respir Dis* 1984, 130(1):29–32.

36. Reich JM, Johnson RE: Course and prognosis of sarcoidosis in a nonreferral setting: analysis of 86 patients observed for 10 years. *Am J Med* 1985, 78(1):61–67.

37. Baughman RP, Teirstein AS, Judson MA, *et al*. Clinical characteristics of patients in a case control study of sarcoidosis. *Am J Respir Crit Care Med* 2001, 164(10 Pt 1):1885–1889.

38. Raghu G: Interstitial lung disease: a diagnostic approach: are CT scan and lung biopsy indicated in every patient? *Am J Respir Crit Care Med* 1995, 151(3 Pt 1):909–914.

39. Gossot D, Toledo L, Fritsch S, Celerier M: Mediastinoscopy vs thoracoscopy for mediastinal biopsy: results of a prospective nonrandomized study. *Chest* 1996, 110(5):1328–1331.

40. Gilman MJ, Wang KP: Transbronchial lung biopsy in sarcoidosis: an approach to determine the optimal number of biopsies. *Am Rev Respir Dis* 1980, 122(5):721–724.

41. Descombes E, Gardiol D, Leuenberger P: Transbronchial lung biopsy: an analysis of 530 cases with reference to the number of samples. *Monaldi Arch Chest Dis* 1997, 52(4):324–329.

42. Uemura A, Morimoto S, Hiramitsu S, *et al.*: Histologic diagnostic rate of cardiac sarcoidosis: evaluation of endomyocardial biopsies. *Am Heart J* 1999, 138(2 Pt 1):299–302.

43. Devaney K, Goodman ZD, Epstein MS, *et al.*: Hepatic sarcoidosis: clinicopathologic features in 100 patients. *Am J Surg Pathol* 1993, 17(12):1272–1280.

44. Judson MA, Baughman RP, Teirstein AS, *et al.*: Defining organ involvement in sarcoidosis: the ACCESS proposed instrument. ACCESS Research Group. A Case Control Etiologic Study of Sarcoidosis. *Sarcoidosis Vasc Diffuse Lung Dis* 1999, 16(1):75–86.

45. Mana J, Salazar A, Manresa F: Clinical factors predicting persistence of activity in sarcoidosis: a multivariate analysis of 193 cases. *Respiration* 1994, 61(4):219–225.

46. Costabel U, Hunninghake GW. ATS/ERS/WASOG statement on sarcoidosis. Sarcoidosis Statement Committee. American Thoracic Society. European Respiratory Society. World Association for Sarcoidosis and Other Granulomatous Disorders. *Eur Respir J* 1999, 14(4):735–737.

47. Arcasoy SM, Christie JD, Pochettino A, *et al.*: Characteristics and outcomes of patients with sarcoidosis listed for lung transplantation. *Chest* 2001, 120(3):873–880.

48. James DG, Carstairs LS, Trowell J, Sharma OP: Treatment of sarcoidosis: report of a controlled therapeutic trial. *Lancet* 1967, 2(7515):526–528.

49. Israel HL, Fouts DW, Beggs RA: A controlled trial of prednisone treatment of sarcoidosis. *Am Rev Respir Dis* 1973, 107(4):609–614.

50. Eule H, Roth I, Ehrke I, Weinecke W: Corticosteroid therapy of intrathoracic sarcoidosis stages I and II—results of a controlled clinical trial. *Z Erkr Atmungsorgane* 1977, 149(1):142–147.

51. Selroos O, Sellergren TL: Corticosteroid therapy of pulmonary sarcoidosis: a prospective evaluation of alternate day and daily dosage in stage II disease. *Scand J Respir Dis* 1979, 60(4):215–221.

52. Zaki MH, Lyons HA, Leilop L, Huang CT: Corticosteroid therapy in sarcoidosis: a five-year, controlled follow-up study. *N Y State J Med* 1987, 87(9):496–499.

53. Pietinalho A, Tukiainen P, Haahtela T, *et al.*: Oral prednisolone followed by inhaled budesonide in newly diagnosed pulmonary sarcoidosis: a double-blind, placebo-controlled multicenter study. Finnish Pulmonary Sarcoidosis Study Group. *Chest* 1999, 116(2):424–431.

54. Paramothayan NS, Lasserson TJ, Jones PW: Corticosteroids for pulmonary sarcoidosis. *Cochrane Database Syst Rev* 2005(2):CD001114.

55. Baughman RP, Lower EE: Evidence-based therapy for cutaneous sarcoidosis. *Clin Dermatol* 2007, 25(3):334–340.

INTERSTITIAL LUNG DISEASE

Joseph P. Lynch III and Jeffrey L. Myers

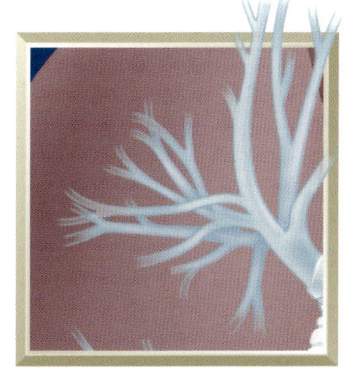
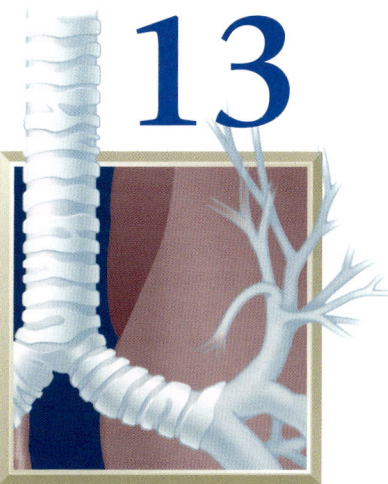
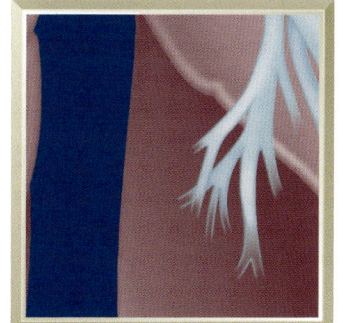

Interstitial lung disease (ILD) is a heterogeneous group of diseases characterized by a spectrum of inflammatory and fibrotic changes affecting alveolar walls and airspaces [1–5]. Clinical manifestations are protean, but progressive cough, dyspnea, parenchymal infiltrates on chest radiographs, loss of pulmonary function, and histopathologic features of inflammation and fibrosis in the lung parenchyma are characteristic [1,2].

Chest radiographs are often the first clue to the presence of ILD. Parenchymal infiltrates, cystic radiolucencies, nodules, or reduced lung volumes are present in most patients with ILDs [6]. The distribution and pattern of radiographic lesions may suggest specific ILDs. Although chest radiographs are nonspecific, serial chest radiographs are invaluable in assessing chronicity or evolution of ILDs. In this context, review of old films is critical, even in patients with newly diagnosed ILD.

High-resolution CT scanning, using 1- to 2-mm thin sections of the lung parenchyma, more clearly demarcates honeycombing, cystic changes, alveolar opacities, and interstitial disease, compared with standard chest radiographs [6,7]. High-resolution CT is far superior to conventional chest radiography in depicting fine parenchymal details, in identifying the nature and extent of the pulmonary disease, and in discriminating between end-stage fibrosis (*eg*, honeycombing) and potentially reversible disease [6]. More than 150 causes of ILD have been identified, and these include disorders in which specific agents or antigens are known (*eg*, pneumoconioses, asbestosis, silicosis, berylliosis, granulomatous infections, hypersensitivity pneumonia) and disorders in which the etiologic factors (or inciting stimuli) are unknown [1–3].

A discussion of these myriad disorders is beyond the scope of this chapter. A few ILDs, such as sarcoidosis, connective tissue disorders, pulmonary vasculitis, and cryptogenic organizing pneumonia, are discussed elsewhere in this book. This chapter limits the discussion to a few rare ILDs, each of which has distinctive characteristics but shares overlapping clinical, radiographic, and physiologic features with other ILDs.

Etiology of Interstitial Lung Disorders

Known Causes	Inherited Causes	Unknown Causes
Granulomatous infections (eg, tuberculosis, fungal infections)	Hermanszky-Pudlak syndrome	Cryptogenic organizing pneumonia
Hypersensitivity pneumonitis (eg, farmer's lung, bird fancier's disease)	Neurofibromatosis	Idiopathic pulmonary fibrosis
Malignant neoplasms (eg, lymphangitic carcinomatosis, lymphoproliferative neoplasms, bronchoalveolar cell carcinomas)	Metabolic storage disorders	Collagen vascular disease–associated pulmonary fibrosis
Pneumoconiosis (eg, asbestosis, silicosis, berylliosis, hard metal pneumoconiosis)	Hypocalciuric hypercalcemia	Langerhans' cell histiocytosis
Respiratory bronchiolitis (caused by cigarette smoking)	Tuberous sclerosis	Eosinophilic pneumonia (chronic or acute)
Toxic pneumonitis (eg, drugs, fumes, chemicals, radiation therapy)	Familial (eg, subsets of idiopathic pulmonary fibrosis, sarcoidosis)	Lymphangioleiomyomatosis
		Pulmonary alveolar proteinosis (alveolar phospholipidosis)
		Pulmonary vasculitis (eg, Wegener's granulomatosis, alveolar hemorrhage syndromes)
		Sarcoidosis

Figure 13-1. Etiology of interstitial lung disorders.

Diagnostic Evaluation of Interstitial Lung Disease

- Careful occupational, exposure, drug, and family histories, and risk factors
- Conventional chest radiographs (compare with old films)
- Pulmonary function tests
  - Spirometry, flow-volume loop, lung volumes, diffusing capacity for carbon monoxide (DL_{co}), oximetry (rest, exercise)
  - Formal cardiopulmonary exercise tests (arterial cannulation) for selected patients
- Serologies for selected patients (eg, collagen vascular disease profile, complement fixation for fungi, serum angiotensin-converting enzyme, hypersensitivity pneumonitis screen)
- High-resolution thin-section CT
- Lung biopsy for selected patients
- Fiberoptic bronchoscopy with transbronchial lung biopsies and bronchoalveolar lavage
- Video-assisted thoracoscopic lung biopsy (when fiberoptic bronchoscopy is nondiagnostic, and no contraindications to surgical biopsy exist)

Figure 13-2. Diagnostic evaluation of interstitial lung disorders. In addition to myriad interstitial lung disorders (ILDs) of known etiology, a group of chronic fibrosing interstitial pneumonias of unknown etiology have been described [5,8]. Idiopathic pulmonary fibrosis (IPF) (also termed cryptogenic fibrosing alveolitis) is the most common of these idiopathic interstitial pneumonias (IIPs), comprising 47% to 71% of cases [2,5,8,9]. IPF is a specific clinicopathological syndrome associated with the histopathological pattern of usual interstitial pneumonia (UIP) [2,7,8]. Salient clinical features of IPF include onset at greater than 50 years of age, dry cough, dyspnea, end-inspiratory velcro rales, diffuse parenchymal infiltrates on chest radiographs, hypoxemia (at rest or with exercise), a restrictive ventilatory defect on pulmonary function tests, an indolent but progressive course, and poor prognosis (mean survival is approximately 3 years following diagnosis) [2,7,8]. No pharmacological therapy has been shown to be efficacious [7]. For severe cases, lung transplant is the best therapeutic option [7]. Although UIP is the distinctive histological lesion observed in IPF [2,7], this histological pattern can also be found in other diseases (eg, connective tissue disorders; asbestosis; diverse occupational, environmental, or drug exposures) [1,2]. The diagnosis of IPF is established only when these and other alternative etiologies have been excluded. Other IIPs share clinical, physiologic, and radiographic features with IPF/UIP but display different histopathologic patterns (eg, desquamative interstitial pneumonia [2,5,7,8], respiratory bronchiolitis interstitial lung disease [4,5,10], nonspecific interstitial pneumonia/fibrosis [9], acute interstitial pneumonia [11], and lymphocytic interstitial pneumonia [1,12]. These entities are distinct from UIP/IPF and exhibit marked differences in prognosis and in responsiveness to therapy. Because of small sample size and disease heterogeneity, transbronchial lung biopsies (TBBs) are not adequate to diagnose UIP or other IIPs. A definitive diagnosis of IPF/UIP or other IIPs requires surgical lung biopsy (SLBx) [7]. However, high-resolution CT (HRCT) can substantiate the diagnosis of UIP with confidence in some patients, provided the salient features are present [7,13]. Further, the combination of TBBs, bronchoalveolar lavage (BAL), and HRCT can affirm the diagnosis of hypersensitivity pneumonia, provided clinical features are compatible [14]. In addition, TBBs and BAL are often helpful in diagnosing other ILDs (eg, sarcoidosis, pulmonary alveolar proteinosis, malignancy, granulomatous infections, Langerhans' cell histiocytosis, cryptogenic organizing pneumonia, chronic eosinophilic pneumonia), thus obviating the need for SLBx. Because SLBx is invasive and has potential morbidity, it is reserved primarily for patients manifesting atypical or indeterminate patterns on HRCT [6,13]. The risks and benefits of SLBx and the therapeutic options available must be assessed carefully in individual patients.

IDIOPATHIC PULMONARY FIBROSIS

High-Resolution CT Features of Idiopathic Pulmonary Fibrosis

Typical Findings	Late Findings
Predilection for the basilar and subpleural regions	Anatomic distortion, severe volume loss
Patchy involvement, with areas of intervening normal lung	Traction bronchiectasis or bronchiolectasis
Honeycomb cysts (4–20 mm in diameter)	Dilated pulmonary arteries
Coarse reticular (linear) opacities; thick septal lines	
Patchy ground glass opacities (mild or absent)	
Possible coexisting zones of emphysema in smokers	

Figure 13-3. High-resolution CT (HRCT) features of idiopathic pulmonary fibrosis. HRCTs are superior to conventional chest radiographs in depicting salient parenchymal aberrations (eg, honeycomb cysts, alveolar or reticular opacities, distortion) and in demarcating the extent and distribution of the disease [6,13]. Salient HRCT features of idiopathic pulmonary fibrosis and usual interstitial pneumonia are outlined here.

Prognostic Value of High-Resolution CT Pattern in Idiopathic Interstitial Pneumonias

Pattern of HRCT Scans

Ground glass (alveolar) opacities
  Usually associated with alveolitis and a favorable response to therapy
  In some cases, ground glass opacities represent irreversible fibrosis involving intralobular and alveolar septae
Reticular pattern (intersecting fine or coarse lines)
  May reflect fibrosis or inflammation
  The prognosis of reticular or mixed ground glass/reticular patterns is less favorable than predominant ground glass patterns
  Regression occurs with therapy in some patients

Honeycomb cysts

Indicates end-stage, irreversible fibrosis
Traction bronchiectasis and distortion also indicate irreversible fibrosis

Extent of Abnormality of HRCT Scans

Quantitative scoring systems assessing the extent and pattern of HRCT have prognostic value

Figure 13-4. Prognostic value of high-resolution CT (HRCT) patterns in idiopathic interstitial pneumonias. The extent of disease visible on HRCT correlates roughly with the severity of functional impairment [15]. Specific HRCT patterns may help to distinguish early alveolar inflammation (alveolitis) from fibrosis, and may have prognostic value [7,15].

Histologic Patterns or Variants in Idiopathic Interstitial Pneumonias

Usual Interstitial Pneumonia

Patchy, heterogeneous involvement; lack of uniformity
Minimal intra-alveolar component
Interstitial inflammatory infiltrate
Destruction of alveolar walls
Fibrosis, honeycombing, destruction of the alveolar architecture
Fibroblastic foci

Desquamative Interstitial Pneumonia

Uniform process throughout all fields
Filling of the alveolar spaces with alveolar macrophages
Interstitial infiltration (less striking than usual interstitial pneumonia)
Prominent type II pneumocytes
Intact alveolar walls
Preservation of alveolar architecture
Mild or absent fibrosis or honeycombing

Nonspecific Interstitial Pneumonia/Fibrosis

Foci of fibrosis and inflammation (intra-alveolar and interstitial)
Temporally uniform
Features overlap with usual interstitial pneumonia and desquamative interstitial pneumonia
Foci of bronchiolitis obliterans organizing pneumonia
± Collections of intra-alveolar macrophages
± Loosely formed granulomas

Acute Interstitial Pneumonia

Acute and organizing alveolar damage
Hyaline membranes
Fibrinous exudates
Epithelial cell necrosis
Interstitial and intra-alveolar edema

Figure 13-5. The histologic pattern of usual interstitial pneumonia (UIP). The term *UIP* describes the typical histopathologic features seen in idiopathic pulmonary fibrosis [7]. Histologic features of UIP include patchy involvement and temporal heterogeneity; areas of relatively uninvolved lung parenchyma; varying degrees of inflammation and fibrosis of alveolar walls and spaces; prominent fibroblastic foci; excessive collagen and extracellular matrix within the alveolar walls; distortion and destruction of the alveolar architecture; reduced airspace volume; and honeycomb change [5]. Among patients with idiopathic interstitial pneumonias, the finding of UIP on a surgical lung biopsy (SLBx) is a robust measure and is the single most important factor influencing mortality [7,13,16]. However, among patients with histologically-confirmed UIP, the prognostic value of other specific histologic features is controversial. Surprisingly, neither the extent of alveolar inflammation nor fibrosis on SLBx predicts survival in UIP [17,18].

USUAL INTERSTITIAL PNEUMONIA

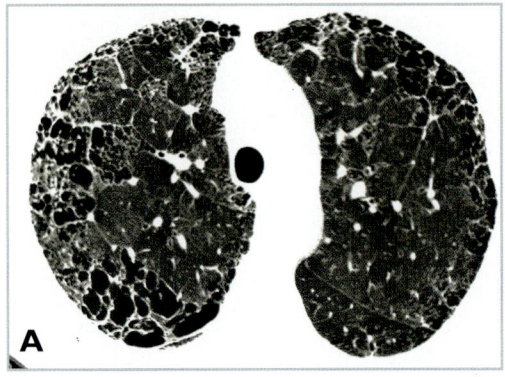
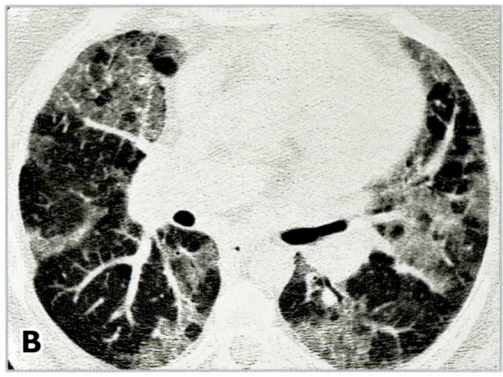
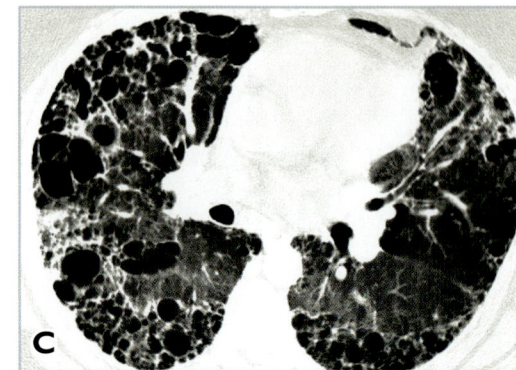

Figure 13-6. High-resolution CTs showing a usual interstitial pneumonia pattern. **A,** Thin section cuts from mid-portions of lower lobes show focal honeycomb cysts distributed in a peripheral (subpleural) distribution. **B,** Thin section cuts from extreme bases of lower lobes of another patient show evidence of foci of alveolar opacification (ground glass) in a patchy distribution. No definite honeycomb cysts are evident. **C,** Thin section cuts from lower lobes of a third patient reveal extensive honeycomb cysts. Note the predominantly peripheral (subpleural) distribution.

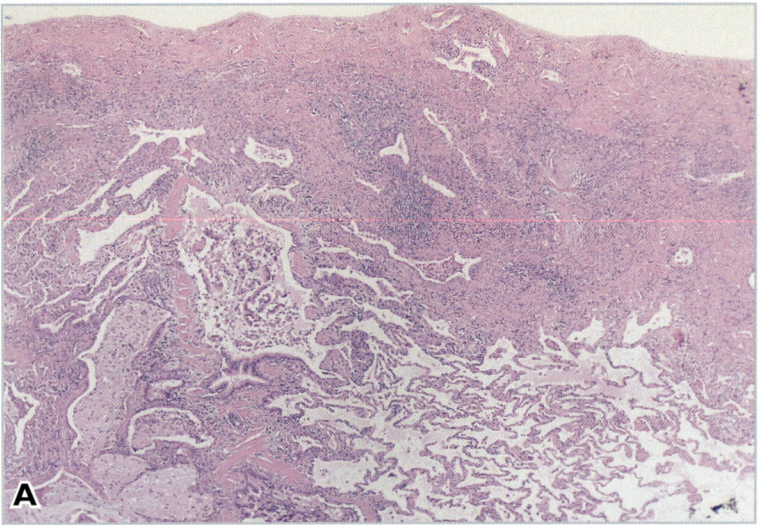
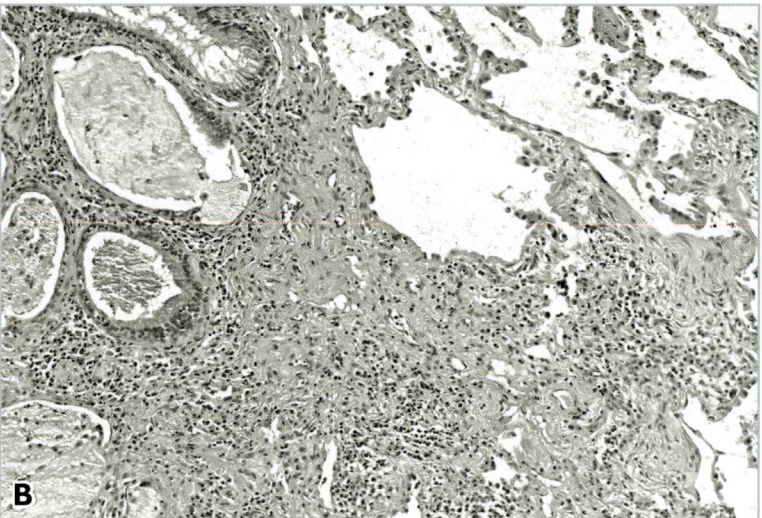

Figure 13-7. Surgical lung biopsy specimens showing usual interstitial pneumonia. **A,** Low-magnification photomicrograph showing patchy irregular interstitial thickening as a result of inflammation and fibrosis. The changes are accentuated in peripheral subpleural parenchyma and include areas of early honeycomb change. **B,** Higher magnification showing inflammation and fibrosis. The fibrosis includes dense eosinophilic collagen deposition and foci of fibroblast proliferation. An area of honeycomb change is present on the left and comprises cystically dilated fibrotic air spaces lined by bronchiolar-type epithelium.

DESQUAMATIVE INTERSTITIAL PNEUMONIA

Desquamative interstitial pneumonia (DIP), observed primarily among cigarette smokers, is characterized by dense filling of alveolar spaces with macrophages containing a finely granular pigment that stains for hemosiderin [4,5,10]. Varying degrees of fibrosis and chronic inflammation may be present, but honeycomb change (HC) or fibroblastic foci are absent or minimal [4,5]. High-resolution CTs show dense ground glass opacities with minimal or no HC [4,10]. Clinical presentation is usually insidious, with cough and dyspnea developing over weeks or months [4,10]. Following cessation of cigarette smoking, the course stabilizes in most patients, but radiological abnormalities often persist [4,10]. Sustained improvement is uncommon [10]. Progression to fibrosis occurs in a minority of patients; mortality rates attributable to DIP range from 0% to 26% [4,10].

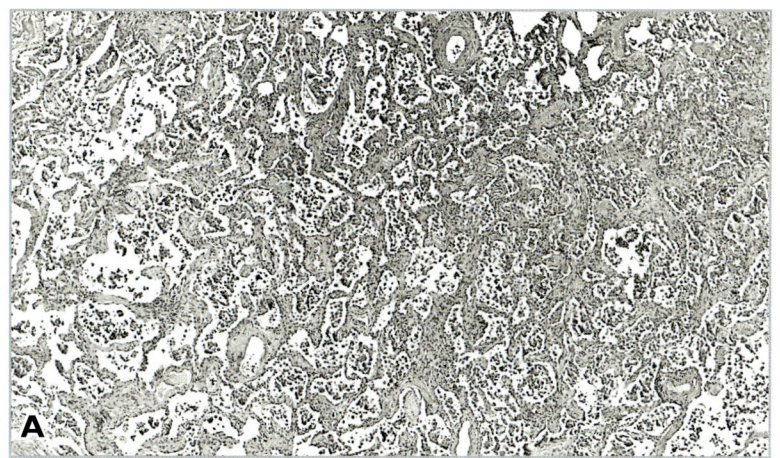
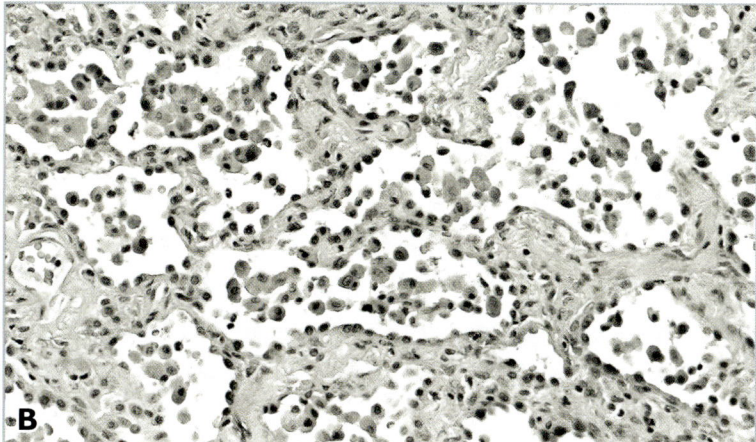
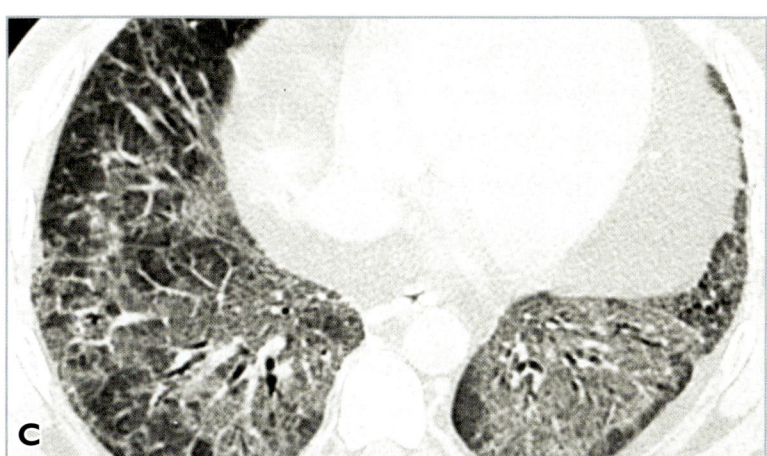

Figure 13-8. Surgical lung biopsy specimens showing desquamative interstitial pneumonia. **A,** Low-magnification photomicrograph showing uniform alveolar septal thickening, which is associated with prominent clusters of lightly pigmented alveolar histiocytes. **B,** Higher magnification depicting relatively uniform alveolar septal thickening caused by mild inflammatory infiltrate, fibrosis, and hyperplasia of alveolar lining cells. Alveolar spaces contain lightly pigmented "smoker's" macrophages. **C,** High-resolution CT showing desquamative interstitial pneumonia. Bilateral ground glass opacities are associated with minimal architectural distortion.

RESPIRATORY BRONCHIOLITIS INTERSTITIAL LUNG DISEASE

Respiratory bronchiolitis–associated interstitial lung disease (RB-ILD) occurs nearly exclusively (> 90%) in smokers and is characterized by accumulation of pigmented macrophages within terminal and respiratory bronchioles [4,5,10]. In contrast to desquamative interstitial pneumonia (DIP), which is distributed within the alveolar ducts and spaces, RB-ILD is bronchocentric; extension to the alveolar ducts or spaces is minimal or lacking [4,5]. Furthermore, there is greater interstitial fibrosis, more lymphoid follicles, and more eosinophilic infiltrates in DIP than in RB-ILD [4,5,10]. Clinical expression varies; some patients are asymptomatic, but dyspnea or cough is present in most patients [4,10]. Pulmonary function tests demonstrate reduced diffusing capacity of lung for carbon monoxide (DL_{CO}) in more than 80% of cases; restrictive or obstructive defects may be present in 50% [10,19]. High-resolution CTs show bronchial wall thickening, centrilobular nodules, and ground glass opacities; honeycomb change is absent or minimal [10,19]. Following cessation of cigarette smoking, prognosis of RB-ILD is good, with low mortality rates at 5 years (< 5%) [10,19]. However, clinical or physiological improvement occurs in a minority of patients, and disease progression may occur [19]. Corticosteroids and immunosuppressive agents have been used, but they are of unproven benefit [4,10,19].

NONSPECIFIC INTERSTITIAL PNEUMONIA

Nonspecific interstitial pneumonia (NSIP) represents a subset of idiopathic interstitial pneumonias (IIPs) [5,9]. Defining histological criteria include temporal homogeneity, varying degrees of interstitial inflammation and/or fibrosis, relative preservation of the alveolar architecture, and the absence of features of other IIPs (eg, usual interstitial pneumonia [UIP], desquamative interstitial pneumonia [DIP], respiratory bronchiolitis interstitial lung disease [RB-ILD], acute interstitial pneumonia [AIP], lymphocytic interstitial pneumonia [LIP]) [5,9]. Additional features distinguish NSIP from UIP. Honeycomb change and fibroblastic foci are prominent features of UIP, but are rare or absent in NSIP [5,9]. Clinical features of NSIP overlap with those of UIP [7,9]. However, in contrast to UIP, high-resolution CTs in NSIP patients typically demonstrate ground glass opacities and minimal or no honeycomb change [6,9]. Most importantly, NSIP exhibits a better prognosis and a better responsiveness to corticosteroid or immunosuppressive therapies [9,13]. Importantly, both UIP and NSIP patterns may be present in individual patients [9], and the matter of whether NSIP progresses to UIP is controversial [7].

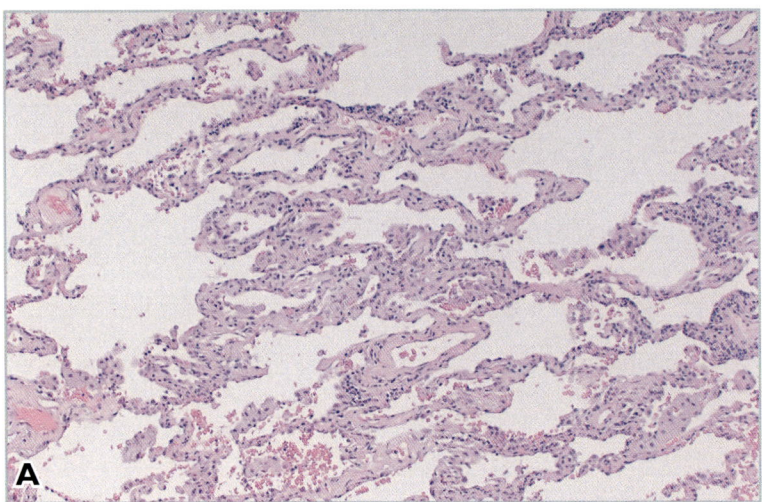 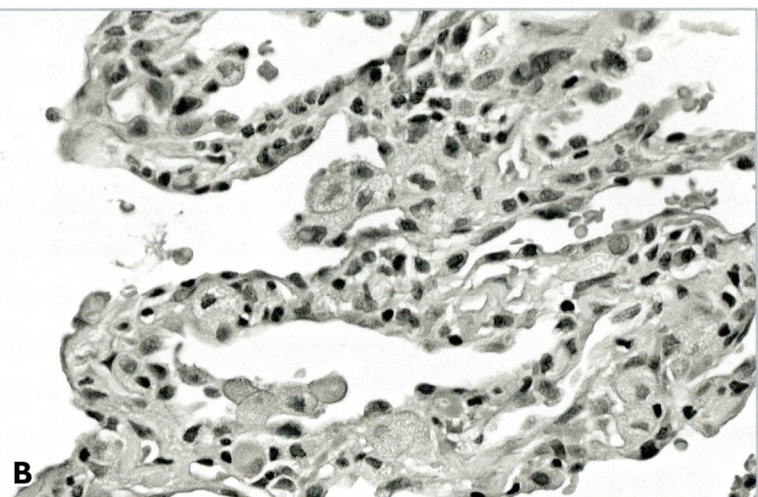

Figure 13-9. Surgical lung biopsy specimens showing nonspecific interstitial pneumonia. A, Low-magnification photomicrograph illustrating temporally uniform interstitial thickening. The pattern contrasts sharply with the more heterogeneous, variegated pattern seen in classic usual interstitial pneumonia (see Fig. 13-7A). B, Higher magnification showing uniform expansion of alveolar septa by a combination of inflammation and fibrosis in nonspecific interstitial pneumonia.

LYMPHOCYTIC INTERSTITIAL PNEUMONIA

Associated Disorders of Lymphoid Interstitial Pneumonia

- HIV infection (particularly infants and children)
- Miscellaneous immunodeficiency or immunologic disorders
    - Sjögren's syndrome
    - Dysproteinemias (eg, hypogammaglobulinemia, monoclonal gammopathies)
    - Allogeneic bone marrow transplant recipients
    - Systemic lupus erythematosus
    - Myasthenia gravis
    - Common variable immunodeficiency syndrome
    - Primary biliary cirrhosis

Figure 13-10. Associated disorders of lymphoid interstitial pneumonia (LIP). LIP is a rare disorder characterized by dense infiltration of alveolar septa by small lymphocytes and plasma cells with relative sparing of airways [1,20]. The pathogenesis is not known, but viral infections may play a role [20]. LIP usually occurs in patients infected with human immunodeficiency virus (HIV) (particularly children) [12] and occurs less commonly in HIV-negative patients with diverse underlying immunologic disorders [20]. In HIV-negative patients, LIP typically affects adults older than 40 and rarely affects children; women are affected twice as often as men [1,20]. High-resolution CT typically reveals ground glass opacities and poorly defined centrilobular nodules; a few cysts may also be found [21]. The clinical course is extremely varied [20]. LIP patients are usually treated with corticosteroids (alone or with cytotoxic agents); excellent remissions may be observed [20], but data are limited.

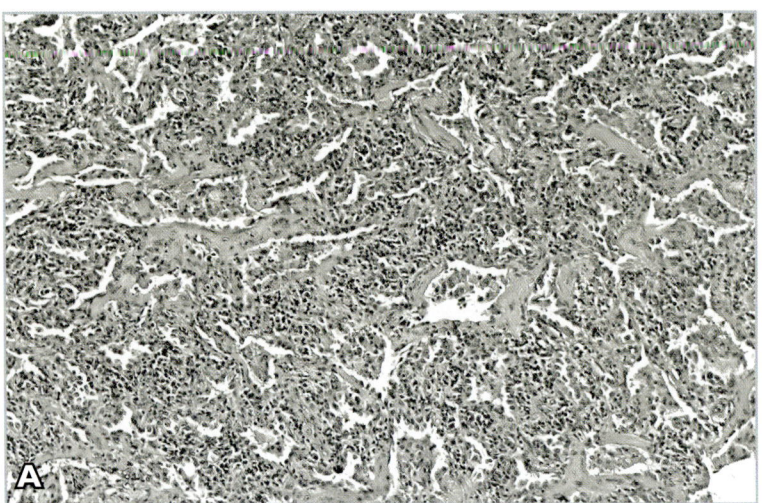 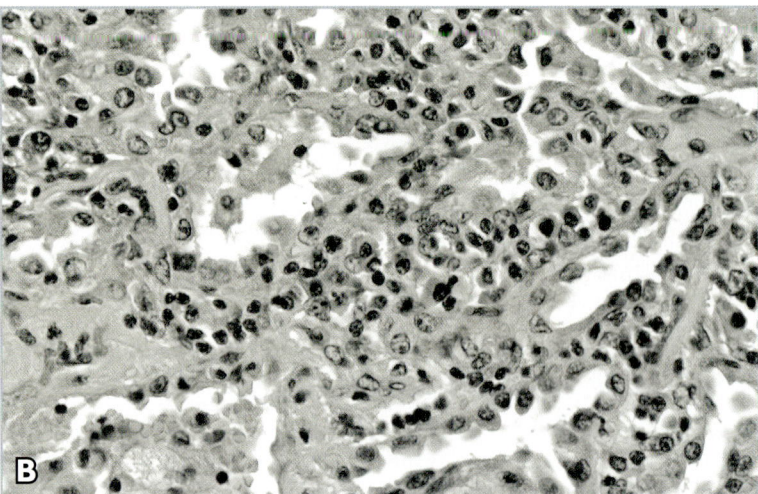

Figure 13-11. Surgical lung biopsy specimens showing lymphocytic interstitial pneumonia. A, Low-magnification photomicrograph presenting an interstitium that is expanded markedly by a dense infiltrate of lymphocytes and plasma cells. B, Higher magnification showing dense alveolar septal infiltrate of lymphocytes and plasma cells.

HYPERSENSITIVITY PNEUMONIA

Selected Causes of Hypersensitivity Pneumonitis

Disease Syndrome	Source	Offending Antigen
Farmer's lung	Moldy hay or corn	Thermophilic actinomycetes
Ventilator lung	Air conditioner, humidifier	Thermophilic actinomycetes
Bagassosis	Moldy sugar cane	Thermophilic actinomycetes
Mushroom worker's lung	Moldy compost	Thermophilic actinomycetes
Hot tub lung	Mold on ceiling	*Cladosporium* spp
Suberosis	Moldy cork	*Penicillium* spp
Maple bark stripper's disease	Contaminated maple	*Cryptostroma corticale*
Malt worker's lung	Contaminated barley	*Aspergillus clavatus*
Tobacco worker's lung	Mold on tobacco	*Aspergillus* spp
Wine grower's disease	Mold on grapes	*Aspergillus* spp
Wood pulp worker's disease	Wood pulp	*Alternaria* spp
Japanese summer house hypersensitivity pneumonia	House dust	*Trichosporon cutaneum*
Pigeon breeder's disease	Excreta or feathers	Avian antigens
Laboratory worker's lung	Rat fur	Rat urine protein
Pituitary snuff	Pituitary powder	Vasopressin
Miller's lung	Grain weevils in wheat flour	*Sitophilius granarius* proteins
Toluene diisocyanate hypersensitivity pneumonia	Toluene diisocyanate	Altered proteins
Trimellitic anhydride hypersensitivity pneumonia	Trimellitic anhydride	Altered proteins

Figure 13-12. Selected causes of hypersensitivity pneumonia. Hypersensitivity pneumonia (HP) (also termed extrinsic allergic alveolitis) is a cell-mediated response to a variety of inhaled organic dusts or inorganic chemicals [14,22–26]. Exposure in the workplace environs (*eg*, in agricultural or textile occupations), exposure to woods, hobbies (*eg*, raising birds) [27,28], and home features (*eg*, humidifiers, hot tubs) [29] may elicit the syndrome. The prototype of HP is "farmer's lung," which is caused by inhalation of thermophilic actinomycetes spores from moldy hay and occurs in 1% to 8% of exposed farmers [22]. Other syndromes elicited by thermophilic actinomycetes in occupational settings include "air conditioner (humidifier) lung," "mushroom worker's lung," and bagassosis. In Mexico, domestic exposure to pigeon antigens ("pigeon breeder's lung") is the most common cause of HP [27]. This occurs in 6% to 15% of pigeon breeders [23,27]. In Japan, summer-type pneumonitis due to *Cryptococcus albidus* or *Tricophorin cutaneum* is the most common type of HP [24]. More than 50 different occupational and environmental sources of antigen associated with HP have been described [22,23]. (*Adapted from* Curtis and Schuyler [10].)

HP is classified into three phases: acute, subacute, and chronic [22,26]. Acute HP presents abruptly with dyspnea and wheezing within a few hours after heavy antigenic exposure in a sensitized patient [22,30]. Subacute HP is caused by intermittent or continuous exposure to low doses of antigen [22,30]. Chronic HP results from persistent or chronic low-grade exposure, leading to fibrosis or emphysema (and sometimes death) [25,31]. Following removal of the antigenic source, acute HP is usually self-limited. Corticosteroids may be efficacious for severe cases [22]. Subacute or chronic HP may result in progressive fibrosis [22,30]. The role of corticosteroids in subacute or chronic HP is controversial [25,31].

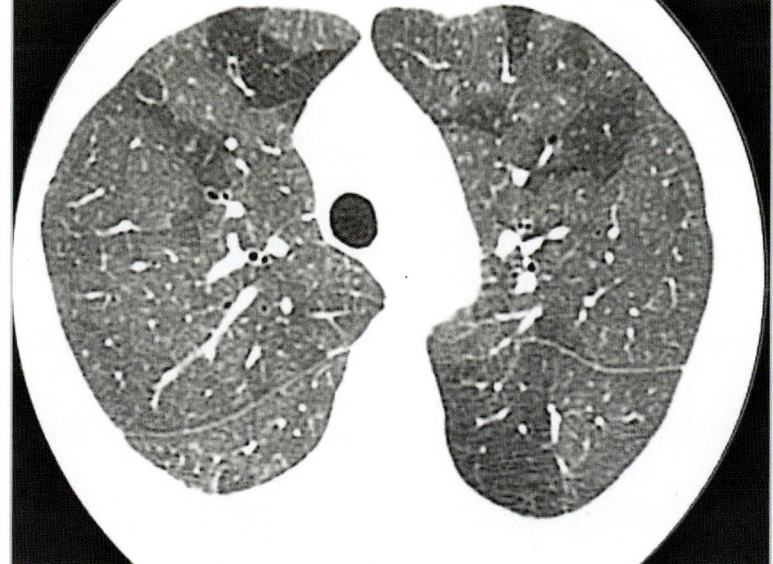

Figure 13-13. High-resolution CT showing hypersensitivity pneumonia. CT features of acute hypersensitivity pneumonia (HP) include centrilobular micronodules, ground glass opacities, a peribronchiolar distribution, focal areas of organizing pneumonia, a predilection for middle or upper lung zones, and variable areas of attenuation (a mosaic pattern) [22,30]. With subacute or chronic HP, reticulation, bronchiectasis, and bronchiolectasis may develop [30]. With end-stage chronic HP, fibrosis and areas of emphysema may be severe [30]. Although CT features of chronic HP overlap with those of usual interstitial pneumonia (UIP) and fibrotic nonspecific interstitial pneumonia (NSIP), the centrilobular nodules, lobular areas of air trapping, and mosaic pattern commonly observed in chronic HP are not found in UIP or in NSIP [30].

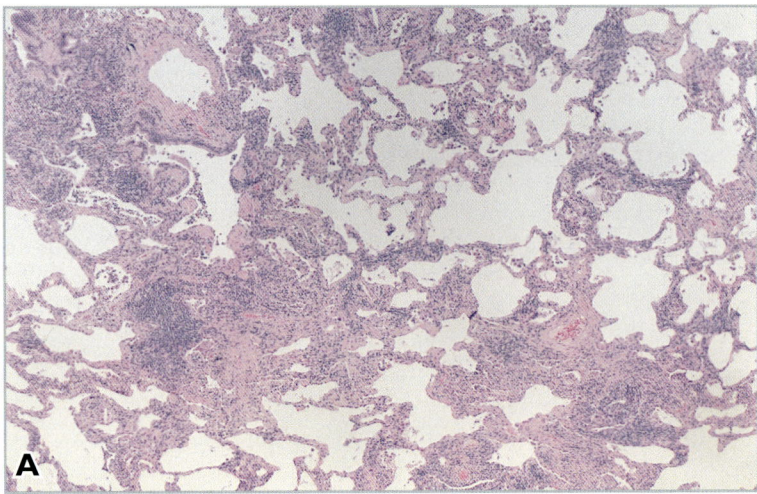
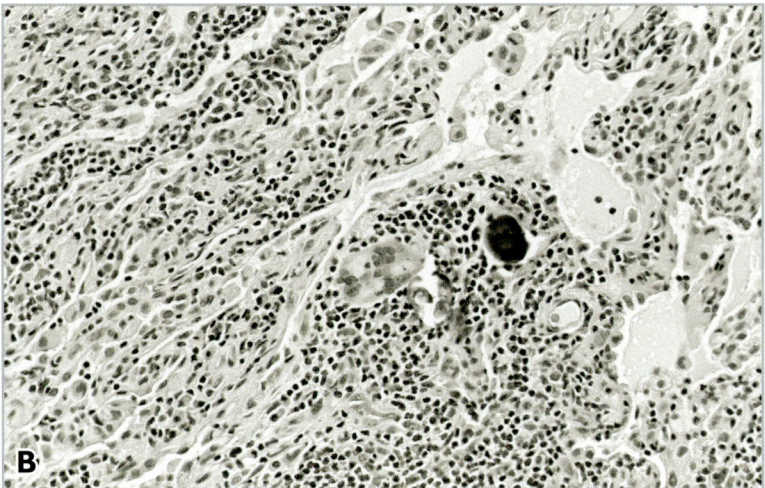

Figure 13-14. Surgical lung biopsy specimens showing hypersensitivity pneumonia (extrinsic allergic alveolitis). **A,** Low-magnification photomicrograph showing a patchy, cellular interstitial pneumonia accentuated around bronchioles. **B,** Higher magnification showing a combination of lymphocytes and isolated multinucleated giant cells in hypersensitivity pneumonia. The giant cells contain a variety of nonspecific calcified and noncalcified cytoplasmic inclusions.

CHRONIC EOSINOPHILIC PNEUMONIA

Chronic eosinophilic pneumonia (CEP) is a rare disorder of uncertain etiology characterized by coughing, wheezing, migratory alveolar infiltrates, constitutional symptoms, and peripheral blood eosinophilia [32,33]. Lung biopsies demonstrate dense aggregates of eosinophils, histiocytes, and multinucleated giant cells; fibrosis or parenchymal necrosis are rare [32]. Chest radiographs demonstrate patchy, subpleural alveolar infiltrates, with a predilection for the upper lobes [32,33]. High-resolution CTs (HRCTs) depict the alveolar nature and peripheral distribution of CEP but are nonspecific [32,33]. Corticosteroids are highly efficacious. Responses are usually dramatic (within 24 to 72 hours), but chronic low-dose prednisone is usually required to prevent late relapses [32,33].

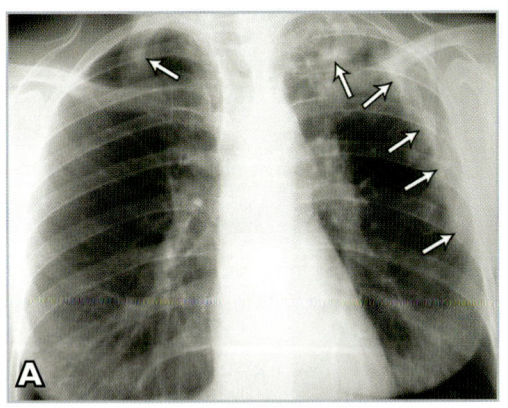
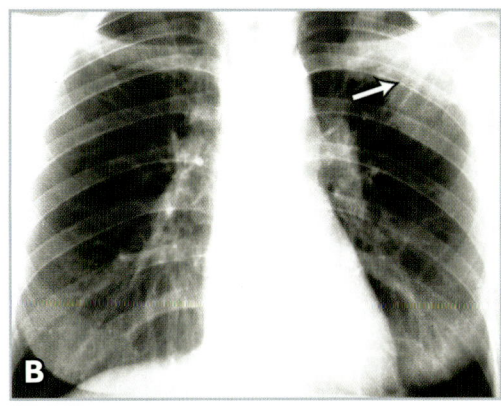
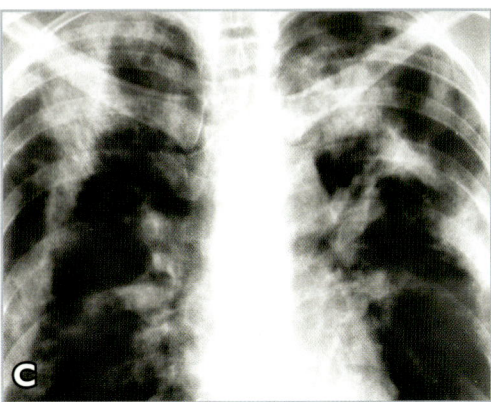
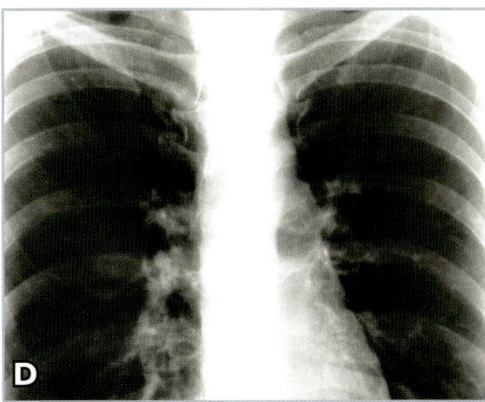

Figure 13-15. Chronic eosinophilic pneumonia [32]. **A,** Posteroanterior chest radiograph from a 37-year-old woman demonstrating focal peripheral alveolar infiltrates (*arrows*). Transbronchial lung biopsies showed aggregates of eosinophils and scattered multinucleated giant cells. Symptoms and chest radiographs normalized with corticosteroid therapy. **B,** Posteroanterior chest radiograph from the same patient 5 years later demonstrating a peripheral alveolar infiltrate in the apical region of the left upper lobe (*arrow*). Symptoms of cough, malaise, and wheezing improved promptly, and chest radiographs normalized with intensification of corticosteroid therapy. **C,** Posteroanterior chest radiograph from a 33-year-old woman with dyspnea, wheezing, and blood eosinophilia demonstrating focal alveolar infiltrates. Bronchoalveolar lavage revealed intense eosinophilia (> 30%). Prednisone 60 mg daily was initiated. **D,** Posteroanterior chest radiograph from the same patient 5 days later demonstrating nearly complete resolution of infiltrates. (*Panel B from* Lynch and Flint [34]; with permission.)

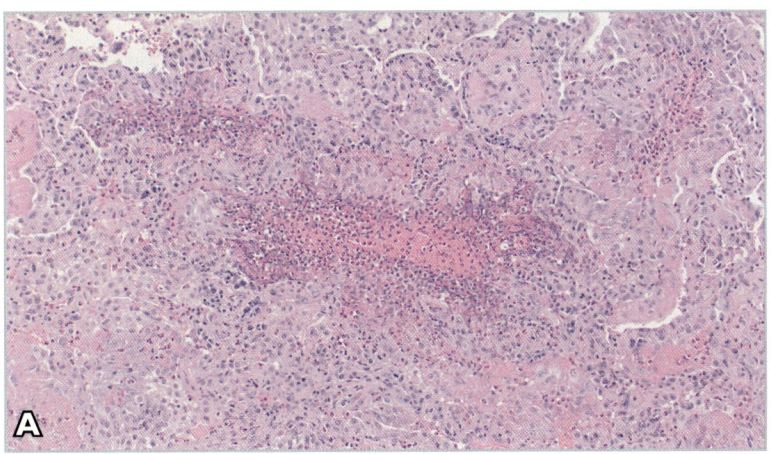
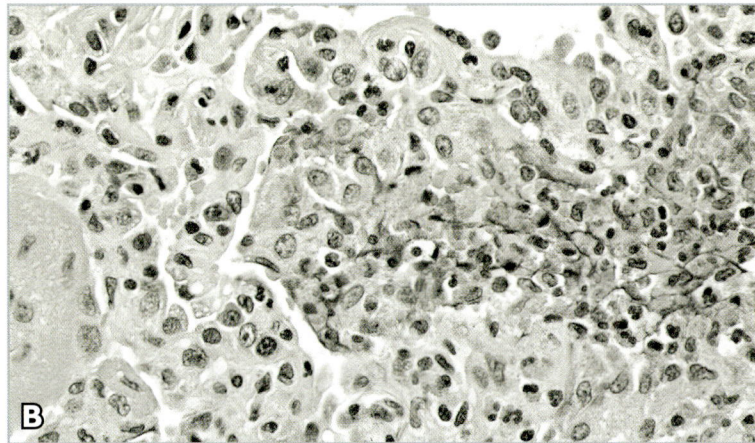

Figure 13-16. Surgical lung biopsy specimens showing chronic eosinophilic pneumonia. **A,** Low-magnification photomicrograph depicting a partially necrotic air space exudate. The necrotic zones represent eosinophilic abscesses, a finding characteristic of chronic eosinophilic pneumonia. **B,** Higher magnification photomicrograph showing an air space exudate of eosinophils and histiocytes.

IDIOPATHIC PULMONARY ALVEOLAR PROTEINOSIS

Idiopathic pulmonary alveolar proteinosis (iPAP) is a rare autoimmune disease in which circulating antibodies against the granulocyte macrophage colony-stimulating factor (GM-CSF) result in abnormal surfactant clearance from the alveoli [35,36]. Histologically, the alveolar spaces are filled with granular, eosinophilic material composed of surfactant apoproteins [35]. Salient findings include dyspnea, hypoxemia, bilateral alveolar infiltrates, and elevated serum lactate dehydrogenase (LDH) [35,36]. Anti–GM-CSF antibodies impair surfactant homeostasis and inhibit alveolar macrophage and neutrophil function [37]. Anti–GM-CSF antibodies in bronchoalveolar lavage fluid may reflect disease severity in iPAP [38]. Whole lung lavage has been the treatment of choice [35], but recent studies have cited improvement with administration of recombinant GM-CSF [36].

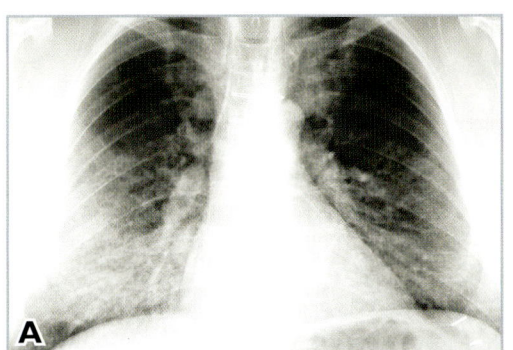
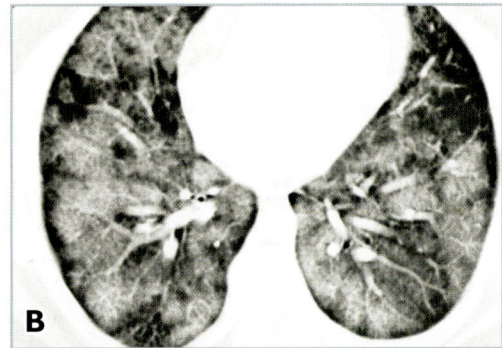

Figure 13-17. Pulmonary alveolar proteinosis [35]. **A,** Posteroanterior chest radiograph demonstrates bilateral, predominantly basilar, alveolar infiltrates in a 50-year-old man with progressive exertional dyspnea. **B,** CT from the same patient shows multiple foci of ground glass opacification throughout the lung parenchyma. Surgical lung biopsy demonstrated classic features of pulmonary alveolar proteinosis. (*From* Lynch and Raghu [3]; with permission.)

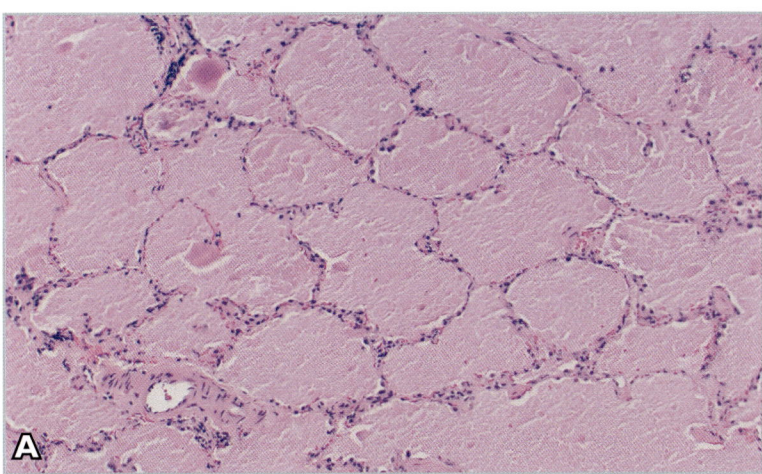
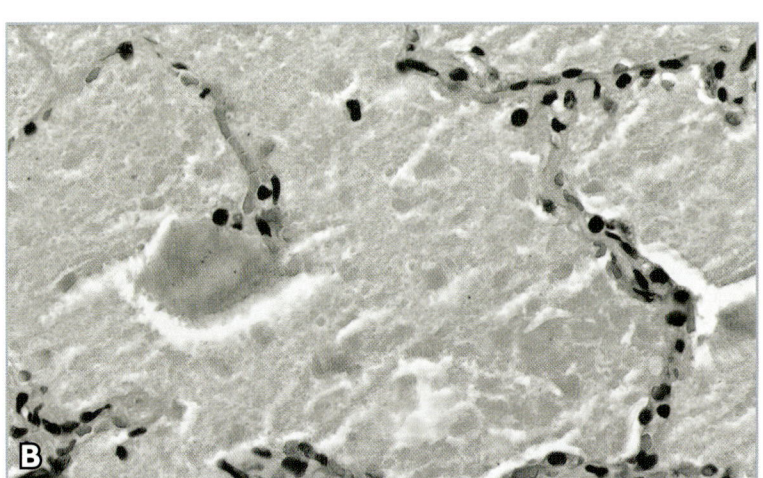

Figure 13-18. Surgical lung biopsy specimens showing pulmonary alveolar proteinosis. **A,** Photomicrograph demonstrating complete filling of alveolar spaces with a dense proteinaceous exudate. The alveolar architecture is preserved. **B,** Higher magnification photomicrograph showing characteristic air space exudate and relatively normal alveolar septa.

PULMONARY LANGERHANS' CELL HISTIOCYTOSIS

Pulmonary Langerhans' cell histiocytosis (also termed Langerhans' cell granulomatosis) is a rare disease of cigarette smokers presenting with pneumothoraces, dyspnea, or cough [39,40]. Extrapulmonary involvement (such as osteolytic lesions of bone or diabetes insipidus) occurs in 15% to 20% of patients [39,40]. High-resolution CTs are distinctive and reveal numerous thin-wall cysts and peribronchiolar nodules, preferentially involving the upper and mid-lung zones [39–41]. The prognosis and natural history are variable. With cessation of smoking, the disease stabilizes or improves in most patients [39–41]. However, fatality rates range from 6% to 25% [39–41].

Differential Diagnosis of Cystic Lesions on High-Resolution CT

	Langerhans' Cell Histiocytosis	Lymphangioleiomyomatosis	Usual Interstitial Pneumonia/Idiopathic Pulmonary Fibrosis
Cysts	Thin-walled; often regular in size	Thin-walled; often regular in size; may coalesce	Less-defined walls; variable size
Location	Upper, mid-lung zones; peribronchiolar; subpleural; spare costophrenic angles	Uniform; all lobes	Peripheral (subpleural); bibasilar; patchy, heterogeneous
Associated findings	Peribronchiolar nodules	Lack nodules	Reticular or alveolar opacities; distortion; traction bronchiolectasis

Figure 13-19. Differential diagnosis of cystic lesions on high-resolution CT. Cysts are highly characteristic of pulmonary Langerhans' cell histiocytosis (formerly termed pulmonary eosinophilic granuloma), lymphangioleiomyomatosis, and usual interstitial pneumonia, but they may be seen in any chronic lung disorder that destroys alveolar walls and distorts the alveolar architecture [39]. Honeycomb cysts may be observed in advanced cases of pulmonary sarcoidosis, chronic hypersensitivity pneumonia, granulomatous infections, connective tissue–associated pulmonary fibrosis, pneumoconioses, and other disorders [42]. In some cases, associated features depict the underlying nature of the disorder. Upper lobe predominance, a predilection for central bronchovascular bundles and lymphatics, concomitant nodules, alveolar opacities, distortion, or hilar or mediastinal lymphadenopathy may be clues to the diagnosis of sarcoidosis [43]. In chronic obstructive pulmonary disease caused by cigarette smoking, emphysematous "cysts" are more irregular in size, lack well formed walls, and are more extensive in the upper lobes.

Histologic Features of Langerhans' Cell Histiocytosis

- Combination of cystic, nodular, and fibrotic lesions
- Bronchocentric distribution
- Intervening zones of normal lung parenchyma
- Stellate pattern of fibrosis (low-power magnification)
- Cellular granulomatous lesions (high-power magnification)
- Proliferation of atypical histiocytes (Langerhans' cells)
  - Moderately large, ovoid histiocytes
  - Pale eosinophilic cytoplasm
  - Indented (grooved nuclei), inconspicuous nucleoli
  - Positive staining for S100 protein or common thymocyte antigen (OKT6)
  - Intracytoplasmic rod, or racquet-shape inclusions 42–45 nm in thickness (electron microscopy)
- Destruction of bronchioles and alveolar parenchyma
- Blebs, subpleural cysts, honeycomb lung (late features)

Figure 13-20. Histologic features of pulmonary Langerhans' cell histiocytosis. Histologically, pulmonary Langerhans' cell histiocytosis is characterized by inflammatory, cystic, nodular, and fibrotic lesions distributed in a bronchocentric fashion [39–41]. Langerhans' cells (also termed histiocytosis X cells) are the cornerstone of the diagnosis and can usually be identified by hematoxylin–eosin stains. In equivocal cases, immunohistochemical stains (such as those of the S100 protein or the common thymocyte antigen [OKT6 or CD1a]) may substantiate the identity of Langerhans' cells [41,39].

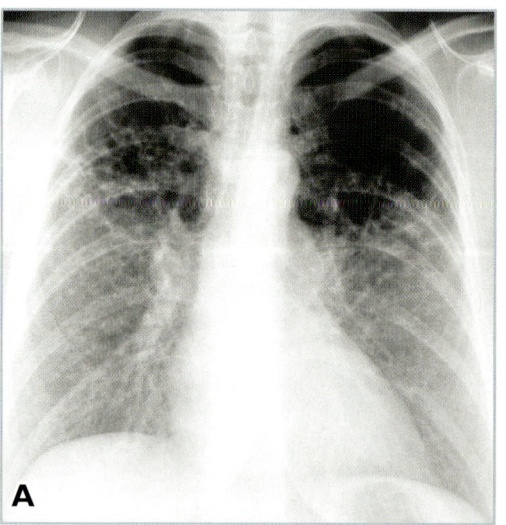

Figure 13-21. Pulmonary Langerhans' cell histiocytosis. **A,** Posteroanterior chest radiograph demonstrating diffuse reticular and cystic changes. Note that the upper lobes are hyperlucent, reflecting extensive cystic destruction of the lung parenchyma.

Continued on the next page

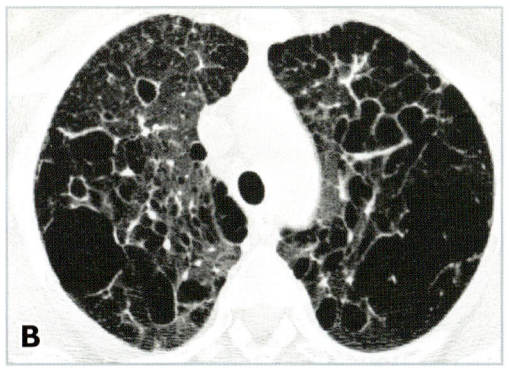
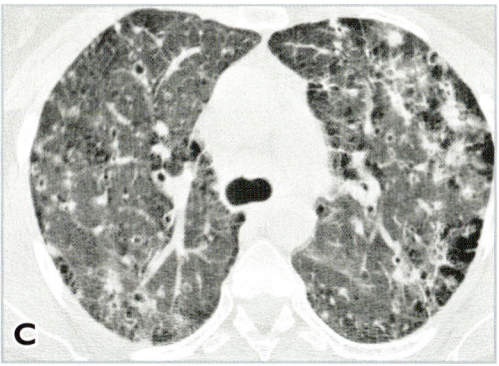

Figure 13-21. *(Continued)* **B,** A high-resolution CT (HRCT) from the same patient illustrating cuts from the upper lobes, demonstrating multiple cystic spaces, with coalescence. A nodular component is not obvious. **C,** An HRCT from the same patient (lower lobes) reveals multiple well defined cystic spaces. Peribronchiolar infiltrates and a slight nodular component are also evident.

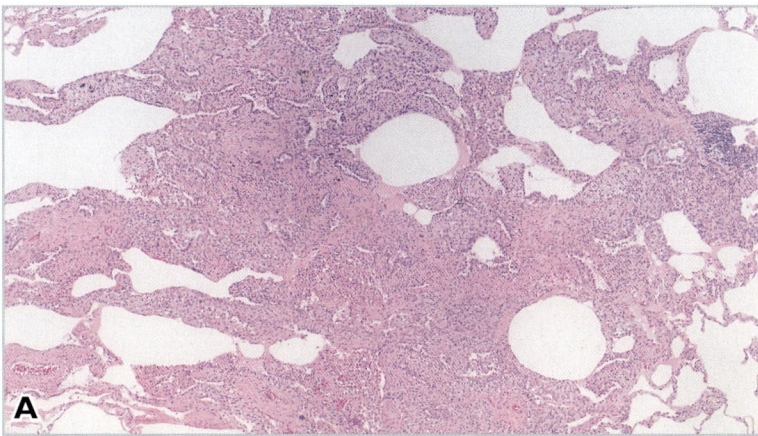
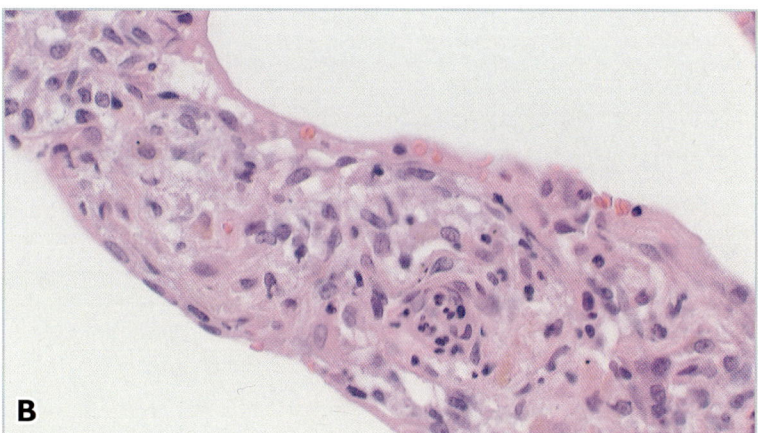

Figure 13-22. Surgical lung biopsy specimens showing Langerhans' cell histiocytosis. **A,** A low-magnification photomicrograph shows a stellate bronchiolocentric nodule. There is associated paracictricial airspace enlargement ("scar emphysema"), which accounts for the frequent finding of cystic change. **B,** A higher magnification photomicrograph shows a polymorphic inflammatory infiltrate in Langerhans' cell histiocytosis, which includes diagnostic Langerhans' cells with highly convoluted nuclear contours.

LYMPHANGIOLEIOMYOMATOSIS

Lymphangioleiomyomatosis (LAM) is a rare disease of unknown etiology affecting only women (primarily premenopausal), with predominant manifestations of progressive airflow obstruction, pneumothoraces, and chylothorax or chylous ascites [44]. High-resolution CTs demonstrating innumerable thin-walled cysts without predilection for any particular lobe; nodules are not found [44]. Extrapulmonary involvement is common. Abdominal CT reveals cysts or angiomyolipomas in kidney, spleen, abdominal or retroperitoneal lymph nodes, uterus, and ovaries in up to 60% of patients with LAM [44]. The prognosis for LAM (with or without therapy) is poor, with inexorable progression over 5 to 15 years [44]. Strategies to ablate estrogen are used but are of unproven value [44]. Lung transplantation is an option for patients with life-threatening respiratory insufficiency caused by LAM [44].

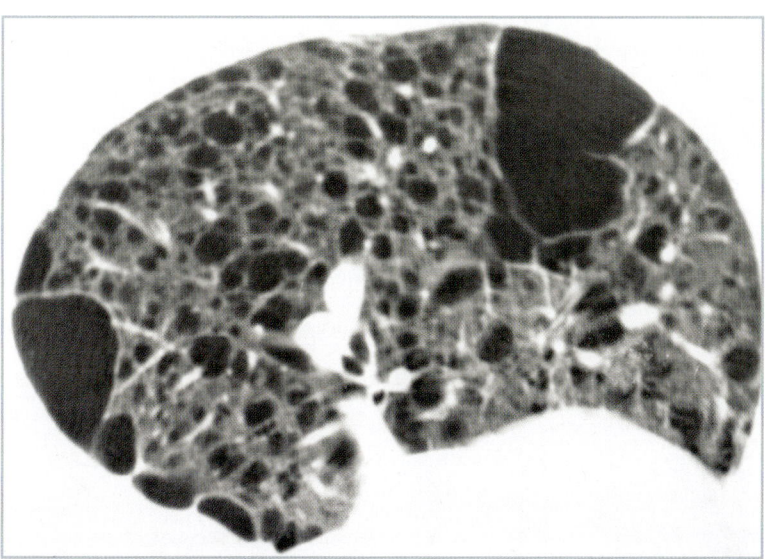

Figure 13-23. High-resolution CT of a 44-year-old woman with lymphangioleiomyomatosis demonstrating multiple, thin-walled cystic radiolucencies bilaterally [44]. Note the two large lesions, representing confluent cysts. (*From* Lynch and Raghu [3]; with permission.)

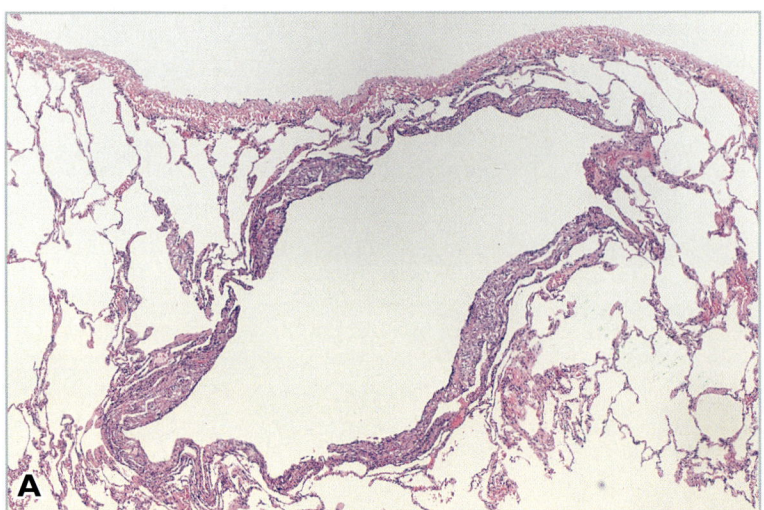
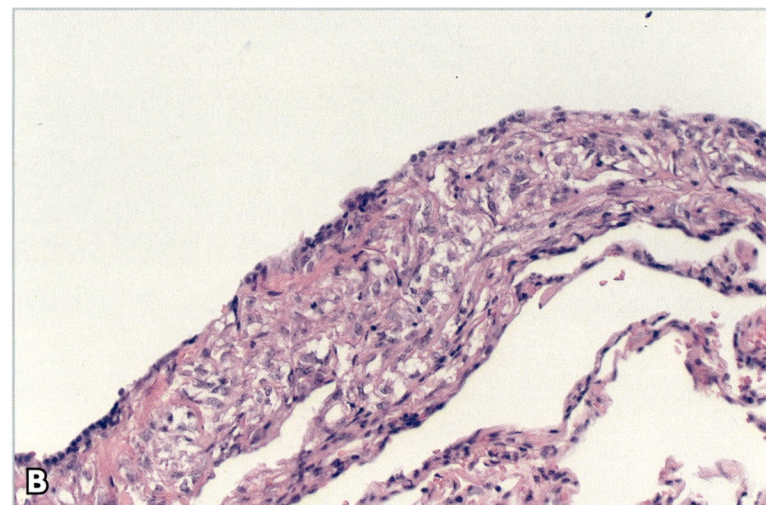

Figure 13-24. Surgical lung biopsy specimens showing lymphangioleiomyomatosis (LAM). **A,** Low-magnification photomicrograph illustrating characteristic cysts in LAM. **B,** Higher magnification photomicrograph showing characteristic smooth muscle cells in LAM.

REFERENCES

1. American Thoracic Society/European Respiratory Society: American Thoracic Society/European Respiratory Society international multidisciplinary consensus classification of the idiopathic interstitial pneumonias. *Am J Respir Crit Care Med* 2002, 165(2):277–304.

2. American Thoracic Society: Idiopathic pulmonary fibrosis: diagnosis and treatment. International consensus statement. American Thoracic Society (ATS), and the European Respiratory Society (ERS). *Am J Respir Crit Care Med* 2000, 161(2 Pt 1):646–664.

3. Lynch J III, Raghu G: Major disease syndromes of unknown etiology. In *Textbook of Pulmonary Diseases,* 6th ed. Edited by Baum GA, Crapo J, Celli B, Karlinsky J. Philadelphia: Lippincott-Raven; 1998:431–476.

4. Caminati A, Harari S: Smoking-related interstitial pneumonias and pulmonary Langerhans' cell histiocytosis. *Proc Am Thorac Soc* 2006, 3(4):299–306.

5. Lai CK, Wallace WD, Fishbein MC: Histopathology of pulmonary fibrotic disorders. *Semin Respir Crit Care Med* 2006, 27(6):613–622.

6. Elliot TL, Lynch DA, Newell JD Jr, et al.: High-resolution computed tomography features of nonspecific interstitial pneumonia and usual interstitial pneumonia. *J Comput Assist Tomogr* 2005, 29(3):339–345.

7. Lynch JP III, Saggar R, Weigt SS, et al.: Usual interstitial pneumonia. *Semin Respir Crit Care Med* 2006, 27(6):634–651.

8. Kim DS, Collard HR, King TF Jr: Classification and natural history of the idiopathic interstitial pneumonias. *Proc Am Thorac Soc* 2006, 3(4):285–292.

9. Flaherty KR, Martinez FJ: Nonspecific interstitial pneumonia. *Semin Respir Crit Care Med* 2006, 27(6):652–658.

10. Ryu JH, Myers JL, Capizzi SA, et al.: Desquamative interstitial pneumonia and respiratory bronchiolitis–associated interstitial lung disease. *Chest* 2005, 127(1):178–184.

11. Swigris JJ, Brown KK: Acute interstitial pneumonia and acute exacerbations of idiopathic pulmonary fibrosis. *Semin Respir Crit Care Med* 2006, 27(6):659–667.

12. Travis WD, Fox CH, Devaney KO, et al.: Lymphoid pneumonitis in 50 adult patients infected with the human immunodeficiency virus: lymphocytic interstitial pneumonitis versus nonspecific interstitial pneumonitis. *Hum Pathol* 1992, 23(5):529–541.

13. Flaherty KR, Thwaite EL, Kazerooni EA, et al.: Radiological versus histological diagnosis in UIP and NSIP: survival implications. *Thorax* 2003, 58(2):143–148.

14. Lacasse Y, Selman M, Costabel U, et al.: Clinical diagnosis of hypersensitivity pneumonitis. *Am J Respir Crit Care Med* 2003, 168(8):952–958.

15. Wells A: HRCT in the diagnosis of diffuse lung disease. *Semin Respir Crit Care Med* 2003, 24:347–356.

16. Flaherty KR, Toews GB, Travis WD, et al.: Clinical significance of histological classification of idiopathic interstitial pneumonia. *Eur Respir J* 2002, 19(2):275–283.

17. Flaherty KR, Colby TV, Travis WD, et al.: Fibroblastic foci in usual interstitial pneumonia: idiopathic versus collagen vascular disease. *Am J Respir Crit Care Med* 2003, 167(10):1410–1415.

18. Nicholson AG, Fulford LG, Colby TV, et al.: The relationship between individual histologic features and disease progression in idiopathic pulmonary fibrosis. *Am J Respir Crit Care Med* 2002, 166(2):173–177.

19. Portnoy J, Veraldi KL, Schwarz MI, et al.: Respiratory bronchiolitis–interstitial lung disease: long-term outcome. *Chest* 2007, 131(3):664–671.

20. Nicholson AG: Lymphocytic interstitial pneumonia and other lymphoproliferative disorders in the lung. *Semin Respir Crit Care Med* 2001, 22(4):409–422.

21. Do KH, Lee JS, Seo JB, et al.: Pulmonary parenchymal involvement of low-grade lymphoproliferative disorders. *J Comput Assist Tomogr* 2005, 29(6):825–830.

22. Selman M: Hypersensitivity pneumonitis: a multifaceted deceiving disorder. *Clin Chest Med* 2004, 25(3):vi,531–547.

23. Schuyler M, Cormier Y: The diagnosis of hypersensitivity pneumonitis. *Chest* 1997, 111(3):534–536.

24. Miyagawa T, Hamagami S, Tanigawa N: Cryptococcus albidus induced summer-type hypersensitivity pneumonitis. *Am J Respir Crit Care Med* 2000, 161(3 pt 1):961–966.

25. Sahin H, Brown KK, Curran-Everett D, et al.: Chronic hypersensitivity pneumonitis: CT features comparison with pathologic evidence of fibrosis and survival. *Radiology* 2007, 244(2):591–598.

26. Churg A, Muller NL, Flint J, Wright JL: Chronic hypersensitivity pneumonitis. *Am J Surg Pathol* 2006, 30(2):201–208.

27. Perez-Padilla R, Salas J, Chapela R, et al.: Mortality in Mexican patients with chronic pigeon breeder's lung compared with those with usual interstitial pneumonia. *Am Rev Respir Dis* 1993, 148(1):49–53.

28. Ohtani Y, Saiki S, Kitaichi M, et al.: Chronic bird fancier's lung: histopathological and clinical correlation: an application of the 2002 ATS/ERS consensus classification of the idiopathic interstitial pneumonias. *Thorax* 2005, 60(8):665–671.

29. Marras TK, Wallace RJ Jr, Koth LL, et al.: Hypersensitivity pneumonitis reaction to *Mycobacterium avium* in household water. *Chest* 2005, 127(2):664–671.

30. Silva CI, Churg A, Muller NL: Hypersensitivity pneumonitis: spectrum of high-resolution CT and pathologic findings. *AJR* 2007, 188(2):334–344.

31. Vourlekis JS, Schwarz MI, Cherniack RM, *et al.*: The effect of pulmonary fibrosis on survival in patients with hypersensitivity pneumonitis. *Am J Med* 2004, 116(10):662–668.

32. Cottin V, Cordier JF: Eosinophilic pneumonias. *Allergy* 2005, 60(7):841–857.

33. Marchand E, Cordier JF: Idiopathic chronic eosinophilic pneumonia. *Semin Respir Crit Care Med* 2006, 27(2):134–141.

34. Lynch J III, Flint A: Sorting out the pulmonary eosinophilic syndromes. *J Respir Dis* 1984, 5:61–78.

35. Trapnell BC, Whitsett JA, Nakata K: Pulmonary alveolar proteinosis. *N Engl J Med* 2003, 349(26):2527–2539.

36. Venkateshiah SB, Yan TD, Bonfield TL, *et al.*: An open-label trial of granulocyte macrophage colony stimulating factor therapy for moderate symptomatic pulmonary alveolar proteinosis. *Chest* 2006, 130(1):227–237.

37. Uchida K, Beck DC, Yamamoto T *et al.*: GM-CSF autoantibodies and neutrophil dysfunction in pulmonary alveolar proteinosis. *N Engl J Med* 2007, 356(6):567–579.

38. Lin FC, Chang GD, Chern MS, *et al.*: Clinical significance of anti-GM-CSF antibodies in idiopathic pulmonary alveolar proteinosis. *Thorax* 2006, 61(6):528–534.

39. Tazi A: Adult pulmonary Langerhans' cell histiocytosis. *Eur Respir J* 2006, 27(6):1272–1285.

40. Vassallo R, Ryu JH, Schroeder DR, *et al.*: Clinical outcomes of pulmonary Langerhans'-cell histiocytosis in adults. *N Engl J Med* 2002, 346(7):484–490.

41. Vassallo R, Ryu JH, Colby TV, *et al.*: Pulmonary Langerhans'-cell histiocytosis. *N Engl J Med* 2000, 342(26):1969–1978.

42. Koyama M, Johkoh T, Honda O, *et al.*: Chronic cystic lung disease: diagnostic accuracy of high-resolution CT in 92 patients. *AJR* 2003, 180(3):827–835.

43. Lynch J III: Computed tomographic scanning in sarcoidosis. *Semin Respir Crit Care Med* 2003, 24:393–418.

44. Johnson SR: Lymphangioleiomyomatosis. *Eur Respir J* 2006, 27(5):1056–1065.

CONNECTIVE TISSUE DISEASE

Maureen Heldmann, Nicole Elizabeth Vignes, and Seth Mark Berney

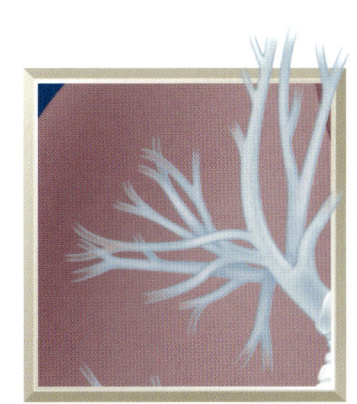
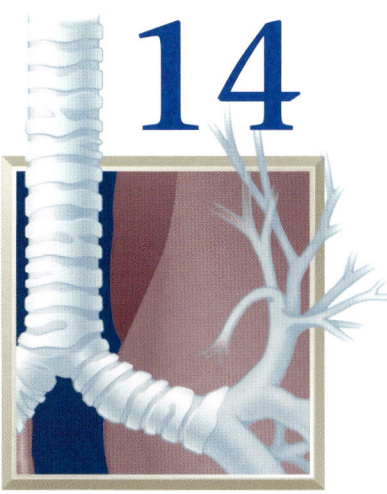
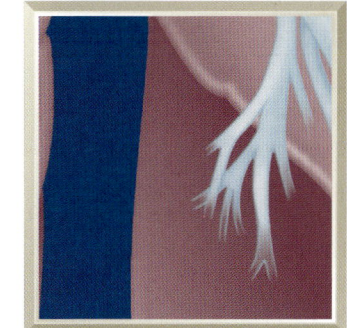

Many autoimmune connective tissue diseases involve the lungs either directly or as a complication of treatment. Rheumatoid arthritis, systemic lupus erythematosus, scleroderma, polymyositis and dermatomyositis, ankylosing spondylitis, and Sjögren's syndrome are all systemic autoimmune disorders of unknown etiology that cause pulmonary pathology. This chapter highlights the pulmonary manifestations of the most common of such disorders (see Chapter 15 for a discussion of pulmonary vasculitis).

Rheumatoid arthritis affects 1% to 2% of the world's population. The peak age of onset is 25 to 55 years with a female-to-male ratio of 2.5:1 [1,2]. Rheumatoid arthritis is characterized by symmetric polyarthritis, circulating autoantibodies (rheumatoid factor and anticyclic citrullinated peptide [CCP] antibody), inflammatory laboratory abnormalities (*eg*, elevated erythrocyte sedimentation rate, anemia of chronic disease, thrombocytosis, and increased inflammatory cytokines), and extra-articular manifestations. Genetics appear to play a role in the development or severity of disease; HLA-DR4 (DRB10401) and -DR1 (DRB10101) frequently occur in patients with more severe cases [3]. Extra-articular manifestations typically occur in patients who have severe joint disease and high-titer rheumatoid factor and include subcutaneous or pulmonary nodules, vasculitis, pleuropericarditis, pneumonitis, bronchiolitis, episcleritis, or scleritis. Rheumatologists treat patients aggressively with disease-modifying antirheumatic drugs, which include hydroxychloroquine, methotrexate, gold, sulfasalazine, D-penicillamine, and biologics (the tumor necrosis factor-α inhibitors adalimumab [Humira; Abbott Laboratories, Abbott Park, IL], etanercept [Enbrel; Immunex, Thousand Oaks, CA], and infliximab [Remicade; Centocor, Malvern, PA], and the interleukin-1 inhibitor anakinra [Kineret; Amgen, Thousand Oaks, CA]); the T-cell costimulator blocker abatacept (Orencia; Bristol-Myers Squibb, Princeton, NJ); and the anti–B-cell antibody rituximab (Rituxan; Genentech, South San Francisco, CA). Cytotoxic therapy (azathioprine, cyclophosphamide, and chlorambucil) and immunomodulators (cyclosporine and FK-506) are reserved for resistant synovitis and potentially life-threatening extra-articular manifestations. In addition, because of their multitude of adverse side effects, systemic steroids (whether administered orally, intramuscularly, or intravenously) are reserved for potentially life-threatening extra-articular manifestations.

Systemic lupus erythematosus affects approximately one of every 2000 individuals. The peak age of onset is 15 to 40 years, and the ratio of females to males affected is 5:1 [4]. Lupus is characterized by immune complex deposition, circulating autoantibodies, arthritis, cerebritis, cytopenias, nephritis, rash, and vasculitis. Genetics plays an important role in the development of the disease, as evident in the increased frequency of HLA-DR2 and HLA-DR3 in white patients who have systemic lupus erythematosus [5]. However, other undetermined genetic or environmental factors are also important. The nature of therapy depends on the severity of the disease; systemic steroids and cytotoxic agents are reserved for potentially life-threatening or major-organ manifestations.

Progressive systemic sclerosis (diffuse scleroderma) and limited scleroderma (formerly known as CREST syndrome [calcinosis, Raynaud phenomenon, esophageal dysmotility, sclerodactyly, and telangiectasia]) affect approximately one of every 5000 to 20,000 individuals. The peak age of onset is 40 to 60 years, with women more commonly affected [6,7].

Scleroderma manifests with circulating autoantibodies and fibrosis of the skin, vasculature, lungs, kidneys, heart, and gastrointestinal tract. Treatment is restricted to aggressive angiotensin-converting enzyme inhibitor therapy, which decreases renal crises and subsequent renal failure; angiotensin receptor blockers and vasodilators for Raynaud's phenomenon [8]; systemic steroids and cytotoxics for inflammatory organ involvement (for example, cyclophosphamide in patients with scleroderma-related interstitial lung disease or active alveolitis) [9]; and epoprostenol sodium (Flolan; GlaxoSmithKline, Philadelphia, PA), bosentan (Tracleer; Actelion, San Francisco, CA), treprostinil sodium (Remodulin; GlaxoSmithKline, Philadelphia, PA), iloprost (Ventavis; Actelion, San Francisco, CA), sildenafil citrate (Revatio; Pfizer, New York, NY), and ambrisentan (Letairis; Gilead Sciences, Westminster, CO) for pulmonary hypertension.

Polymyositis and dermatomyositis are inflammatory myopathies that affect one in every 100,000 to 200,000 individuals—predominantly women [10]. Although its cause is also unknown, dermatomyositis affecting individuals older than 50 to 60 years of age may be paraneoplastic. Up to 10% of these patients are diagnosed with a malignancy within 1 year of the onset of their myositis symptoms [11]. Polymyositis and dermatomyositis cause lymphocyte infiltration of proximal skeletal muscle, manifesting as proximal weakness but sparing sensation and facial/distal extremity muscles. The disease also affects the lungs, heart, skin, esophagus, joints, and vasculature. The mainstay of therapy is systemic steroids. If the disease is steroid-resistant or involves vital organs, doctors have found methotrexate, cytotoxics, or intravenous immunoglobulin (IV IgG) to often be effective.

Ankylosing spondylitis is a systemic inflammatory arthropathy that primarily affects the axial skeleton. This disease is strongly associated with HLA-B27 and is three times more common in men. Onset usually occurs before 40 years of age [12]. Ankylosing spondylitis manifests as sacroiliitis and spondylitis, causing fused sacroiliac joints and the classic bamboo spine. Uncommon extra-axial manifestations include peripheral arthritis, anterior uveitis, aortic root dilation, apical lung fibrosis, and cauda equina syndrome. Treatment includes physical therapy, nonsteroidal anti-inflammatory drugs, sulfasalazine, TNF-alpha inhibitors, and, if necessary, ophthalmic immunosuppressants and orthopedic, cardiothoracic, or spinal surgery.

Sjögren's syndrome is a systemic autoimmune disease of the exocrine glands that affects one of every 1250 individuals (among whom middle-aged women are at greatest risk) but can also complicate rheumatoid arthritis, systemic lupus erythematosus, progressive systemic sclerosis, and myositis (considered secondary Sjögren's) [13]. Sjögren's syndrome manifests as autoantibody formation, keratoconjunctivitis sicca (dry eyes), and xerostomia (dry mouth), which are caused by lymphocytic infiltration of lacrimal and salivary glands. Other organ systems affected include the musculoskeletal, renal, integumentary, pulmonary, gastrointestinal, hematologic, and peripheral and central nervous systems. Treatment includes replenishment of deficient hormones (thyroid, insulin, artificial tears, and artificial saliva), as well as immunosuppression when life-threatening or major organ involvement occurs.

A — Pulmonary Manifestations of Connective Tissue Diseases

Disease	Parenchymal	Serosal	Vascular	Neuromuscular	Airway	Other
Systemic lupus erythematosus	Infectious pneumonia	Pleurocarditis	Pulmonary hypertension	Shrinking lung syndrome	—	—
	Pneumonitis	Pericarditis	Thrombosis			
	Diffuse alveolar hemorrhage		Thromboembolism			
	Acute reversible hypoxemia syndrome					
Rheumatoid arthritis	Interstitial pneumonitis	Pleuritis	Arteritis	—	Bronchiolitis obliterans and organizing pneumonia	—
	Interstitial fibrosis					
	Nodulosis					
Progressive systemic sclerosis	Interstitial pneumonitis	Pleurocarditis	Pulmonary hypertension	—	—	Respiratory restriction secondary to skin tightness
	Interstitial fibrosis	Pericarditis				Dilated esophagus
Polymyositis/ dermatomyositis	Interstitial pneumonitis	—	Pulmonary hypertension	Respiratory muscle weakness	—	—
	Interstitial fibrosis			Pharyngeal muscle weakness with recurrent aspiration		
Ankylosing spondylitis	Apical fibrosis	—	—	—	—	Respiratory restriction secondary to loss of thoracic expansion
						Bamboo spine
						Aortic root dilation
Sjögren's syndrome	Interstitial pneumonitis	—	—	—	—	—

B — Pulmonary Side Effects of Commonly Used Antirheumatic Medication

Cyclophosphamide
  Interstitial fibrosis
Gold
  Interstitial pneumonitis
  Alveolar pneumonitis
Methotrexate
  Interstitial pneumonitis
  Alveolar pneumonitis
  Interstitial fibrosis
Sulfasalazine
  Interstitial pneumonitis

Figure 14-1. **A,** Pulmonary manifestations of connective tissue diseases. **B,** Noninfectious pulmonary side effects of commonly used antirheumatic medications.

SYSTEMIC LUPUS ERYTHEMATOSUS

Classification Criteria for Systemic Lupus Erythematosus

S	Serositis	Pleuritis or pericarditis
O	Oral ulcers	Oral or nasopharyngeal ulcerations (usually painless)
A	Arthritis	Nonerosive arthritis involving two or more peripheral joints with synovitis
P	Photosensitivity	Skin rash from ultraviolet light/radiation exposure
B	Blood dyscrasias	Coombs-positive hemolytic anemia with reticulocytosis or
		Leukopenia < 4000/mm^3 leukocytes on two or more occasions or
		Lymphopenia < 1500/mm^3 on two or more occasions or
		Thrombocytopenia < 100,000/mm^3 on two or more occasions
R	Renal disorder	Persistent proteinuria > 0.5 g/d or cellular (erythrocytes or leukocytes) casts
A	Antinuclear antibody	Anti-double-stranded DNA (ds-DNA) antibody or
		Anti-Smith (Sm) antibody or
I	Immunologic disorder	Antiphospholipid antibody based on one of the following:
		Abnormal serum IgG or IgM anticardiolipin antibody or
		Positive lupus anticoagulant or
		False-positive rapid plasma reagin or Venereal Disease Research Laboratory tests known positive for ≥ 6 mo and confirmed by *Treponema pallidum* immobilization or fluorescent treponemal antibody absorption test
N	Neurologic disorder	Seizures or psychosis
M	Malar rash	Fixed erythema, flat or raised, over the malar eminences, sparing the nasolabial folds
D	Discoid rash	Erythematous raised patches with scaling and follicular plugging; atrophic scarring may occur in older lesions

Figure 14-2. Systemic lupus erythematosus classification criteria. Four of the 11 manifestations listed in the figure are required for classification of systemic lupus erythematosus. The mnemonic is SOAP BRAIN MD. (*Adapted from* Hochberg [14] and Tan *et al.* [15].)

Pulmonary Manifestations of Systemic Lupus Erythematosus

Manifestation	Incidence	Comments
Pleuro- and pericarditis	50%–80% [16]	—
Infection	Unknown	Most common cause of infiltrate in systemic lupus erythematosus: typical (especially encapsulated organisms) and opportunistic (especially nocardia, fungal)
Interstitial lung disease	25% [17]	—
Pulmonary hypertension	9% [18]	—
Acute pneumonitis	1%–9% [19–21]	Patient is acutely ill with hypoxemia; chest radiograph has diffuse bibasilar infiltrates with or without effusions [19–21]
Diffuse alveolar hemorrhage	1%–2% [22,23]	—
Thrombosis and thromboembolism	Unknown	Hypercoagulability state secondary to nephrosis or antiphospholipid antibody syndrome
Shrinking lung syndrome	Unknown	Secondary to respiratory muscle dysfunction with atelectasis and diaphragm elevation
Acute reversible hypoxemia syndrome	Unknown	—

Figure 14-3. The most common pulmonary manifestations of systemic lupus erythematosus.

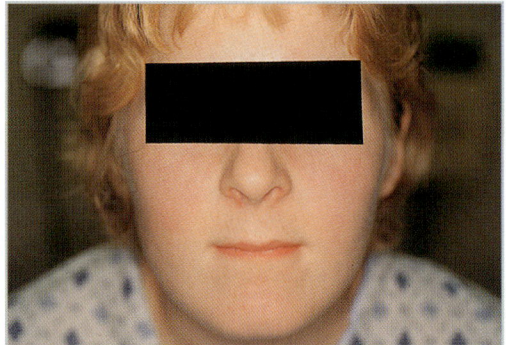

Figure 14-4. Malar rash. The classic malar (butterfly) rash typically spares the nasolabial folds and is commonly precipitated by solar irradiation.

Atlas of Pulmonary Medicine

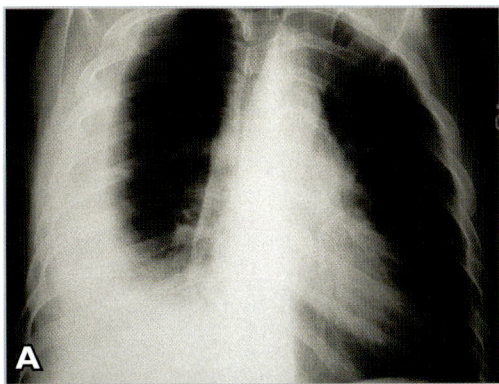
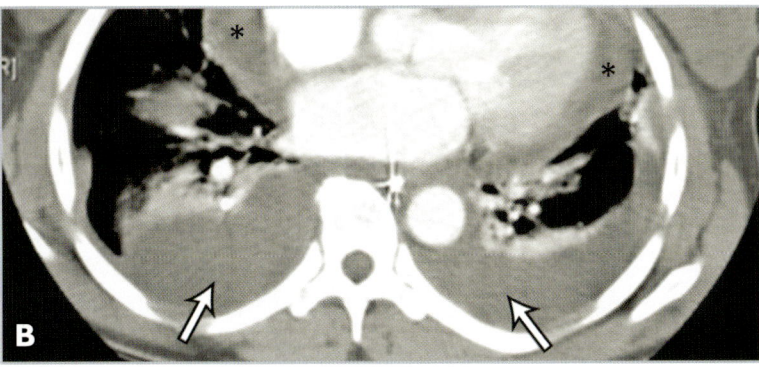
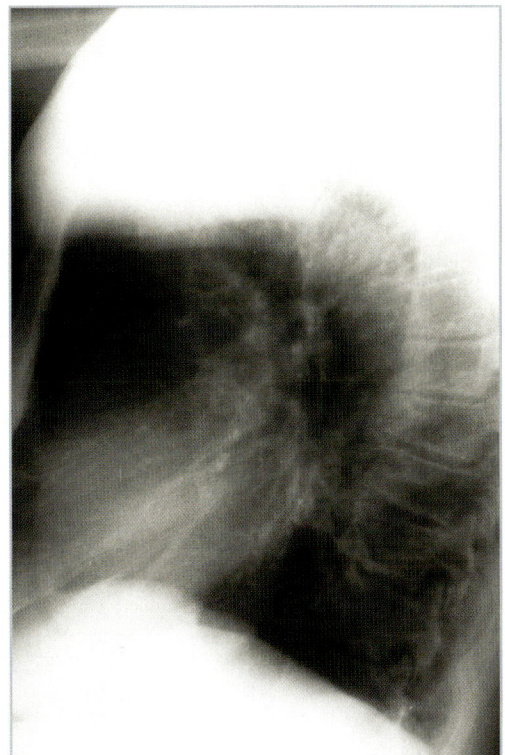
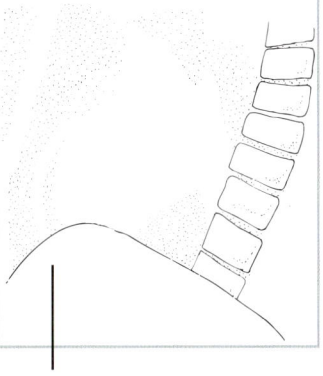

Figure 14-5. **A,** Right lateral decubitus chest radiograph revealing a free-flowing right pleural effusion. **B,** Enhanced CT at systemic lupus erythematosus (SLE) presentation. Bilateral pleural (*arrows*) and pericardial effusions (*asterisks*) resolved promptly with therapy. Lupus pleural fluid is exudative, with a leukocyte count of less than 10,000 (monocytes/lymphocytes); the glucose level is normal; and the pH is greater than 7.35. Pleural fluid lupus erythematosus cell detection is insensitive but specific for SLE. Pleural fluid antinuclear antibody and complement levels are not specific for SLE and have been found in patients with empyema and malignancy. Their presence has not been tested extensively in other autoimmune diseases, and, as a result, routine measurements of antinuclear antibodies and C3/C4 are not helpful [24].

Figure 14-6. The presence of pericardial effusion from systemic lupus erythematosus illustrated by a lateral chest radiograph showing separation of the epicardial fat pad from the sternum. The heart is normally closely applied to the posterior sternum. This separation suggests the presence of a substance (usually fluid) between the epicardium and pericardium.

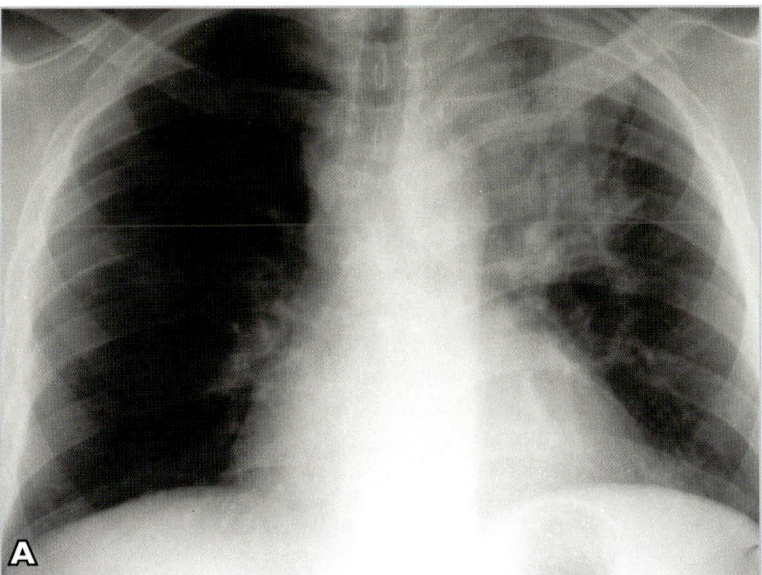
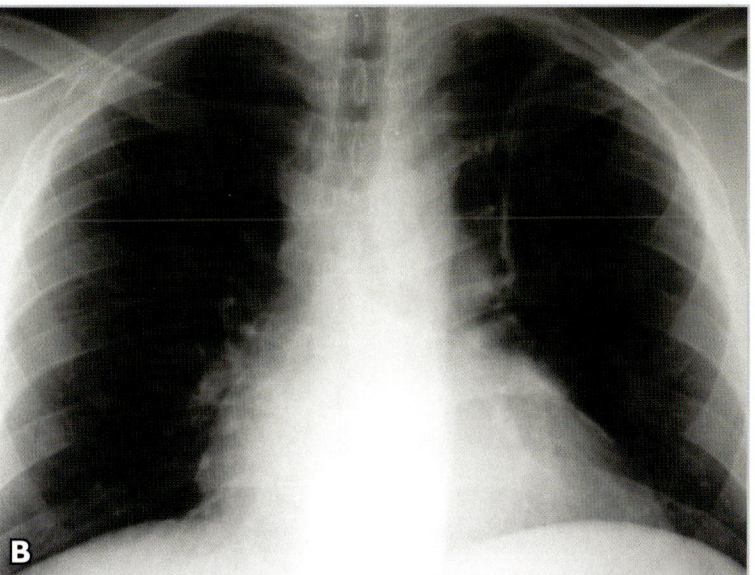

Figure 14-7. **A,** Erect posteroanterior chest radiograph of a patient with lupus demonstrating left upper lobe consolidation, with associated air bronchogram. During treatment for glomerulonephritis with cyclophosphamide and prednisone, this patient developed fever, dyspnea, and a slightly purulent cough. Sputum culture revealed blastomycosis, which responded to decreases in his immunosuppression and beginning itraconazole. **B,** Chest radiograph after therapy, revealing a small scar.

RHEUMATOID ARTHRITIS

Classification Criteria for Rheumatoid Arthritis

- Morning stiffness in and around joints lasting ≥ 1 h before maximal improvement
- Soft-tissue swelling of three or more joint areas observed by a physician (PIP, MCP, wrist, elbow, knee, ankle, MTP)
- Swelling of the PIP, MCP, or wrist joints
- Symmetric joint swelling
- Subcutaneous nodules over bony prominence or extensor surface or in juxta-articular regions
- Positive test result for rheumatoid factor
- Radiographic erosions or periarticular osteopenia in hand or wrist joints

Figure 14-8. Classification criteria for rheumatoid arthritis. Four of the seven manifestations listed must be present for classification as rheumatoid arthritis [25]. MCP—metacarpophalangeal; MTP—etatarsophalangeal; PIP—proximal interphalangeal.

Pulmonary Manifestations of Rheumatoid Arthritis

Manifestation	Incidence	Comments
Pleural disease	20%–40% [26,27]	Pleurisy with or without effusion (very low glucose)
Interstitial pneumonitis	5%–10% [28]	Interstitial infiltrate with predilection for lung bases and periphery
Nodulosis	≤ 1% [29]	Solitary or multiple with or without pneumoconiosis (Caplan's syndrome); more common in men with high-titer rheumatoid factor, subcutaneous nodules, active rheumatoid arthritis; upper and midlung zone predominance
Interstitial fibrosis	Unknown	Basal predilection
Bronchiolitis obliterans and organizing pneumonia	Rare	—
Arteritis	Rare	Usually occurs in setting of diffuse alveolar hemorrhage

Figure 14-9. The most common pulmonary manifestations of rheumatoid arthritis.

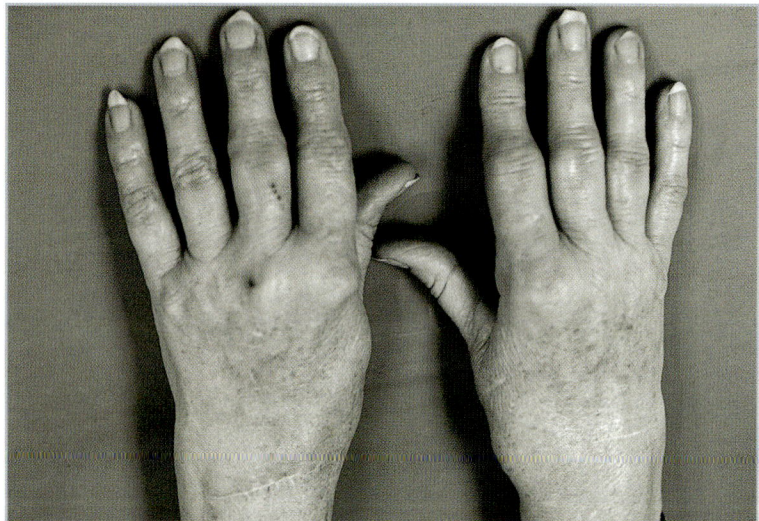

Figure 14-10. Synovitis. This patient with rheumatoid arthritis has synovitis of both wrists and several metacarpophalangeal and proximal interphalangeal joints. This patient also had rupture of the left wrist extensor tendon, which was repaired (evidenced by left wrist scar).

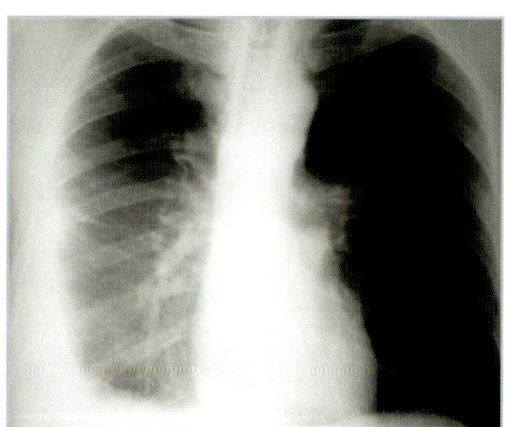

Figure 14-11. Erect posteroanterior chest radiograph showing rheumatoid pleural disease with effusion. In this patient, the disease is represented by a moderate-sized right pleural-based density. Rheumatoid pleural fluid is exudative with a pH of less than 7.2, a glucose level of 30 mg/dL or less, and a leukocyte count of 15,000 or less. Because the pleural rheumatoid factor is found in tuberculosis, malignancy, and other infections, this test is unhelpful [28].

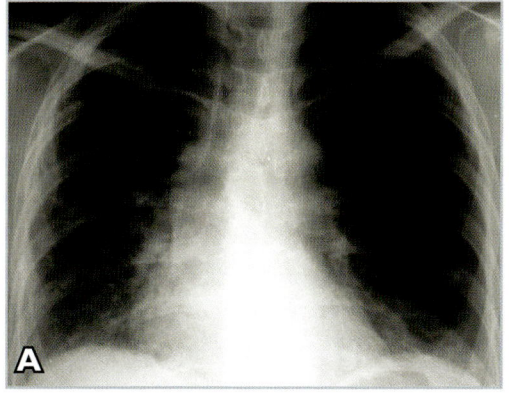
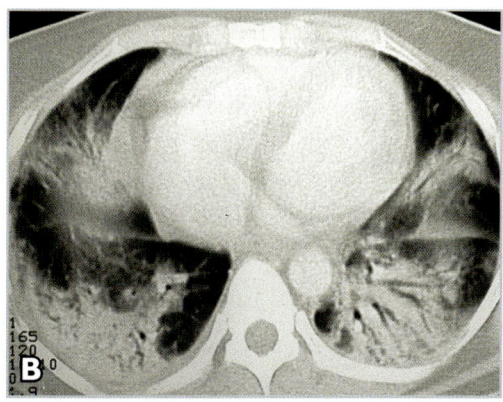
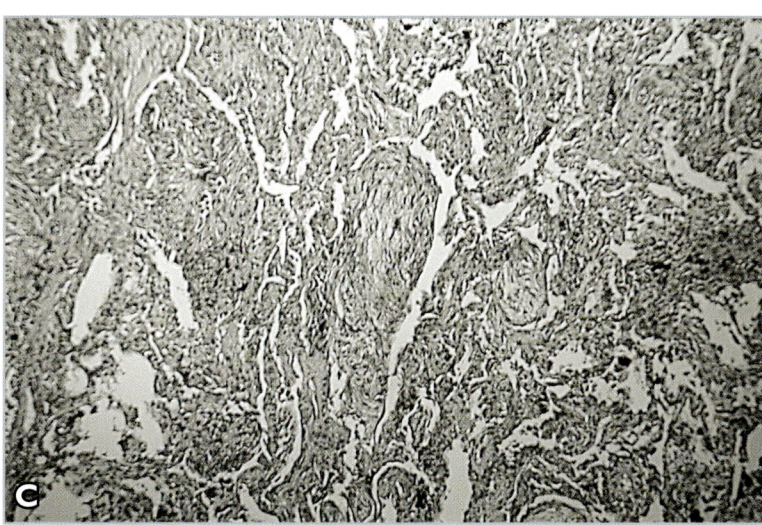

Figure 14-12. Erect posteroanterior chest radiograph (**A**) and lung window chest CT (**B**) demonstrating patchy bibasilar areas of consolidation. These areas are notably peribronchiolar in distribution and are associated with mild bronchiolar dilation in affected areas, which are common findings in bronchiolitis obliterans organizing pneumonia (BOOP). (**C**) Lung biopsy specimen from the same patient, containing balls of fibroblasts within a respiratory bronchiole and surrounding air spaces consistent with BOOP. (*Panel C courtesy of* WD Grafton, MD.)

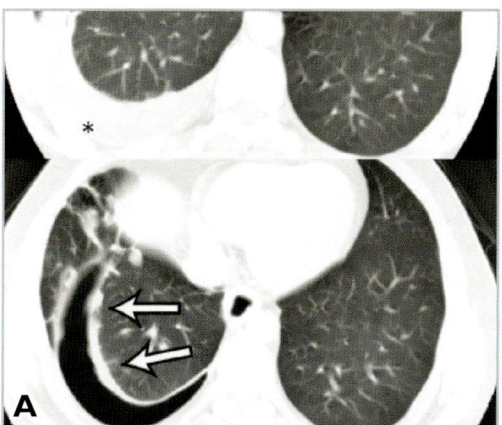
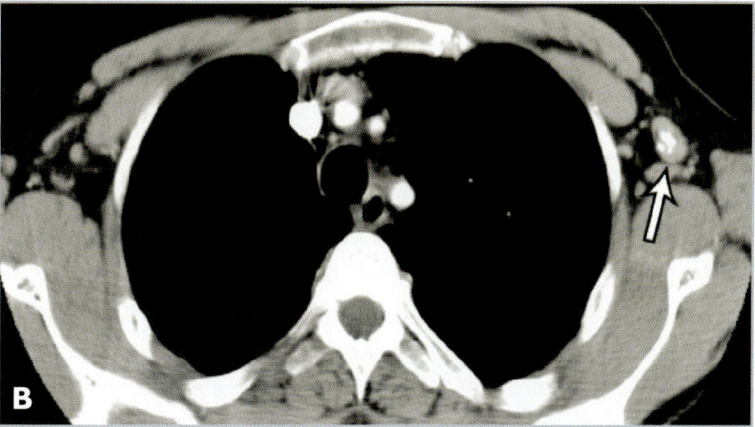

Figure 14-13. Composite lung window chest CTs taken 3 years apart. **A,** Pleural and parenchymal necrobiotic nodules (*arrows*) remained stable, but interval cavitation resulted in chronic pneumothorax (*asterisk*). **B,** Soft-tissue window CT image of the same patient demonstrates accumulation of high-density material in a left axillary node (*arrow*) thought to be related to therapeutic administration of gold salts.

PROGRESSIVE SYSTEMIC SCLEROSIS

Classification Criteria for Progressive Systemic Sclerosis

Major Criterion

Proximal scleroderma
  Symmetric thickening, tightening, and induration of the skin of the fingers and the skin proximal to the metacarpophalangeal or metatarsophalangeal joints
  The changes may affect the entire extremity, face, neck, and trunk

Minor Criteria

Sclerodactyly
  Skin changes listed under major criterion limited to the fingers
Digital pitting scars or loss of substance from the finger pad
  Depressed areas at tips of fingers or loss of digital pad tissue as a result of ischemia
Bibasilar pulmonary fibrosis
  Bilateral reticular or reticular pattern or reticulonodular densities most pronounced in basilar portions of the lungs on standard chest radiograph; may assume appearance of diffuse mottling or "honeycomb lung"; these changes should not be attributable to primary lung disease

Figure 14-14. Classification criteria for progressive systemic sclerosis (scleroderma). One major or two minor criteria are needed for classification [30].

Pulmonary Manifestations of Progressive Systemic Sclerosis

	Incidence	
	Diffuse, %	Limited, %
Interstitial pneumonitis—alveolar effusions (ground glass appearance)	30–90	30–90
Interstitial fibrosis	35	35
Pulmonary hypertension	≤ 1	10
Dilated esophagus	75	75
Pleuro- and pericarditis	40	?
Respiratory restriction secondary to chest wall skin tightness	?	0

Figure 14-15. Pulmonary manifestations of diffuse and limited (formerly known as CREST [calcinosis, Raynaud phenomenon, esophageal dysmotility, sclerodactyly, and telangiectasia]) scleroderma [31].

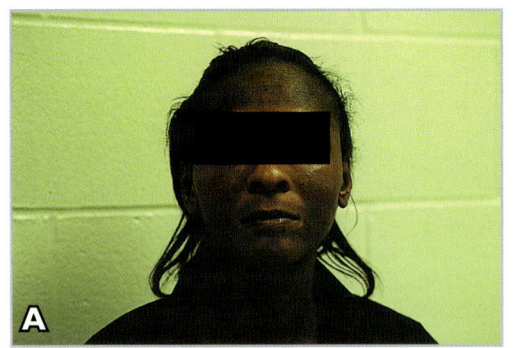 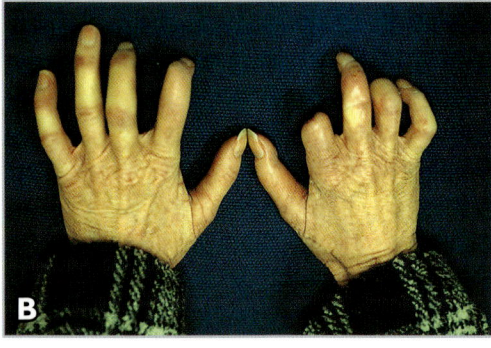

Figure 14-16. Sclerodactyly in a patient with scleroderma. **A,** This patient with scleroderma has tight skin (*ie,* lack of wrinkles), which has caused a decreased oral aperture. **B,** This patient with Raynaud's phenomenon of the fingers has autoamputation of right index and ring fingers and areas of blanching and cyanosis.

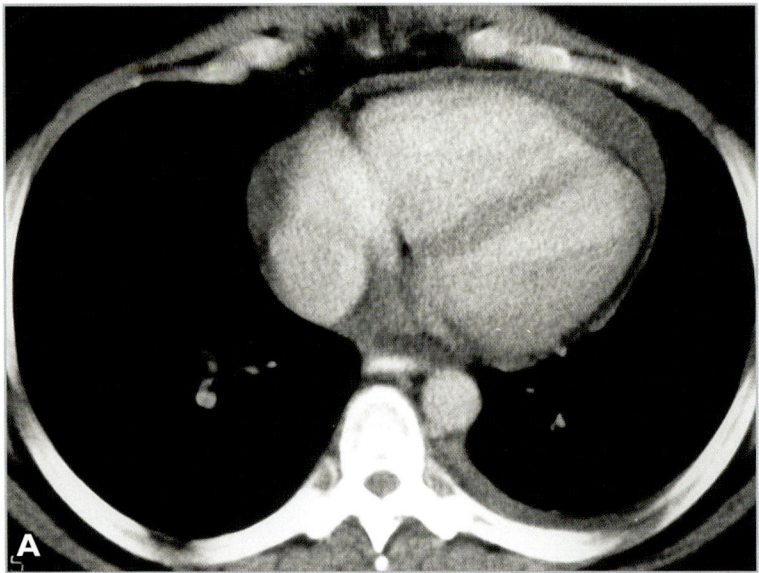 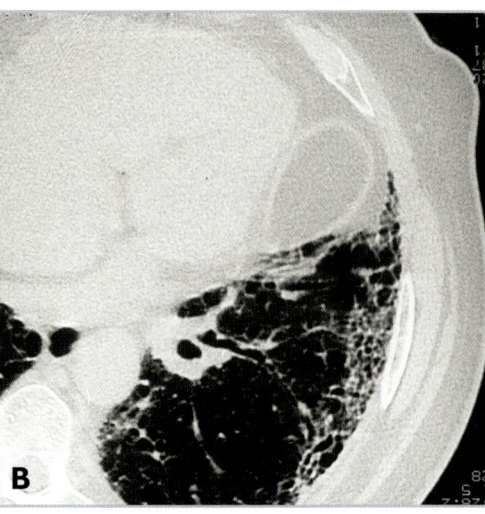

Figure 14-17. A, CT showing small left pleural and pericardial effusions in a patient with scleroderma. **B,** High-resolution CT of a different patient demonstrates typical subpleural honeycombing with lower zonal posterior predominance of pulmonary fibrosis.

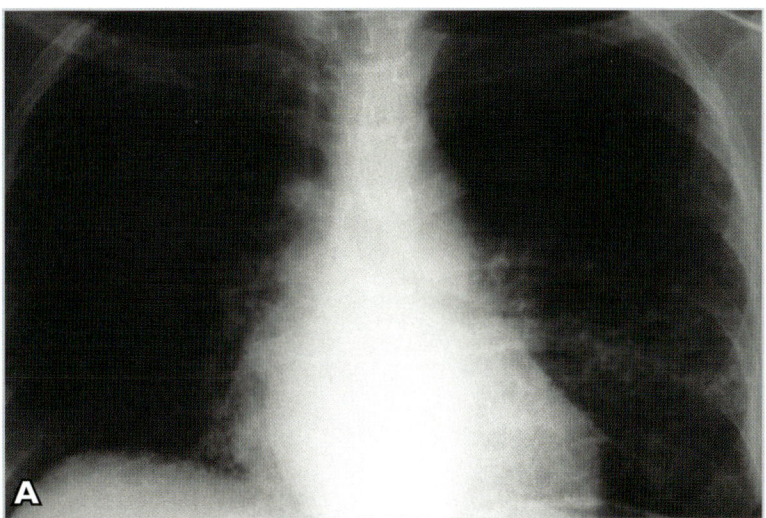
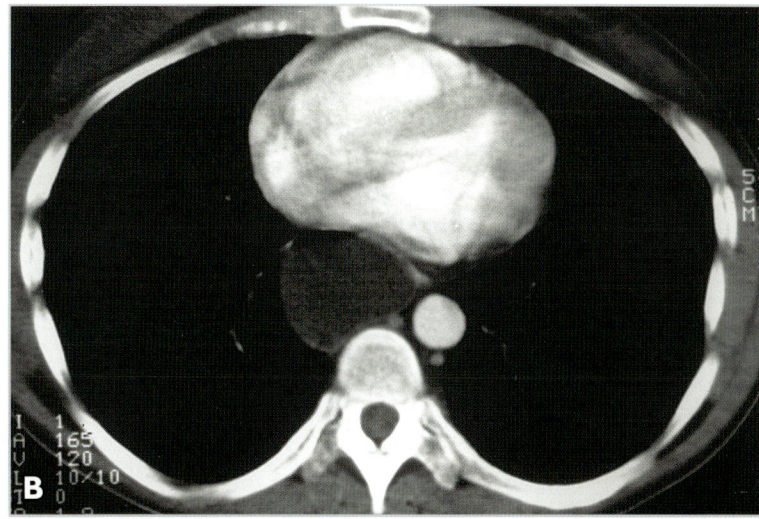
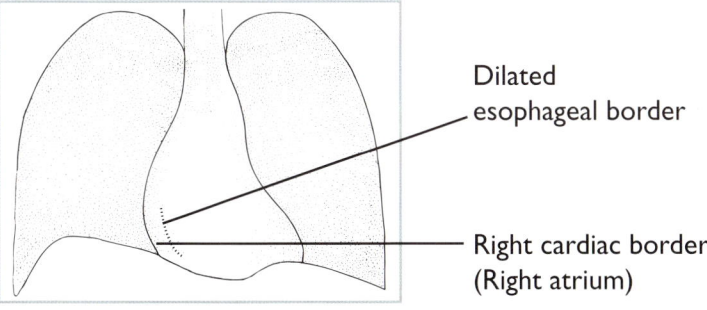
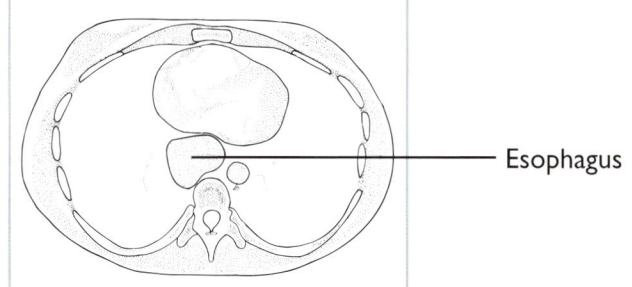
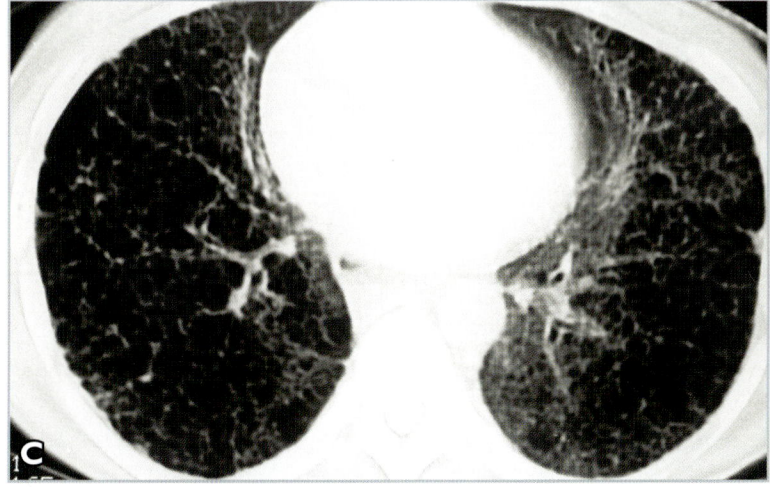

Figure 14-18. A, Erect posteroanterior chest radiograph showing lower and midzonal coarse reticular interstitial disease in a patient with scleroderma. Note the double density of the right cardiac border. **B,** Chest CT displays the same density as in A, which represents a dilated, fluid-filled esophagus. **C,** Lung window CT of the same patient illustrates honeycomb, end-stage lung disease.

POLYMYOSITIS AND DERMATOMYOSITIS

Classification Criteria for Polymyositis and Dermatomyositis

Symmetric proximal muscle weakness (limb girdle and anterior neck muscles) ± tenderness
Elevated serum muscle enzymes (creatine phosphokinase, lactate dehydrogenase, aldolase, aspirate aminotransferase, alanine aminotransferase)
Myopathic changes on electromyography manifested as the triad of
  Short, small polyphasic motor units
  Fibrillations, positive waves, and insertional irritability
  Bizarre high-frequency discharges
Muscle biopsy specimen demonstrating inflammation (muscle fiber necrosis/regeneration/atrophy in a perifascicular distribution with an inflammatory exudate)
Skin rash
  Heliotrope (lilac-colored) discoloration of eyelids with periorbital edema
  Scaly, erythematous dermatitis over the dorsa of the hands (especially over the metacarpophalangeal and proximal interphalangeal joints [Gottron's sign]) and involvement of the knees, elbows, medial malleoli, face, neck, and upper torso

Figure 14-19. Classification criteria for polymyositis and dermatomyositis. (*Adapted from* Wortmann [32] and Bohan and Peter [33].)

Polymyositis and Dermatomyositis Antisynthetase Antibody Syndrome

Polymyositis/dermatomyositis with the following:
  Relatively acute onset
  Interstitial lung disease
  Fever
  Arthritis
  Raynaud's phenomenon
  "Mechanic's hands" (darkened or dirty-appearing cracking and fissuring of the lateral and palmar aspects of the fingers)
Presence of the myositis-specific antisynthetase antibodies to
  Histidyl-tRNA synthetase (Jo-1)
  Threonyl-tRNA synthetase (PL-7)
  Alanyl-tRNA synthetase (PL-12)
  Glycyl-tRNA synthetase (EJ)
  Isoleucyl-tRNA synthetase (OJ)

Figure 14-20. Polymyositis and dermatomyositis antisynthetase antibody syndrome. (*Adapted from* Wortmann [32].)

Pulmonary Manifestations of Polymyositis and Dermatomyositis

Manifestation	Incidence, %
Interstitial lung disease (but increased in patients with antisynthetase antibody)	5–30 [34,35]
Interstitial fibrosis (but increased in patients with antisynthetase antibody)	5–10 [36]
Diaphragm/respiratory muscle weakness	≤ 5 [37]
Pharyngeal muscle weakness with recurrent aspiration	> 50 [38]
Pulmonary hypertension	Unknown

Figure 14-21. Pulmonary manifestations of polymyositis and dermatomyositis.

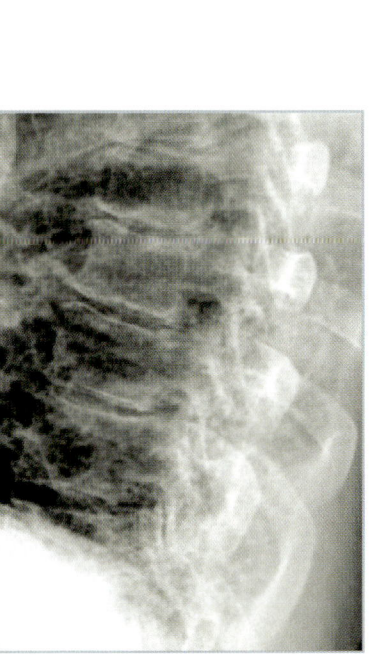

Figure 14-22. Magnification lateral-view chest radiograph showing lower zonal reticular interstitial lung disease.

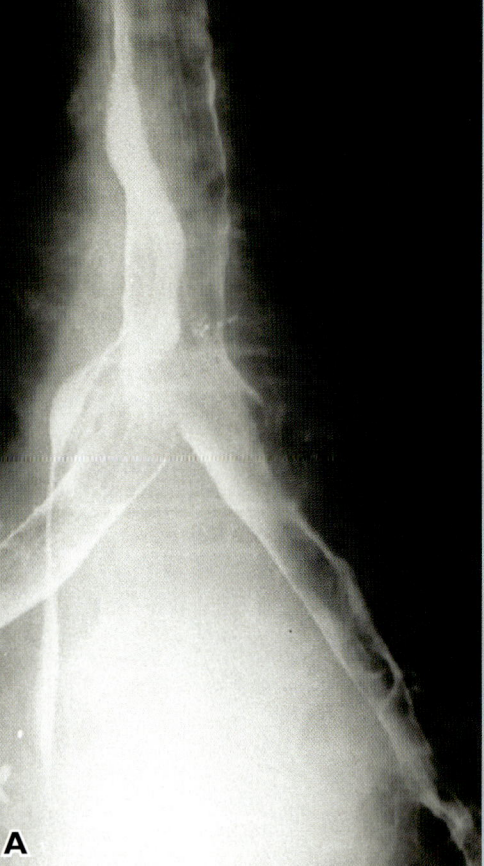
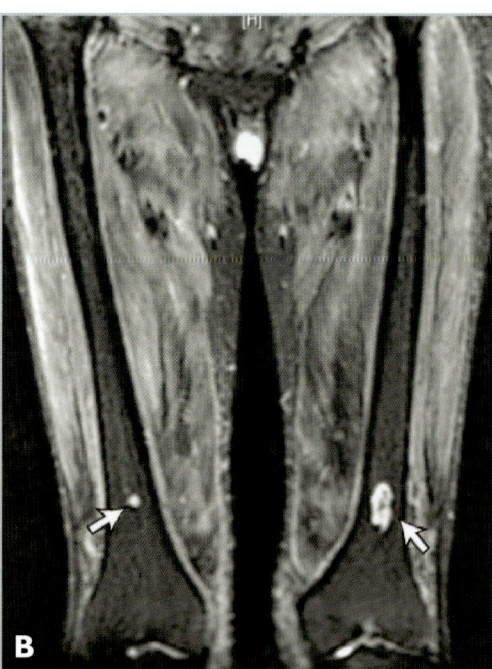

Figure 14-23. A, Upper gastrointestinal examination of a patient with dermatomyositis. Pharyngeal dysmotility predisposes to aspiration, as seen by contrast material coating the trachea and proximal bronchi. Barium pools in the pyriform sinuses, with only a small amount traversing the esophagus. **B,** Coronal inversion recovery MRI of the thighs. Muscle signal is abnormally bright, consistent with active myositis. Small medullary infarcts (*arrows*) are present in both femora from prior steroid therapy. Creatine phosphokinase at the time was 11,000 U/L.

ANKYLOSING SPONDYLITIS

Thoracic and Pulmonary Manifestations of Ankylosing Spondylitis

Manifestation	Incidence
Bamboo spine and chest wall fixation	Develops in many patients
Apical fibrosis (which may cavitate and become infected with *Aspergillus* spp or mycobacteria)	< 2% [39]
Aortic root dilation and aortic valve regurgitation	3.5% in ankylosing spondylitis >15 y [40]

Figure 14-24. Thoracic and pulmonary manifestations of ankylosing spondylitis.

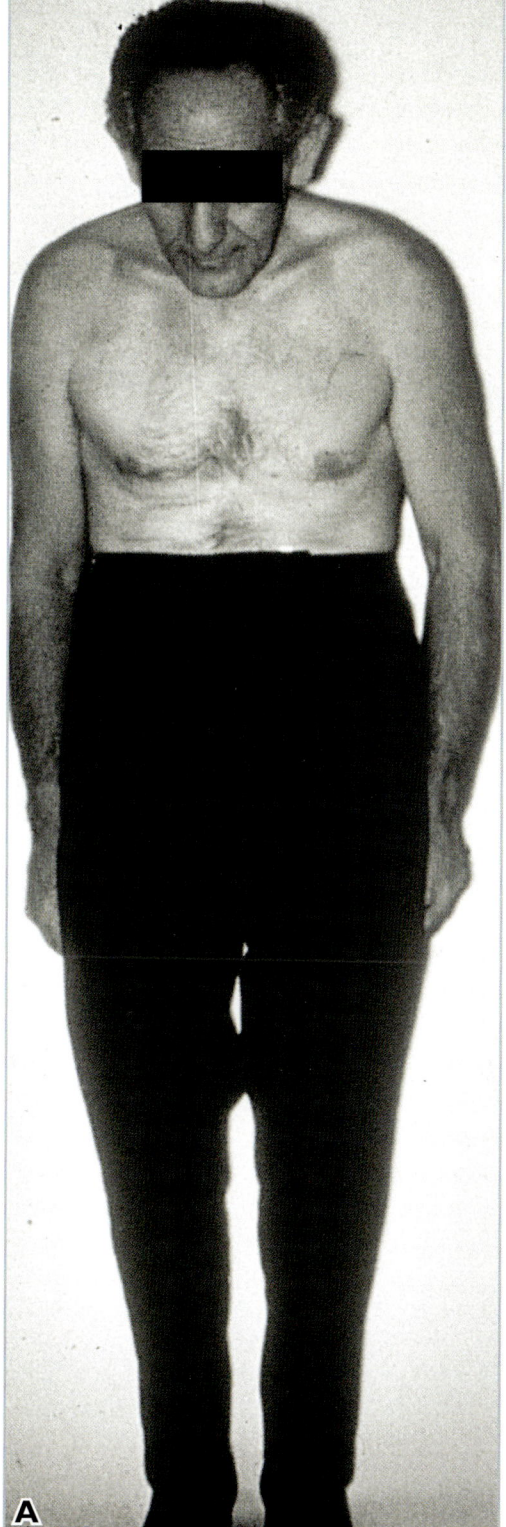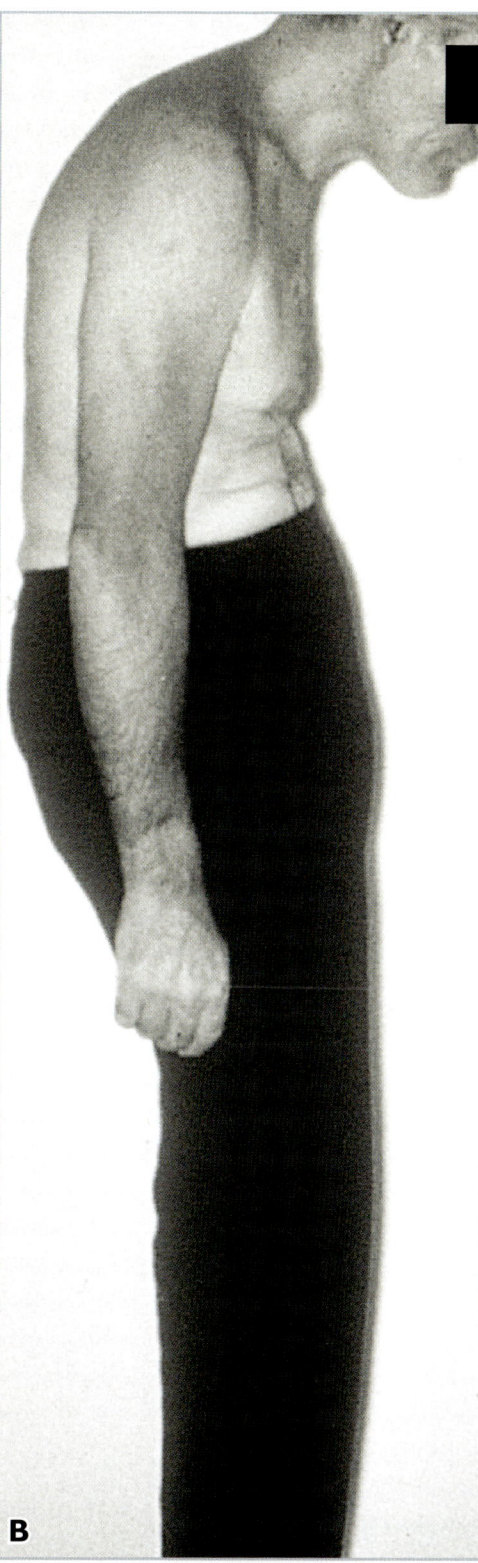

Figure 14-25. Frontal (**A**) and side (**B**) views of a patient with advanced ankylosing spondylitis. The patient maintains fixed forward protrusion of the head, thoracic kyphosis, and loss of normal lumbar lordosis. (*From* the Visual Aids Subcommittee of the Professional Education Committee of the Arthritis Foundation [41]; with permission.)

| *Connective Tissue Disease* |

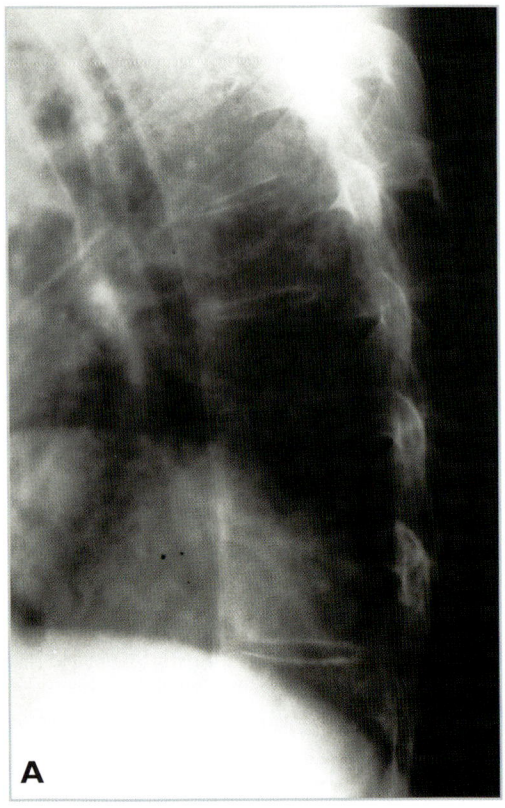
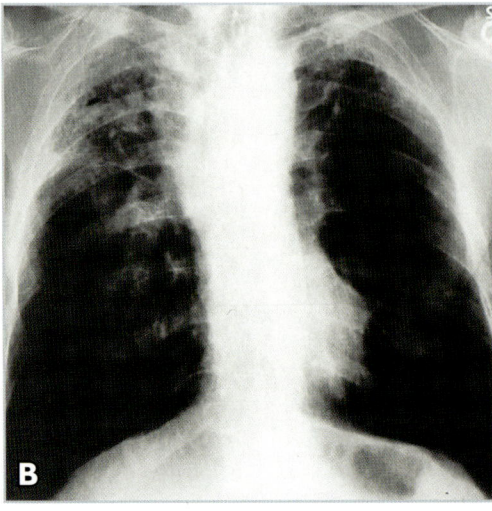

Figure 14-26. **A**, Lateral thoracic spine radiograph revealing flowing ossification of the paraspinal soft tissues producing the classic bamboo spine of ankylosing spondylitis. **B**, Chest radiograph of patient with ankylosing spondylitis and bilateral upper-zone fibronodular infiltrates. (*Panel B from Schwarz [28]; with permission.*)

A   Drug Toxicity

Drug	Manifestations	Description	Treatment
Methotrexate	Alveolar/interstitial infiltrate	Frequently acute onset with fever, dyspnea	Drug withdrawal or in severe cases prednisone (1 mg/kg) [42,43]
		1%–11% incidence in rheumatoid arthritis	
		May be a hypersensitive reaction and may result in fibrosis	
Gold	Alveolar/interstitial infiltrate with upper lung predominance	Dyspnea, cough, fever, peripheral eosinophilia	Drug withdrawal or in severe cases prednisone (1 mg/kg)
Cyclophosphamide	Interstitial pulmonary fibrosis	—	—
Sulfasalazine	Diffuse interstitial infiltrate	Hypersensitivity lung disease with cough, fever, and dyspnea	Drug withdrawal or in severe cases prednisone (1 mg/kg)

B   Rheumatologic Drugs That May Predispose to Infection

- Abatacept (Orencia; Bristol-Myers Squibb, Prinecton, NJ)
- Adalimumab (Humira; Abbott Laboratories, Abbott Park, IL)
- Anakinra (Kineret; Amgen, Thousand Oaks, CA)
- Azathioprine (Imuran; GlaxoSmithKline, Philadelphia, PA)
- Cyclophosphamide (Cytoxan; Mead Johnson Oncology Products, Princeton, NJ)
- Cyclosporin A
- Etanercept (Enbrel; Immunex, Thousand Oaks, CA)
- Glucocorticoids (prednisone, Solu-Medrol [Pharmacia & Upjohn, Kalamazoo, MI])
- Infliximab (Remicade; Centocor, Malvern, PA)
- Methotrexate
- Mycophenolate mofetil (CellCept; Hoffmann-LaRoche, Nutley, NJ)
- Rituximab (Rituxan; Genentech, South San Francisco, CA)

Figure 14-27. **A**, Toxicity of common antirheumatic medications. **B**, Rheumatologic drugs that may predispose to infection.

Atlas of Pulmonary Medicine

Autoantibodies and Their Incidences in Connective Tissue Disease

Autoantibody	Rheumatoid Arthritis	Systemic Lupus Erythematosus	Sjögren's Syndrome	PSS (Scleroderma)	Polymyositis/ Dermatomyositis	Ankylosing Spondylitis
Rheumatoid factor	Common*	Common	Common	Common	Rare†	Undetectable
Antinuclear antibody	Common	Common	Common	Common	Rare	Undetectable
Double-stranded DNA	Undetectable	Diagnostic	Undetectable	Undetectable	Undetectable	Undetectable
Smith antibody	Undetectable	Diagnostic	Undetectable	Undetectable	Undetectable	Undetectable
Ro(SSA)/La(SSB) ("Sjögren's antibodies")	Uncommon‡ (associated with Sjögren's)	Uncommon (associated with Sjögren's)	Common	Uncommon	Rare	Undetectable
Centromere	Undetectable	Undetectable	Rare	Common in limited PSS	Rare	Undetectable
SCL-70 (topoisomerase I)	Undetectable	Undetectable	Rare	Common in diffuse PSS	Rare	Undetectable
Jo-1 (synthetase)	Undetectable	Undetectable	Undetectable	Rare	Common in patients with interstitial lung disease	Undetectable
Antineutrophil cytoplasmic antibody	Rare	Rare	Uncommon	Undetectable	Uncommon	Undetectable

* > 25% of patients.
† < 5% of patients.
‡ 5%–25% of patients.

Figure 14-28. Autoantibodies and their incidence in connective tissue disease. PSS–progressive systemic sclerosis. (*Adapted from* Froelich et al. [44] and Gross [45].)

REFERENCES

1. Kellgren JH: Epidemiology of rheumatoid arthritis. *Arthritis Rheum* 1966, 9:658–674.

2. Chan KA, Felson DT, Yood RA, Walker AM: Incidence of rheumatoid arthritis in central Massachusetts. *Arthritis Rheum* 1993, 36:1691–1696.

3. Weyand CM, Hicok KC, Conn DL, et al.: The influence of HLA-DRB1 genes on disease severity in rheumatoid arthritis. *Ann Intern Med* 1992, 118:801–806.

4. Fessel WJ: Systemic lupus erythematosus in the community: incidence, prevalence, outcome and first symptoms; the high prevalence in black women. *Arch Intern Med* 1974, 134:1027–1035.

5. Howard PF, Hochberg MC, Bias WB, et al.: Relationship between C4 null genes, HLA-D region antigens, and genetic susceptibility to systemic lupus erythematosus in Caucasian and Black Americans. *Am J Med* 1986, 81:187–193.

6. Tamaki T, Mori S, Takehara K: Epidemiological study of patients with systemic sclerosis in Tokyo. *Arch Dermatol Res* 1991, 283:366–371.

7. Maricq HR, Weinrich MC, Keil JE, et al.: Prevalence of scleroderma spectrum disorders in the general population of South Carolina. *Arthritis Rheum* 1989, 32:998–1006.

8. Dziadzio M, Denton CP, Smith R, et al. Losartan therapy for Raynaud's phenomenon and scleroderma: clinical and biochemical findings in a fifteen-week, randomized, parallel-group, controlled trial. *Arthritis Rheum* 1999; 42(12): 2646–2655.

9. Tashkin DP, Elashoff R, Clements P, et al.: Cyclophosphamide versus placebo in scleroderma lung disease. *N Engl J Med* 2006; 354: 2655–2666.

10. Oddis CV, Conte CG, Steen VD, et al.: Incidence of polymyositis-dermatomyositis: a 20-year study of hospital diagnosed cases in Allegheny County, PA 1963–1982. *J Rheumatol* 1990, 17:1329–1334.

11. Sigurgeirsson B, Lindelof B, Edhag O, et al.: Risk of cancer in patients with dermatomyositis or polymyositis: a population-based study. *N Engl J Med* 1992, 326:363–367.

12. Khan MA, van der Linden SM: Ankylosing spondylitis and associated diseases. *Rheum Dis Clin North Am* 1990, 16:551–579.

13. Youinou P, Moutsopoulos HM, Pennec YL: Clinical features of Sjögren's syndrome. *Curr Opin Rheumatol* 1990, 2:687–693.

14. Hochberg MD: Updating the American College of Rheumatology revised criteria for the classification of systemic lupus erythematosus. *Arthritis Rheum* 1997, 40:1725.

15. Tan EM: The 1982 revised criteria for the classification of systemic lupus erythematosus. *Arthritis Rheum* 1982, 25:1271–1277.

16. Gross M, Esterley R, Earle RH: Pulmonary alterations in systemic lupus erythematosus. *Am Rev Respir Dis* 1972, 105:572–577.

17. Boulware DW, Hedgpeth MT: Lupus pneumonitis and anti-SSA(Ro) antibodies. *J Rheumatol* 1989, 16:479–481.

18. Badui E, Garcia-Rubi D, Robles E, et al.: Cardiovascular manifestations in systemic erythematosus: prospective study of 100 patients. *Angiology* 1985, 36:431–440.

19. Estes D, Christian CL: The natural history of systemic lupus erythematosus by prospective analysis. *Medicine* 1971, 50:85–95.

20. Bulgrin JG, Dubois EL, Jacobson G: Chest roentgenographic changes in systemic lupus erythematosus. *Radiology* 1960, 74:42–49.

21. Matthay RA, Schwartz MI, Petty TL, et al.: Pulmonary manifestations of systemic lupus erythematosus: review of twelve cases of acute lupus pneumonitis. *Medicine* 1975, 54:397–409.

22. Abud-Mendoza C, Diaz-Jouanen E, Alarcon-Segovia D: Fetal pulmonary hemorrhage in systemic lupus erythematosus: occurrence without hemoptysis. *J Rheumatol* 1985, 12:558–561.

23. Marino CT, Pertschuk LP: Pulmonary hemorrhage in systemic lupus erythematosus. *Arch Intern Med* 1981, 141:201–203.

24. Khare V, Baethge B, Lang S, et al.: Antinuclear antibodies in pleural fluid. *Chest* 1994, 106:866–871.

25. Arnett FC, Edworthy SM, Bloch DA, et al.: The American Rheumatism Association 1987 revised criteria for the classification of rheumatoid arthritis. *Arthritis Rheum* 1988, 31:315–324.

26. Jurik AG, Graudal H: Pleurisy in rheumatoid arthritis. *Scand J Rheumatol* 1983, 12:75–80.

27. Jurik AG, Davidsen D, Graudal H: Prevalence of pulmonary involvement in rheumatoid arthritis and its relationship to some characteristics of the patients: a radiological and clinical study. *Scand J Rheumatol* 1982, 11:217–224.

28. Schwarz MI: Pulmonary manifestations of the collagen vascular diseases. In *Fishman's Pulmonary Diseases and Disorders*, edn 3. Edited by Fishman AP, Elias JA, Fishman JA, et al. New York: McGraw-Hill; 1998:1115–1132.

29. Walker WC, Wright V: Pulmonary lesions and rheumatoid arthritis. *Medicine* 1968, 47:501–520.

30. Masi AT, Rodnan GP, Medsger TA Jr, et al.: Preliminary criteria for the classification of systemic sclerosis (scleroderma). *Arthritis Rheum* 1980, 23:581–590.

31. Medsger TA, Steen V: Systemic sclerosis and related syndromes: clinical features and treatment. In *Primer on the Rheumatic Diseases*, edn 10. Edited by Schumacher HR Jr, Klippel JH, Koopman WJ. Atlanta: Arthritis Foundation; 1993:120–127.

32. Wortmann RL: Inflammatory diseases of muscle. In *Textbook of Rheumatology*, edn 5. Edited by Kelley WN, Harris ED Jr, Ruddy S, Sledge CB. Philadelphia: WB Saunders; 1997:1177.

33. Bohan A, Peter JB: Polymyositis and dermatomyositis (first of two parts). *N Engl J Med* 1975, 292:344.

34. Bernstein RM, Morgan SH, Chapman J, et al.: Anti-Jo-1 antibody: a marker for myositis with interstitial lung disease. *BMJ* 1984, 289:151–152.

35. Schwarz MI, Matthay RA, Sahn SA, et al.: Interstitial lung disease in polymyositis-dermatomyositis: analysis of 6 cases and review of the literature. *Medicine* 1976, 55:89–104.

36. Tazelaar HD, Viggiano RW, Pickergill J, Colby TV: Interstitial lung disease in polymyositis and dermatomyositis: clinical features and prognosis as correlated with histologic findings. *Am Rev Respir Dis* 1990, 14:272.

37. Schwarz MI: Pulmonary and cardiac manifestations of polymyositis-dermatomyositis. *J Thorac Imaging* 1992, 7:46–54.

38. Dickey BF, Myers AR: Pulmonary disease in polymyositis-dermatomyositis. *Semin Arthritis Rheum* 1984, 14:60–76.

39. Boushea DK, Sundstrom WR: The pleuropulmonary manifestations of ankylosing spondylitis. *Semin Arthritis Rheum* 1989, 18:277–281.

40. Carette S, Graham DC, Little HA, et al.: The natural disease course of ankylosing spondylitis. *Arthritis Rheum* 1983, 26:186–190.

41. The Visual Aids Subcommittee of the Professional Education Committee of the Arthritis Foundation: Clinical Slide Collection of the Rheumatic Diseases. New York: The Arthritis Foundation; 1995.

42. Carroll GJ, Thomas R, Phatouros CC, et al.: Incidence, prevalence, and possible risk factors for pneumonitis in patients with rheumatoid arthritis receiving methotrexate. *J Rheumatol* 1994, 21:51–54.

43. Hargreaves MR, Mowat AG, Benson MK: Acute pneumonitis associated with low dose methotrexate treatment for rheumatoid arthritis: report of five cases and review of published reports. *Thorax* 1992, 47:628–633.

44. Froelich CJ, Wallman J, Skosey JL, Teodorescu M: Clinical value of an integrated ELISA system for the detection of 6 autoantibodies (ssDNA, dsDNA, Sm, RNP/Sm, SSA, and SSB). *J Rheumatol* 1990, 17:192–200.

45. Gross WL: Antineutrophil cytoplasmic autoantibody testing in vasculitides. In *Rheumatic Disease Clinics of North America—Vasculitis*, vol 21. Edited by Hunder GG. Philadelphia: WB Saunders; 1995:997.

PULMONARY VASCULITIS

Talmadge E. King Jr and Cyrus Shariat

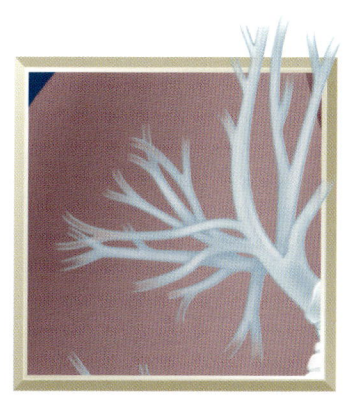
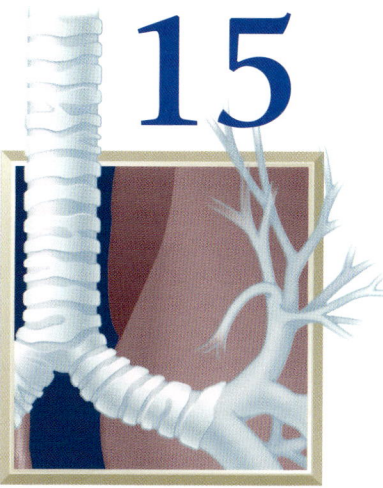
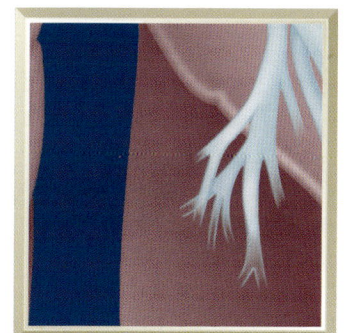

Vasculitis—the inflammation of the walls of arteries and/or veins—is found in many clinical settings. Often, the resulting syndromes are separated into primary and secondary forms [1]. The primary vasculitidies consist of a heterogeneous group of syndromes of unknown cause. Most are thought to be immune mediated and are often responsive to immunosuppressive therapy. Secondary vasculitis is caused by or associated with another well-defined underlying illness that usually precedes the diagnosis of the complicating vasculitis, eg, systemic lupus erythematosus. This chapter concentrates on the most common primary vasculitides affecting the lungs: Wegener's granulomatosis, microscopic polyangiitis, and Churg-Strauss syndrome.

Despite attempts to clarify the nomenclature, identification, and diagnosis of the primary vasculitidies, controversy remains and physicians still experience confusion in their efforts to manage patients with these illnesses [2–9]. Often the vasculitides are grouped according to the size of the affected vessel, the presence or absence of antineutrophil cytoplasmic antibodies (ANCA), the pathogenesis (immune complex–associated, antibody-associated, endothelium/cell–mediated), or the intensity of the inflammatory cell infiltrate of the artery wall (angiitis). In 1992 an international consensus conference developed a nomenclature that took into account many of these features—including the size of vessels involved and the association with ANCA titers—and acknowledged that the clinical presentation of vasculitis could change over time [10].

WEGENER'S GRANULOMATOSIS

Wegener's granulomatosis is a necrotizing granulomatous vasculitis with an age of onset of 30 to 50 years; it affects men and women equally [11]. A triad of involved tissue characterizes this disease: upper respiratory tract, lower respiratory tract, and kidney. Disease involvement in these sites represents the classic presentation; however, incomplete forms are common, making the diagnosis more difficult. A "limited" form, with clinical findings isolated to the upper respiratory tract or the lungs, occurs in approximately one fourth of cases. The key manifestations include nasal or oral inflammation (painful or painless oral ulcers or purulent or bloody nasal discharge); abnormal chest imaging showing nodules (which may cavitate), alveolar opacities, pleural opacities, or diffuse hazy opacities (which may reflect alveolar hemorrhage); and abnormal urinary sediment (microscopic hematuria with or without red cell casts). Skin lesions include palpable purpura, ulcers, vesicles, papules, and subcutaneous nodules. Nearly all patients with active systemic Wegener's granulomatosis test positive for antineutrophil cytoplasmic antibodies (range, 65% to >90%). However, it is advisable that a tissue biopsy be performed for confirmation of the diagnosis. Biopsy of a nasopharyngeal lesion (if present) is preferred because it is relatively noninvasive. If there is no lesion in the upper respiratory tract, the next step is biopsy of an affected organ such as the kidney or lung. Kidney biopsy is preferred because it is easier to perform and is more often diagnostic. Kidney biopsy typically reveals a segmental necrotizing glomerulonephritis with little or no immunoglobulin deposition (pauci-immune) on immunofluorescence or electron microscopy. In the lung, the typical histopathologic finding is vasculitis and granulomatous inflammation.

MICROSCOPIC POLYANGIITIS

Microscopic polyangiitis affects men somewhat more often than it does women (an imbalance of 1.5:1) and has an age of onset of 40 to 60 years [12]. The clinical characteristics of microscopic polyangiitis include kidney (rapidly progressive glomerulonephritis), skin, peripheral nerve, gastrointestinal, and lung involvement [13]. Alveolar hemorrhage is the most common (and most life-threatening) manifestation. This disorder is thought by some investigators to represent part of a clinical spectrum that includes Wegener's granulomatosis, because both are associated with the presence of antineutrophil cytoplasmic antibodies (ANCA) and similar histologic changes outside the respiratory tract [14,15]. In this case, granulomatous involvement of the respiratory tract and the presence of c-ANCA favor the diagnosis of Wegener's granulomatosis. A distinction is often made between microscopic polyangiitis and polyarteritis nodosa. Microscopic polyangiitis is a pauci-immune vasculitis affecting mostly small vessels, including glomerular capillaries (ie, glomerulonephritis), which is not seen with polyarteritis nodosa [10]. In addition, ANCA titers are found in more than 85% of patients with microscopic polyangiitis with a predominance of MPO-ANCA (p-ANCA), but their presence is rare in patients with polyarteritis nodosa [16–18]. There are also differences in the natural history of these diseases. Microscopic polyangiitis tends to relapse, but polyarteritis nodosa does not [16].

CHURG-STRAUSS SYNDROME

Churg-Strauss syndrome affects small to medium-sized arteries, has an age of onset of 15 to 75 years (mean, 38 y), and afflicts men twice as often as women [12,19]. This disease is characterized by three phases: 1) allergic rhinitis and/or asthma, 2) peripheral and tissue eosinophilia (infiltrative eosinophilia such as eosinophilic pneumonia or gastroenteritis), and 3) granulomatous vasculitis and angiitis. No laboratory tests are specific for Churg-Strauss syndrome. The patient's asthma often subsides as the vasculitis appears, and constitutional symptoms may herald the onset of systemic disease. The development of Churg-Strauss syndrome has been associated with the use of the leukotriene receptor antagonists: zafirlukast, montelukast, and pranlukast. Patients with asthma treated with these medications developed a Churg-Strauss-like syndrome as their physicians tapered their systemic corticosteroids [20]. Surveillance of postmarketing data and studies of patient cohorts have failed to provide compelling evidence for a causal relationship [1]. The diagnosis of Churg-Strauss syndrome is suggested by clinical findings and then confirmed by lung biopsy or by biopsy of other clinically affected tissues.

MANAGEMENT OF VASCULITIS

Aggressive immunosuppressive therapy remains the mainstay of treatment for the vasculitides. The use of such aggressive immunotherapy is justified because survival in untreated generalized vasculitis is extremely poor, with up to 90% of patients with Wegener's granulomatosis dying within 2 years, usually of respiratory or renal failure. Despite the improved survival among treated patients with a systemic vasculitis, unfortunately, there remains a significantly higher death rate among patients with systemic vasculitis compared to the general population [16], and treatment-related complications have a major negative impact on these patients' quality of life.

Treatment goals are focused on reducing disease-related morbidity and minimizing treatment-related complications. The severity of disease dictates the intensity and choice of the initial treatment [1,21]. An initial remission-induction phase is followed by a maintenance phase during which less intensive therapy is used. The transition to maintenance therapy should be made when clinical remission occurs, which is generally within 3 to 6 months after the onset of therapy [22]. It is important to closely monitor the patient on therapy to identify disease flare, infection, or drug toxicity, all of which can present with nonspecific signs and symptoms. Clinical trials currently under way will address specific treatment-related issues including the potential benefits of daily oral cyclophosphamide over pulsed intravenous dosing, the ideal duration of maintenance therapy, and the efficacy of novel investigational agents.

Red Flags of Vasculitis

- Fever of unknown origin
- Unexplained multisystem disease
- Unexplained inflammatory arthritis
- Unexplained myositis
- Unexplained glomerulonephritis
- Unexplained cardiac/gastrointestinal/central nervous system ischemia
- Mononeuritis multiplex
- Suspicious rash:
  - Palpable purpura
  - Maculopapular
  - Nodules
  - Ulcers
  - Livedo reticularis

Figure 15-1. Red flags of vasculitis. (*Adapted from* Calabrese [23].)

Necrotizing Vasculitides Grouped According to Affected Vessel Size/Vasculitis

	Vasculitic lung involvement	ANCA findings	Estimated annual incidence*	5-year survival, %**
Large				
Giant cell arteritis	Rare	No	13	> 90
Takayasu arteritis	Frequent	No	2.6	> 90
Medium				
Polyarteritis nodosa	Rare	Rare	9	80
Small				
Wegener's granulomatosis	Frequent	PR3-ANCA	8.5–10.3	75
Microscopic polyangiitis	Frequent	MPO-ANCA or PR3-ANCA	6.8–8.9	74
Churg-Strauss syndrome	Frequent	MPO-ANCA or PR3-ANCA	1.5–3.7	75

*Data on incidence per million adult population adapted from Specks [1].
**The prognosis for patients diagnosed with vasculitis has dramatically improved since the advent of glucocorticoids, and the inclusion of cyclophosphamide has further improved patient survival [1,14,15,17,23–28].

Figure 15-2. Necrotizing vasculitides grouped according to affected vessel size following the nomenclature recommended by the 1992 Chapel Hill International Consensus Conference [10]. The vasculitides are defined by the presence of leukocytes in the vessel wall with reactive damage to mural structures, leading to tissue ischemia and necrosis [14]. The exact mechanisms underlying these disorders are unclear. ANCA—antineutrophil cytoplasmic antibodies; MPO—myeloperoxidase; PR3—proteinase 3.

Distinguishing Features of Necrotizing Vasculitis

	Patients, %		
	Wegener's granulomatosis	Microscopic polyangiitis	Churg-Strauss syndrome
System			
Cutaneous	40	40	60
Renal	80	90	45
Pulmonary	90	50	70
Ear/nose/throat	90	35	50
Musculoskeletal	60	60	50
Neurologic	50	30	70
Gastrointestinal	50	50	50
ANCA	90*	90**	70**
Asthma and eosinophilia	—	—	Diagnostic
Granuloma formation	100	0	100

*Most patients have cytoplasmic ANCA antibody against proteinase 3
**Most patients have perinuclear ANCA antibody against myeloperoxidase

Figure 15-3. Distinguishing features of necrotizing vasculitis. ANCA—antineutrophil cytoplasmic antibodies. (*Adapted from* Jennette and Falk [29].)

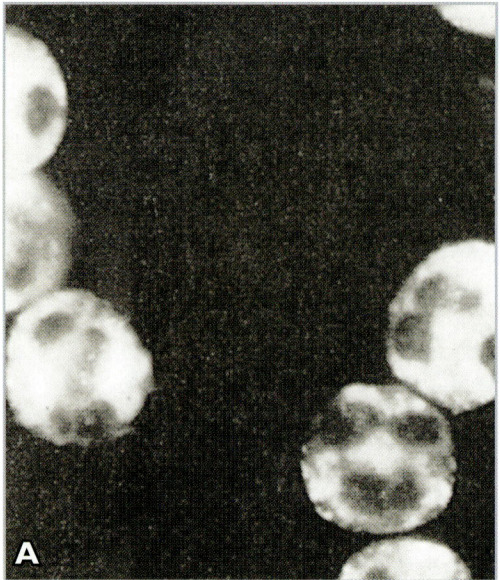
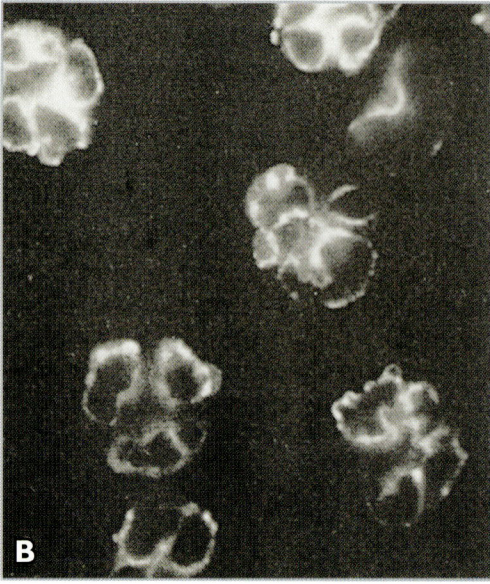

Figure 15-4. Fluorescence patterns of antineutrophil cytoplasmic antibodies. **A,** Cytoplasmic antineutrophil cytoplasmic antibodies (c-ANCA) causes a cytoplasmic fluorescence. More than 90% of c-ANCA is directed against the neutrophil alpha granule enzyme proteinase [3]. It is known that c-ANCA is associated strongly with Wegener's granulomatosis. **B,** Perinuclear ANCA (p-ANCA) causes a perinuclear fluorescence. More than 70% of p-ANCA is directed against the neutrophil alpha granule enzyme myeloperoxidase. Other p-ANCA antigens include cathepsin G, human leukocyte elastase, and lactoferrin. (*From* Gross [30]; with permission.)

Clinical Manifestatinos of Wegener's Granulomatosis

System	Manifestation
Pulmonary	70%–90% of patients (dyspnea, cough, hemoptysis, chest pain)
Ear/nose/throat	90% of patients experience epistaxis, nasal ulcers, sinusitis, oropharyngeal pain/ulcers, otitis media (which can injure facial nerve), or hearing impairment
Renal	Glomerulonephritis is found in 20% of patients at presentation; however, 80% of patients eventually develop renal abnormalities of proteinuria, hematuria, erythrocyte casts, or renal insufficiency; hypertension is uncommon
Musculoskeletal	60% of patients experience arthralgias, mild nondestructive arthritis, or myalgias
Ocular	50% of patients; orbital involvement frequently occurs secondary to extension from sinusitis; proptosis, conjunctivitis, scleritis, episcleritis, uveitis, and ophthalmoplegia can occur
Nervous	50% of patients develop peripheral neuropathy with or without mononeuritis multiplex (30%), cranial neuropathy, headaches, seizures, cerebritis, or cerebrovascular accident symptoms
Gastrointestinal	50% of patients develop vasculitis, which causes abdominal pain, distention, hematemesis, or melena
Cutaneous	40% of patients develop subcutaneous nodules, purpura, or skin infarction (lower > upper extremities)
Cardiac	Uncommon, but dysrhythmias, pericarditis, and coronary arteritis have been observed
Constitutional	15%–45% experience fever, weight loss, malaise

Figure 15-5. Clinical manifestations of Wegener's granulomatosis. The manifestation of specific organ involvement represents the overall frequency throughout the course of illness. In addition, most patients develop constitutional signs or symptoms, including fatigue, weight loss, and low-grade fever. (*Adapted from* Jennette and Falk [29]; Hoffman *et al.* [11].)

Pulmonary and Airway Manifestations of Wegener's Granulomatosis

Upper airway

Tracheobronchial lesions (subglottic stenosis, bronchial stenosis, endobronchial lesions)—5% of adults, 50% of children
Nasal/palatal ulcerations with or without destruction
Destructive sinusitis
Saddle nose deformity

Lower airway

Unilateral or bilateral nodules with or without cavitation—60%
Interstitial opacities—65%
Pleuritis with or without effusions—28%
Alveolar capillaritis resulting in diffuse alveolar hemorrhage (less fixed and more irregular opacities)—8%

Figure 15-6. Pulmonary and airway manifestations of Wegener's granulomatosis [11,31].

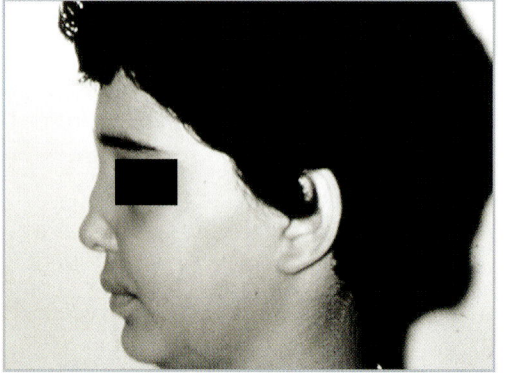

Figure 15-7. Saddle nose deformity in a patient with Wegener's granulomatosis. Saddle nose deformity, which eroded nasal cartilage in this patient, can also occur in relapsing polychondritis, sarcoidosis, and congenital syphilis. (*From* the Visual Aids Subcommittee of the Professional Education Committee of the Arthritis Foundation [32]; with permission.)

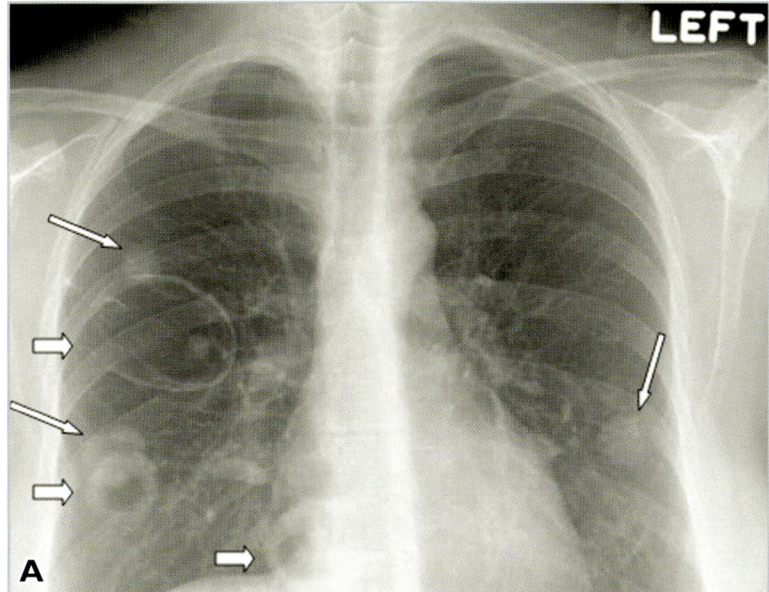
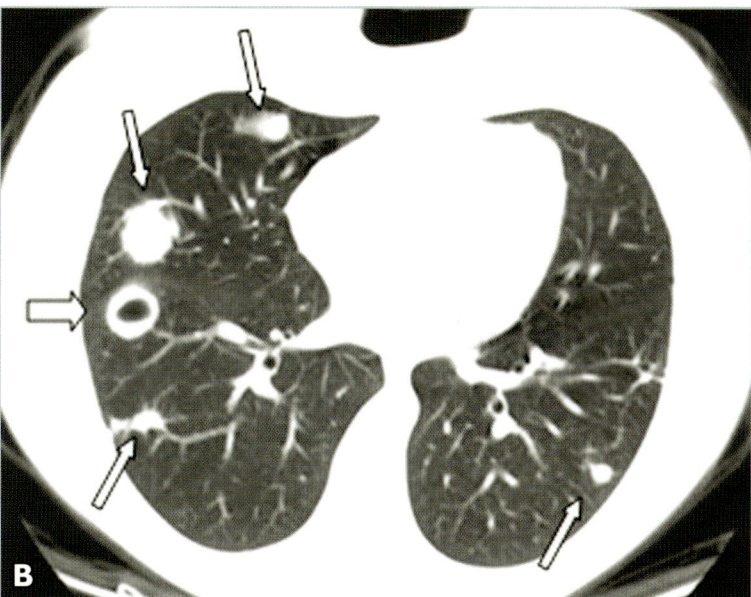

Figure 15-8. Wegener's granulomatosis. **A,** Posteroanterior chest radiograph reveals multiple well-defined nodules (*long, narrow arrows*), some of which have cavitated (*broad arrows*).

B, Lung window CT shows multiple lesions, from defined nodules (*long, narrow arrows*) to cavitary nodules (*broad arrow*). (**A** and **B** *courtesy of* WR Webb, MD.)

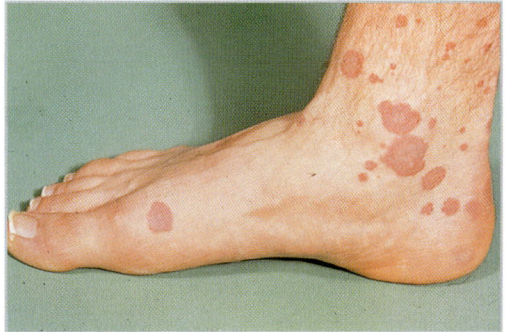

Figure 15-9. Wegener's granulomatosis. Cutaneous vasculitis manifesting as palpable purpura. (*Courtesy of* D. Hogan, MD.)

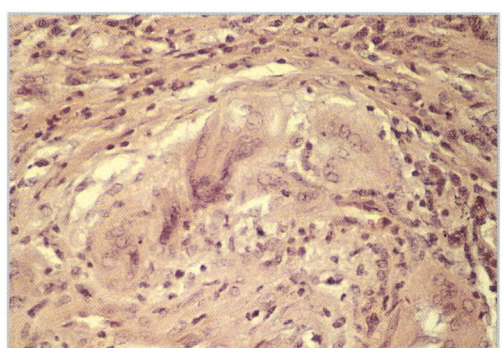

Figure 15-10. Lung biopsy specimen from a patient with Wegener's granulomatosis demonstrating multiple granulomas with central necrosis and multinucleated giant cells. (*Courtesy of* F. Abreo, MD.)

Clinical Manifestations of Microscopic Polyangiitis

System	Manifestation
Constitutional	70%–80% of patients develop fever, chills, weight loss
Renal	90%–100% of patients develop rapidly progressive glomerulonephritis
Musculoskeletal	70% of patients experience myalgias, arthralgias, and a nondeforming arthritis
Pulmonary	25%–50% of patients develop pulmonary manifestations
Gastrointestinal	50% of patients develop vasculitis manifested as abdominal pain
Cutaneous	50% of patients manifest as palpable purpura
Nervous	30% of patients have involvement of the nervous system primarily as peripheral neuropathy
Cardiac	15% of patients develop pericarditis or coronary arteritis

Figure 15-11. Clinical manifestations of microscopic polyangiitis. Most patients develop constitutional symptoms, including fatigue, weight loss, and low-grade fever. (*Adapted from* Guillevin *et al.*[13]; Lhote *et al.*[12] and [33].)

Pulmonary Manifestations of Microscopic Polyangiitis

Manifestation	Incidence
Diffuse alveolar hemorrhage	11%–30% of patients develop hemorrhage manifesting as hemoptysis or rapid anemia
Pleurisy (with or without effusion)	6%–15%
Pneumonitis	11%

Figure 15-12. Pulmonary manifestations of microscopic polyangiitis [13,15].

| *Pulmonary Vasculitis* |

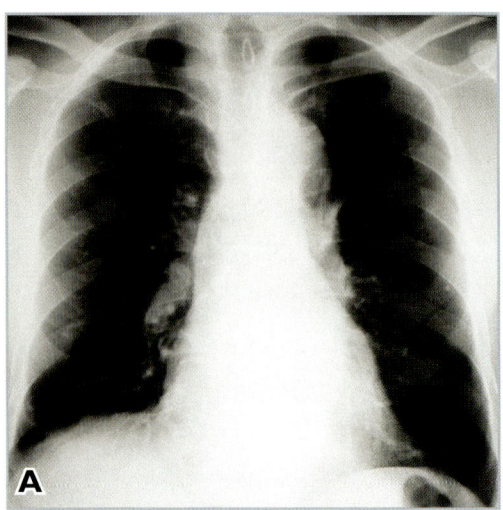 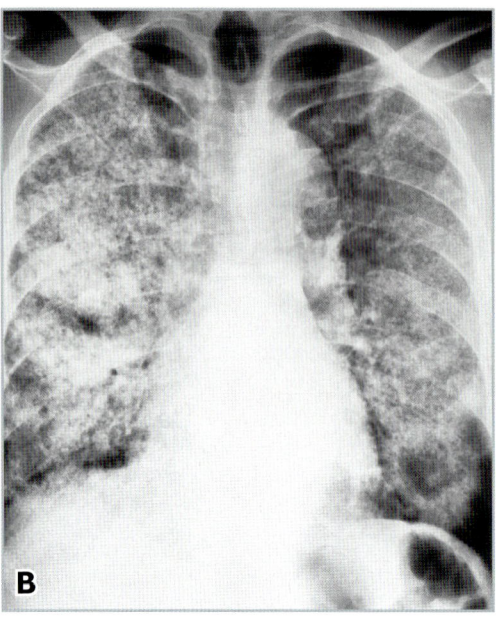

Figure 15-13. Microscopic polyangiitis. **A,** Erect posteroanterior chest radiograph of a 62-year-old man. **B,** Erect posteroanterior radiograph from the same patient 1 month later. The patient developed diffuse pulmonary hemorrhage manifesting as airspace consolidation, sparing only the apices and costophrenic angles.

Clinical Manifestations of Churg-Strauss Syndrome

System	Manifestation
Constitutional	70%–80% have fever, chills, weight loss
Pulmonary	100% of patients have asthma; 70% of patients may have interstitital opacities, nodular lesions, or pleural disease on chest imaging studies
Paranasal sinusitis	61% of patients
Nervous	70% of patients have peripheral nervous system manifestations (mononeuritis multiplex or polyneuropathy)
Cutaneous	60% of patients develop subcutaneous nodules, petechia, purpura, skin infarction
Cardiac	14%–50% of patients develop coronary arteritis; congestive heart failure; peri-, myo-, endocarditis
Gastrointestinal	33%–50% of patients develop vasculitis, which causes abdominal pain, diarrhea, distention, hematemesis, or melena
Musculoskeletal	50% of patients experience arthralgia or nondestructive arthritis
Renal	26%–45% of patients develop glomerulonephritis; however, renal failure and nephrotic syndrome are infrequent
Prostate and lower genitourinary tract	Eosinophilic granulomatosis is unique to Churg-Strauss syndrome

Figure 15-14. Clinical manifestations of Churg-Strauss syndrome. Most patients develop constitutional symptoms, including fatigue, weight loss, and low-grade fever. (*Adapted from* Jennette and Falk [29]; Chumbley *et al.*[34]; Lanham *et al.*[35]; Guillevin *et al.*[36]; Brown [1].)

Classification Criteria for Churg-Strauss Syndrome

- Asthma
- Eosinophilia > 10% leukocytes
- Mononeuropathy or polyneuropathy
- Transitory pulmonary opacities
- Paranasal sinus abnormality
- Biopsy specimen showing extravascular eosinophils

Figure 15-15. Classification criteria for Churg-Strauss syndrome. The patient must have four of the six criteria to meet the classification requirements [5].

Pulmonary Manifestations of Churg-Strauss Syndrome

Upper airway
  Sinusitis
  Nasal inflammation/polyps
Lower airway—chest radiographs are abnormal in 40% of patients and show
  Patchy, shifting interstitial opacities
  Massive bilateral nodular opacities without cavitation
  Diffuse interstitial disease (suggesting eosinophilic pneumonia)
  Pleural effusions
Thin-section CT
  Bilateral, multifocal peripheral air-space opacifications that may be consolidative or ground-glass are located predominantly at the lung bases
  Centrilobular nodules (frequently observed within areas of ground-glass opacification)
  Areas of ground-glass opacity in the periphery of larger nodules, or lobular consolidations
  Bronchial wall thickening
  Increased vessel caliber

Figure 15-16. Pulmonary manifestations of Churg-Strauss syndrome [5,12,35]. (*Adapted from* Marten *et al.*[37]; Choi *et al.*[38].)

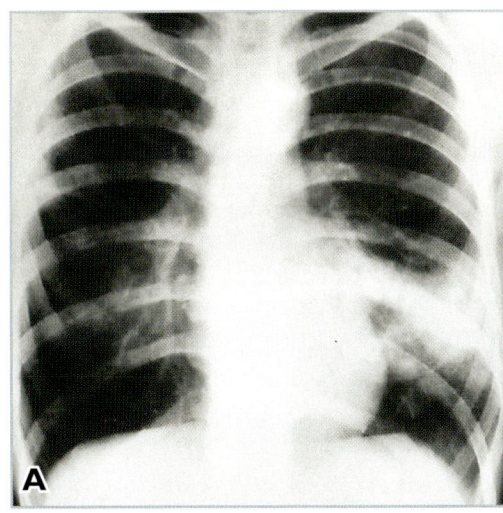 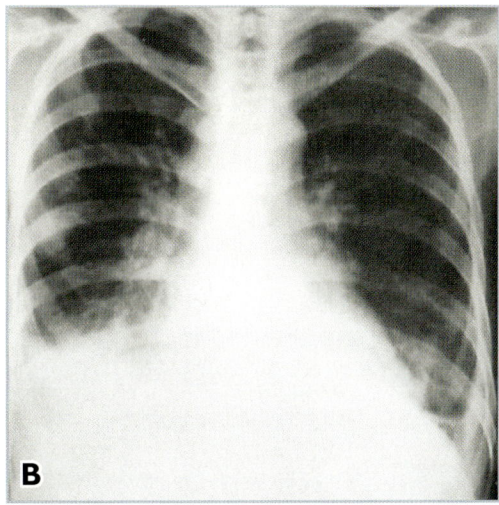 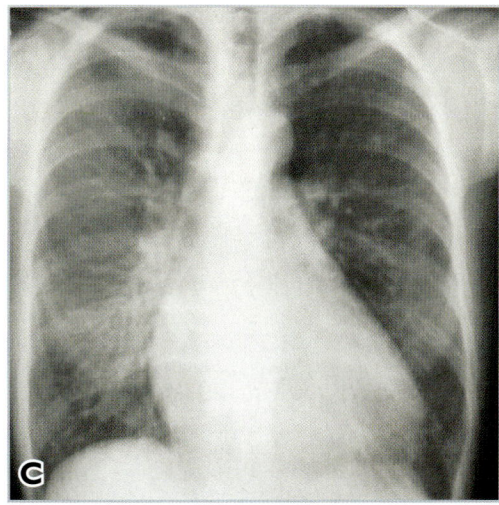

Figure 15-17. Churg-Strauss syndrome. A 28-year-old woman with asthma had peripheral eosinophilia (10.3×10^9/L) and original right upper lung consolidation. **A,** Chest radiograph showing left lower lung zone consolidation. **B,** Chest radiograph 6 months later showing that the patient developed bilateral pleural effusions. **C,** Chest radiograph from the same patient 1 year later revealing the development of cardiomyopathy. (*From* Wilson [39]; with permission.)

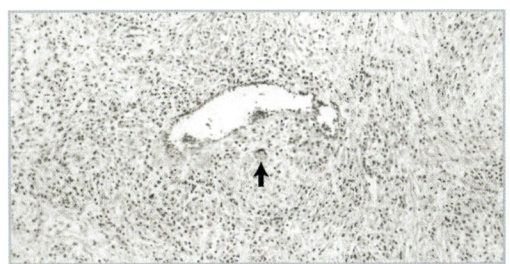

Figure 15-18. Lung biopsy specimen from a patient with Churg-Strauss syndrome showing mixed inflammatory cell infiltrate with numerous eosinophils. A small pulmonary vessel is focally necrotic and is being destroyed by this process. Note the multinucleated giant cell in the wall of the vessel (*arrow*). (*From* Winterbauer [40]; with permission.)

European Vasculitis Study Group Grading of Disease Severity and First-line Treatment Options for Induction Therapy

Disease classification	Constitutional symptoms	Renal function	Threatened organ function	Treatment options for induction	Level of evidence
Limited	No	Serum creatinine < 120 µmol/L (1.4 mg/dL)	No	Corticosteroids OR methotrexate OR azathioprine	Expert opinion
Early, generalized	Yes	Serum creatinine < 120 µmol/L (1.4 mg/dL)	No	Cyclophosphamide + corticosteroids OR methotrexate + corticosteroids	Randomized prospective trials
Active, generalized	Yes	Serum creatinine < 500 µmol/L (5.7 mg/dL)	Yes	Cyclophosphamide + corticosteroids	Expert opinion; nonrandomized prospective trials
Severe	Yes	Serum creatinine > 500 µmol/L (5.7 mg/dL) or receiving dialysis	Yes	Cyclophosphamide + corticosteroids + plasma exchange	Randomized prospective trials
Refractory	Yes	Any	Yes	Consider investigational or compassionate use agents	Expert opinion; nonrandomized prospective trials

Figure 15-19. European Vasculitis Study Group Grading of Disease Severity and First-line Treatment Options for Induction Therapy. The European Vasculitis Study Group has devised a clinically useful grading system in which the patient's disease is categorized as 1) limited (localized disease of the upper airways with no systemic symptoms, end-organ function is not threatened, no renal involvement); 2) early, generalized; 3) active, generalized; 4) severe (presence of severe renal involvement [creatinine concentration, diffuse alveolar hemorrhage, or other life-threatening disease]); and 5) refractory (patients who have not responded to cytotoxic agents, high-dose corticosteroids, or plasma exchange). (*Adapted from* Brown [1]; Frankel *et al.* [21]; European Community Study Group [41]; Jayne [42].)

REFERENCES

1. Brown KK: Pulmonary vasculitis. *Proc Am Thorac Soc* 2006, 3:48–57.

2. Leavitt RY, Fauci AS, Bloch DA, *et al*.: The American College of Rheumatology 1990 criteria for the classification of Wegener's granulomatosis. *Arthritis Rheum* 1990, 33:1101–1107.

3. Calabrese LH, Michel BA, Bloch DA, *et al*.: The American College of Rheumatology 1990 criteria for the classification of hypersensitivity vasculitis. *Arthritis Rheum* 1990, 33:1108–1113.

4. Hunder GG, Bloch DA, Michel BA, *et al*.: The American College of Rheumatology 1990 criteria for the classification of giant cell arteritis. *Arthritis Rheum* 1990, 33:1122–1128.

5. Masi AT, Hunder GG, Lie JT, *et al*.: The American College of Rheumatology 1990 criteria for the classification of Churg-Strauss syndrome (allergic granulomatosis and angiitis). *Arthritis Rheum* 1990, 33:1094–1100.

6. Arend WP, Michel BA, Bloch DA, *et al*.: The American College of Rheumatology 1990 criteria for the classification of Takayasu arteritis. *Arthritis Rheum* 1990, 33:1129–1134.

7. Mills JA, Michel BA, Bloch DA, *et al*.: The American College of Rheumatology 1990 criteria for the classification of Henoch-Schonlein purpura. *Arthritis Rheum* 1990, 33:1114–1121.

8. Bruce IN, Bell AL: A comparison of two nomenclature systems for primary systemic vasculitis. *Br J Rheumatol* 1997, 36:453–458.

9. Sorensen SF, Slot O, Tvede N, Petersen J: A prospective study of vasculitis patients collected in a five year period: evaluation of the Chapel Hill nomenclature. *Ann Rheum Dis* 2000, 59:478–482.

10. Jennette J, Falk R, Andrassy K, *et al*.: Nomenclature of systemic vasculitides: proposal of an international consensus conference. *Arthritis Rheum* 1994, 37:187–192.

11. Hoffman GS, Kerr GS, Leavitt RY, *et al*.: Wegener granulomatosis: an analysis of 158 patients. *Ann Intern Med* 1992, 116:488–498.

12. Lhote F, Guillevin L: Polyarteritis nodosa, microscopic polyangiitis, and Churg-Strauss syndrome: clinical aspects and treatment. *Rheum Dis Clin North Am* 1995, 21:911–947.

13. Guillevin L, Durand-Gasselin B, Cevallos R, *et al*.: Microscopic polyangiitis: clinical and laboratory findings in eighty-five patients. *Arthritis Rheum* 1999, 42:421–430.

14. Hunder GG: Classification of and approach to the vasculitides in adults. In *UpToDate*. Edited by Rose BD. Wellesley, MA: UpToDate; 2008.

15. Savage COS, Winearls CG, Evans DJ, *et al*.: Microscopic polyarteritis: presentation, pathology and prognosis. *Q J Med* 1985, 56:467–483.

16. Gayraud M, Guillevin L, le Toumelin P, *et al*.: Long-term followup of polyarteritis nodosa, microscopic polyangiitis, and Churg-Strauss syndrome: analysis of four prospective trials including 278 patients. *Arthritis Rheum* 2001, 44:666–675.

17. Specks U: Pulmonary vasculitis. In *Interstitial Lung Diseases*, edn 4. Edited by Schwarz MI, King TE, Jr. Hamilton, Ontario, Canada: BC Decker, Inc.; 2003:599–631.

18. Guillevin L, Visser H, Noel LH, *et al*.: Antineutrophil cytoplasm antibodies in systemic polyarteritis nodosa with and without hepatitis B virus infection and Churg-Strauss syndrome—62 patients. *J Rheumatol* 1993, 20:1345–1349.

19. King TE Jr: Churg-Strauss syndrome (allergic granulomatosis and angiitis). In *UpToDate*. Edited by Rose BD. Wellesley, MA: UpToDate; 2008.

20. Wechsler ME, Pauwels R, Drazen JM: Leukotriene modifiers and Churg-Strauss syndrome: adverse effect or response to corticosteroid withdrawal? *Drug Saf* 1999, 21:241–251.

21. Frankel SK, Cosgrove GP, Fischer A, *et al*.: Update in the diagnosis and management of pulmonary vasculitis. *Chest* 2006, 129:452–465.

22. Stone JH, Kaplan AA, Rose BD: Initial and maintenance therapy of Wegener's granulomatosis and microscopic polyangiitis. In *UpToDate*. Edited by Rose BD. Wellesley, MA: UpToDate; 2008.

23. Calabrese LH: Vasculitis. In *New York Rheumatism Association—Rheumatology Board Review Course;* New York: September 27, 1996.

24. Fauci AS, Katz P, Haynes BF, Wolff SM: Cyclophosphamide therapy of severe systemic necrotizing vasculitis. *N Engl J Med* 1979, 301:235–238.

25. Guillevin L, Guittard T, Bletry O, *et al*.: Systemic necrotizing angiitis with asthma: causes and precipitating factors in 43 cases. *Lung* 1987, 165:165–172.

26. Hall S, Barr W, Lie JT, *et al*.: Takayasu arteritis: a study of 32 North American patients. *Medicine* (Baltimore) 1985, 64:89–99.

27. Nordborg E, Nordborg C, Malmvall BE, *et al*.: Giant cell arteritis. *Rheum Dis Clin North Am* 1995, 21:1013–1026.

28. Kerr GS: Takayasu's arteritis. *Rheum Dis Clin North Am* 1995, 21:1041–1058.

29. Jennette JC, Falk RJ: Small-vessel vasculitis. *N Engl J Med* 1997, 337:1512–1523.

30. Gross WL: Antineutrophil cytoplasmic autoantibody testing in vasculitides. *Rheum Dis Clin North Am* 1995, 21987–1011.

31. Duna GF, Galperin C, Hoffman GS: Wegener's granulomatosis. *Rheum Dis Clin North Am* 1995, 21:949–986.

32. The Visual Aids Subcommittee of the Professional Education Committee of the Arthritis Foundation: *Clinical Slide Collection of the Rheumatic Diseases*. New York: The Arthritis Foundation; 1995.

33. Alberts WM: Pulmonary manifestations of the Churg-Strauss syndrome and related idiopathic small vessel vasculitis syndromes. *Curr Opin Pulm Med* 2007, 13:445–450.

34. Chumbley LC, Harrison EG Jr, DeRemee RA: Allergic granulomatosis and angiitis (Churg-Strauss syndrome): report and analysis of 30 cases. *Mayo Clin Proc* 1977, 52:477–484.

35. Lanham JG, Elkon KB, Pusey CD, Hughes GR: Systemic vasculitis with asthma and eosinophilia: a clinical approach to the Churg-Strauss syndrome. *Medicine* (Baltimore) 1984, 63:65–81.

36. Guillevin L, Cohen P, Gayraud M, *et al*.: Churg-Strauss syndrome: clinical study and long-term follow-up of 96 patients. *Medicine* (Baltimore) 1999, 78:26–37.

37. Marten K, Schnyder P, Schirg E, *et al*.: Pattern-based differential diagnosis in pulmonary vasculitis using volumetric CT. *Am J Roentgenol* 2005, 720–733.

38. Choi YH, Im JG, Han BK, *et al*. Thoracic manifestation of Churg-Strauss syndrome: radiologic and clinical findings. *Chest* 2000, 117:117–124.

39. Wilson AG: Immunologic diseases of the lungs. In *Imaging of Diseases of the Chest*, edn 2. Edited by Armstrong P, Wilson AG, Dee P, Hansell DM. St. Louis: Mosby; 1995:485–567.

40. Winterbauer RH: Wegener's granulomatosis and other pulmonary granulomatosis vasculitides. In *Pulmonary and Critical Care Medicine*. Edited by Bone RC. St. Louis: Mosby; 1993:1–13.

41. European Community Study Group on Clinical Trials in Systemic Vasculitis (ECSYSVASTRIAL): European therapeutic trials in ANCA-associated systemic vasculitis: disease scoring, consensus regimens and proposed clinical trials. *Clin Exp Immunol* 1995, 101(Suppl 1):29–34.

42. Jayne D: Evidence-based treatment of systemic vasculitis. *Rheumatology* (Oxford, England) 2000, 39:585–595.

HYPERSENSITIVITY PNEUMONITIS

Harold R. Collard and Marvin I. Schwarz

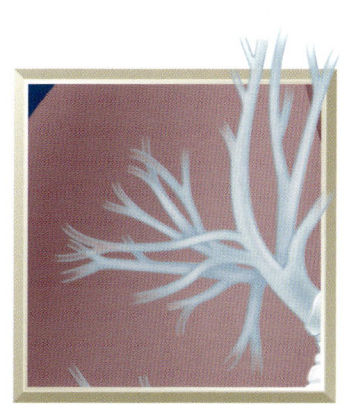
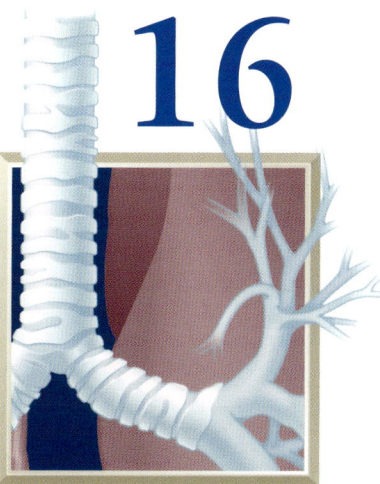
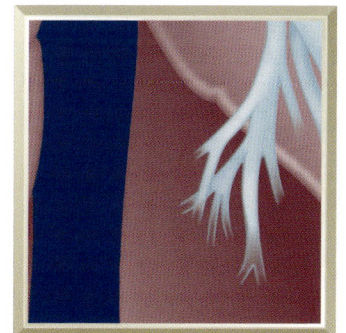

Hypersensitivity pneumonitis (also called extrinsic allergic alveolitis) is an important cause of diffuse parenchymal lung disease characterized by varying degrees of inflammation and fibrosis in the lung. Hypersensitivity pneumonitis is caused by exposure of susceptible individuals to any one of dozens of known organic antigens that initiate inflammation in the distal airways. This process may be abrupt and self-limited (acute hypersensitivity pneumonitis) or more indolent and progressive (chronic hypersensitivity pneumonitis). If it goes unrecognized, hypersensitivity pneumonitis may progress to end-stage lung disease with significant morbidity and mortality.

The cornerstone of treatment of hypersensitivity pneumonitis is removal from or avoidance of the initiating antigen. Critical to the accurate diagnosis and management of suspected hypersensitivity pneumonitis are a high index of suspicion; careful investigation of the occupational, avocational, and home environment; and high-resolution CT scanning of the chest.

Because no single test confirms the diagnosis, hypersensitivity pneumonitis should remain in the differential diagnosis of all patients presenting with signs or symptoms of diffuse parenchymal lung disease until an alternative diagnosis is established.

Typical Features of Hypersensitivity Pneumonitis

1. History of exposure to an antigen known or suspected to cause hypersensitivity pneumonitis
2. Presence of antibodies in the serum (serum precipitins) and/or bronchoalveolar lavage fluid directed against the suspected offending agent
3. History of dyspnea and cough, often exacerbated by exposure to a specific agent or environment
4. Improvement in symptoms on avoidance of the suspected environment
5. Inspiratory crackles on chest examination
6. Reticulonodular changes on chest radiography; centrilobular nodules, ground glass opacities, mosaic perfusion, and air trapping on high-resolution CT of the chest
7. Bronchoalveolar lavage fluid lymphocytosis
8. Predominantly interstitial and bronchiolocentric lymphoplasmacytic inflammation, organization, granulomas, and giant cell formation with or without fibrosis on lung biopsy

Figure 16-1. Typical features of hypersensitivity pneumonitis. Hypersensitivity pneumonitis may be acute, subacute, or chronic. Although diagnostic criteria have been suggested, there are no pathognomonic clinical or radiographic features of this condition [1]. Diagnosis requires a high index of suspicion and, most importantly, an exhaustive search for exposure to a potential etiologic agent, most typically in the home or workplace. Confirmation of exposure by the identification of serum or bronchoalveolar lavage antibody is useful if present, but if absent has a poor negative predictive value for disease. In the setting of an appropriate exposure, the presence of breathlessness; cough; inspiratory crackles on chest examination; micronodules and reticular changes on chest radiography; centrilobular nodules, ground glass opacities, mosaic perfusion, and air trapping on a high-resolution CT of the chest; and a lymphocytic bronchoalveolar lavage strongly suggest the diagnosis [1,2].

Selected Causes of Hypersensitivity Pneumonitis

Disease	Exposure
Fungus/bacteria/amebae	
Farmer's lung	Hay, grain (mold)
Bagassosis	Sugarcane (mold)
Suberosis	Cork (mold)
Humidifier/air conditioner lung	Forced-air systems, water reservoirs
Hot tub lung	Hot tub mist, ceiling mold
Detergent lung	Detergents
Mushroom worker's lung	Mushroom compost (mold)
Sequoiosis	Wood dust (mold)
Woodworker's/wood trimmer's lung	Wood dust and trimmings
Maple bark stripper's lung	Maple bark (mold)
Composter's lung	Compost
Malt worker's lung	Barley (mold)
Paprika slicer's lung	Paprika pods (fungus)
Wine maker's lung	Grapes (mold)
Cheese washer's lung	Cheese (mold)
Summer-type pneumonitis	Old homes
Familial hypersensitivity pneumonitis	Wood dust in building walls
Animal/insect	
Bird fancier's disease	Parakeets, pigeons, chickens, turkeys
Duvet lung	Bird feather–filled bedding, pillows, clothes
Animal handler's lung	Rats, gerbils
Fish meal worker's lung	Fish meal dust
Furrier's lung	Animal pelts
Miller's lung	Insect-contaminated grain
Chemical	
Sodium diazobenzene sulfate	Pauli's reagent (laboratory reagent)
Isocyanates/trimellitic anhydride	Spray paints, polyurethane foam, glue
Copper sulfate (vineyard sprayer's lung)	Bordeaux mixture
Pyrethrum	Pesticide
Phthalic anhydride	Heated epoxy resin
Unknown	
Bible printer's lung	Unknown
Mummy handler's (Coptic) lung	Unknown
Coffee worker's lung	Dried leaves?
Tobacco grower's lung	Dried leaves?
Tea grower's lung	Dried leaves?
Grain measurer's lung	Unknown
Mollusk shell hypersensitivity pneumonitis	Ground-up shells (for industrial purposes)?

Figure 16-2. Selected causes of hypersensitivity pneumonitis. There are many known antigens capable of inducing hypersensitivity pneumonitis, and doubtless many more that remain to be identified. The most common organic antigens are of fungal, bacterial, or animal origin. There are several inorganic chemicals, as well as other occupational exposures, that cause this disease. (*Adapted from* Selman [2].)

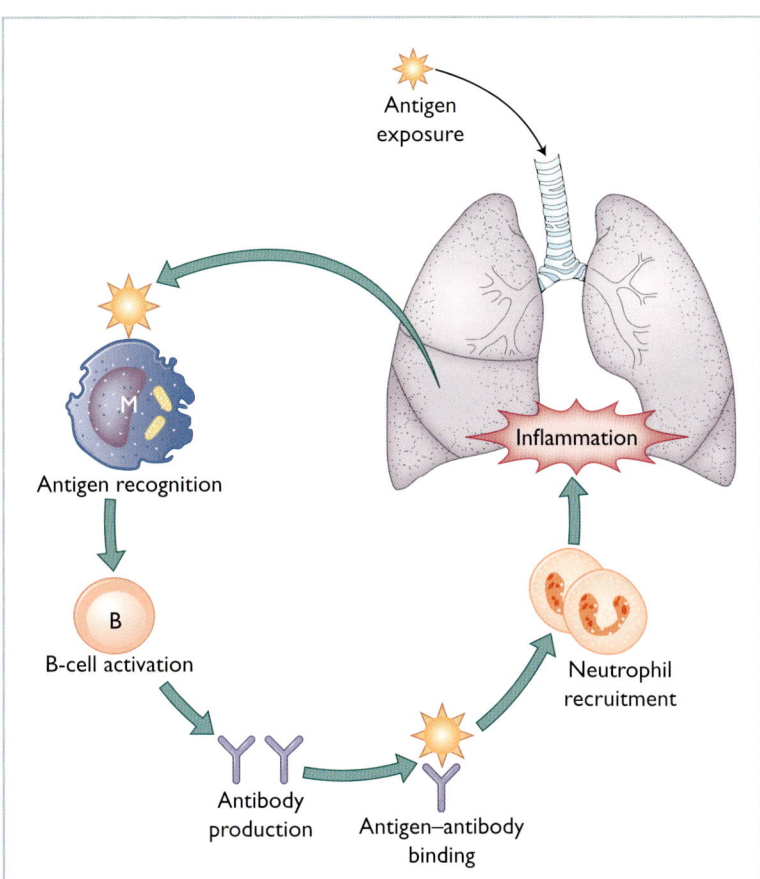

Figure 16-3. Pathophysiologic schema for acute hypersensitivity pneumonitis. Acute hypersensitivity pneumonitis is thought to represent a primarily humoral immune response to an inhaled antigen (to be distinguished from the cellular immune response of the more chronic forms) [2–4]. An inhaled antigen is recognized by antigen-presenting cells such as the alveolar macrophage (M) and presented to B cells (B). This results in B-cell activation, clonal proliferation, and antibody production. Antigen–antibody immune complexes result in complement activation, recruitment of neutrophils, and generation of reactive oxygen species that result in acute inflammation. Equal antigen exposure to potential causative agents does not result in disease in all individuals. It is likely that a genetic variation in individuals' antigen processing is important to disease pathogenesis [5].

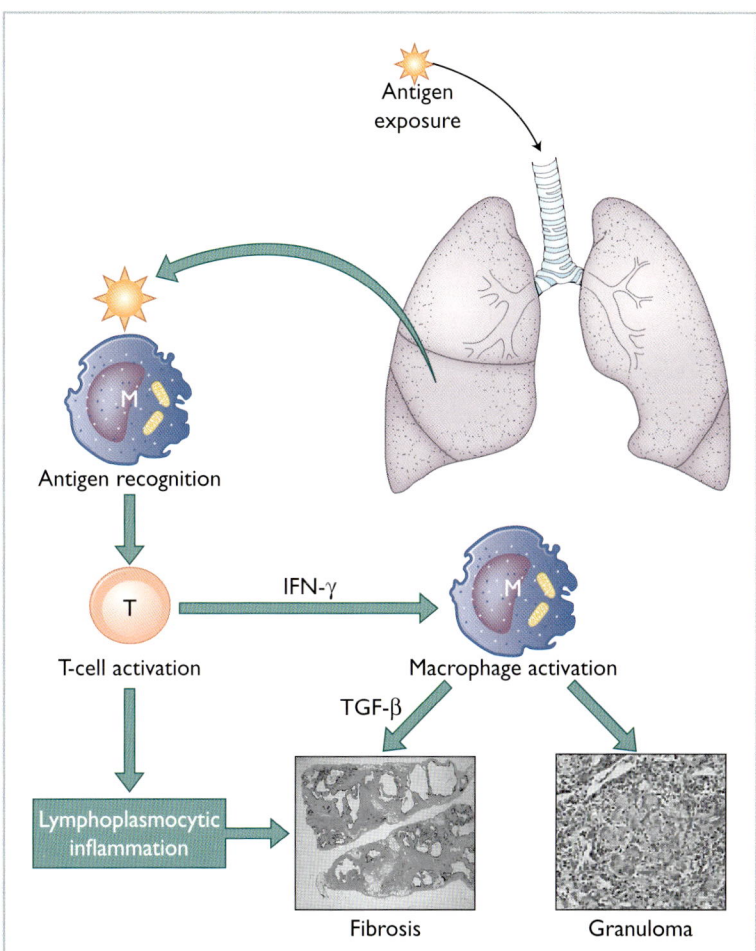

Figure 16-4. Pathophysiologic schema for chronic hypersensitivity pneumonitis. Subacute and chronic hypersensitivity pneumonitis are likely caused by a T-cell–mediated response to an inhaled antigen [6,7]. Antigen presentation leads to activation of CD4+ and CD8+ T-cells. CD4+ cells elaborate T helper-1 cytokines such as interferon (INF)–ψ, which promote macrophage (M) activation and granuloma formation [8]. CD8+ cells are critical to the development of delayed-type hypersensitivity and represent the lymphoplasmacytic inflammation characteristic of this disease. With continued exposure, activated macrophages release proliferative cytokines such as transforming growth factor (TGF)–β. This, in combination with ongoing lymphoplasmacytic inflammation, eventually leads to fibrosis.

Differential Diagnosis of Hypersensitivity Pneumonitis

Acute Hypersensitivity Pneumonitis	Chronic Hypersensitivity Pneumonitis
• Pneumonia	• Sarcoidosis
• Aspiration	• Berylliosis
• Congestive heart failure	• Chronic infection (eg, mycobacteria, fungus)
• Acute lung injury/acute respiratory distress syndrome	• Idiopathic interstitial pneumonia (eg, idiopathic pulmonary fibrosis, nonspecific interstitial pnemonia)
• Diffuse alveolar hemorrhage	
• Acute interstitial pneumonia (Hamman-Rich syndrome)	• Connective tissue–related interstitial lung disease
• Cryptogenic organizing pneumonia (fulminant)	
• Reactive airways dysfunction syndrome	• Pneumoconioses (eg, silicosis, asbestosis)
• Organic dust toxic syndrome	• Chronic eosinophilic pneumonia
• Acute eosinophilic pneumonia	

Figure 16-5. Differential diagnosis of hypersensitivity pneumonitis. The differential diagnosis of hypersensitivity pneumonitis is broad, because signs and symptoms are nonspecific. Acute disease presents with fever, cough, and dyspnea, mimicking a number of conditions, including viral and mycoplasmal pneumonia. Noninfectious causes of acute cough, dyspnea, and radiographic abnormalities must also be considered. Chronic disease is gradual in onset and mimics any number of diffuse parenchymal lung diseases. Granulomatous lung diseases, such as sarcoidosis and berylliosis, may be confused with hypersensitivity pneumonitis both clinically and on lung biopsy. Chronic infection should always be considered. Chronic hypersensitivity pneumonitis may appear clinically, radiographically, and histopathologically identical to idiopathic pulmonary fibrosis; other chronic forms of idiopathic interstitial pneumonia, such as nonspecific interstitial pneumonia; connective tissue–related interstitial lung disease; and some pneumoconioses [2,9,10].

Common Presenting Signs and Symptoms in Hypersensitivity Pneumonitis

Acute Hypersensitivity Pneumonitis*	Chronic Hypersensitivity Pneumonitis†
• Fever	• Malaise
• Myalgia	• Weight loss
• Cough	• Chronic progressive dyspnea
• Dyspnea	• Chronic cough
• Basilar crackles	• Basilar crackles, wheeze
• Leukocytosis	• Hypoxemia

*Generally occur 4–8 h after antigen exposure.
†Generally chronic; a temporal relationship to antigen exposure is not always present.

Figure 16-6. Common presenting signs and symptoms in hypersensitivity pneumonitis. The clinical features of hypersensitivity pneumonitis are often classified as acute, subacute, and chronic, although this distinction is not always clear. Acute disease presents with a flulike illness characterized by fever, myalgia, cough, dyspnea, inspiratory crackles on chest examination, and an elevated leukocyte count. In general, acute hypersensitivity pneumonitis occurs within hours of antigen exposure and usually resolves within a few days if further exposure is avoided. In some cases, symptoms persist and require treatment; such symptoms are generally gradual and insidious in their onset. Nonspecific symptoms such as malaise and weight loss are common. Cough and dyspnea are chronic and progressive. Inspiratory crackles may be heard on chest examination. Finger clubbing is present in up to half of chronic hypersensitivity pneumonitis cases and predicts a poor outcome [11]. Gas exchange abnormalities may be prominent in chronic disease. Interestingly, hypersensitivity pneumonitis occurs far less frequently in active smokers.

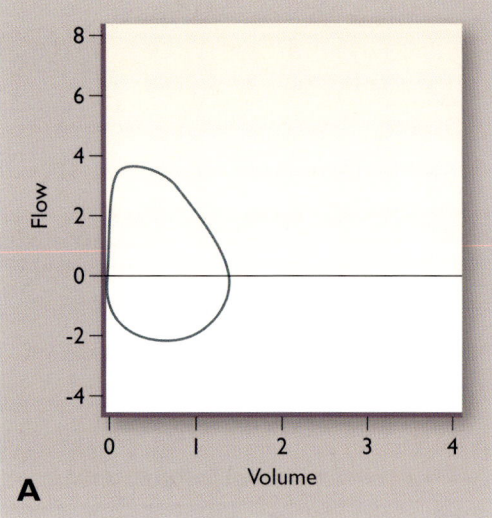
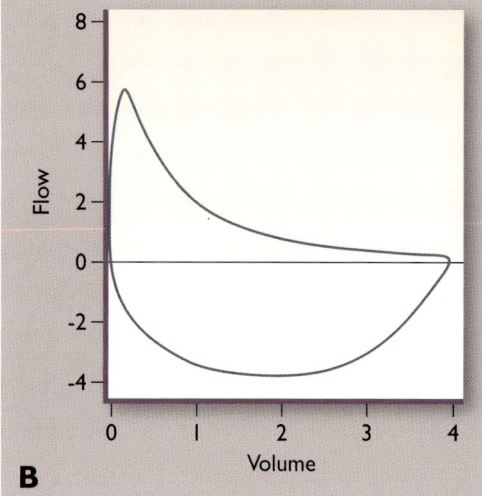

Figure 16-7. Pulmonary function in hypersensitivity pneumonitis. Hypersensitivity pneumonitis is generally considered a restrictive lung disease. **A,** On pulmonary function testing, airflows are preserved for the given lung volume, and there may be an increase in the forced expiratory volume in 1 second (FEV_1)/forced vital capacity (FVC) ratio. Total lung capacity and other measures of lung volume are decreased, as is the diffusing capacity for carbon monoxide. **B,** However, patients with chronic hypersensitivity pneumonitis may also manifest obstructive physiology with airflow limitation (a decrease in FEV_1 and FEV_1/FVC ratio) and hyperinflation [12]. This is thought to occur because of peribronchiolar inflammation and fibrosis, leading to clinical obliterative bronchiolitis.

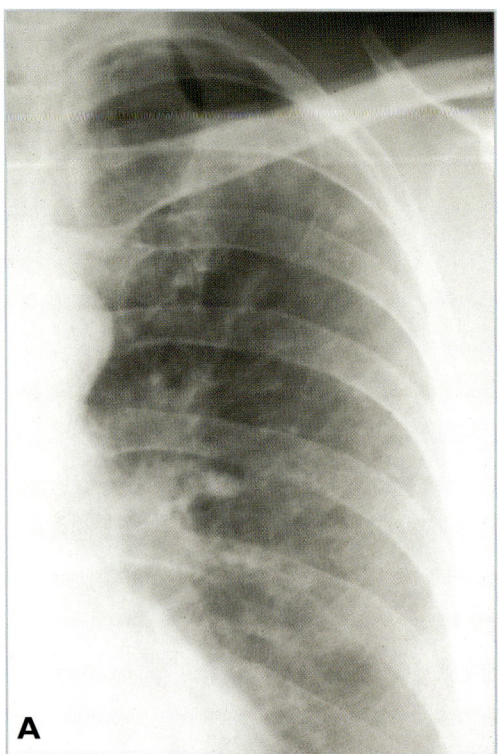
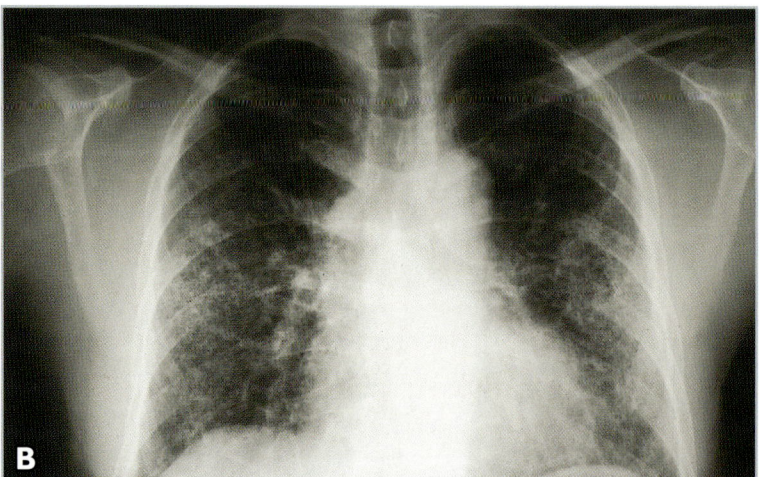

Figure 16-8. Chest radiography in hypersensitivity pneumonitis. The chest radiograph is usually abnormal in hypersensitivity pneumonitis, although there are reports of otherwise typical cases in which the chest radiograph is normal [13]. **A,** The most typical radiographic appearance in acute disease is a diffuse ground-glass abnormality. Chronic disease generally presents with reticular abnormalities and fine nodules. There may be some degree of ground-glass abnormality as well. **B,** More advanced disease will demonstrate diffuse interstitial thickening and cyst formation (honeycombing) that is often indistinguishable from that of other fibrotic lung diseases, such as idiopathic pulmonary fibrosis.

| Atlas of Pulmonary Medicine |

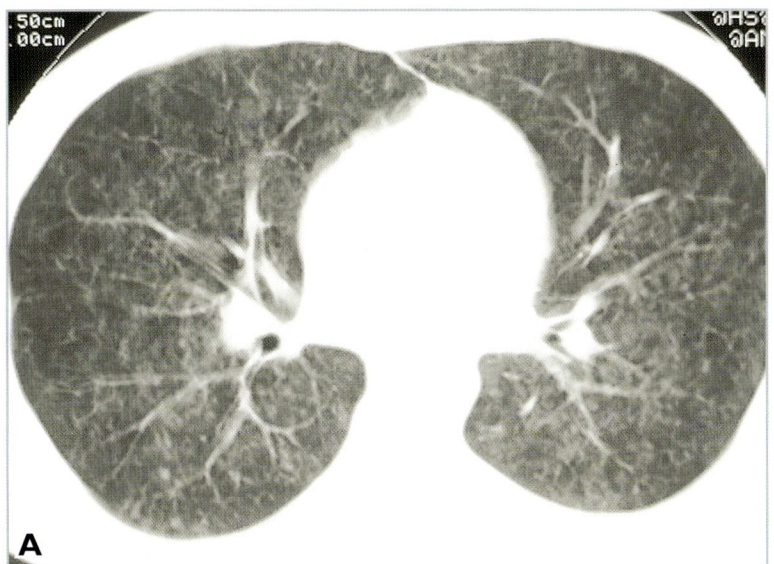
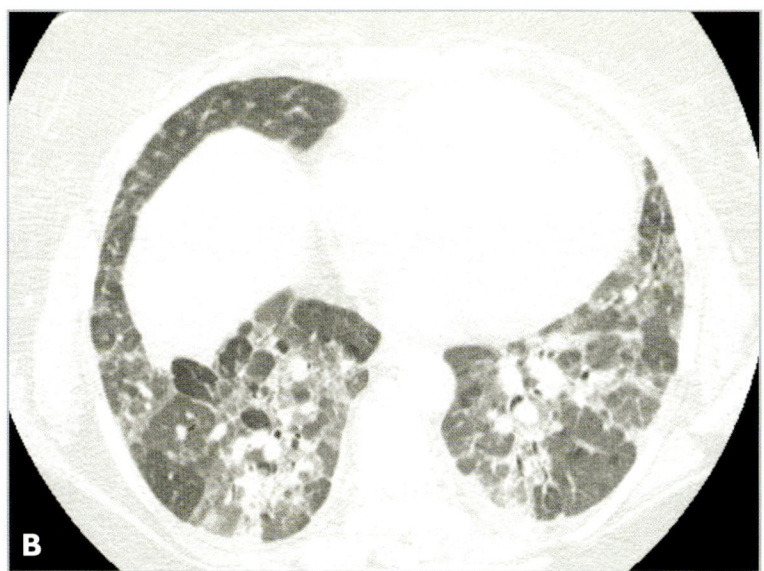
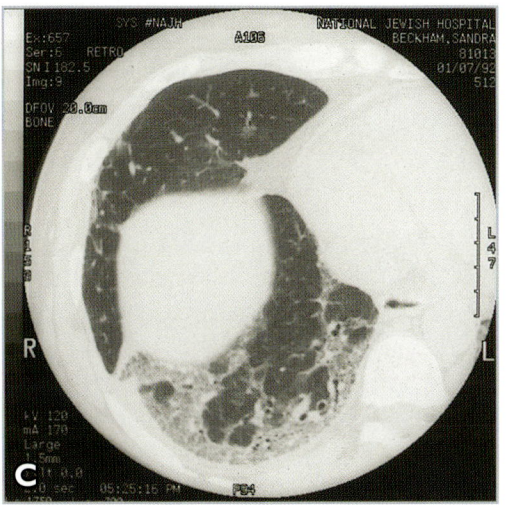

Figure 16-9. High-resolution chest CT in hypersensitivity pneumonitis. High-resolution CT of the chest is more sensitive and specific than chest radiography and should be performed in all patients suspected of having hypersensitivity pneumonitis [14]. **A,** Although acute disease can present with diffuse ground glass abnormality, the more typical presentation is a mixture of diffuse centrilobular nodules and patchy ground glass abnormality, often with an upper lobe predominance. **B,** Mosaic perfusion and airtrapping are manifest radiographically by discrete areas of varying attenuation because of the obstruction of secondary pulmonary lobules. These abnormalities are best appreciated on expiratory images. **C,** In more advanced disease, fibrotic changes with traction bronchiectasis and honeycomb cysts may predominate [15].

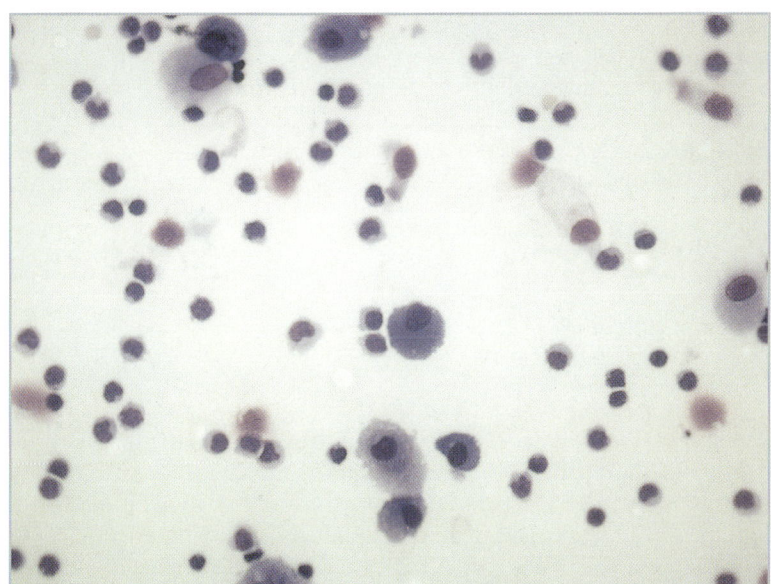

Figure 16-10. Bronchoalveolar lavage in hypersensitivity pneumonitis. The cellular constituency of the bronchoalveolar lavage in hypersensitivity pneumonitis, although not diagnostic, is suggestive. There is a significant increase in total cellularity. Importantly, there is almost always a preponderance of lymphocytes in the lavage, comprising at least 30%—and usually more—of the total cell population. A presence of lymphocytes less than 30% should suggest an alternative diagnosis except in chronic cases [2]. These lymphocytes are largely CD8+ T-cells. In more acute cases, neutrophil and eosinophil percentages are also increased. In more chronic cases, increased numbers of mast cells have been reported and the lymphocyte percentages are often decreased.

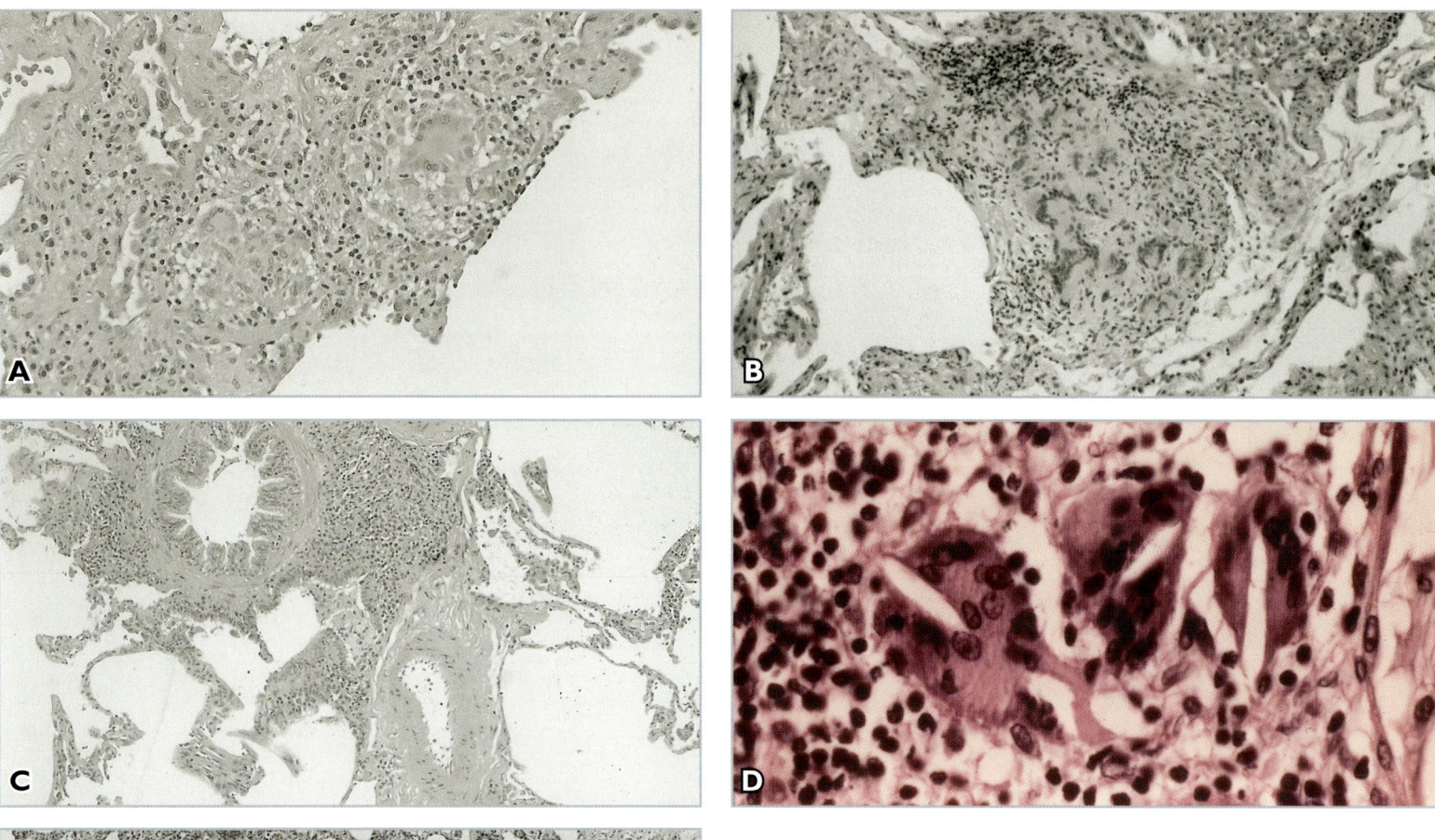

Figure 16-11. Histopathologic appearance of hypersensitivity pneumonitis. **A–C,** The histopathologic hallmarks of hypersensitivity pneumonitis are a lymphoplasmacytic interstitial infiltrate, organizing pneumonia, and nonnecrotizing granulomas [16]. There is often a bronchiolocentric distribution of these findings. **D,** Giant cells with cholesterol clefts, although not diagnostic, are suggestive of the diagnosis. These features are not always present, however, and histopathology may reveal the patterns of nonspecific interstitial pneumonia or usual interstitial pneumonia [9]. **E,** In chronic disease, widespread fibrosis may be seen, along with profound architectural distortion and appearance of honeycomb cysts.

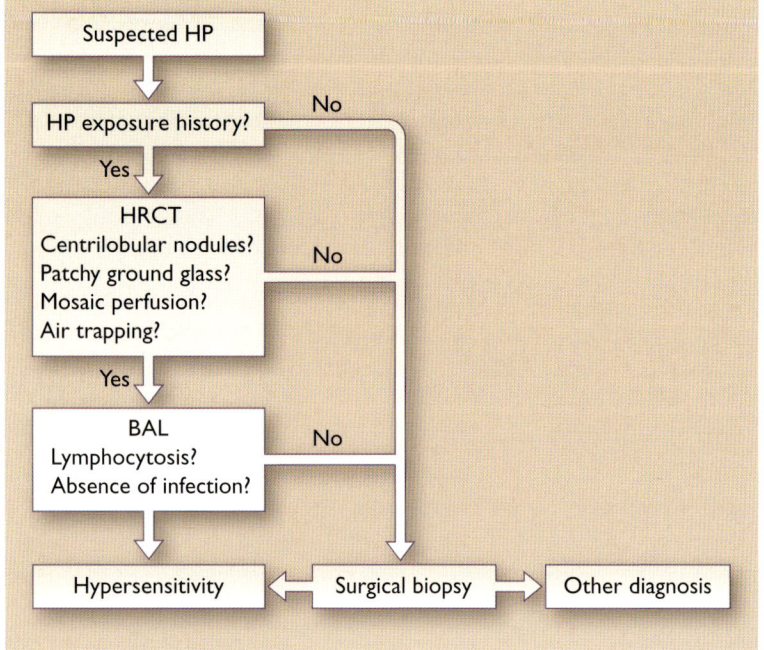

Figure 16-12. Diagnostic algorithm for hypersensitivity pneumonitis (HP). The algorithm represents one approach to establishing the diagnosis of HP. Selected patients may not fit this algorithmic approach, but it serves as a general guide for evaluation. Patients with symptoms that suggest HP (eg, cough and dyspnea) should be carefully questioned about exposure to potential causative agents. A detailed occupational and environmental history is critical. High-resolution CT (HRCT) should be performed on all patients, and bronchoalveolar lavage (BAL) should be performed when HRCT findings suggest the diagnosis. In patients with suspected HP, the presence of a definite exposure to known causative antigens (eg, birds, contaminated water, grain), typical radiographic findings, and more than 30% lymphocytes on BAL establish a presumptive diagnosis. In cases in which one or more of these findings are absent, surgical lung biopsy may be necessary.

Atlas of Pulmonary Medicine

Treatment of Hypersensitivity Pneumonitis

Antigen Avoidance
- Antigen identification is critical
- Removal of offending agent (eg, bird, contaminated water)
- Use of masks and air filters
- Removal of the patient from the antigen's environment

Medications
- Corticosteroids (0.5–1.0 mg/kg/d, tapered slowly)
- Cytotoxic agents (azathioprine, mycophenolate, cyclophosphamide) may be indicated
- Inhaled ß-agonists in select patients

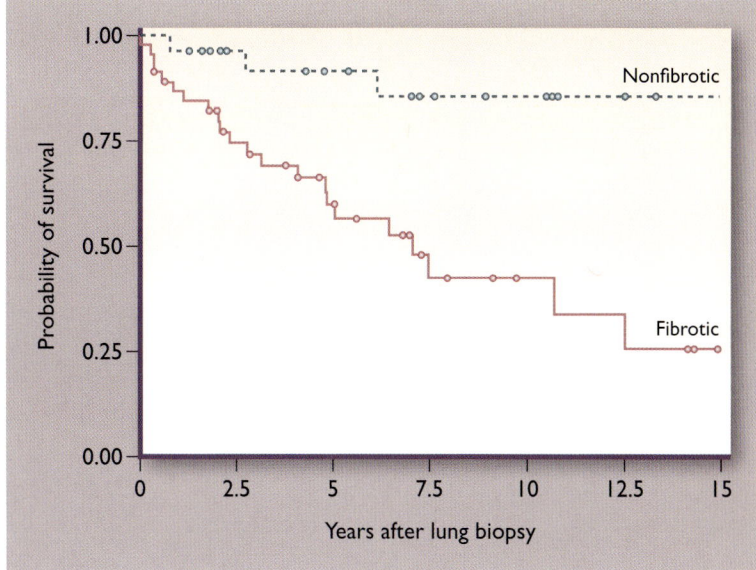

Figure 16-13. Treatment of hypersensitivity pneumonitis. The most effective therapy for hypersensitivity pneumonitis is identification and avoidance of the causative antigen. In acute disease, removing the offending agent from the patient's environment may be the only treatment required. When antigen avoidance is impractical or ineffective, the use of personal protective equipment such as filtered masks may prevent cases of acute disease, but the effectiveness of such devices in subacute and chronic disease is questionable [17]. In persistent or progressive cases, patients must be removed from the responsible home or work environment, and attempts must be made to clean the area. This often requires inspection and cleaning supervised by an environmental engineer—especially in cases in which the antigen exposure is not readily apparent. Oral corticosteroids are usually effective for acute and subacute cases of hypersensitivity pneumonitis [18]. The long-term benefit, however, particularly with persistent antigen exposure, is unproven, underscoring the importance of antigen avoidance as the first line of defense. In resistant cases, cytotoxic agents such as azathioprine, mycophenolate, and cyclophosphamide have had anecdotal success. Patients with airflow limitation may benefit from inhaled bronchodilators.

Figure 16-14. Survival in hypersensitivity pneumonitis. The outcome for acute hypersensitivity pneumonitis is good; the majority of patients respond to removal from exposure and, in certain cases, to corticosteroid therapy. Chronic disease has a worse prognosis—an estimated 5-year survival rate of 75% [19]. Important predictors of survival in this population are the presence of finger clubbing and the degree of fibrosis on lung biopsy. When cases of subacute or chronic hypersensitivity pneumonitis were characterized by the presence or absence of fibrosis on lung biopsy, survival was significantly worse in the fibrotic group [20]. (*Adapted from Vourlekis et al.* [20].)

REFERENCES

1. Lacasse Y, Selman M, Costabel U, et al.: Clinical diagnosis of hypersensitivity pneumonitis. *Am J Respir Crit Care Med* 2003, 168:952–958.

2. Selman M: Hypersensitivity pneumonitis. In *Interstitial Lung Disease*, edn 4. Edited by Schwarz M, King TJ. Hamilton, Ontario: BC Decker Inc; 2003.

3. Fournier E, Tonnel AB, Gosset P, et al.: Early neutrophil alveolitis after antigen inhalation in hypersensitivity pneumonitis. *Chest* 1985, 88:563–566.

4. Ando M, Suga M, Kohrogi H: A new look at hypersensitivity pneumonitis. *Curr Opin Pulm Med* 1999, 5:299–304.

5. Camarena A, Juarez A, Mejia M, et al.: Major histocompatibility complex and tumor necrosis factor-alpha polymorphisms in pigeon breeder's disease. *Am J Respir Crit Care Med* 2001, 163:1528–1533.

6. Salvaggio JE, Millhollon BW: Allergic alveolitis: new insights into old mysteries. *Respir Med* 1993, 87:495–501.

7. Trentin L, Zambello R, Facco M, et al.: Selection of T lymphocytes bearing limited TCR-Vbeta regions in the lung of hypersensitivity pneumonitis and sarcoidosis. *Am J Respir Crit Care Med* 1997, 155:587–596.

8. Patel AM, Ryu JH, Reed CE: Hypersensitivity pneumonitis: current concepts and future questions. *J Allergy Clin Immunol* 2001, 108:661–670.

9. Vourlekis JS, Schwarz MI, Cool CD, et al.: Nonspecific interstitial pneumonitis as the sole histologic expression of hypersensitivity pneumonitis. *Am J Med* 2002, 112:490–493.

10. Lynch DA, Newell JD, Logan PM, et al.: Can CT distinguish hypersensitivity pneumonitis from idiopathic pulmonary fibrosis? *AJR* 1995, 165:807–811.

11. Sansores R, Salas J, Chapela R, et al.: Clubbing in hypersensitivity pneumonitis. Its prevalence and possible prognostic role [see comment]. *Arch Intern Med* 1990, 150:1849–1851.

12. Selman M, Vargas MH: Airway involvement in hypersensitivity pneumonitis. *Curr Opin Pulm Med* 1998, 4:9–15.

13. Epler GR, McLoud TC, Gaensler EA, et al.: Normal chest roentgenograms in chronic diffuse infiltrative lung disease. *N Engl J Med* 1978, 298:934–939.

14. Webb W, Muller N, Naidich D: *High Resolution CT of the Lung*, edn 3. Philadelphia: Lippincott Williams & Wilkins; 2001.

15. Silva CI, Churg A, Muller NL: Hypersensitivity pneumonitis: spectrum of high-resolution CT and pathologic findings. *AJR* 2007, 188:334–344.

16. Coleman A, Colby TV: Histologic diagnosis of extrinsic allergic alveolitis. *Am J Surg Pathol* 1988, 12:514–518.

17. Kusaka H, Ogasawara H, Munakata M, et al.: Two-year follow up on the protective value of dust masks against farmer's lung disease. *Intern Med* 1993, 32:106–111.

18. Kokkarinen JI, Tukiainen HO, Terho EO: Effect of corticosteroid treatment on the recovery of pulmonary function in farmer's lung. *Am Rev Respir Dis* 1992, 145:3–5.

19. Perez-Padilla R, Salas J, Chapela R, et al.: Mortality in Mexican patients with chronic pigeon breeder's lung compared with those with usual interstitial pneumonia. *Am Rev Respir Dis* 1993, 148:49–53.

20. Vourlekis JS, Schwarz MI, Cherniak R, et al.: The effect of pulmonary fibrosis on survival in hypersensitivity pneumonitis. *Am J Med* 2004, 116:662–668.

VENOUS THROMBOEMBOLISM

Nils Kucher and Samuel Z. Goldhaber

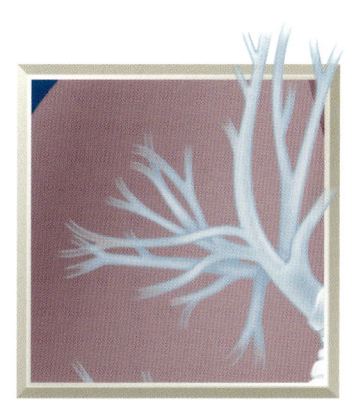
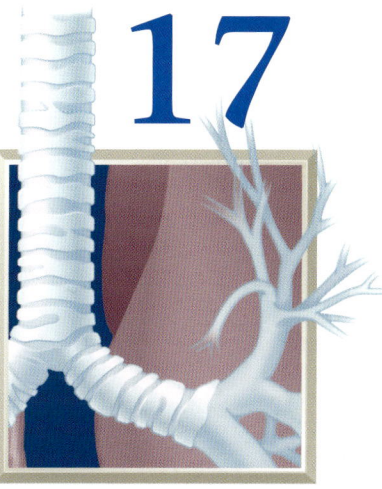
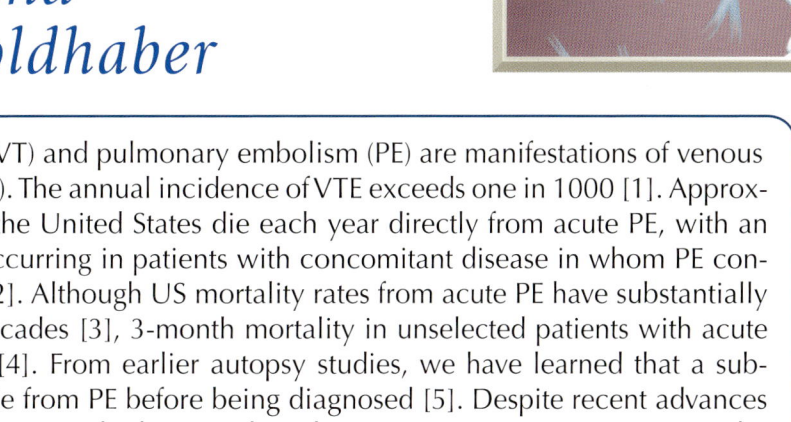
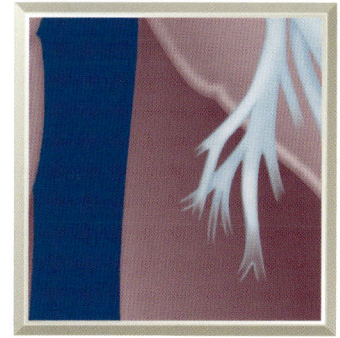

Deep vein thrombosis (DVT) and pulmonary embolism (PE) are manifestations of venous thromboembolism (VTE). The annual incidence of VTE exceeds one in 1000 [1]. Approximately 100,000 patients in the United States die each year directly from acute PE, with an additional 100,000 deaths occurring in patients with concomitant disease in whom PE contributes as a cause of death [2]. Although US mortality rates from acute PE have substantially decreased in the past two decades [3], 3-month mortality in unselected patients with acute PE remains as high as 17% [4]. From earlier autopsy studies, we have learned that a substantial number of patients die from PE before being diagnosed [5]. Despite recent advances in diagnosis and treatment, PE is underdiagnosed, and preventive measures continue to be underutilized. In a registry of 5451 US patients with ultrasound-confirmed DVT, only 42% of the inpatients had received prophylaxis within 30 days prior to diagnosis [6].

The risk of recurrence remains increased after an initial DVT or PE. This is particularly the case in patients with idiopathic VTE, defined broadly as occurring in the absence of surgery or trauma. Recent large-scale randomized, controlled trials proved that patients with idiopathic VTE benefit from long-term anticoagulation with warfarin [7,8].

Anticoagulation with unfractionated heparin or low molecular weight heparin as a "bridge" to warfarin or other oral anti–vitamin K agents is the standard, classical treatment for PE. The pentasaccharide fondaparinux, given subcutaneously in a fixed dose, is at least as effective and safe as continuous-infusion intravenous unfractionated heparin in the initial management of symptomatic, hemodynamically stable PE [9]. Novel direct factor Xa inhibitors, such as rivaroxaban, are promising oral anticoagulants that do not require monitoring when administered in fixed daily doses. After successful completion of the phase II program, the efficacy and safety of rivaroxaban is currently being investigated for the prevention and treatment of VTE.

EPIDEMIOLOGY

Epidemiology of Venous Thromboembolism

US incidence of diagnosed VTE	1.22–1.45 per 1000 per year [1,10,11]
Estimated ratio of diagnosed/undiagnosed VTE	1:3
US population	300 million
US total cases of VTE	1.1–1.3 million per year
30-day mortality DVT	5% [12]
30-day mortality PE	11% [4]
3-month mortality PE	17% [4]

Figure 17-1. Epidemiology of venous thromboembolism. Cohort studies in patients with venous thromboembolism (VTE) show a remarkable consistency in incidence estimates in western populations. DVT—deep vein thrombosis; PE—pulmonary embolism.

Common Acquired Risk Factors for Venous Thromboembolism

- Increasing age
- Immobility
- Trauma/surgery
  - High risk: orthopedic surgery, cancer surgery, especially neurosurgery
- Medical comorbidities
  - Cancer
  - Congestive heart failure
  - Chronic lung disease
  - Hypertension
  - Diabetes mellitus
  - Obesity
  - Inflammatory bowel disease
  - Stroke with extremity paresis
  - Varicose veins
- Prior venous thromboembolism
- Indwelling central venous catheter/pacemaker/defibrillator
- Pregnancy/postpartum
- Oral contraceptives/hormone replacement therapy
- Long-distance airplane travel

Figure 17-2. Common acquired risk factors for venous thromboembolism. In 1856, Virchow proposed his triad of factors leading to intravascular coagulation, including stasis, vessel wall injury, and hypercoagulability. Risk factors for deep vein thrombosis (DVT) are based on these processes. In a large prospective registry of 5451 patients with ultrasound-confirmed DVT [6], the most common comorbidities were arterial hypertension (50%), surgery within 3 months (38%), immobility within 30 days (34%), cancer (32%), and obesity (27%).

Upper-extremity DVT is becoming more important because of an increasing use of pacemakers, implantable defibrillators, and long-term indwelling central venous catheters. It is rarely (< 3%) associated with symptomatic pulmonary embolism (PE) [13].

The proportion of subjects who develop acute PE during or after airplane travel correlates with the flight distance. The risk of PE significantly increases with a flight distance greater than 5000 kilometers (3106.85 miles) [14].

Thrombophilic Risk Factors for Venous Thromboembolism

- Factor V Leiden
- Prothrombin G20210 mutation
- Protein C deficiency
- Protein S deficiency
- Antithrombin III deficiency
- Dysfibrinogenemia
- Disorders of plasminogen
- Antiphospholipid antibody syndrome
- Hyperhomocysteinemia
- Increased levels of factor VIII or XI
- Increased lipoprotein (a)

Figure 17-3. Thrombophilic risk factors for venous thromboembolism. The factor V Leiden mutation, a single base mutation (substitution of A for G at position 506), is a common genetic polymorphism associated with activated protein C resistance. It is present in approximately 4% to 6% of the general population [15]. The relative risk of a first idiopathic deep vein thrombosis (DVT) among men heterozygous for the mutation has been shown to be three- to seven-fold higher than that of those not affected. The prothrombin gene defect, present in 2% to 4% of the general population, increases the risk of DVT by a factor of 2.7 to 3.8 [16]. Homocysteine has potentially thrombogenic effects, including injury to vascular endothelium and antagonism of the synthesis and function of nitric oxide [17]. Interactions between the genetic factors (defects in enzymes such as methylenetetrahydrofolate reductase) that control homocysteine metabolism and nutritional factors (folate, vitamin B6, and vitamin B12 deficiencies) that affect homocysteine metabolism warrant additional investigation with regard to venous thromboembolism.

DIAGNOSIS OF VENOUS THROMBOEMBOLISM

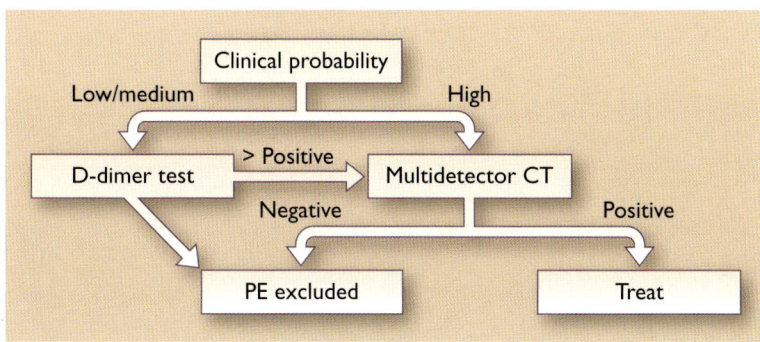

Figure 17-4. Suggested diagnostic strategy. The initial assessment of patients with suspected pulmonary embolism (PE) includes history taking, physical examination, and electrocardiogram to determine the clinical probability of PE. A plasma D-dimer enzyme-linked immunosorbent assay should be obtained for all patients with low or intermediate clinical probability. In hospitalized patients and in outpatients with high clinical probability, contrast-enhanced multidetector-row CT is usually performed without obtaining the D-dimer test. If the D-dimer is below the assay-specific cutoff level, PE is essentially excluded [18]. If D-dimer levels are elevated, we recommend obtaining a contrast-enhanced multidetector-row CT. In patients with severe impairment of renal function or with allergy to contrast agents, ventilation perfusion scanning or MRI may be performed as primary imaging tests.

Ventilation Perfusion Lung Scanning

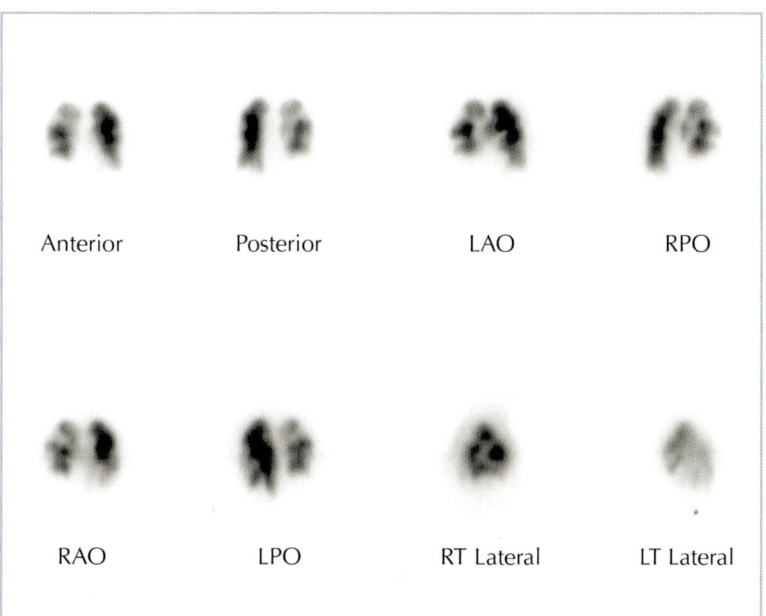

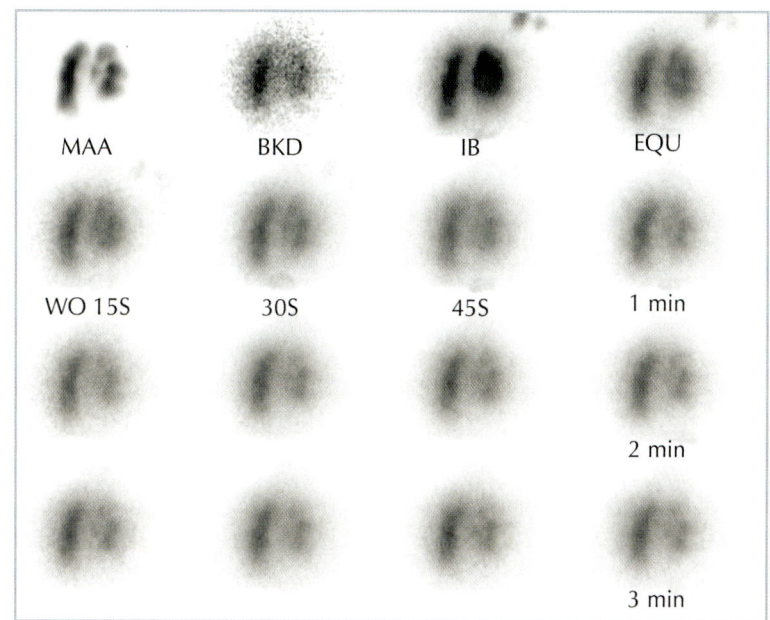

Figure 17-5. Perfusion lung scan of a 65-year-old woman who presented after 3 days of unexplained "gasping for breath" with any activity. She underwent a perfusion lung scan with 5.0 mCi of 99 mTc macroaggregated albumin. The eight standard views were obtained: anterior, posterior, left anterior oblique (LAO), right posterior oblique (RPO), right anterior oblique (RAO), left posterior oblique (LPO), right lateral (RT), and left lateral (LT). The perfusion scan was abnormal and showed multiple peripheral perfusion defects in both lungs. In the presence of a normal chest radiograph, this perfusion scan shows high probability for acute pulmonary embolism.

Figure 17-6. Ventilation lung scan of the patient in Figure 17-5. The scan taken in the right posterior oblique (RPO) position demonstrates a "mismatch" between abnormal perfusion and normal ventilation of the right lung. This ventilation–perfusion mismatch indicates a high probability for acute pulmonary embolism.

The upper left-hand image is the perfusion scan in the RPO position. All of the other images are ventilation scans in the RPO position. The ventilation is normal. The contrast between the abnormal perfusion scan and the normal ventilation scan is best seen by comparing the perfusion scan in the uppermost left image with the ventilation scan seen in the image to its right.

Electrocardiography

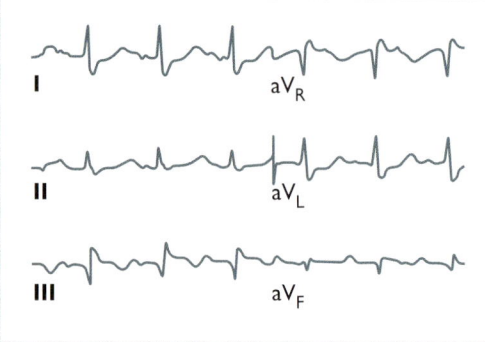

Figure 17-7. Electrocardiogram of a 64-year-old woman who was hospitalized with "atypical chest pain." Her electrocardiogram shows sinus tachycardia, incomplete right bundle branch block, and an S1Q3TIII pattern with an S wave in lead I, a Q wave in lead III, and an inverted T wave in lead III—findings indicative of right ventricular strain [19].

Echocardiography

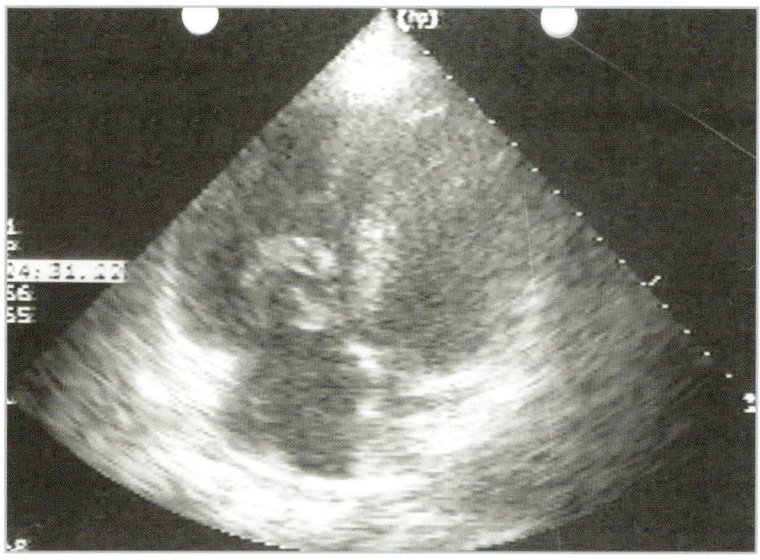

Figure 17-8. Echocardiogram of the patient in Figure 17-7. In the apical four-chamber view, the right ventricle is abnormally dilated. This is apparent because the right ventricle is larger than the left ventricle, whereas normally, the right ventricle should be smaller than (*ie,* no more than 0.6 times the size of) the left ventricle.

A 3 by 4 cm round mass is observed in the right ventricle, just below the tricuspid valve. This mass turned out to be a giant curled-up venous thrombus, which embolized to the pulmonary arteries and caused massive acute pulmonary embolism.

Pulmonary Angiography

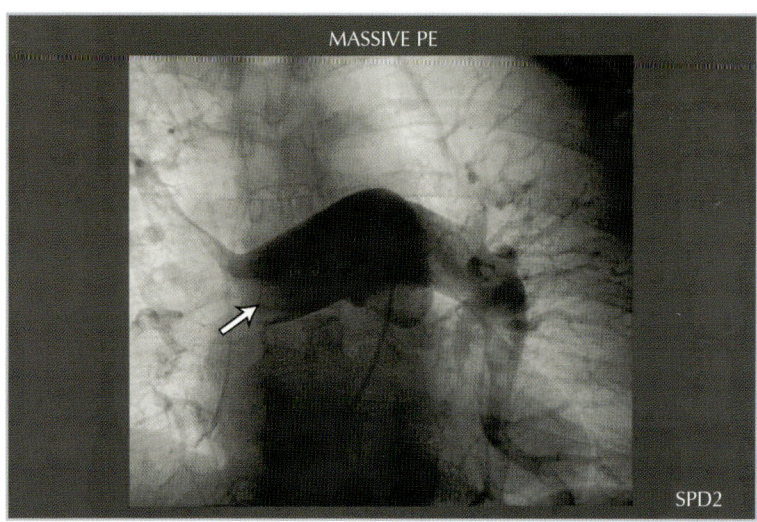

Figure 17-9. Contrast pulmonary angiogram of the patient in Figures 17-7 and 17-8. A massive bilateral saddle embolism is present. The *white arrow* indicates the thrombus in the right main pulmonary artery.

Atlas of Pulmonary Medicine

SPIRAL CT OF THE CHEST

First-Generation Scanner

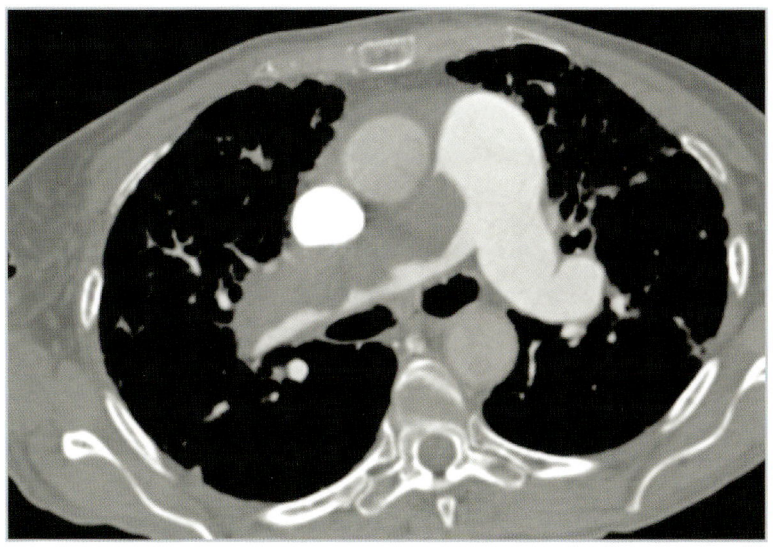

Figure 17-10. CT of a 59-year-old woman with advanced sarcoidosis who underwent evaluation for possible lung transplantation. The CT with contrast demonstrated a previously unsuspected, large defect filling the right pulmonary artery. The thrombus extends from the right main pulmonary artery into the right upper and right lower lobe pulmonary arteries.

First-generation scanners are accurate for the diagnosis of large clots in the central and lobar pulmonary arteries. The overall sensitivity and specificity for pulmonary embolism (PE) are about 70% and 90%, respectively [20]. First-generation scanners lack sensitivity for segmental and subsegmental PE. Spiral chest CTs are also useful in detecting alternative diagnoses, such as aortic dissection, pneumonia, and pericardial tamponade [21].

Third-Generation Scanner

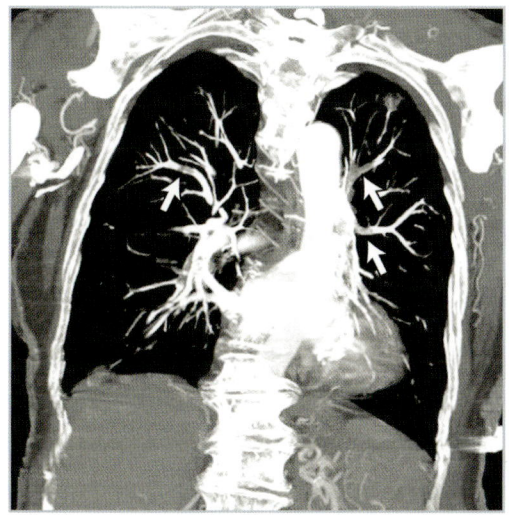

Figure 17-11. Bilateral segmental pulmonary embolism in a patient with atypical chest pain (*arrows*). Newer-generation scanners involve continuous movement of the patient through the scanner, with concurrent scanning by a constantly rotating gantry and detector system. Rapid, continuous volume acquisitions can be obtained during a single breath, thereby facilitating imaging of critically ill patients. Multidetector CT scanners permit image acquisition of the entire chest with 1-mm resolution and a breath hold of less than 10 seconds. They reveal emboli in the main, lobar, or segmental pulmonary arteries with greater than 90% sensitivity and specificity [22].

Autopsy

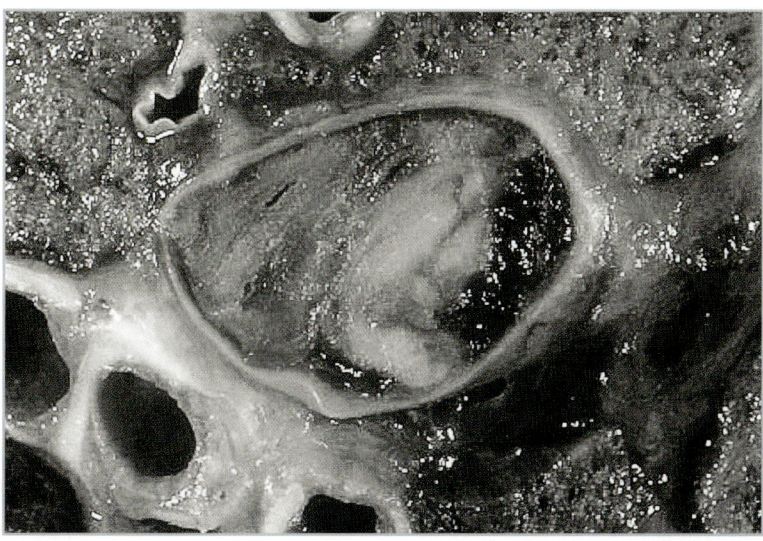

Figure 17-12. Thrombus. The patient shown in Figure 17-11 suffered a cardiac arrest and died 3 days later, despite maximal resuscitative efforts. At autopsy, the right main pulmonary artery, seen in cross-section, was filled with thrombi of varying ages.

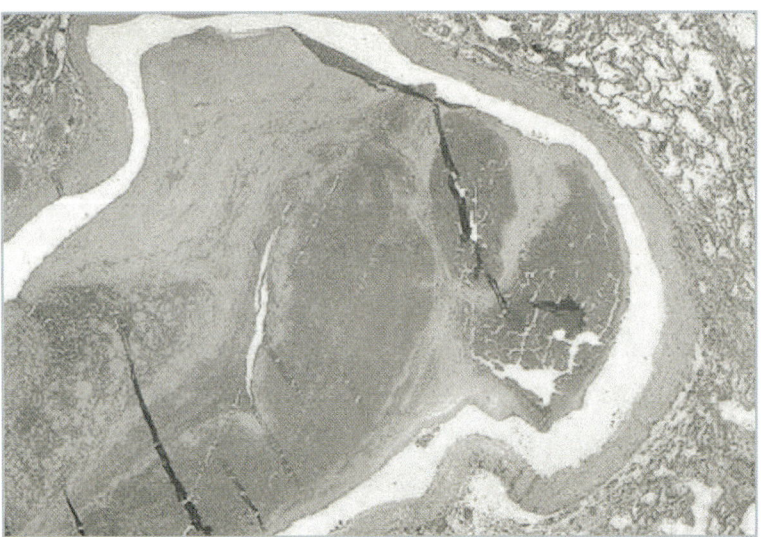

Figure 17-13. Microscopy of a right segmental pulmonary artery showing a red fibrin clot filling most of the vessel.

THERAPY OF VENOUS THROMBOEMBOLISM

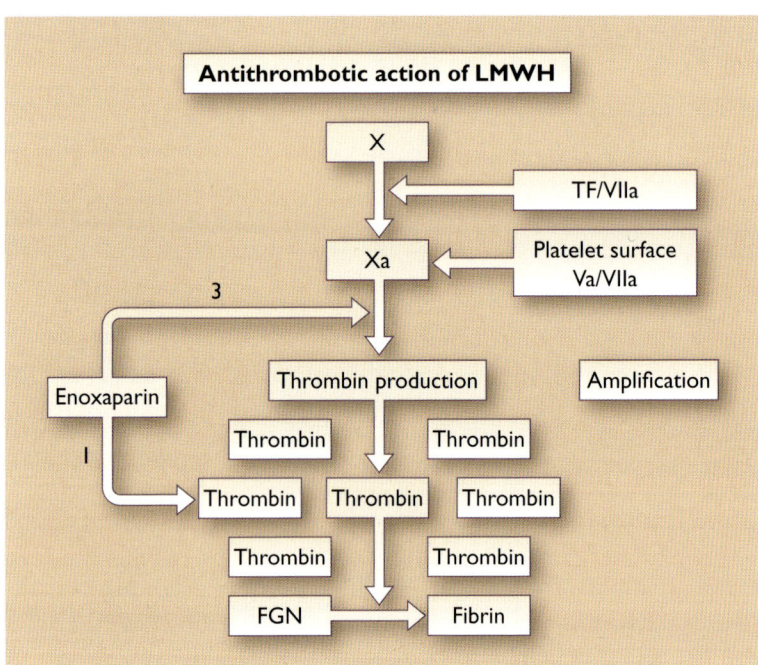

Figure 17-14. Low molecular weight heparin. Although the ratio of anti-Xa to antithrombin of unfractionated heparin is 1:1, the low molecular weight heparins (LMWHs) have significantly higher ratios (eg, enoxaparin, 3:1). In addition, other anticoagulant properties, such as stimulation of tissue factor pathway–inhibitor release, appear to be responsible for the effect of these agents.

LMWHs have several advantages over unfractionated heparin. They exhibit less binding to plasma proteins and to endothelial cells than unfractionated heparin. Consequently, LMWHs tend to have a more predictable dose response, a more dose-independent mechanism of clearance, and a longer plasma half-life than unfractionated heparin. Furthermore, osteoporosis and heparin-induced thrombocytopenia appear to be less common with LMWH than with unfractionated heparin.

Two trials have shown that therapy with LMWH is as safe and effective as therapy with unfractionated heparin in hemodynamically stable patients with acute pulmonary embolism (PE) [23,24]. The Food and Drug Administration has approved enoxaparin for outpatient treatment of symptomatic deep vein thrombosis with or without PE, as a bridge to warfarin. Two dosing regimens exist: 1 mg/kg subcutaneously every 12 hours for both outpatients and inpatients, and 1.5 mg/kg subcutaneously once daily for inpatients. FGN—fibrinogen; TF—tissue factor. (*Courtesy of* Elliott M. Antman, MD.)

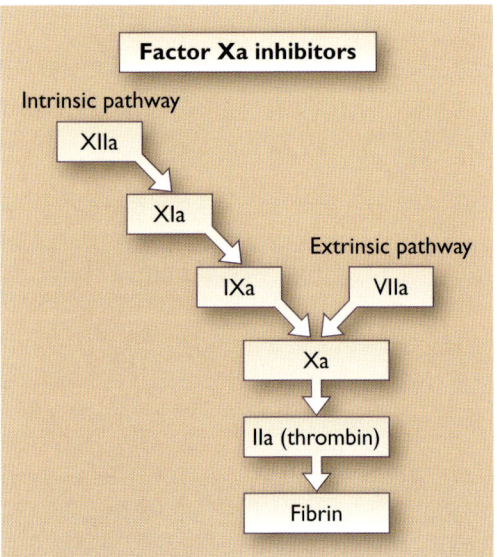

Figure 17-15. Pentasaccharides, such as fondaparinux: effective factor Xa inhibitors for the prevention and treatment of venous thromboembolism. These pentasaccharides produce an irreversible conformational change in antithrombin, which binds and inhibits factor Xa. For prevention of venous thromboembolism (VTE), fondaparinux is administered subcutaneously in a fixed low dose. The dosage for fondaparinux is 2.5 mg once daily [25].

Atlas of Pulmonary Medicine

MATISSE-PE		
Outcome	Fondaparinux (n = 1103), %	UFH (n = 1110), %
Recurrence	3.8	5.0
Major bleed	2.0	2.4
Death	5.2	4.4

Figure 17-16. Fondaparinux. MATISSE-PE was a randomized, open-label trial involving 2213 hemodynamically stable patients with acute pulmonary embolism (PE) to compare the efficacy and safety of fondaparinux with unfractionated heparin [9]. Patients received either fondaparinux (5.0, 7.5, and 10.0 mg in patients weighing < 50, 50 to 100, and > 100 kg, respectively) subcutaneously once daily or a continuous intravenous infusion of unfractionated heparin (UFH) (ratio of the activated partial thromboplastin time to a control value, 1.5:2.5), both given for at least 5 days and until the use of vitamin K antagonists resulted in an international normalized ratio above 2.0. Fondaparinux was at least as effective and as safe as unfractionated heparin in the initial treatment of patients with acute PE, as shown by similar rates of venous thromboembolism recurrence, major bleeding, and death.

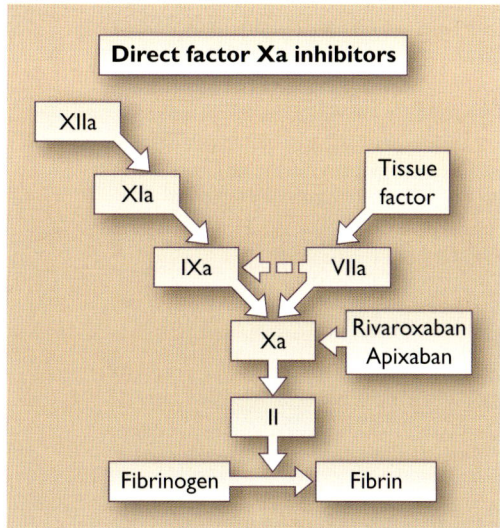

Figure 17-17. Direct factor Xa inhibitors. Novel direct factor Xa inhibitors, such as rivaroxaban or apixaban, are a class of oral synthetic anticoagulants that directly and selectively bind factor Xa, independently of antithrombin III levels. Rivaroxaban has a rapid onset of action, no apparent drug–drug interactions, and no need for anticoagulation monitoring with fixed daily dosing. It is in advanced clinical development for the prevention and treatment of venous thromboembolism.

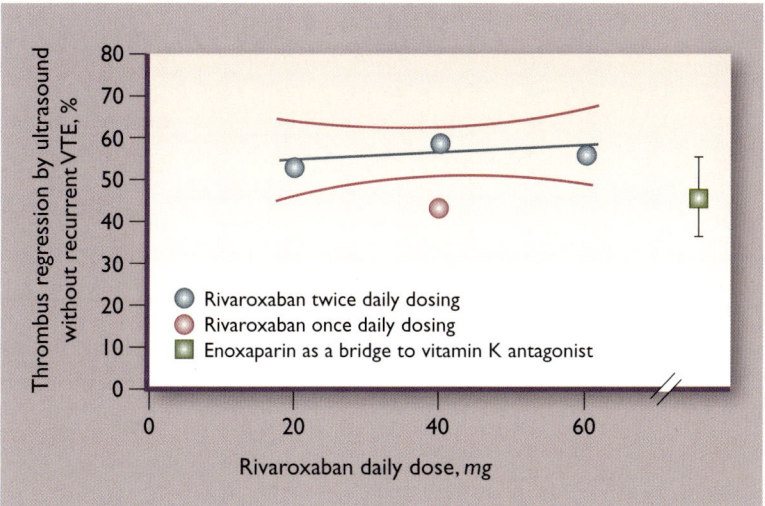

Figure 17-18. ODIXa-DVT: rivaroxaban dose–response relationship for efficacy. In a randomized controlled dose-finding study of fixed-dose oral rivaroxaban, efficacy was measured by identifying the proportion of patients with improvement in thrombus burden by ultrasound and without clinical recurrence at day 21 in comparison to standard therapy with enoxaparin as a bridge to vitamin K antagonists. In this phase II study, no dose–response relationship was found regarding the efficacy of rivaroxaban, and there was no difference in efficacy in comparison with standard therapy. The rate of bleeding complications was low and did not differ between the treatment groups [26]. VTE—venous thromboembolism.

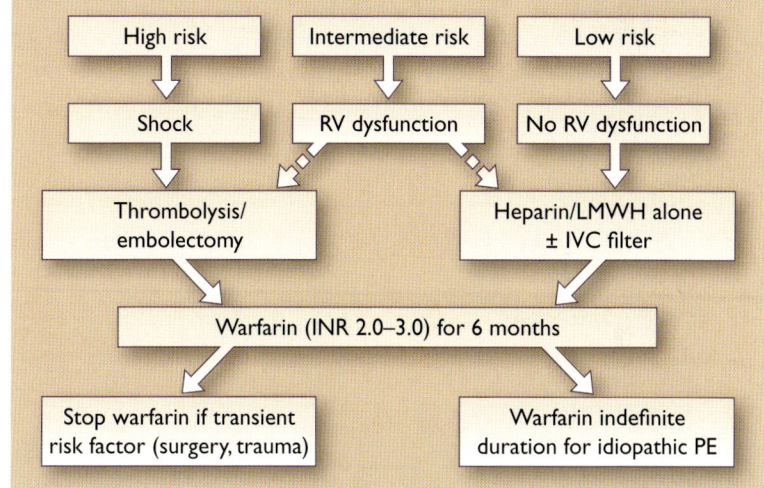

Figure 17-19. Suggested pulmonary embolism management strategy. Treatment decisions in acute pulmonary embolism (PE) are based on the hemodynamic presentation of the patient. Although high-risk patients with massive PE and cardiogenic shock should be treated rapidly with a reperfusion regimen (thrombolysis, catheter embolectomy, or surgical embolectomy), the decision to treat a patient with preserved systemic arterial pressure remains controversial; it depends mostly on the presence of right ventricular dysfunction (intermediate risk). Low-risk patients with preserved systemic arterial pressure and normal right ventricular function will benefit from anticoagulation alone and should not be treated with thrombolysis.

PE patients should be treated with full-dose anticoagulation for at least 6 months. Anticoagulation is usually discontinued after 6 months in patients with transient venous thromboembolism risk factors such as surgery or trauma within 90 days. INR—international normalized ratio; IVC—inferior vena cava; LMWH—low molecular weight heparin; RV—right ventrical.

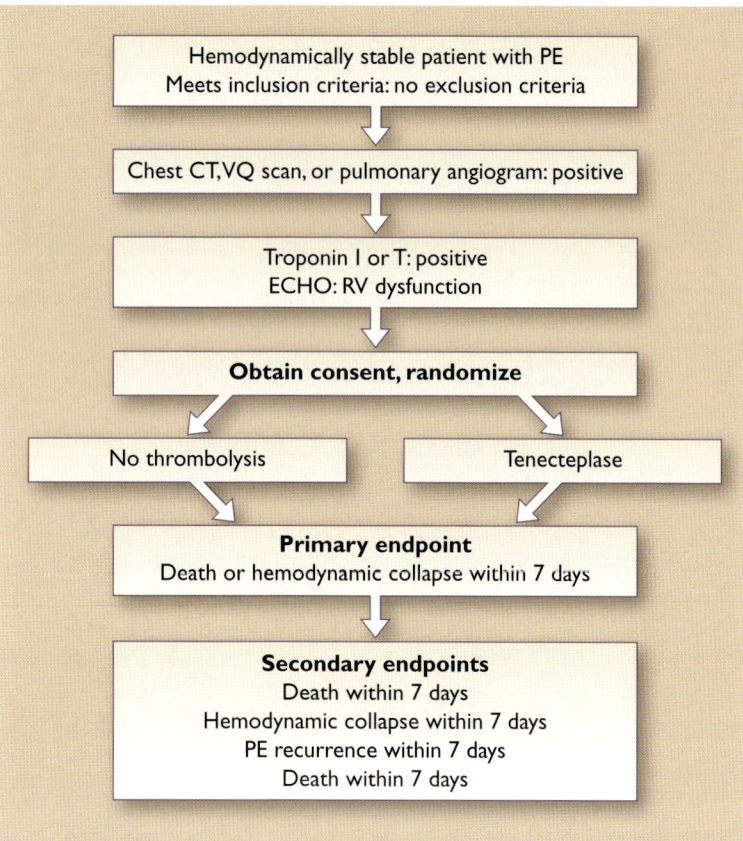

Figure 17-20. Thrombolysis and high risk patients. There is a 30-year-long debate about the efficacy and safety of thrombolysis in hemodynamically stable pulmonary embolism (PE) patients with preserved systolic systemic pressure but clinical signs of acute right ventricular failure. In these patients, acute right ventricular involvement can be confirmed by echocardiographic evidence of right ventricular dysfunction and a positive troponin test. A large, randomized, controlled trial is currently ongoing to determine whether or not thrombolysis should be used for these high-risk patients. RV—right ventricle; VQ—ventilation-perfusion.

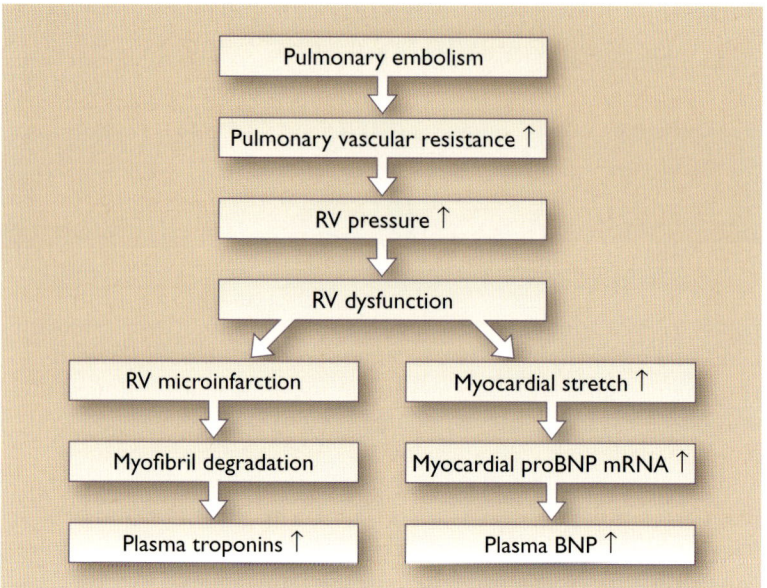

Figure 17-21. Cardiac biomarkers for risk stratification. Echocardiography has emerged as the most important tool for risk assessment and treatment guidance in patients with acute pulmonary embolism (PE) [27]. New, promising tools for risk assessment include cardiac troponins I and T [28,29] as well as N-terminal pro-brain natriuretic peptide [30] and brain natriuretic peptide (BNP) [31–33]. Myocardial ischemia due to alterations in oxygen supply and demand of the failing right ventricle probably plays a major role in the pathogenesis of troponin release. The stimulus for BNP synthesis and secretion is cardiomyocyte stretch of the right ventricle. Increases in troponins and BNP are both related to the extent of right ventricular dysfunction. These cardiac biomarkers are similarly accurate in identifying low-risk PE patients through their high negative predictive value for in-hospital death, ranging from 97% to 100%. mRNA—mitochondrial RNA; proBNP—pro-brain natriuretic peptide; RV—right ventricle.

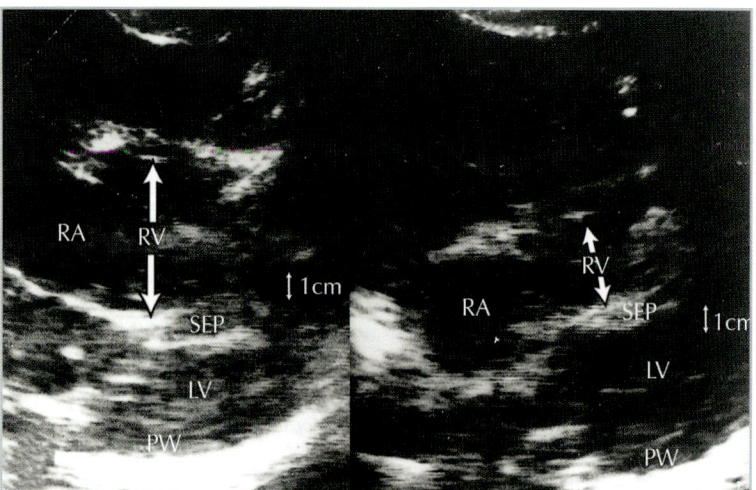

Figure 17-22. Thrombolysis. Systemic thrombolysis is lifesaving and is considered standard therapy in patients with massive pulmonary embolism (PE) and cardiogenic shock. The only contemporary Food and Drug Administration–approved thrombolytic regimen is a continuous intravenous infusion of 100 mg alteplase over 2 hours. The figure shows successful thrombolysis to reverse right heart failure, including right ventricular hypokinesis, right ventricular dilatation, and tricuspid regurgitation. The *left panel* is a subcostal image from a patient who presented with congestive heart failure, and who was diagnosed with acute PE after this echocardiogram—which looked suspicious for PE rather than for left-heart failure—led to further work-up, including contrast pulmonary angiography. The right ventricle (RV) is markedly enlarged, and the diameter of the left ventricle (LV) is reduced. After receiving 2 hours of peripherally administered intravenous tissue plasminogen activator, a remarkable decrease in RV size and a corresponding increase in LV size are apparent (*right panel*).

In the Management Strategies and Prognosis of Pulmonary Embolism (MAPPET-3) study, the largest thrombolysis study to have been conducted thus far, heparin plus alteplase given as a continuous infusion over 2 hours was compared with heparin alone [34]. Compared to heparin alone, thrombolysis markedly reduced adverse clinical outcomes from 25% to 11%; adverse outcomes were defined as the need for cardiopulmonary resuscitation, mechanical ventilation, administration of pressors, secondary "rescue" thrombolysis, or surgical embolectomy. There was no significant increase in major bleeding, and there was no intracranial bleeding with alteplase among these carefully selected PE patients. However, use of thrombolysis remains controversial in patients with preserved arterial pressure because a mortality benefit has not been demonstrated when compared with anticoagulation alone. PW—posterior wall; RA—right atrium; SEP—interventricular septum.

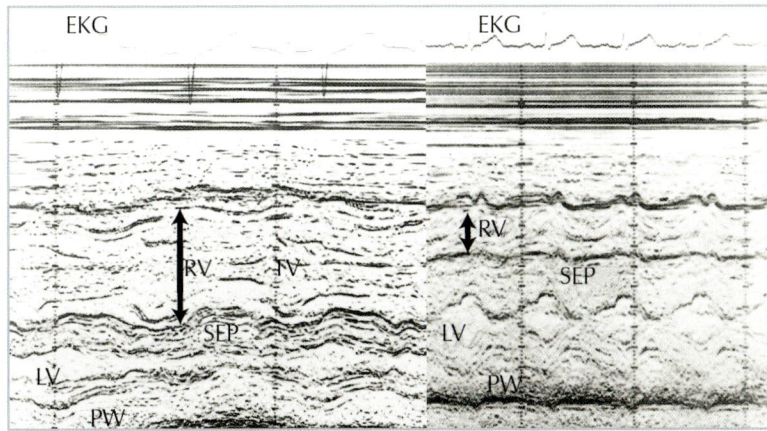

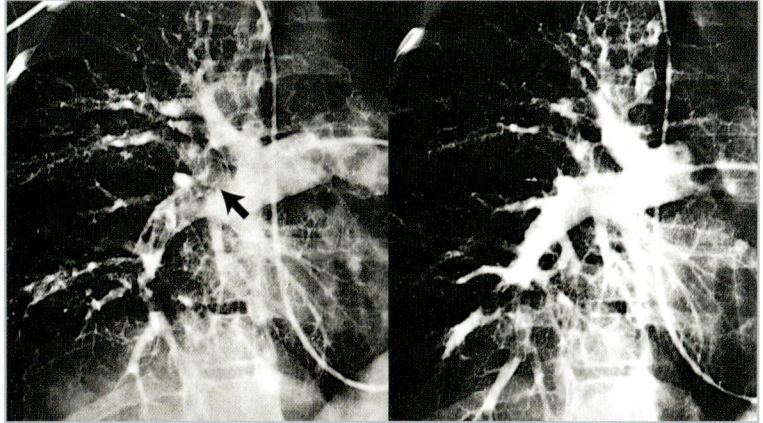

Figure 17-23. M-mode echocardiographic recordings of the right ventricle and left ventricle from a subcostal transducer position in the patient in Figure 17-22. Before thrombolysis (*left panel*), the right ventricle (RV) was markedly enlarged, and the left ventricle (LV) chamber size was reduced. The interventricular septum (SEP) moved paradoxically. The RV wall motion was markedly hypokinetic. After thrombolysis (*right panel*), the RV became much smaller, and the LV became larger. Paradoxical motion of the SEP was no longer present, and right ventricular wall motion normalized. PW—posterior wall; TV—tricuspid valve.

Figure 17-24. Peripheral intravenous administration of alteplase given as a continuous infusion over 2 hours. In the *left panel*, at baseline, there is a massive right pulmonary artery thromboembolism (*arrow*). Immediately after thrombolysis, a follow-up contrast pulmonary angiogram (*right panel*) shows marked clot lysis.

Thrombolysis can be immediately lifesaving by rapidly reversing right heart failure, the usual cause of death from acute pulmonary embolism. In addition, thrombolysis may preserve the normal hemodynamic response to exercise over the long term, and may prevent recurrence of venous thromboembolism and the development of chronic pulmonary hypertension.

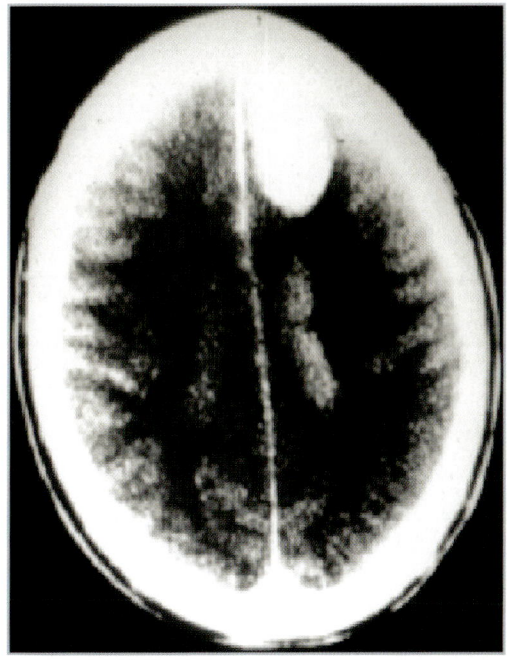

Optimal Duration and Intensity of Anticoagulation in Patients with Idiopathic Venous Thromboembolism

Trial	Treatment	Control	Recurrent VTE
PREVENT [7]	Warfarin	Placebo	RRR 64% in the treatment group
	INR 1.5–2.0		
ELATE [8]	Warfarin	Warfarin	RRR 78% in the treatment group
	INR 2.0–3.0	INR 1.5–1.9	

Figure 17-25. CT of a large front intracranial hemorrhage. The biggest disadvantage of thrombolysis is the potential for intracranial hemorrhage. About half of the intracranial hemorrhages are fatal. Among those who survive this complication, about half have major, permanent neurologic deficits. In the International Cooperative Pulmonary Embolism Registry, 3.0% of patients who received thrombolytic therapy developed intracranial bleeding [4]. In a meta-analysis of trials in patients with pulmonary embolism, thrombolysis was associated with a twofold increase in major hemorrhage in comparison with treatment with heparin alone [35].

Figure 17-26. Optimal duration and intensity of anticoagulation in patients with idiopathic venous thromboembolism (VTE). In the two cited studies, patients with idiopathic VTE were enrolled after an average of 6-month, full-intensity (target international normalized ratio [INR] 2.0–3.0) anticoagulation with warfarin. In these trials, no difference in major bleeding events between the treatment and control arms was observed. ELATE—Extended Low-Intensity Anticoagulation for Thrombo-Embolism Investigators; PREVENT—Prevention of Recurrent Venous Thromboembolism; RRR—relative risk reduction.

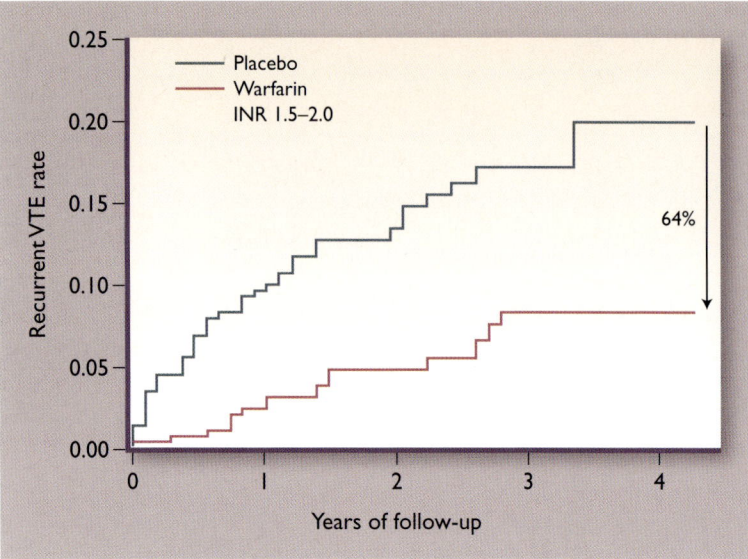

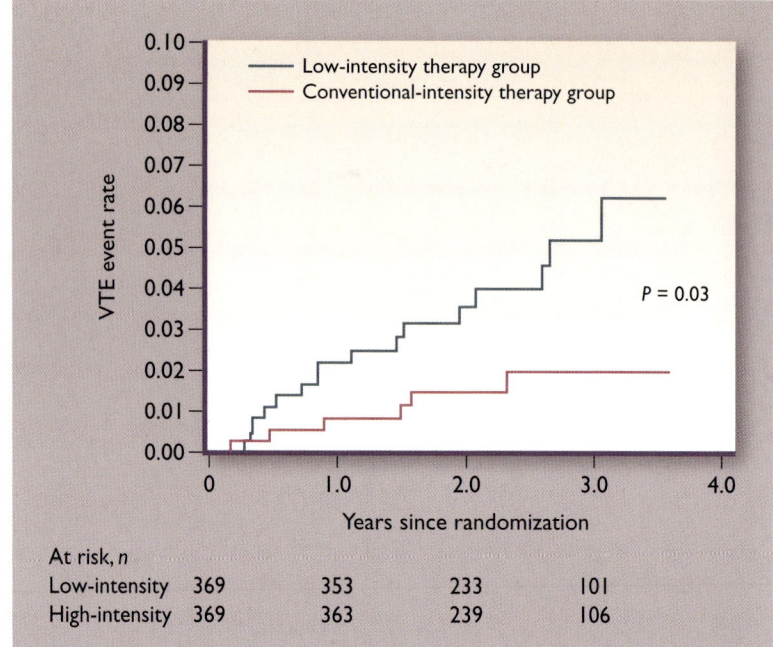

Figure 17-27. Indefinite-duration, low-intensity oral anticoagulation. In Prevention of Recurrent Venous Thromboembolism (PREVENT) [7], a double-blind, randomized, controlled trial of idiopathic venous thromboembolism (VTE) patients who had completed an average of 6 months of full-intensity warfarin, and then low-intensity warfarin (target international normalized ratio [INR] of 1.5–2.0) for an average of 2 years, patients' recurrence rate was reduced by two thirds. Patients required INR testing only once every 8 weeks. The strategy of long-term low-intensity warfarin was highly effective in preventing recurrence in all subgroups, even those with factor V Leiden or the prothrombin gene mutation.

Figure 17-28. Indefinite-duration, full-intensity oral anticoagulation. In the Extended Low-Intensity Anticoagulation for Thrombo-Embolism Investigators (ELATE) study of 739 patients with idiopathic venous thromboembolism (VTE) who had completed an average of 6 months of full-intensity warfarin, indefinite-duration full-intensity warfarin (target international normalized ratio [INR] 2–3) was more effective and was as safe as indefinite-duration low-intensity warfarin therapy (target INR 1.5–1.9) [8].

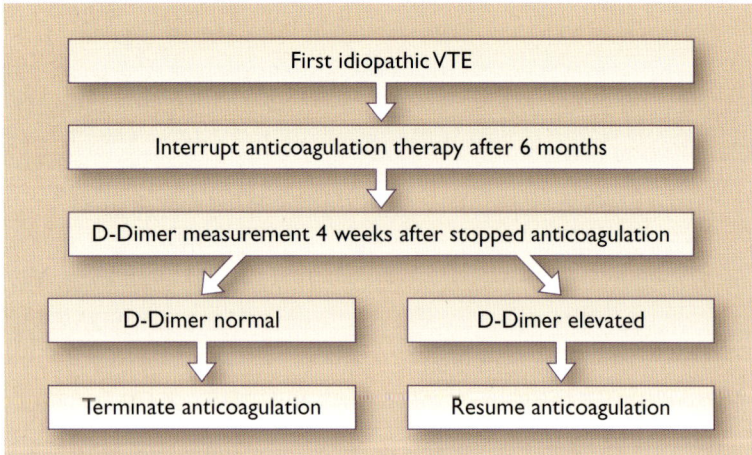

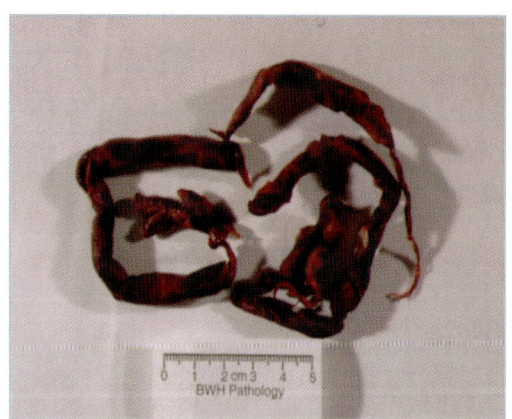

Figure 17-29. Duration of anticoagulant therapy: guidance with D-dimer levels. D-dimer testing is an established method for excluding pulmonary embolism and may also be useful for deciding the duration of anticoagulation in patients with a first unprovoked venous thromboembolic event. With this strategy, anticoagulation therapy is administered for the duration of 6 months. D-dimer testing is then performed 4 weeks after stopped anticoagulation. If the D-dimer level is low, then anticoagulation therapy is terminated. If the D-dimer level is elevated, then anticoagulation therapy is resumed.

In a randomized controlled study of 608 patients with a first event of idiopathic venous thromboembolism (VTE), the recurrence rate was 15.0% in the patients with abnormal D-dimer levels randomized to terminate anticoagulation, 2.9% in patients with abnormal D-dimer levels randomized to resume anticoagulation, and 6.2% in patients with normal D-dimer levels and stopped anticoagulation [36]. The proposed strategy needs confirmation in a larger trial.

Figure 17-30. Surgical embolectomy. Extensive thrombi were removed during surgical embolectomy in a patient with acute massive pulmonary embolism (PE).

Surgical embolectomy in massive PE is indicated in the setting of 1) a high bleeding risk from thrombolysis, 2) failed thrombolysis, 3) the presence of large right heart thrombi, or 4) an atrial septal defect with or without paradoxic embolism. In a cohort study of 29 patients presenting with massive PE, the survival rate after emergency embolectomy was 89% [37]. In a recent meta-analysis of 1300 reported pulmonary embolectomy cases, the mortality rate was 30% [38].

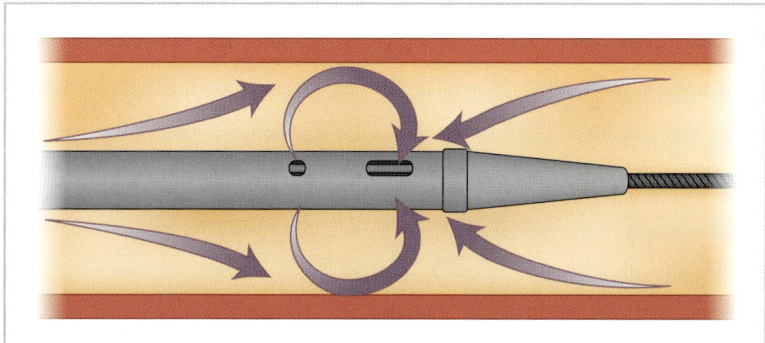
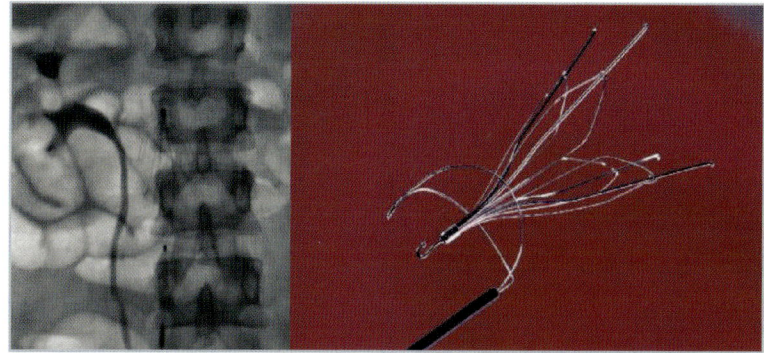

Figure 17-31. Catheter embolectomy in pulmonary embolism. Interventional thrombus fragmentation with or without embolectomy is an alternative to surgical embolectomy [39]. Successful interventions have been performed using suction devices (Greenfield catheter) [40], a pigtail rotational catheter [41], a high-speed impeller rotational device (Amplatz; Microvena, White Bear Lake, MN) [42], and rheolytic catheters [43]. The AngioJet thrombectomy catheter (Possis Medical; Minneapolis, MN) is shown here; it achieves clot fragmentation and embolectomy via a high-pressure saline injection (Venturi effect). The clinical outcome of catheter embolectomy may be comparable to the clinical outcome of surgical embolectomy. In a meta-analysis of more than 300 reported catheter intervention cases, the mortality rate ranged between 0% and 25% [44]. The efficacy of catheter techniques for improving hemodynamic parameters and clinical outcomes is difficult to assess because adjunctive local or systemic thrombolytic therapy was administered in the majority of the reported patients.

Figure 17-32. Vena cava interruption. The two principal indications for vena caval filter placement are major contraindications to anticoagulation and recurrent embolism, despite adequate therapy. There was an extraordinarily high rate (24%) of vena caval filter use for secondary prevention in patients with pulmonary embolism in a large prospective registry [6]. Filters are not recommended in the absence of clear indications because patients with filters are more than twice as likely as those without filters to require rehospitalization for deep vein thrombosis (DVT) due to formation of thrombi proximal to the filter or on the proximal tip of the filter [45].

Temporary filters have been placed in individuals deemed at extremely high risk for DVT yet unable to receive anticoagulant prophylaxis, such as certain trauma patients [46]. Retrievable filters, such as the Guenther vena cava retrievable filter (Cook; Bloomington, IN) shown in the figure, can be removed within 2 weeks after placement, or can remain permanently if necessary.

PREVENTION OF VENOUS THROMBOEMBOLISM

Prevention of Venous Thromboembolism	
Indication	**Prophylaxis Strategy**
General surgery	Enoxaparin, 40 mg qd Dalteparin, 2500 or 5000 U qd Unfractionated heparin, 5000 U bid/tid
Total hip/knee replacement	Enoxaparin, 40 mg qd Fondaparinux, 2.5 mg qd Warfarin (for hip replacement only)
Neurosurgery	Graduated compression stockings and intermittent pneumatic compression PLUS unfractionated heparin, 5000 U bid, or enoxaparin, 40 mg qd, PLUS predischarge venous ultrasound in patients with brain tumor
Trauma (not brain)	Enoxaparin, 40 mg qd
Thoracic surgery	Graduated compression stockings, intermittent pneumatic compression, and unfractionated heparin, 5000 U tid
Medical patients	Unfractionated heparin, 5000 U subcutaneously tid Graduated compression stockings and/or intermittent pneumatic compression Enoxaparin, 40 mg qd Dalteparin, 5000 U qd

Figure 17-33. Pharmacologic and mechanical measures. bid—twice daily; qd—once daily; tid—three times daily.

REFERENCES

1. Goldhaber SZ, Elliot CG: Acute pulmonary embolism: part I. epidemiology, pathophysiology, and diagnosis. *Circulation* 2003, 108:2726–2729.
2. White RH: The epidemiology of venous thromboembolism. *Circulation* 2003, 107(Suppl 1):4–8.
3. Horlander KT, Mannino DM, Leeper KV: Pulmonary embolism mortality in the United States, 1979–1998: an analysis using multiple-cause mortality data. *Arch Intern Med* 2003, 163:1711–1717.
4. Goldhaber SZ, Visani L, De Rosa M: Acute pulmonary embolism: clinical outcomes in the International Cooperative Pulmonary Embolism Registry (ICOPER). *Lancet* 1999, 353:1386–1389.

5. Lindblad B, Eriksson A, Bergquist D: Autopsy-verified pulmonary embolism in a surgical department: analysis of the period from 1951 to 1988. Br J Surg 1991, 78:849–852.

6. Goldhaber SZ, Tapson VF: A prospective registry of 5451 patients with confirmed deep vein thrombosis. Am J Cardiol 2004, 93:259–262.

7. Ridker PM, Goldhaber SZ, Danielson E, et al.: Long-term, low-intensity warfarin therapy for the prevention of recurrent venous thromboembolism. N Engl J Med 2003, 348:1425–1434.

8. Kearon C, Ginsberg JS, Kovacs MJ, et al.: Comparison of low-intensity warfarin therapy with conventional-intensity warfarin therapy for long-term prevention of recurrent venous thromboembolism. N Engl J Med 2003, 349:631–639.

9. Buller HR, Davidson BL, Decousus H, et al.: Subcutaneous fondaparinux versus intravenous unfractionated heparin in the initial treatment of pulmonary embolism. N Engl J Med 2003, 349:1695–1702.

10. Oger E. Incidence of venous thromboembolism: a community-based study in Western France. EPI-GETBP Study Group. Groupe d'Etude de la Thrombose de Bretagne Occidentale. Thromb Haemost 2000, 83:657–660.

11. Tsai AW, Cushman M, Rosamond WD, et al.: Cardiovascular risk factors and venous thromboembolism incidence: the longitudinal investigation of thromboembolism etiology. Arch Intern Med 2002, 162:1182–1189.

12. Heit JA, Silverstein MD, Mohr DN, et al.: Predictors of survival after deep vein thrombosis and pulmonary embolism: a population-based cohort study. Arch Intern Med 1999, 159:445–453.

13. Joffe HV, Kucher N, Tapson VF, Goldhaber SZ: Upper-extremity deep vein thrombosis: a prospective registry of 592 patients. Circulation 2004, 110:1605–1611.

14. Lapostolle F, Surget V, Borron SW, et al.: Severe pulmonary embolism associated with air travel. N Engl J Med 2001, 345:779–783.

15. Ridker PM, Hennekens CH, Lindpaintner K, et al.: Mutation in the gene coding for coagulation factor V and the risk of myocardial infarction, stroke, and venous thrombosis in apparently healthy men. N Engl J Med 1995, 332:912–917.

16. Hillarp A, Zoller B, Svensson PJ, Dahlback B: The 20210A of the prothrombin gene is a common risk factor among Swedish outpatients with verified deep venous thrombosis. Thromb Haemost 1997, 78:990–992.

17. Ridker PM, Hennekens CH, Selhub J, et al.: Interrelation of hyperhomocysteinemia, factor V Leiden, and risk of future venous thromboembolism. Circulation 1997, 95:1777–1782.

18. Dunn KL, Wolf JP, Dorfman DM, et al.: Normal D-dimer levels in emergency department patients suspected of acute pulmonary embolism. J Am Coll Cardiol 2002, 40:1475–1478.

19. Kucher N, Walpoth N, Wustmann K, et al.: QR in V1—an ECG sign associated with right ventricular dysfunction and adverse clinical outcome in pulmonary embolism. Eur Heart J 2003, 24:1113–1119.

20. Perrier A, Howarth N, Didier D, et al.: Performance of helical computed tomography in unselected outpatients with suspected pulmonary embolism. Ann Intern Med 2001, 135:88–97.

21. Schoepf UJ, Goldhaber SZ, Costello P: Spiral computed tomography for acute pulmonary embolism. Circulation 2004, 109:2160–2167.

22. Schoepf UJ, Holzknecht N, Helmberger TK, et al.: Subsegmental pulmonary emboli: improved detection with thin-collimation multi-detector row spiral CT. Radiology 2002, 222:483–490.

23. Simonneau G, Sors H, Charbonnier B, et al.: A comparison of low-molecular-weight heparin with unfractionated heparin for acute pulmonary embolism. N Engl J Med 1997, 337:663–669.

24. The Columbus Investigators: Low-molecular-weight heparin in the treatment of patients with venous thromboembolism. N Engl J Med 1997, 337:657–662.

25. Lassen MR, Bauer KA, Eriksson BI, Turpie AG: Postoperative fondaparinux versus preoperative enoxaparin for prevention of venous thromboembolism in elective hip-replacement surgery: a randomised double-blind comparison. Lancet 2002, 359:1715–1720.

26. Agnelli G, Gallus A, Goldhaber SZ, et al.: Treatment of proximal deep-vein thrombosis with the oral direct factor Xa inhibitor rivaroxaban (BAY 59-7939): the ODIXa-DVT (Oral Direct Factor Xa Inhibitor BAY 59-7939 in Patients With Acute Symptomatic Deep-Vein Thrombosis) study. Circulation 2007, 116:180-187.

27. Goldhaber SZ: Echocardiography in the management of pulmonary embolism. Ann Intern Med 2002, 136:691–700.

28. Konstantinides S, Geibel A, Olschewski M, et al.: Importance of cardiac troponins I and T in risk stratification of patients with acute pulmonary embolism. Circulation 2002, 106:1263–1268.

29. Kucher N, Wallmann D, Windecker S, et al.: Incremental prognostic value of troponin I and echocardiography in patients with acute pulmonary embolism. Eur Heart J 2003, 24:1651–1656.

30. Kucher N, Printzen G, Doernhoefer T, et al.: Low pro-brain natriuretic peptide levels predict benign clinical outcome in acute pulmonary embolism. Circulation 2003, 107:1576–1578.

31. ten Wolde M, Tulevski II, Mulder JW, et al.: Brain natriuretic peptide as a predictor of adverse outcome in patients with pulmonary embolism. Circulation 2003, 107:2082–2084.

32. Kucher N, Printzen G, Goldhaber SZ: Prognostic role of brain natriuretic peptide in acute pulmonary embolism. Circulation 2003, 107:2545–2547.

33. Kucher N, Goldhaber SZ: Cardiac biomarkers for risk stratification of patients with acute pulmonary embolism. Circulation 2003, 108:2191–2194.

34. Konstantinides S, Geibel A, Heusel G, et al.: Heparin plus alteplase compared with heparin alone in patients with submassive pulmonary embolism. N Engl J Med 2002, 347:1143–1150.

35. Thabut G, Thabut D, Myers RP, et al.: Thrombolytic therapy of pulmonary embolism: a meta-analysis. J Am Coll Cardiol 2002, 40:1660–1667.

36. Palareti G, Cosmi B, Legnani B, et al.: D-dimer testing to determine the duration of anticoagulation therapy. N Engl J Med 2006, 355:1780–1789.

37. Aklog L, Williams CS, Byrne JG, Goldhaber SZ: Acute pulmonary embolectomy: a contemporary approach. Circulation 2002, 105:1416–1419.

38. Stein PD, Alnas M, Beemath A, et al.: Pulmonary embolectomy. Am J Cardiol 2007, 99:421–423.

39. Goldhaber SZ: Integration of catheter thrombectomy into our armamentarium to treat acute pulmonary embolism. Chest 1998, 114:1237–1238.

40. Greenfield LJ, Proctor MC, Williams DM, et al.: Long-term experience with transvenous catheter pulmonary embolectomy. J Vasc Surg 1993, 18:450–458.

41. Schmitz-Rode T, Janssens U, Duda SH, et al.: Massive pulmonary embolism: percutaneous emergency treatment by pigtail rotation catheter. J Am Coll Cardiol 2000, 36:375-380.

42. Uflacker R, Strange C, Vujic I: Massive pulmonary embolism: preliminary results in treatment with the Amplatz thrombectomy device. J Vasc Interv Radiol 1996, 7:519-528.

43. Koning R, Cribier A, Gerber L, et al.: A new treatment for pulmonary embolism: percutaneous rheolytic thrombectomy. Circulation 1997, 96:2498–2500.

44. Skaf E, Beemath A, Siddiqui T, et al.: Catheter-tip embolectomy in the management of acute pulmonary embolism. Am J Cardiol 2007, 99:415–420.

45. White RH, Zhou H, Kim J, Romano PS: A population-based study of the effectiveness of inferior vena cava filter use among patients with venous thromboembolism. Arch Intern Med 2000, 160:2033–2041.

46. Offner PJ, Hawkes A, Madayag R, et al.: The role of temporary inferior vena cava filters in critically ill surgical patients. Arch Surg 2003, 138:591–594.

IDIOPATHIC PULMONARY ARTERIAL HYPERTENSION

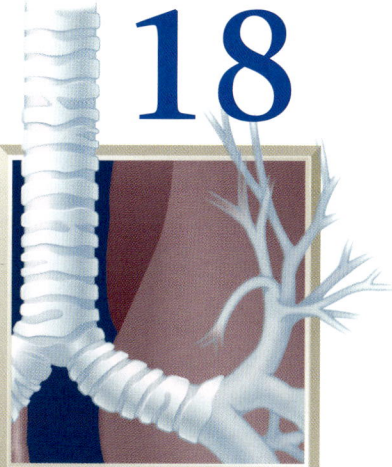

Victor F. Tapson and Jaspal Singh

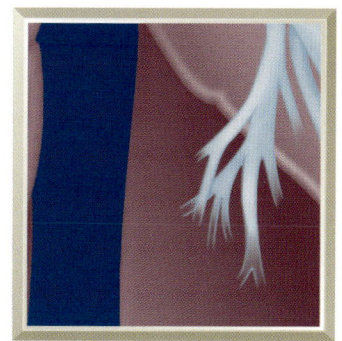

Idiopathic pulmonary arterial hypertension (IPAH) is a rare disease characterized by an unexplained elevation in pulmonary artery pressure. Since the description of the disease by Dresdale over a half-century ago, it has been characterized by a relentless progression to death from right ventricular failure [1]. However, over the past two decades, there have been considerable advances in our understanding of the pathology and pathogenesis of this disorder and commensurate advances in treatment [2,3].

IPAH is defined as a mean pulmonary artery pressure (mPAP) greater than 25 mm Hg at rest or 30 mm Hg with exercise in the absence of any cause identifiable in a thorough investigation [4]. This disorder is rare, with an incidence of approximately 1 to 2 per million per year when all possible causative factors are eliminated. The reported female-to-male ratio is 1.7:1 [4], although at many centers it appears to be at least 3:1. The mean age at diagnosis is 37 years [4,5]; however, the age range of affected individuals may be increasing, perhaps because of improved longevity from advances in therapy [6].

Pathologic findings in IPAH have been reported in pulmonary arterial, capillary, and venous circulation [7,8]. Although lung biopsy is rarely performed in pulmonary arterial hypertension (PAH), specific patterns may have therapeutic relevance because epoprostenol use in pulmonary veno-occlusive disease has been associated with the development of fatal pulmonary edema [9]. IPAH is primarily an arteriopathy with four types of lesions described: isolated medial hypertrophy, plexiform lesions, thrombotic pulmonary arteriopathy, and isolated pulmonary arteritis [7]. Although the plexiform lesion was once considered pathognomonic of IPAH, it is recognized that these lesions are seen in other forms of PAH and that IPAH can be diagnosed in its absence.

As with other causes of severe PAH, the most frequent symptoms in this disease are dyspnea and fatigue, and the physical findings are those of pulmonary hypertension and right heart failure. A loud P2 and tricuspid murmur are typical, and a pulmonic insufficiency murmur may be present when pressures are more severely elevated. The nonspecific nature of the symptoms and the absence of right ventricular failure until late in the disease likely account for the mean delay of 2 years from symptom onset to diagnosis [3,4].

The diagnostic evaluation focuses on the exclusion of other potential causes of pulmonary hypertension primarily underlying cardiopulmonary disease. Chest radiography, pulmonary function testing, arterial blood gas determination, and echocardiography should be performed. Although chest CT is generally more useful in characterizing pulmonary parenchymal disease, ventilation–perfusion scanning is more sensitive in detecting potential chronic thromboembolic pulmonary hypertension (CTEPH). CT may show specific findings of CTEPH; many pulmonary hypertension specialists order both examinations. If the ventilation–perfusion scan is high probability, or the CT suggests CTEPH, standard pulmonary arteriography is still the most appropriate conformational test. This disease is crucial to rule out, because it is potentially curable surgically. Although electrocardiography is commonly performed in suspected pulmonary hypertension, it almost never changes the diagnostic or therapeutic plan and may not even suggest pulmonary hypertension [10].

Extensive laboratory studies are initially ordered, because liver disease, HIV, and connective tissue disease may be implicated in the cause of pulmonary hypertension. Polysomnography may be ordered if obesity, snoring, daytime hypersomnolence, or hypercapnia suggest a need. The presence and severity of pulmonary hypertension is usually first documented noninvasively by two-dimensional echocardiography, offering an estimate of the right ventricular systolic pressure as well as the size and function of the right ventricle. Finally, 6-minute distance walked aids in both prognostication and treatment.

Right heart catheterization remains the gold standard for establishing the presence of pulmonary hypertension and determining its severity. Cardiac catheterization provides diagnostic, therapeutic, and prognostic information. An elevated pulmonary capillary wedge pressure may reflect pulmonary venous hypertension and thus suggest that pulmonary hypertension is caused by underlying left-sided cardiac disease. If an adequate wedge pressure tracing cannot be obtained, the left ventricular end-diastolic pressure should be measured. Pulmonary artery pressure, right atrial pressure, and cardiac index quantify disease severity; the last two have particular implications for anticipated mortality. A vasodilator trial should be considered at the time of initial cardiac catheterization. Intravenous epoprostenol or adenosine or inhaled nitric oxide are commonly used for this purpose. The consensus definition of a positive vasodilator response is a reduction of mPAP by at least 10 mm Hg to a value of 40 mm Hg or less; patients with this response are most likely to have a beneficial hemodynamic and clinical response to treatment with calcium channel blockers [11,12]. Although it has been suggested that approximately 20% of patients may be responders, the response rate appears to be even lower [11–13]. Patients in whom calcium channel blockers would not be considered as therapy, such as those with functional class IV symptoms, overt right heart failure, or advanced hemodynamics (markedly elevated right atrial pressure or reduced cardiac index), are unlikely to benefit from vasodilator testing.

Certain supportive therapy should be considered in patients with IPAH. Because of the development of in situ thrombi, most experts agree that all patients without contraindications should receive anticoagulant therapy. Two studies suggest that warfarin improves survival [5,12]. Although IPAH patients are often anticoagulated with a target international normalized ratio of about 1.5 to 2.5 (less than for other anticoagulant indications), no prospective, randomized, clinical trials have identified a clearly superior target value. Symptomatic right ventricular failure is addressed with diuretic therapy. Oxygen is prescribed in patients with an oxygen saturation of less than 90%. As with other cardiopulmonary diseases, oxygen with exercise and at night often precedes the need for full-time oxygen. Digoxin is prescribed by some specialists for some patients with concomitant right ventricular failure based upon favorable hemodynamic data [14], but no randomized trials have been conducted that support long-term efficacy and safety.

Research over the past 20 years has led to the development of other therapeutic modalities. The most aggressive and effective form of therapy for patients with advanced IPAH is continuous intravenous prostacyclin. Patients having World Health Organization functional class III or IV symptoms despite maximal therapy may be considered for this approach. Epoprostenol appears to improve survival both in "responders" and in nonvasodilator responders [15–16]. Another prostacyclin, treprostinil, is also FDA approved; this drug can be administered by either the continuous subcutaneous or the intravenous route in patients with PAH and class II–IV symptoms [17–19]. Pain at the subcutaneous infusion site has proven to be a limitation in some patients when the drug is administered by this route. Iloprost, a prostacyclin delivered by inhalation six to nine times daily, is approved for use and is effective in IPAH, with symptomatic and hemodynamic benefits, although it is inconvenient [20].

The development and incorporation of endothelin antagonists into the PAH armamentarium has had a substantial impact on the approach to treating this disease. Two oral endothelin receptor antagonists, bosentan and (most recently) ambrisentan, are FDA approved for patients with IPAH and PAH caused by underlying connective tissue disease. Symptomatic improvement in 6-minute walk and hemodynamic benefits have been demonstrated for both drugs [21–23]. Bosentan, a nonselective endothelin antagonist, also has favorable 1-year follow-up hemodynamic and exercise data [24] and survival data [25]. Ambrisentan is an endothelin A receptor-specific drug; it is unclear if such receptor specificity offers advantages over dual receptor antagonism. Liver function testing must be monitored monthly in patients treated with either of these drugs; preliminary data suggest that the incidence of liver test abnormalities may be lower with ambrisentan [23]. The final class of drugs approved for use in PAH is the phosphodiesterase-5 inhibitor class; sildenafil has proven effective in a large, prospective, placebo-controlled trial, with improvement in 6-minute-walk distance and hemodynamics [26]. Recent data indicate that sildenafil is beneficial in patients already on epoprostenol [27]. Combination therapy with bosentan and epoprostenol and with inhaled iloprost and bosentan also appear promising [28,29]. Overall, the choice of therapy for IPAH depends upon the severity of the disease and is best made by physicians experienced in the treatment of PAH. A recent update to the American College of Chest Physicians's recommendations for therapy has recently been published [30]. Case reports suggest that other classes of drugs, such as tyrosine kinase inhibitors, may offer benefits, particularly in cases of IPAH that are refractory to approved, aggressive therapy regimens [31,32].

When patients fail pharmacologic therapy, lung or heart-lung transplantation can be considered. As with other end-stage cardiopulmonary disease candidates for transplantation, IPAH patients must meet age, weight, and renal function criteria and be screened thoroughly at a center performing the procedures. Atrial septostomy is best considered a bridge to transplantation and is only performed by clinicians who have significant experience with the procedure. This offers the possibility of improvement in right ventricular function at the expense of compromised oxygenation [33].

Patients diagnosed with IPAH must be cautious when exercising. Although no clinical trials indicate the safest, most ideal exercise regimen, physical activity is encouraged in all patients capable of engaging in it. Walking or stationary bicycle riding are perhaps the most appropriate forms. Exercise should be immediately ceased upon the onset of lightheadedness, dizziness, or extreme dyspnea. Weight lifting and other isometric exercises should be avoided. High-altitude travel and unpressurized airplane cabins should be avoided. The hemodynamic changes of pregnancy are not well tolerated by patients with IPAH, and peripartum and postpartum deaths have been reported. Although effective birth control is important, oral contraceptives should be avoided, if possible, because of their potential prothrombotic properties. Appropriate anticoagulation is expected to lower this risk, however.

Based upon the National Institutes of Health registry, without treatment, the median survival for IPAH was 2.8 years from the time of diagnosis, with survival rates of 68%, 48%, and 34% at 1, 3, and 5 years, respectively [34]. In the epoprostenol era, observed survival with epoprostenol therapy at 1, 2, and 3 years has been shown to be 87.8%, 76.3%, and 62.8% [35]. Therapeutic advances continue.

CLASSIFICATION

Revised Clinical Classification of Pulmonary Hypertension

1. Pulmonary arterial hypertension
   1.1. Idiopathic
   1.2. Familial
   1.3. Associated with
      1.3.1. Connective tissue disease
      1.3.2. Congenital systemic-to-pulmonary shunts
      1.3.3. Portal hypertension
      1.3.4. HIV infection
      1.3.5. Drugs and toxins
      1.3.6. Other (thyroid disorders, glycogen storage disease, Gaucher disease, hereditary hemorrhagic telangiectasia, hemoglobinopathies, myeloproliferative disorders, splenectomy)
   1.4. Associated with significant venous or capillary involvement
      1.4.1. Pulmonary veno-occlusive disease
      1.4.2. Pulmonary capillary hemangiomatosis
   1.5. Persistent pulmonary hypertension of the newborn
2. Pulmonary hypertension with left heart disease
   2.1. Left-sided atrial or ventricular heart disease
   2.2. Left-sided valvular heart disease
3. Pulmonary hypertension associated with lung diseases and/or hypoxemia
   3.1. Chronic obstructive pulmonary disease
   3.2. Interstitial lung disease
   3.3. Sleep disordered breathing
   3.4. Alveolar hypoventilation disorders
   3.5. Chronic exposure to high altitude
   3.6. Developmental abnormalities
4. Pulmonary hypertension caused by chronic thrombotic and/or embolic disease
   4.1. Thromboembolic obstruction of proximal pulmonary arteries
   4.2. Thromboembolic obstruction of distal pulmonary arteries
   4.3. Nonthrombotic pulmonary embolism (tumor, parasites, foreign material)
5. Miscellaneous: sarcoidosis, histiocytosis X, lymphangiomatosis, compression of pulmonary vessels (adenopathy, tumor, fibrosing mediastinitis)

Figure 18-1. Classification of pulmonary hypertension. In 1998, the World Health Organization World Symposium on Primary Pulmonary Hypertension took place in Evian, France, and significant changes to the nomenclature and pathologic classification of pulmonary hypertension were made [36]. Subsequently, a modification to this classification (here presented) was developed at the Third World Symposium on Pulmonary Arterial Hypertension in Venice, Italy, in June 2003, and subsequently published [37].

Pathologic Classification of Pulmonary Vascular Disease

Vasculature
  Vessels
    Arteries
    Capillaries
    Veins
    Lymphatics
    Bronchial vessels
  Components
    Intima
    Media
    Adventitia
    Complex vascular lesions
    Inflammatory cells
    Quantification

Lung tissue
  Components
    Airway
    Alveoli
    Interstitium
    Pleura

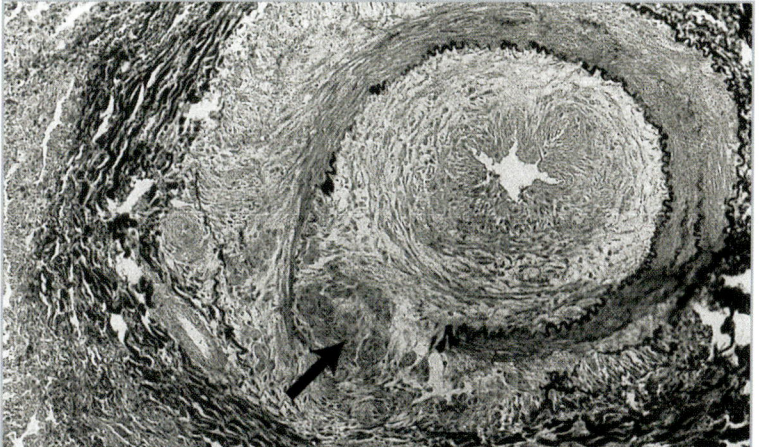

Figure 18-2. Pathologic classification of pulmonary hypertension. The pathologic classification adopted by the World Health Organization shifts the focus from a graded classification method to a descriptive system in which the structures listed in this figure are described comprehensively. It is recommended that the percentage of abnormal vessels and the changes in cellular components, pattern (*ie*, eccentric, concentric), and matrix be made explicit. In addition, the occurrence of complex vascular lesions, such as plexiform lesions, and the presence and location of inflammatory cells should be detailed. Although the entire pulmonary circulation—from artery to vein—may be involved in idiopathic pulmonary arterial hypertension (IPAH), most patients have an arteriopathy. No diagnostic histologic lesions are unique to IPAH [7,8].

Figure 18-3. The plexiform lesion. Pathologic lesions in idiopathic pulmonary arterial hypertension (IPAH) have been reported in pulmonary arterial, capillary, and venous circulation. However, IPAH is primarily an arteriopathy with four reported lesions: plexiform lesions, isolated medial hypertrophy, thrombotic pulmonary arteriopathy, and isolated pulmonary arteritis. The plexiform lesions in IPAH, unlike those seen in pulmonary hypertension related to other conditions, represent monoclonal endothelial cell expansion. This monoclonal cell growth may be a consequence of abnormal growth or of apoptosis gene expression in endothelial cells [38,39]. The *arrow* points to an early plexiform lesion. (*Adapted from* Pietra [7].)

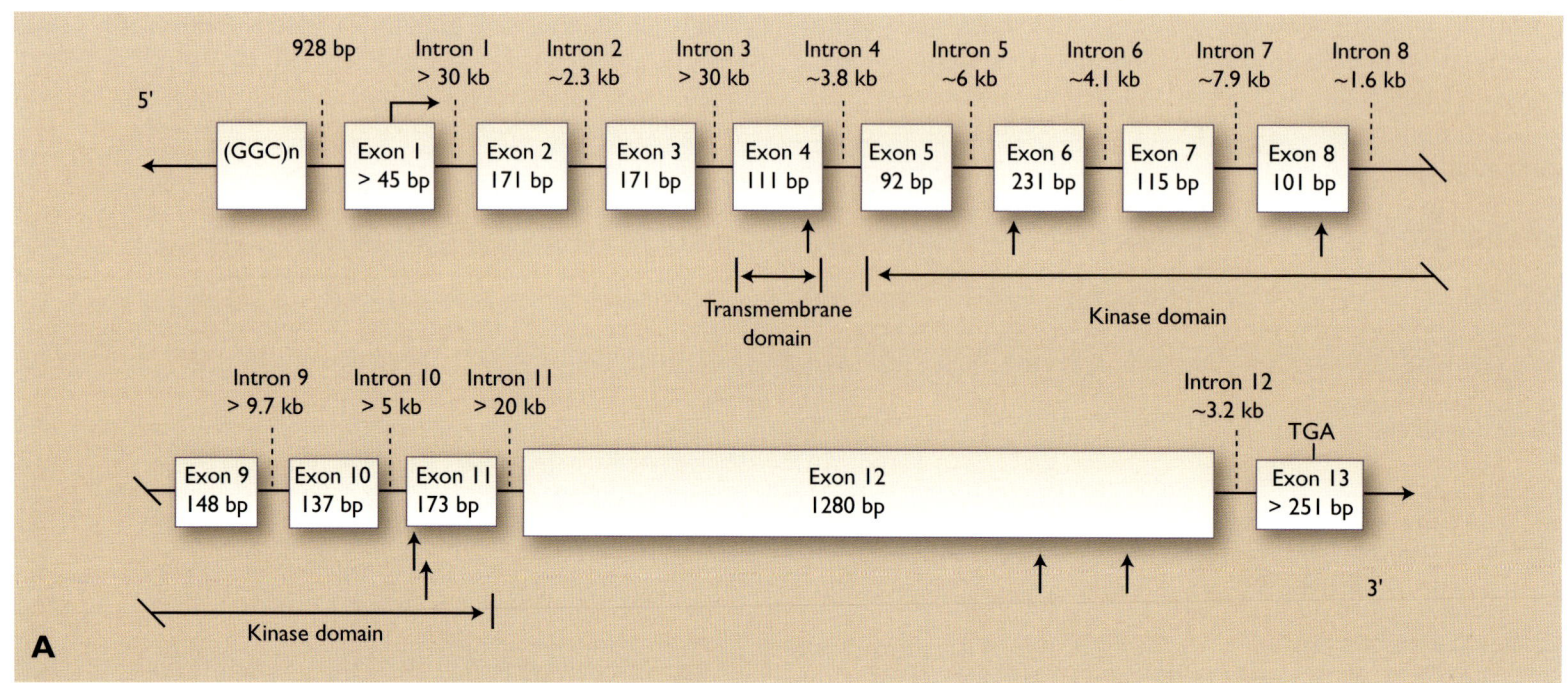

Figure 18-4. Genetics of idiopathic pulmonary arterial hypertension. Idiopathic pulmonary arterial hypertension (IPAH) occurs in familial and sporadic forms. At least 6% of patients in the National Institutes of Health registry had one or more family members affected with IPAH. Familial IPAH is an autosomal-dominant disease with incomplete penetrance and genetic anticipation. It has been mapped to locus *PPH1* on chromosome 2q33. Familial IPAH results from mutations in *BMPR2*, which encodes for a transforming growth factor-b type II receptor, bone morphogenetic protein receptor type II. The sporadic form of the disease is associated with similar mutations in more than 25% of cases [40–42]. **A,** Intron/exon structure of the human *BMPR2* gene with sizes as indicated. *Filled arrows* indicate mutation sites that cause premature termination of *BMPR2*; *unfilled arrows* denote mutations in exon 11 resulting in a change in the amino acid sequence. **B,** Resulting DNA sequence variations from mutations. (*Adapted from* Deng et al. [41].)

Resulting DNA Sequence Variations from Mutations

Family	Exon	DNA Sequence Variation
PPH001, 008, 021	11	1471 → T
PPH010	8	1099-1103delGGGGA
PPH015	12	2579delT
PPH017	4	507-410delCTTTinsAAA
PPH018	12	2617C → T
PPH019	11	1472G → A
PPH022	6	690-691delAinsT

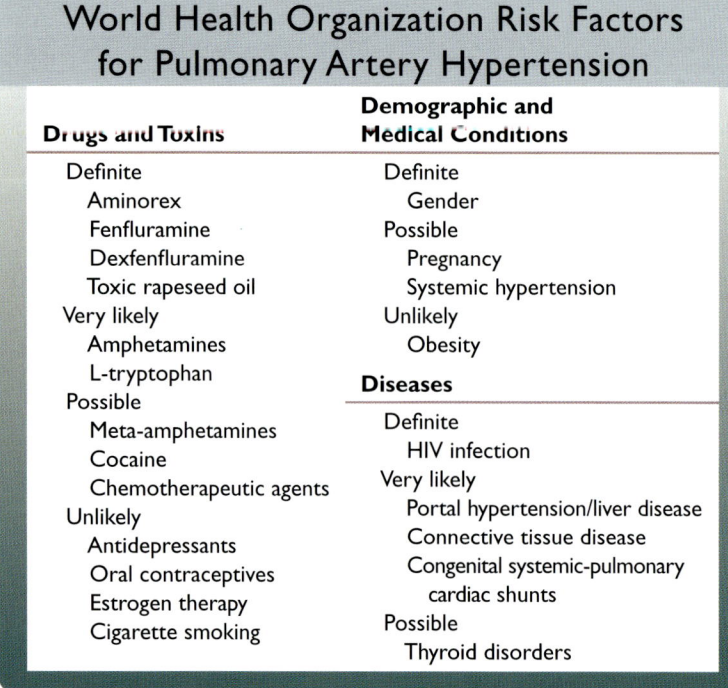

World Health Organization Risk Factors for Pulmonary Artery Hypertension

Drugs and Toxins	Demographic and Medical Conditions
Definite	Definite
Aminorex	Gender
Fenfluramine	Possible
Dexfenfluramine	Pregnancy
Toxic rapeseed oil	Systemic hypertension
Very likely	Unlikely
Amphetamines	Obesity
L-tryptophan	**Diseases**
Possible	Definite
Meta-amphetamines	HIV infection
Cocaine	Very likely
Chemotherapeutic agents	Portal hypertension/liver disease
Unlikely	Connective tissue disease
Antidepressants	Congenital systemic-pulmonary
Oral contraceptives	cardiac shunts
Estrogen therapy	Possible
Cigarette smoking	Thyroid disorders

Figure 18-5. Risk factors for pulmonary arterial hypertension. Numerous agents and conditions have been suggested as having a causal or facilitating role in pulmonary arterial hypertension (PAH). Appetite suppressants in particular have been implicated in several outbreaks. Fenfluramine and dexfenfluramine may cause PAH through effects on potassium channels [43]. The mechanisms for many of the other listed conditions are unknown. It is likely that genetic susceptibility plays a major causal role in many, if not most, patients [40,41].

PATHOGENESIS

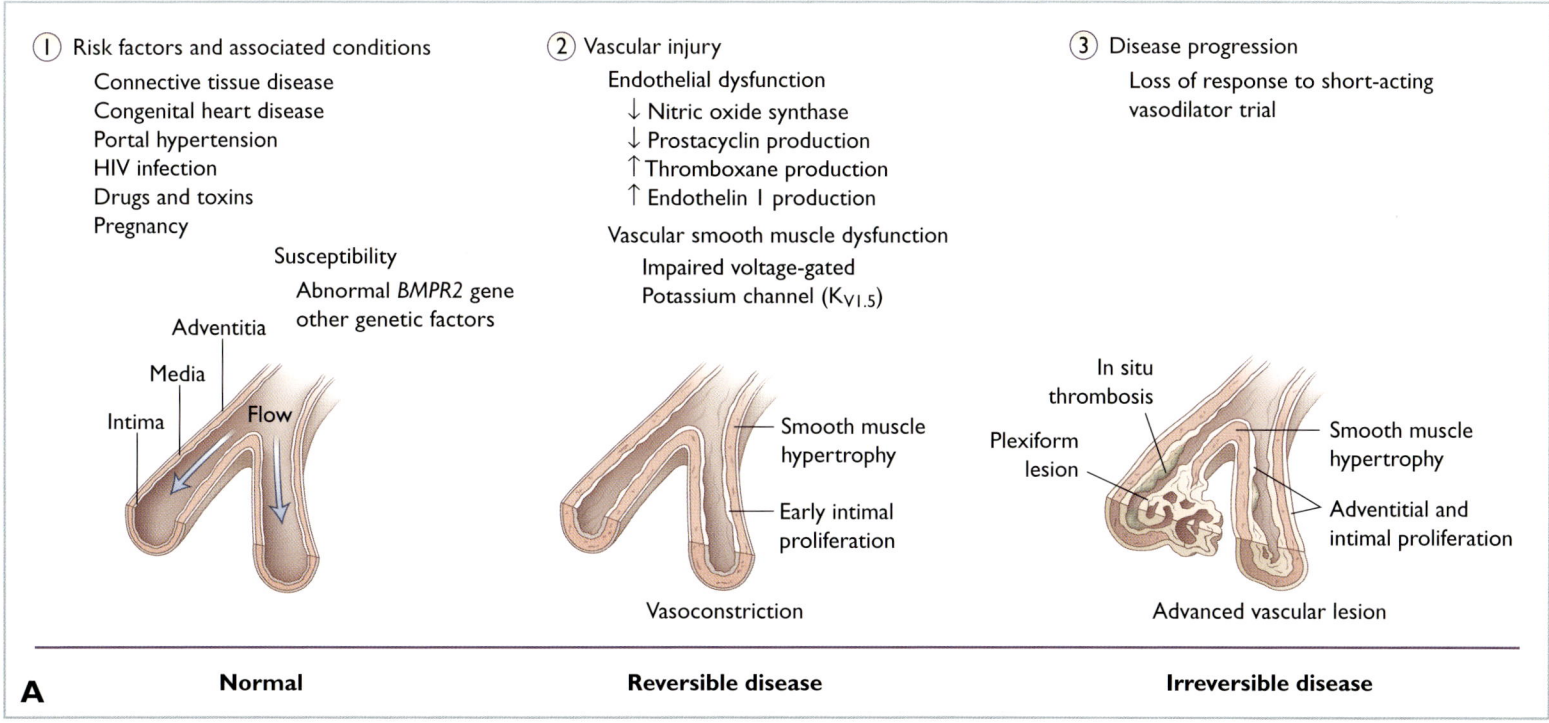

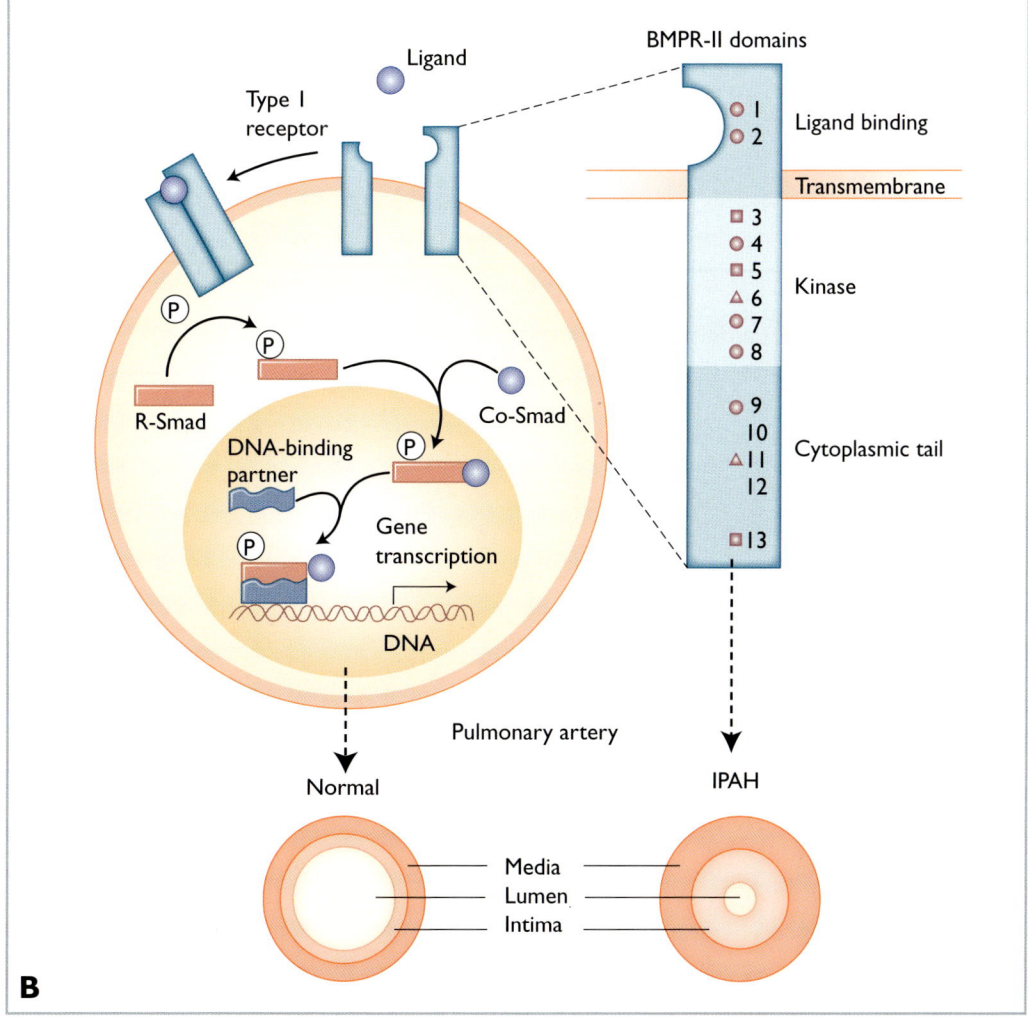

changes characteristic of this disorder. An alteration in the levels or actions of molecules that regulate pulmonary vascular tone and endothelial or smooth muscle cell growth may be involved. Increased vascular tone and vascular remodeling may be joined events responding to the same molecular signals. For example, factors responsible for enhanced vascular tone may also increase smooth muscle mitogenesis (eg, endothelin-1), and vasodilators may inhibit smooth muscle growth (eg, nitric oxide). An imbalance in the levels of these competing processes may contribute to the development of idiopathic pulmonary arterial hypertension (IPAH) [43–49]. **B,** The precise mechanism by which defects in the transforming growth factor-beta (TGF-β) signaling pathway lead to the vascular lesions characteristic of primary pulmonary hypertension are unclear. The TGF-β family of peptides regulates numerous cellular functions in many tissues; in vascular endothelial cells, one of their actions is growth inhibition. Loss of this inhibitory action confers a growth advantage with dysregulated cellular proliferation. In this pathway, a ligand binds to BMPR-II, which then forms a heteromeric complex with a type I receptor on the cell surface. The type II receptors activate the type I receptor serine kinases, which then causes the phosphorylation of a group of intracellular signal mediators called Smads. The Smad complex regulates transcription in target genes. The numbers 1 to 13 refer to mutation sites in BPMR-II [40–42,50]. (*Panel A adapted from* Gaine [44]; *panel B adapted from* Thomson et al. [40].)

Figure 18-6. The pathogenesis of idiopathic pulmonary arterial hypertension is not completely understood. **A,** Injury to the pulmonary vasculature (*eg,* from anorexigens, scleroderma, left-to-right cardiac shunts) in susceptible individuals seems to progress to the extreme pathologic

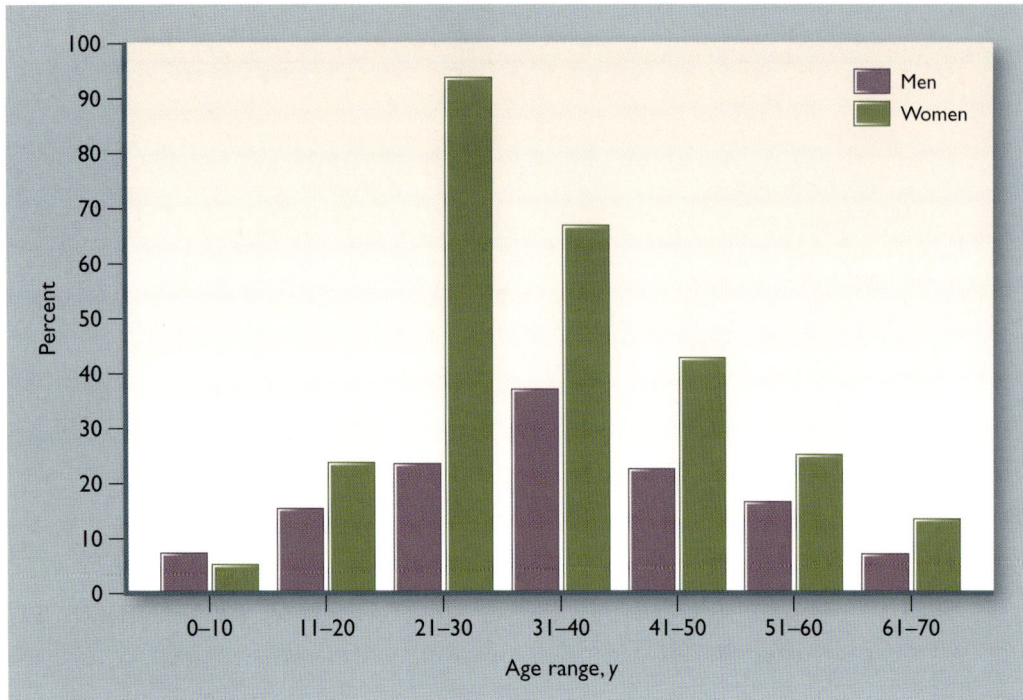

Figure 18-7. Patient distribution. Three large US reports show similar age and gender distributions for patients with idiopathic pulmonary arterial hypertension (PAH) [4,5]. The mean age at diagnosis ranged from 29.8 to 36.4 years. The National Institutes of Health patient registry reported a female-to-male ratio of 1.7:1 and a racial distribution similar to that of the general population [4,5]. The female-to-male ratio, however, appears higher than that reported above. A large PAH registry (REVEAL) is currently under way and will help in updating the demographics of PAH.

DIAGNOSIS

Symptoms in Patients with Idiopathic Pulmonary Arterial Hypertension

Symptom	Initial Symptoms, %	Symptoms Present at Diagnosis, %
Dyspnea	60	98
Fatigue	19	73
Syncope	8	36
Chest pain	7	47
Near syncope	5	41
Palpitations	5	33
Peripheral edema	3	37

Figure 18-8. Symptoms in patients with idiopathic pulmonary arterial hypertension. The most common reason patients with this disease seek medical advice is dyspnea, a nearly universal symptom as the disease progresses. The mechanism for this symptom is unclear. Near-syncope and syncope, often related to activity, result from inadequate cardiac output [3,4]. Other occasional complaints not listed here include cough, hoarseness, and hemoptysis. Seventy-five percent of female patients and 64% of male patients were in the New York Heart Association functional class III or IV on enrollment in the National Institutes of Health patient registry [4]. (*Data from* Rich *et al.* [4].)

Physical Findings in Patients with Idiopathic Pulmonary Arterial Hypertension

Findings	Patients, %
Increase in P2	93
Tricuspid regurgitation murmur	40
Right-sided S4	38
Peripheral edema	32
Right-sided S3	23
Cyanosis	20
Pulmonic insufficiency murmur	13

Figure 18-9. Physical findings in patients with idiopathic pulmonary arterial hypertension. The physical examination is nonspecific, revealing signs of pulmonary hypertension and right ventricular failure. In the National Institutes of Health study, the presence of an S3 gallop and tricuspid regurgitation were associated with an increase in right atrial pressure and a decrease in cardiac index; the finding of pulmonic valve insufficiency was associated with a higher mean pulmonary artery pressure [4]. The physical examination helps exclude secondary causes of pulmonary hypertension by an absence of crackles, wheezes, and clubbing. (*Data from* Rich *et al.* [4].)

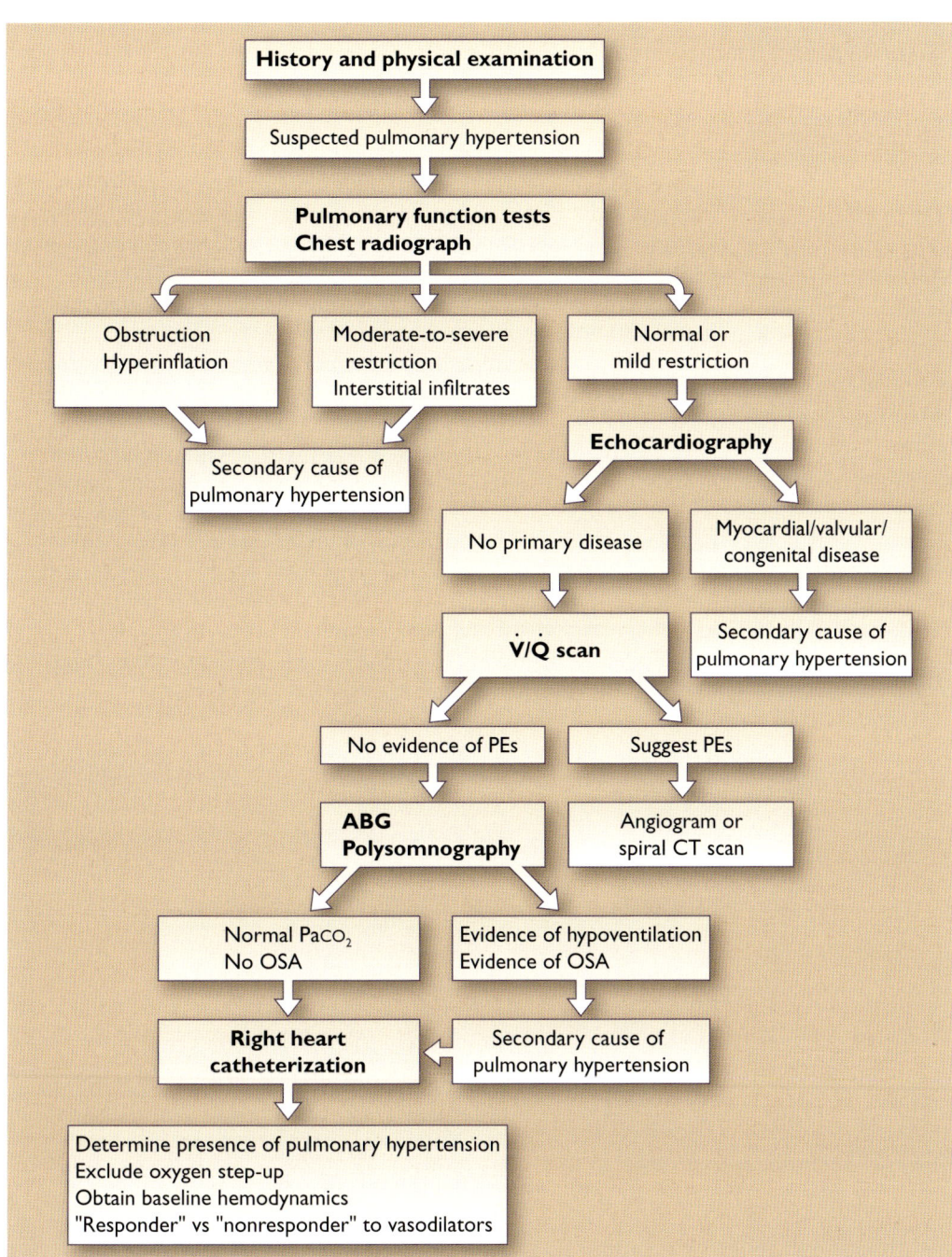

Figure 18-10. Diagnostic evaluation. Idiopathic pulmonary arterial hypertension is a diagnosis of exclusion arrived at through a series of studies. The exact order of tests is not as important as excluding underlying heart and lung disease. Echocardiography is the central noninvasive study when pulmonary hypertension is suspected because it can be used to estimate systolic pulmonary artery pressure and to exclude valvular and myocardial disease. If significant parenchymal lung disease is present, it is likely to be the cause of or a contributor to pulmonary hypertension. If the degree of pulmonary hypertension is disproportionate to the amount of lung disease present, the latter may not serve as a sufficient explanation of the former. Pulmonary artery catheterization is required to establish the diagnosis and to indicate its severity with certainty. ABG—arterial blood gases; OSA—obstructive sleep apnea; PE—pulmonary edema; V/Q—ventilation–perfusion.

Abnormal Findings in Common Tests for Patients with Idiopathic Pulmonary Arterial Hypertension

Chest radiograph	Prominent main pulmonary artery, enlarged hilar vessels, decreased peripheral vessels (pruning)
Pulmonary function tests	Mild restriction, decreased Dlco
Arterial blood gases	Hypoxemia, hypocarbia
Electrocardiogram	RAD, RVH
V/Q scan	Normal or small patchy abnormalities
Pulmonary arteriogram	Dilated proximal vessels, which taper rapidly; pruning of distal vessels
Doppler echocardiography	RAE, RVE+H, tricuspid regurgitation, pulmonary insufficiency, paradoxic septal motion, partial systolic closure of pulmonary valve
Exercise test	Decreased VO_2 max, high VE, low anaerobic threshold, decreased max O_2 pulse, increased A–a difference
Serology	ANA, anti-Ku antibodies

Figure 18-11. Abnormal findings in common tests for patients with idiopathic pulmonary arterial hypertension. The chest radiograph is abnormal in most patients, showing cardiac enlargement, prominent central vessels, and diminished peripheral vessels [4,5]. In chest radiographs of patients with veno-occlusive disease, basilar vascular markings and septal lines may be increased [51]. The concomitant presence of prominent main and hilar pulmonary vessels and decreased peripheral vessels is associated with a higher mean pulmonary artery pressure and a decreased cardiac index [4]. Pulmonary function studies are useful primarily for excluding obstructive or severe restrictive lung disease [4,10]. Exercise capacity correlates with pulmonary hemodynamics and may be used as an independent predictor of survival [14,52]. A–a—alveolar–arterial; ANA—antinuclear antibodies; Dl_{co}—diffusing capacity of lung for carbon monoxide; RAD—right access deviation; RAE—right arterial enlargement; RVE+H—right ventricular enlargement and hypertrophy; RVH—right ventricular hypertrophy; VE—minute ventilation; VO_2 max—maximum oxygen consumption; V/Q—ventilation–perfusion.

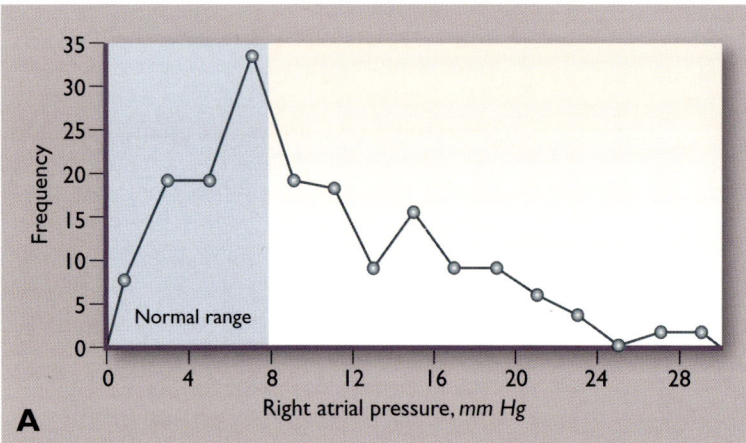
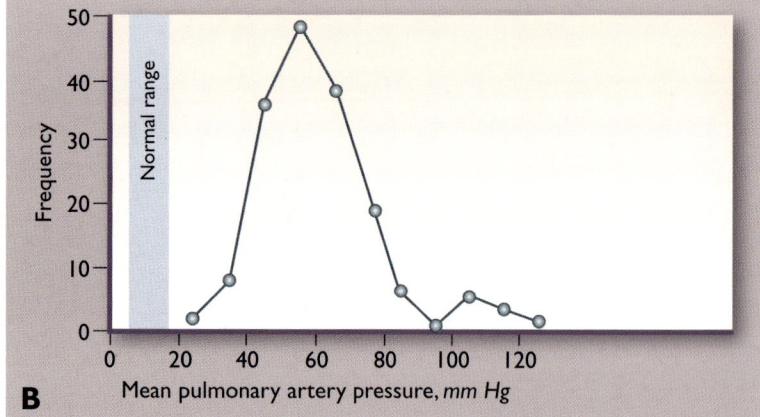
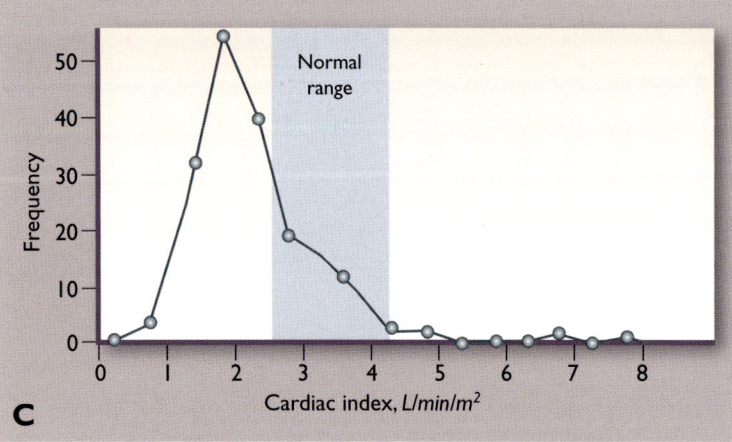
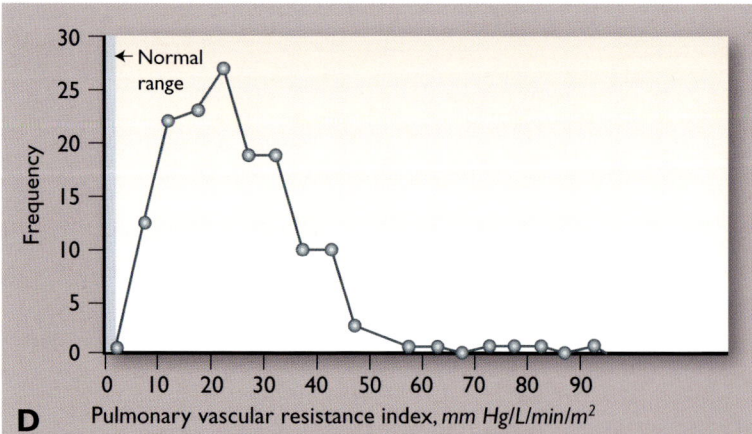

Figure 18-12. A–D, Hemodynamics. By the time patients are diagnosed with idiopathic pulmonary arterial hypertension, their hemodynamic variables are profoundly altered. The mean pulmonary artery pressure is elevated severalfold; higher pressures and right ventricular failure are associated with increasingly disabling symptoms and a worse prognosis [4,5,34]. In the National Institutes of Health registry, the pulmonary vascular resistance was increased 15-fold on average; on average the right atrial pressure was increased in 72% of patients, and the cardiac index was decreased in 71% of patients [4]. Although left-sided filling pressures are usually normal, profound dilation of the right ventricle can increase left ventricular filling pressures. In addition, the pulmonary capillary wedge pressure can be variable and can be elevated in patients with pulmonary veno-occlusive disease. (*Adapted from Rich et al.* [4].)

TREATMENT

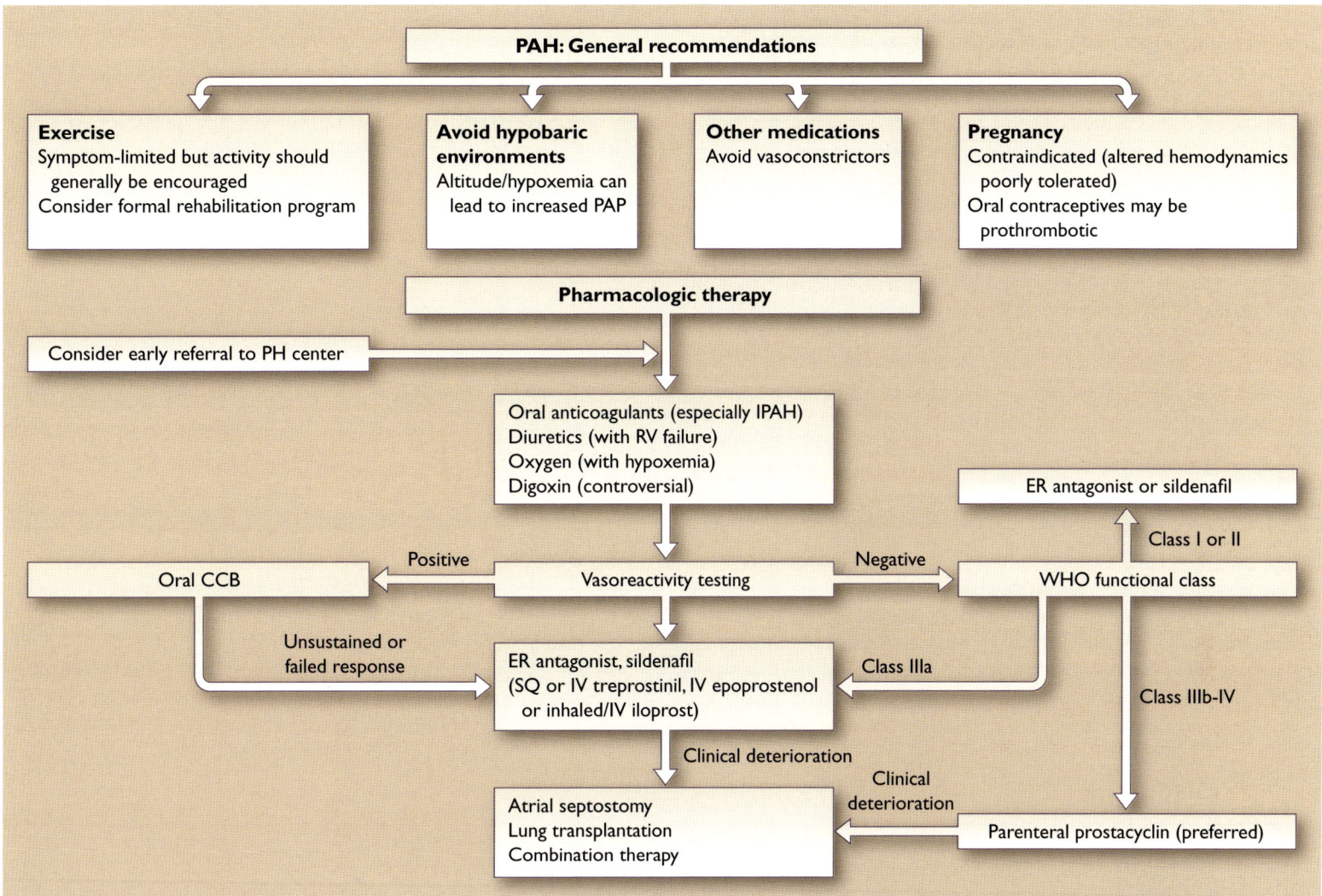

Figure 18-13. Treatment of pulmonary hypertension. Warfarin therapy should be undertaken in patients with idiopathic pulmonary arterial hypertension (IPAH) and chronic thromboembolic pulmonary hypertension if deemed safe [5,12]. Other patients, such as those with connective tissue disease, are sometimes anticoagulated when severe, but no strong supportive data exist. The generally accepted international normalized ratio (INR) range is 1.5 to 2.5. Diuretics and oxygen are used on an individual basis. There may be short-term benefit from digoxin in some patients [14].

Right-heart catheterization is essential in determining initial (and often subsequent) therapy. This, together with World Health Organization (WHO) classification, physical examination, echocardiographic data, exercise testing, N-terminal pro–brain natriuretic peptide levels, and rate of progression affect treatment decisions. The rate at which symptoms are progressing may play a role in the level of aggressiveness of therapy. The majority of patients with pulmonary arterial hypertension (PAH) present with class III symptoms. The terms IIIa and IIIb denote early, stable class III patients and advanced class III patients, respectively, although the precise definition or implications of these subclasses have not been validated prospectively.

Unresponsive class I–II patients are individualized; one option is enrollment in clinical research trials, as in class IIIa. Vasoreactivity refers to a decrease in mean pulmonary artery pressure (PAP) of at least 10 mm Hg and to below 40 mm Hg, in response to inhaled nitric oxide or intravenous epoprostenol or adenosine. For such vasoreactive patients, calcium channel blockers (CCB) alone may be appropriate. Even in this setting, many clinicians will consider adding an additional oral agent. Although high doses of CCB therapy have been shown to be effective in improving survival and in inducing long-term PAP reduction [12,53], such dosing may be difficult to achieve because of associated systemic hypotension, bradycardia, or other adverse effects. There does not appear to be a clear advantage of one CCB over another [12,13].

In patients who respond to CCB, although suboptimally, or in those who respond but clinically worsen, an oral endothelin receptor (ER) antagonist—such as oral bosentan or ambrisentan—can be considered, as can oral sildenafil [21–25]. Oral therapies are generally used in clinically stable patients without significantly elevated right atrial pressures and without markedly reduced cardiac indices. Of these drugs, sildenafil [26,27] is preferred in settings involving liver disease, and endothelin antagonists are favored in settings involving ischemic heart disease in a patient who is on nitrates. Although the algorithm suggests several therapeutic options for functional class IIIa patients (either oral or parenteral therapy), all available data must be considered to make an appropriate decision.

Treprostinil is a prostacyclin analogue delivered by continuous subcutaneous or intravenous infusion (approved for class II–IV PAH) [17–19], and iloprost is a prostacyclin analogue delivered either by inhalation [20] or intravenously. Other investigational agents may be considered in stable class II–III patients in the setting of clinical research trials.

Continued on the next page

Figure 18-13. (Continued) Epoprostenol is a US Food and Drug Administration–approved intravenous prostacyclin for class III–IV patients and is generally reserved for patients having the most severe PAH [15,16]. The endothelin antagonists are appropriate for most class IIIa patients prior to considering epoprostenol, but in class IIIb–IV patients, the parenteral prostacyclins are preferred. The distinction between class IIIb and class IV is essentially arbitrary as these patients are generally handled in the same manner. The relative roles of endothelin antagonists and sildenafil are less well defined in this more severely ill population. Some data are available for combination therapy, including parenteral or inhaled prostanoids, together with bosentan or sildenafil [27–29], and larger, randomized clinical trials are ongoing.

Very few centers have extensive experience with atrial septostomy. When used, it is intended to serve as a bridge to transplantation. The timing of lung transplant referral is individualized at different centers. This depends in part upon the waiting time at the listing institution. Pulmonary hypertension (PH) centers in some areas of the world where drug therapy and transplantation are less available may rely more on septostomy in cases of advanced disease [33]. IV—intravenous; RV—right ventricle; SQ—subcutaneous.

A Assessment of Vasodilator Responsiveness

Mean pulmonary artery pressure	Decreases by ≥ 10 mm Hg and to ≤ 40 mm Hg
Pulmonary vascular resistance	Decreases by > 30%–35%
Cardiac output	Increases
Mean arterial pressure	Minimally decreases
Systemic arterial oxygen saturation	Remains unchanged or improves

B Vasodilators Used to Test for Acute Responsiveness

Epoprostenol (IV infusion)	2–20 ng/kg/min
Adenosine (IV infusion)	50–350 ug/kg/min
Inhaled nitric oxide	5–40 ppm

Figure 18-14. Acute testing: defining vasodilator responsiveness and drug regimens. Calcium channel blocker use should be limited to patients with a favorable acute hemodynamic response. The desired pattern is a reduction in pulmonary artery pressure and pulmonary vascular resistance accompanied by an increase in cardiac output and no deterioration in gas exchange or decrease in systemic blood pressure [54–57]. **A,** The mean pulmonary artery pressure and pulmonary vascular resistance should decrease by at least 10 mm Hg (and to less than 40 mm Hg to be considered a responder) [11]. **B,** Acute hemodynamic testing with invasive monitoring is performed with short-acting vasodilators that include inhaled nitric oxide, epoprostenol, or adenosine. Strong consideration should be given to sending patients to specialized centers experienced with these tests.

PROGNOSIS

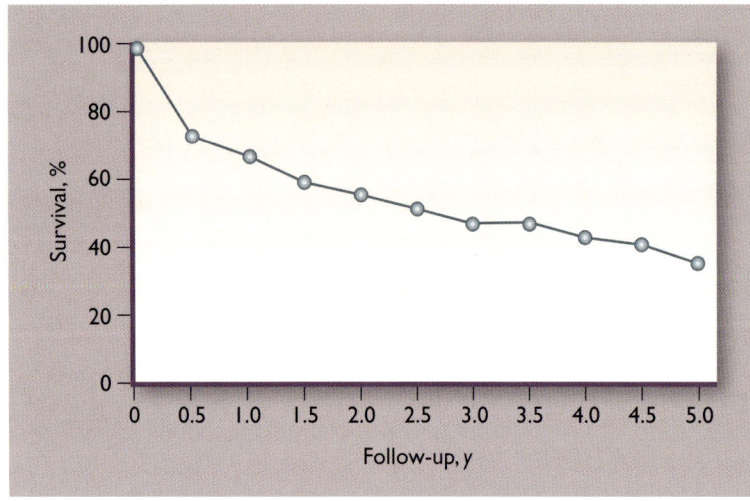

Figure 18-15. Survival of patients with idiopathic pulmonary arterial hypertension (primary pulmonary hypertension). In the National Institutes of Health patient registry, the estimated median survival was 2.8 years. Patients may live longer, particularly when engaged in more aggressive medical therapy [34]. The majority of deaths were from progressive right ventricular failure; a significant number of patients had sudden death. (*Adapted from* D'Alonzo *et al.* [34].)

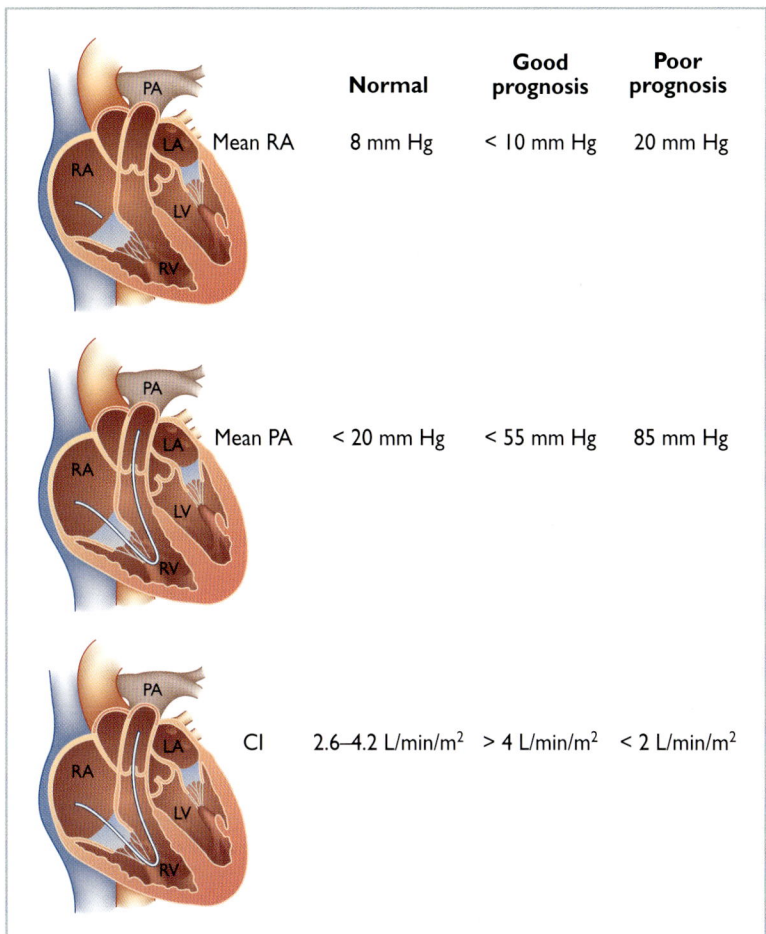

Figure 18-16. Hemodynamic predictors of survival. Hemodynamic, clinical, and therapeutic variables can be used to predict patient survival. The probabilities of survival duration are related to mean right atrial (RA) and pulmonary arterial (PA) pressures and to the cardiac index (CI). The patient's WHO functional class, exercise tolerance, and response to vasodilators also correlate with survival [3,12,34]. LA—left atrium; LV—left ventricle; RV—right ventricle.

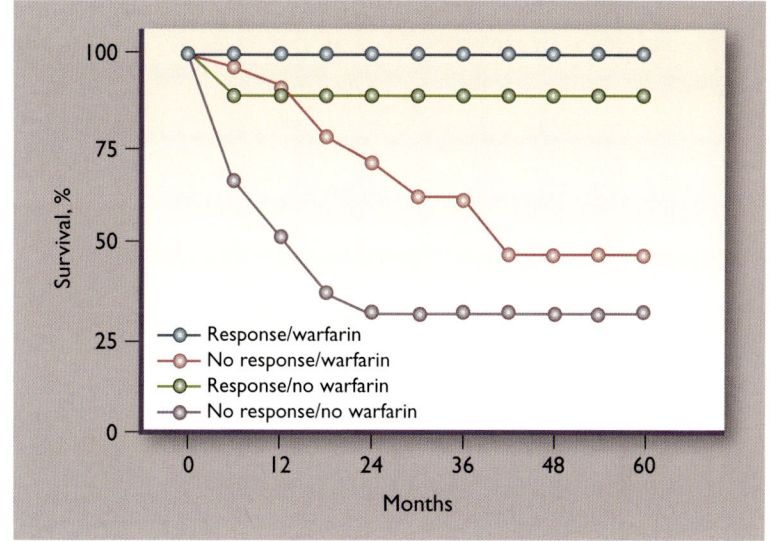

Figure 18-17. Effect of calcium channel blocker therapy and anticoagulation therapy on survival. Long-term treatment with nifedipine or diltiazem can enhance survival if high doses can be achieved. Anticoagulation, regardless of the patient's response to vasodilators, improves survival; this effect is even more pronounced in the nonresponder group [5,12]. (*Adapted from* Rich et al. [12].)

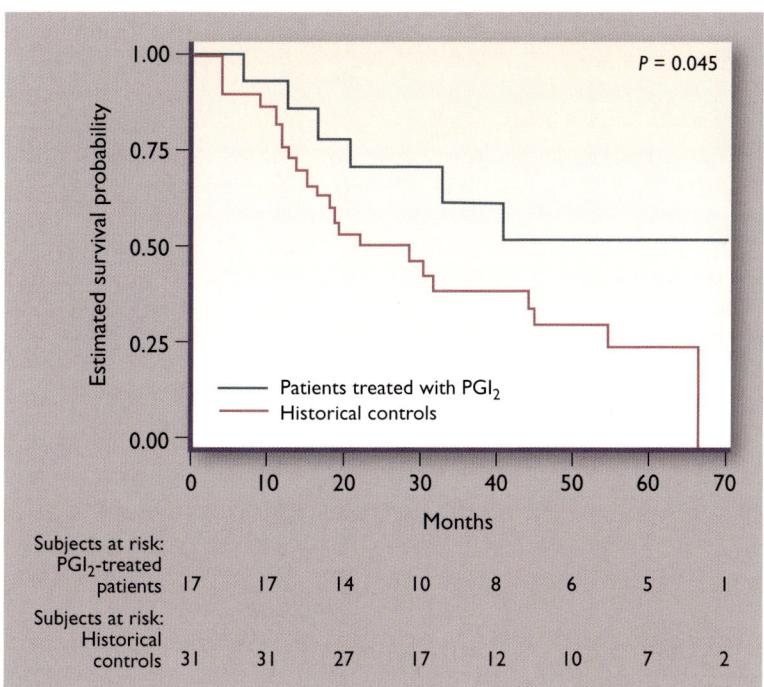

Figure 18-18. Effect of epoprostenol on survival. Treatment with continuous intravenous epoprostenol improves exercise tolerance, pulmonary hemodynamics (an effect that is sustained over time), and survival [15,16]. The long-term effects on pulmonary hemodynamics are seen even in patients without an acute response to vasodilators [15,16,25]. This suggests that the effect of epoprostenol may be mediated through a mechanism other than vasodilation, such as inhibiting platelet aggregation or altering vascular remodeling. PGI_2—prostaglandin. (*Adapted from* Barst et al. [15,16,25].)

| Idiopathic Pulmonary Arterial Hypertension |

Figure 18-19. Hemodynamic effects of long-term epoprostenol. Long-term treatment (ie, >12 weeks) with intravenous epoprostenol improves right ventricular hemodynamic indices [16,58]. Over time, increasing doses of epoprostenol are required. The major limitation of this therapy relates to side effects from the delivery system, which include line infection, sepsis, thrombosis, and inadvertent cessation of delivery due to mechanical malfunctions [15,16]. Aerosolization of prostacyclin and an analog, iloprost, has been described and may offer an alternative delivery method in the future [20]. Although significant progress has been made in treating patients with idiopathic pulmonary arterial hypertension (IPAH), therapeutics have limitations. Case reports suggest that other classes of drugs, such as tyrosine kinase inhibitors, may offer benefits—particularly in cases of IPAH that are refractory to approved, aggressive therapy regimens [31,32]. Drug side effects, systemic vascular actions, and complications from delivery systems carry significant morbidity, but increasing knowledge in the pathogenesis of IPAH continues to offer new avenues for medical intervention.

Hemodynamic Effects of Long-Term Epoprostenol

Variable	Baseline	Epoprostenol*
Mean arterial pressure	102 ± 18	87 ± 10
Right atrial pressure	15 ± 6	9 ± 7
Mean pulmonary artery pressure	67 ± 10	52 ± 12
Pulmonary vascular resistance	16.7 ± 5.4	7.9 ± 3.8
Cardiac output	3.76 ± 1.19	6.29 ± 1.97
Systemic arterial oxygen saturation	91 ± 5	93 ± 6
Mixed venous oxygen saturation	53 ± 8	64 ± 10

*Significant difference compared with baseline.

REFERENCES

1. Dresdale DT, Schultz M, Michtom RJ: Primary pulmonary hypertension: a clinical and hemodynamic study. *Am J Med* 1951, 11:686–705.

2. Fishman AP: A century of primary pulmonary hypertension. In *Primary Pulmonary Hypertension: Lung Biology in Health and Disease,* vol 99. Edited by Rubin LJ and Rich S. New York: Marcel Dekker; 1997:1–17.

3. Rubin LJ: Primary pulmonary hypertension. *N Engl J Med* 1997, 336:111–117.

4. Rich S, Dantzker DR, Ayres SM, et al.: Primary pulmonary hypertension: a national prospective study. *Ann Intern Med* 1987, 107:216–223.

5. Fuster V, Steele PM, Edwards WD, et al.: Primary pulmonary hypertension: natural history and the importance of thrombosis. *Circulation* 1984, 70:580–587.

6. Shapiro BP, McGoon MD, Redfield MM: Unexplained pulmonary hypertension in elderly patients. *Chest* 2007, 131:94–100.

7. Pietra GG: The pathology of primary pulmonary hypertension. In *Primary Pulmonary Hypertension: Lung Biology in Health and Disease,* vol 99. Edited by Rubin LJ and Rich S. New York: Marcel Dekker; 1997:19–61.

8. Pietra GG: Histopathology of primary pulmonary hypertension. *Chest* 1994, 105:2S–6S.

9. Palmer SM, Robinson LJ, Wang A, et al.: Massive pulmonary edema and death after prostacyclin infusion in a patient with pulmonary veno-occlusive disease. *Chest* 1998, 113:237–240.

10. Ahearn GS, Tapson VF, Rebeiz A, Greenfield JC Jr: Electrocardiography to define clinical status in primary pulmonary hypertension and pulmonary arterial hypertension secondary to collagen vascular disease. *Chest* 2002, 122:524–527.

11. Sitbon O, Humbert M, Jais X, et al.: Long-term response to calcium channel blockers in idiopathic pulmonary arterial hypertension. *Circulation* 2005, 111:3105–3111.

12. Rich S, Kaufmann E, Levy PS: The effect of high doses of calcium-channel blockers on survival in primary pulmonary hypertension. *N Engl J Med* 1992, 327:76–81.

13. Rich S, Kaufmann E: High dose titration of calcium channel blocking agents for primary pulmonary hypertension: guidelines for short-term drug testing. *J Am Coll Cardiol* 1991, 18:1323–1327.

14. Rich S, Seiditz M, Dodin E, et al.: The short-term effects of digoxin in patients with right ventricular dysfunction from pulmonary hypertension. *Chest* 1998, 114:787–792.

15. Barst RJ, Rubin LJ, Long WA, et al.: A comparison of continuous intravenous epoprostenol (prostacyclin) with conventional therapy for primary pulmonary hypertension. *N Engl J Med* 1996, 334:296–301.

16. Barst RJ, Rubin LJ, McGoon MD, et al.: Survival in primary pulmonary hypertension with long-term continuous intravenous prostacyclin. *Ann Intern Med* 1994, 121:409–415.

17. Simonneau G, Barst RJ, Galie N, et al.: Continuous subcutaneous infusion of treprostinil, a prostacyclin analogue, in patients with pulmonary arterial hypertension: a double-blind, randomized, placebo-controlled trial. *Am J Respir Crit Care Med* 2002, 165:800–804.

18. Tapson VF, Gomberg-Maitland M, McLaughlin VV, et al.: Safety and efficacy of IV treprostinil for pulmonary arterial hypertension: a prospective, multicenter, open-label, 12-week trial. *Chest* 2006, 129:683–688.

19. Gomberg-Maitland M, Tapson VF, Benza RL, et al.: Transition from intravenous epoprostenol to intravenous treprostinil in pulmonary hypertension. *Am J Respir Crit Care Med* 2005, 172:1586–1589.

20. Olschewski H, Simonneau G, Galiè N, et al.: Inhaled iloprost for severe pulmonary hypertension. *N Engl J Med* 2002, 347: 322–329.

21. Channick RN, Simonneau G, Sitbon O, et al.: Effects of the dual endothelin-receptor antagonist bosentan in patients with pulmonary hypertension: a randomised placebo-controlled study. *Lancet* 2001; 358:1119–1123.

22. Rubin LJ, Badesch DB, Barst RJ, et al.: Bosentan therapy for pulmonary arterial hypertension. *N Engl J Med* 2002, 346:896–903.

23. Galie N, Badesch DB, Oudiz R, et al.: Ambrisentan therapy for pulmonary arterial hypertension. *J Am Coll Cardiol* 2005, 46:529–535.

24. Sitbon O, Badesch DB, Channick RN, et al.: Effects of the dual endothelin receptor antagonist bosentan in patients with pulmonary arterial hypertension: a one-year follow-up study. *Chest* 124:247–254.

25. McLaughlin V, Sitbon O, Badesch DB, et al.: Survival with first-line bosentan in patients with primary pulmonary hypertension. *Eur Respir J* 2005, 25:244–249.

26. Galie N, Ghofrani HA, Torbicki A, et al.: Sildenafil citrate therapy for pulmonary arterial hypertension 2005, 353:2148–2157.

27. Simonneau G, Rubin LJ, Galie N, et al.: Safety and efficacy of sildenafil-epoprostenol combination therapy in patients with pulmonary arterial hypertension (PAH). *Am J Respir Crit Care Med* 2007, 175:A300.

28. Humbert M, Barst RJ, Robbins IM, et al.: Combination of bosentan with epoprostenol in pulmonary arterial hypertension: BREATHE-2. *Eur Respir J* 2004, 24:353–359.

29. McLaughlin VV, Oudiz RJ, Frost A, et al.: Randomized study of adding inhaled iloprost to existing bosentan in pulmonary arterial hypertension. *Am J Respir Crit Care Med* 2006, 174:1257–1263.

30. Badesch DB, Abman SH, Simonneau G, et al.: Medical therapy for pulmonary arterial hypertension. Updated ACCP evidence-based clinical practice guidelines. 2007, 131:1917–1928.

31. Ghofrani HA, Seeger W, Grimminger F. Imatinib for the treatment of pulmonary arterial hypertension. *N Engl J Med* 2005, 353:1412–1413.

32. Patterson KC, Weissmann A, Ahmadi T, Farber HW: Imatinib mesylate in the treatment of refractory idiopathic pulmonary arterial hypertension. *Ann Intern Med* 2006, 145:152–153.

33. Kuryzna M, Dabrowski M, Bielecki D, *et al.*: Atrial septostomy in treatment of end-stage right heart failure in patients with pulmonary hypertension. *Chest* 2007, 131:977–983.

34. D'Alonzo GE, Barst RJ, Ayres SM, *et al.*: Survival in patients with primary pulmonary hypertension: results from a national prospective registry. *Ann Intern Med* 1991, 115:343–349.

35. McLaughlin VV, Shillington A, Rich S: Survival in primary pulmonary hypertension: the impact of epoprostenol therapy. *Circulation* 2002, 106:1477–1482.

36. Rich S: Primary pulmonary hypertension. Executive Summary from the World Symposium. World Health Organization; 1998.

37. Highlights from the Third World Symposium on Pulmonary Arterial Hypertension, Venice, Italy. June 23–5, 2003 *Adv Pulm Hypertension* 2003, 2:6.

38. Lee S-D, Shroyer KR, Markham NE, *et al.*: Monoclonal endothelial cell proliferation is present in primary but not secondary pulmonary hypertension. *J Clin Invest* 1998, 101:927–934.

39. Yeager ME, Halley GR, Golpon HA, *et al.*: Microsatellite instability of endothelial cell growth and apoptosis genes within plexiform lesions in primary pulmonary hypertension. *Circ Res* 2001, 88:e2–e11.

40. Thomson JR, Machado RD, Pauciulo MW, *et al.*: Sporadic primary pulmonary hypertension is associated with germline mutations of the gene encoding *BMPR-II*, a receptor member of the TGF-b family. *J Med Genet* 2000, 37:741–745.

41. Deng Z, Morse JH, Slager SL, *et al.*: Familial primary pulmonary hypertension (gene *PPH1*) is caused by mutations in the bone morphogenetic protein receptor-II gene. *Am J Hum Genet* 2000, 67:737–744.

42. Lane KB, Machado RD, Pauciulo MW, *et al.*: The International *PPH* Consortium: Heterozygous germline mutations in *BMPR2*, encoding a TGF-b receptor, cause familial primary pulmonary hypertension. *Nat. Genet* 2000, 26:81–84.

43. Weir EK, Reeve HL, Huang JMC, *et al.*: Anorexic agents aminorex, fenfluramine, and dexfenfluramine inhibit potassium current in rat pulmonary vascular smooth muscle and cause pulmonary vasoconstriction. *Circulation* 1996, 94:2216–2220.

44. Gaine S: Pulmonary hypertension. *JAMA* 2000, 284:3160–3168.

45. Voelkel NF, Tuder RM: Cellular and molecular mechanisms in the pathogenesis of severe pulmonary hypertension. *Eur Respir J* 1995, 8:2129–2138.

46. Herve P, Launay J-M, Scrobohaci M-L, *et al.*: Increased plasma serotonin in primary pulmonary hypertension. *Am J Med* 1995, 99:249–254.

47. Giaid A, Yanagisawa M, Langleben D, *et al.*: Expression of endothelin-1 in the lungs of patients with pulmonary hypertension. *N Engl J Med* 1993, 328:1732–1739.

48. Christman BW, McPherson CD, Newman JH, *et al.*: An imbalance between the excretion of thromboxane and prostacyclin metabolites in pulmonary hypertension. *N Engl J Med* 1992, 327:70–75.

49. Egermayer P, Town GI, Peacock AJ: Role of serotonin in the pathogenesis of acute and chronic pulmonary hypertension. *Thorax* 1999, 54:161–168.

50. Zimmerman CM, Padgett RW: Transforming growth factor b signaling mediators and modulators. *Gene* 2000, 249:17–30.

51. Rich S, Pietra GG, Kieras K, *et al.*: Primary pulmonary hypertension: radiographic and scintigraphic patterns of histologic subtypes. *Ann Intern Med* 1986, 105:499–502.

52. Rhodes J, Barst RJ, Garofano RP, *et al.*: Hemodynamic correlates of exercise function in patients with primary pulmonary hypertension. *J Am Coll Cardiol* 1991, 18:1738–1744.

53. Rich S, Brundage BH: High-dose calcium channel-blocking therapy for primary pulmonary hypertension: evidence for long-term reduction in pulmonary arterial pressure and regression of right ventricular hypertrophy. *Circulation* 1987, 76:135–141.

54. Rubin LJ: Primary pulmonary hypertension. *Chest* 1993, 104:236–250.

55. Galie N, Ussia G, Passarelli P, *et al.*: Role of pharmacologic test in the treatment of primary pulmonary hypertension. *Am J Cardiol* 1995, 75:55A–62A.

56. Kneussl MP, Lang IM, Brenot FP: Medical management of primary pulmonary hypertension. *Eur Respir J* 1996, 9:2401–2409.

57. Rich S, D'Alonzo GE, Dantzker DR, Levy PS: Magnitude and implications of spontaneous hemodynamic variability in primary pulmonary hypertension. *Am J Cardiol* 1985, 55:159–163.

58. Shapiro SM, Oudiz RJ, Cao T, *et al.*: Primary pulmonary hypertension: improved long-term effects and survival with continuous intravenous epoprostenol infusion. *J Am Coll Cardiol* 1997, 30:343–349.

LUNG CANCER

Otis B. Rickman and James R. Jett

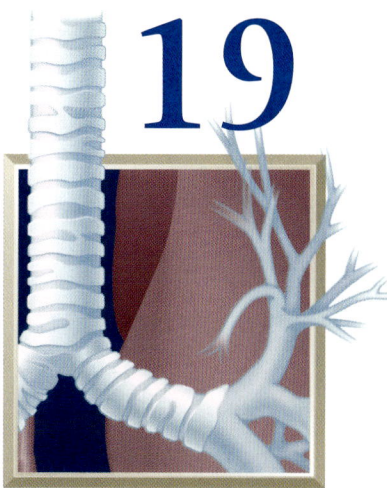
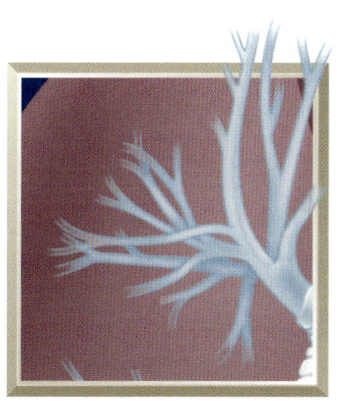
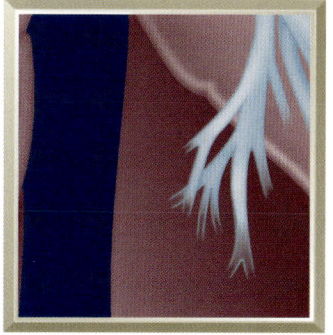

Lung cancer is the leading cause of cancer death in the United States. In 2004, the reported number of cancer deaths from tumors of lung and bronchus was 158,006 (28.5% of all cancer deaths) [1]. This number represents more deaths than the combined totals for the next four leading causes (colorectal, breast, prostate, and pancreas), making lung cancer the third overall leading cause of death in the United States behind only heart disease and the combination of all other forms of cancer [1]. Bronchogenic carcinoma is a worldwide health problem. Successful control of this global epidemic depends on the elimination of tobacco use, the avoidance of environmental and occupational exposure to carcinogens, and a better understanding of the biology of lung cancer. Through the development of primary prevention programs and nicotine control strategies, the elimination of tobacco use, and the development of chemopreventive drugs and improved therapeutic strategies, it may be possible to improve outcomes in this global epidemic.

This chapter reviews lung cancer epidemiology, risk factors, pathology, clinical presentation, diagnostic and staging techniques, the role of screening, prognostic factors, and treatment.

EPIDEMIOLOGY

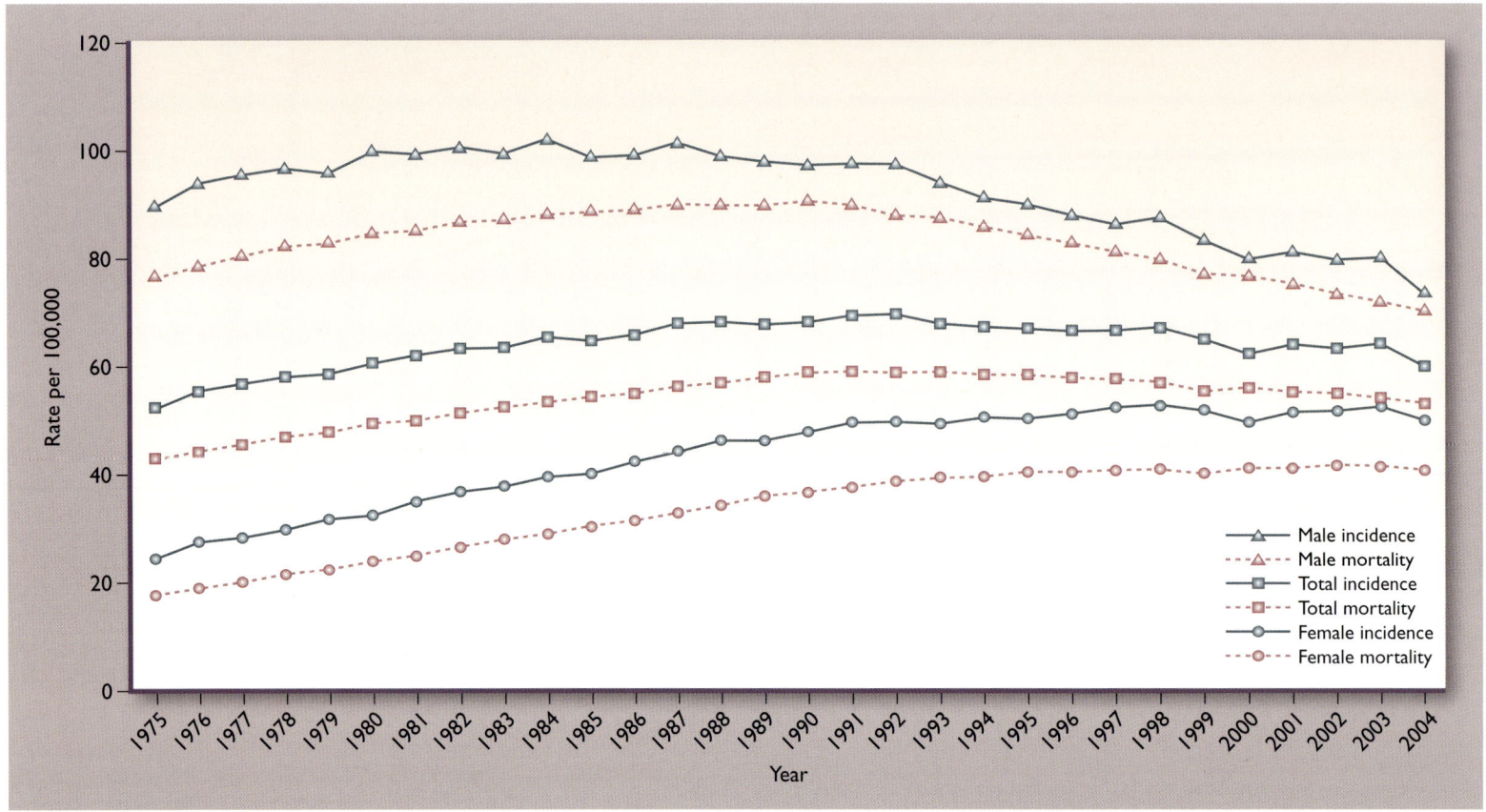

Figure 19-1. Lung cancer incidence and mortality. It is estimated that in 2007 213,380 people (114,760 men and 98,620 women) will be diagnosed with cancer of the lung and bronchus, and 160,390 men and women will die of this disease [1]. The latest data (September 2007) obtained from the Surveillance, Epidemiology, and End Results Program (www.seer.cancer.gov) indicates that the incidence of lung cancer, although still very high, is continuing to decrease. From 1975 to 2000, the age-adjusted incidence rate increased from 52.3 to a peak of 67.3 in 1998 and then declined to 60.0 in the year 2004. During this same period the age-adjusted death rate increased from 42.6 to a peak of 59.1 in 1993 and has now shown a steady decline to 53.3 [2–6].

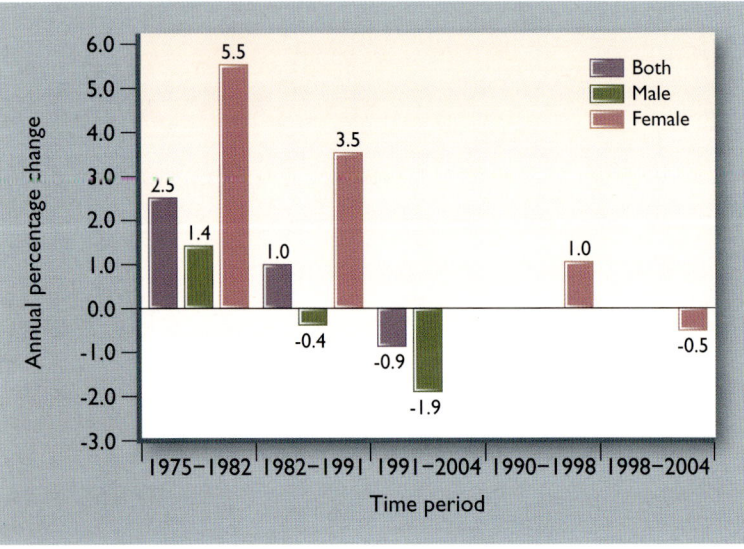

Figure 19-2. Average annual percent change. The annual percent change (APC) is used to measure trends or the change in rates over time. This graph demonstrates the average APC in lung cancer incidence from 1975 to 2004 and shows a continued decrease for men and, finally, a decrease for women [3].

| Atlas of Pulmonary Medicine |

Acquired Risk Factors for Lung Cancer

Tobacco smoke
- Active
- Passive

Environmental factors
- Air pollution
- Radon progeny: natural decay of uranium

Occupational carcinogens
- Proven
  - Arsenic: copper smelters, glass, and pesticide workers
  - Asbestos: insulation workers, textile workers, asbestos users
  - Bischloromethyl ether and chloromethyl methyl ether: textile, paint, chemical, and home insulation workers
  - Chromium: leather, ceramic, and metal workers; tanners
  - Diesel exhaust
  - Ionizing radiation, gamma radiation (x-rays)
  - Mustard gas: soldiers (warfare), production workers
  - Nickel and nickel compounds: nickel refinery, smeltery, and electrolysis workers
  - Radon progeny: uranium miners, fluorspar miners
  - Soot, tar, mineral oils (polycyclic aromatic hydrocarbons): road workers, roofers, coke oven workers, and iron and steel foundry workers
  - Vinyl chloride: plastics workers
- Suspected
  - Acrylonitrile
  - Beryllium
  - Cadmium and cadmium compounds
  - Crystalline silica
  - Electromagnetic fields
  - Formaldehyde
  - Human-made mineral fibers (eg, rock wool or slag wool)
  - Wood dust

Dietary influences
- Vitamin A deficiency
- Vitamin E deficiency
- Vitamin C deficiency
- Selenium deficiency
- High dietary fat/cholesterol intake

Lung diseases
- Peripheral pulmonary scar
- Pulmonary tuberculosis
- Interstitial pulmonary fibrosis
- Scleroderma
- Pneumoconiosis
- Chronic obstructive pulmonary disease

Figure 19-3. Acquired risk factors for lung cancer. There is a broad range of known and proposed acquired risk factors for lung cancer [7]. Chemicals in tobacco smoke are the best known lung carcinogens. Estimates of the proportion of lung cancer attributable to cigarette smoking in developed countries range from 83% to 94% in men and 57% to 80% in women [8]. The risk of developing lung cancer is correlated with the number of cigarettes smoked per day and with length of exposure.

Radon, an inert gas derived from radium-226 during the natural decay of uranium and found in certain soils and rocks, is the second most frequent cause of lung cancer. The incidence of radon-induced lung cancer is increased by smoking [7]. Occupational exposure to carcinogens accounts for about 15% of cases in men and 5% of cases in women. The most common occupational exposure is to asbestos (risk is five times higher than controls); exposure to both asbestos and cigarette smoke increases the risk 90 times. Other potential risk factors include a deficiency in vitamins that are thought to protect against lung cancer and certain chronic lung diseases [7].

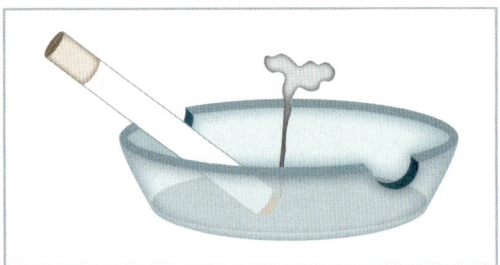

Figure 19-4. Tobacco smoke. At the beginning of the 20th century, lung cancer was among the rarest cancers [7]. There are many anecdotes of surgeons at the turn of the century calling students into operating rooms to see a case of lung cancer, because they might never see it again. In the late 1800s the manufactured cigarette was introduced and mass marketed. The rise in lung cancer paralleled the increase in smoking of manufactured cigarettes. This rise was initially seen in men and was delayed by approximately 20 years. The same rise occurred in the 1960s and 1970s for women who had taken up smoking about 20 years earlier.

It is well known that smoking cigarettes increases the relative risk of lung cancer 20-fold [9]. It is also known that the number of cigarettes smoked and the length of exposure increase risk. Additional factors that affect risk are the depth of inhalation and the amount of tar. Fortunately, the risk for developing lung cancer falls for people who have successfully stopped smoking, approaching that of nonsmokers after about 15 years, but it is also important to note that approximately 50% of all incident cases occur among former smokers. In the United States alone, approximately 90 million adults (> 18 years) classify themselves as current or former smokers. Thus, effective chemopreventive agents will likely provide complementary benefits to smoking cessation programs with respect to reducing the overall lung cancer burden.

PATHOLOGY

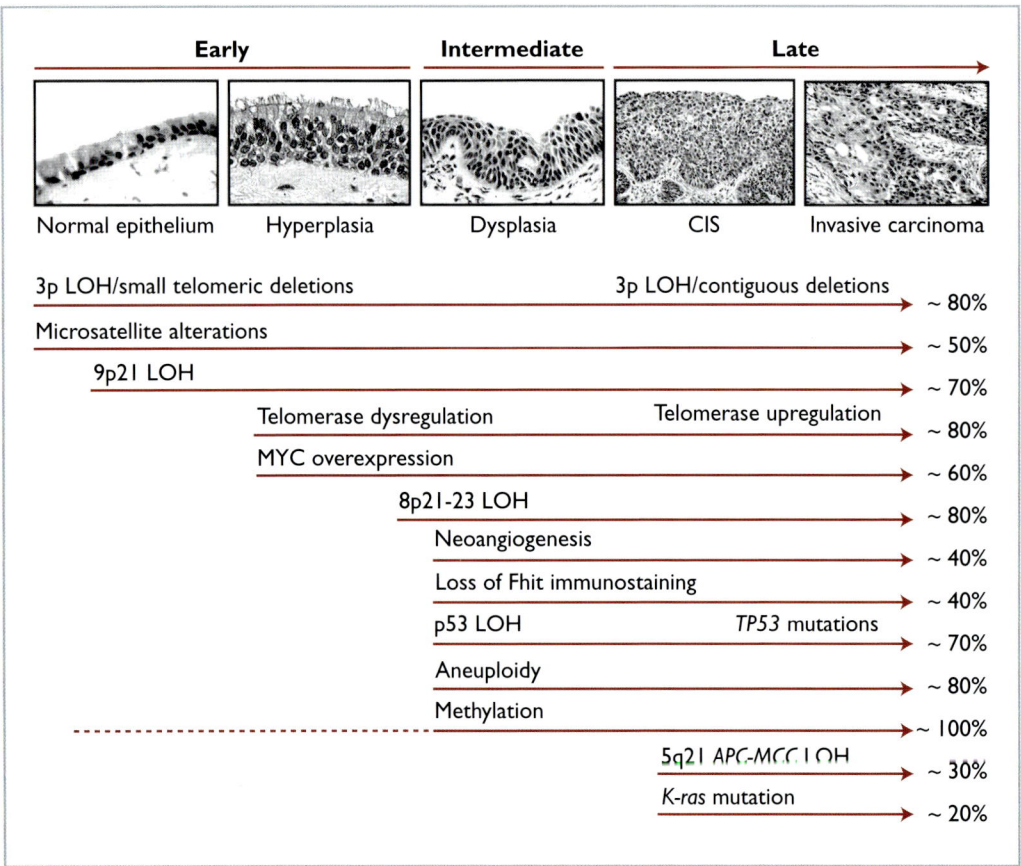

Figure 19-5. Molecular biology of lung cancer. Cellular proliferation is normally controlled by 1) proto-oncogenes, which are crucial for normal cellular functions (including signal transduction and transcription); 2) tumor suppressor genes, which regulate transcription; and 3) antioncogenes, which are recessive growth regulatory genes. Oncogenes and growth factors, and their receptors, play a central role in tumorigenesis. The loss of normal antioncogene expression requires homozygous mutation or deletion; as the number of mutations increases, the neoplasm progresses from a hyperplastic lesion to invasive lung cancer. There are a number of genetic markers associated with lung cancers, and their appearance varies during the neoplastic process. Although usually sequential, these changes can occur anytime during the process. These markers are also found in histologically normal tissue. The "field cancerization" concept proposes that since the entire lung is exposed to carcinogenic damage, the total area exposed is at risk for developing multiple, separate, clonally unrelated foci of neoplasia [10]. This may in part explain the incidence of synchronous primary lung cancers (estimated to range from 0.26% to 1.33%) and the annual incidence of 2% to 5% for second malignancies after resection for stage I non–small cell lung cancer [11]. CIS—carcinoma in situ; LOH—loss of heterozygosity. (*From* Hirsch *et al.* [10]; with permission.)

Molecular Techniques for Investigating Lung Cancer

Technique	Comments
Gene mutations	Widely used technique, especially for p53 and ras genes. Often used to determine the role of a newly discovered gene in the pathogenesis of lung cancer. May be of diagnostic and prognostic significance. Multiple methodologies available.
Allelotyping	Useful as a partial substitute for mutational analysis and for determining the chromosomal locations of putative tumor suppressor genes. Widely used to study multistage pathogenesis. Readily performed on formalin-fixed and microdissected tissues. Increasing use of genotyping using automatic sequencers.
Gene expression at RNA and protein level	Northern blotting and reverse transcription PCR are widely used to investigate gene expression. Western blotting is often used for detection of protein expression. In-situ hybridization for message expression can be performed on paraffin-embedded tissues and thus may be used to investigate multistage pathogenesis. Microarray techniques offer promise of examining all or most of the genome but currently require a relatively large amount of high-quality RNA from purified cell populations. Sage technique is useful for investigation and identification of expressed genes. Similarly, advances in proteomics will permit simultaneous detection of multiple proteins. Numerous immunohistochemical studies of oncogene expression have been used to study multistage pathogenesis. Of particular interest, hnRNP expression on exfoliated epithelial cells in sputum samples may predict development of cancer.
Molecular cytogenetics	In-situ hybridization studies of fixed materials or the use of smears has provided considerable information about numerical and structural changes.
Comparative genomic hybridization	Useful for detection of gene amplifications. Less sensitive for the detection of regions of allelic loss.
Morphometric studies	May be applied to paraffin-embedded tissues. Useful for determining aneuploidy and for measuring a number of nuclear and cytoplasmic parameters.

Figure 19-6. Tumor markers in lung cancer. Recently, advances in molecular biology have provided additional new information regarding diagnosis, prognosis, and treatment. Molecular genetics and immunohistochemical techniques are being studied for their effectiveness in identifying biomarkers of malignancy. Molecular techniques used in the investigation of lung cancer are shown in the table. hnRNP—heterogenous nuclear ribonuclear protein; PCR—polymerase chain reaction. (*Adapted from* Hirsch *et al.* [10].)

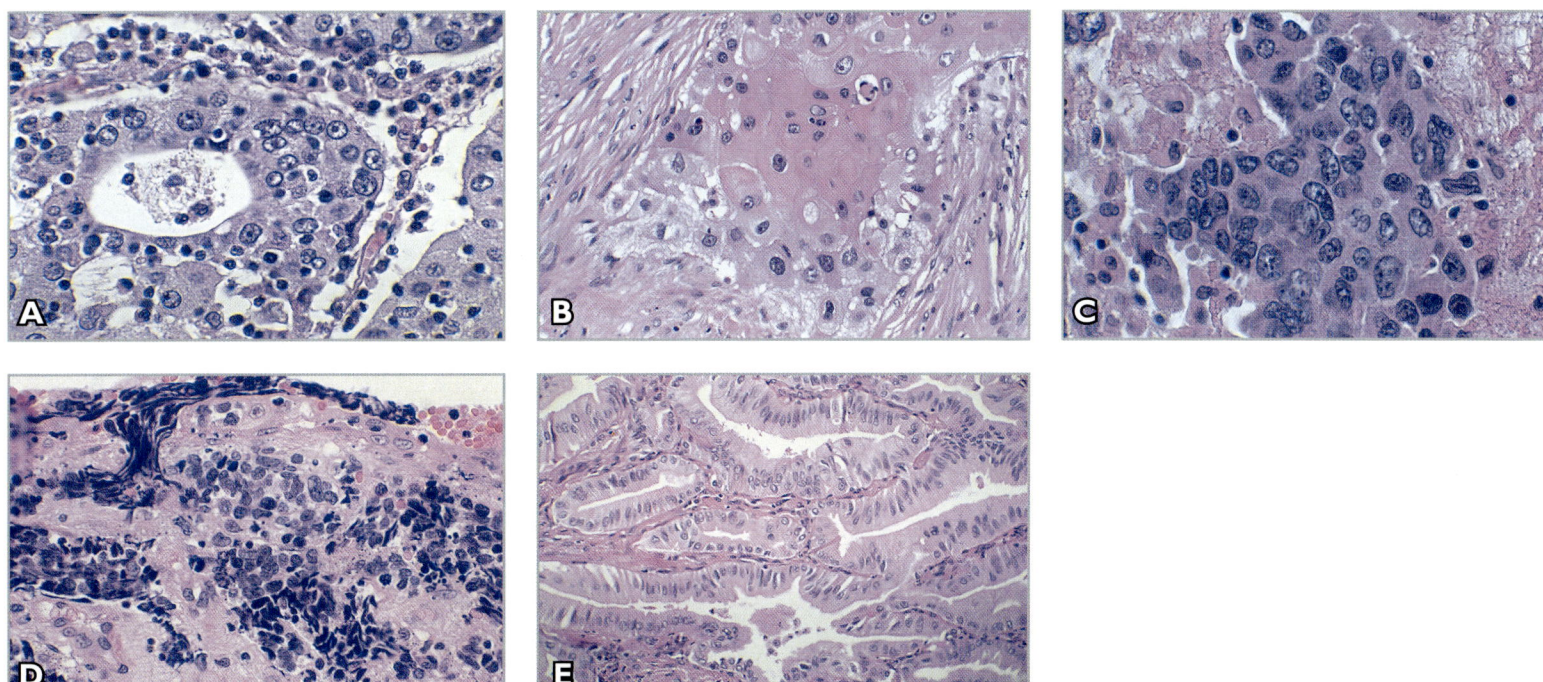

Figure 19-7. Major types of lung cancer. Between 90% and 95% of all lung cancers can be classified under the four major histologic cell types: **A,** Adenocarcinoma is now the leading type and accounts for 30% to 45% of all cases. **B,** Squamous cell carcinoma accounts for 33% of all cases. **C,** Large cell carcinoma accounts for 9% of all cases. **D,** Small cell carcinoma accounts for 20% to 25% of all cases. **E,** Bronchioloalveolar cell carcinoma, a subtype of adenocarcinoma, is less common [12].

The World Health Organization Classification of Malignant Epithelial Lung Tumors [13]

Squamous cell carcinoma	Adenosquamous carcinoma
Papillary	Sarcomatoid carcinomas
Clear cell	Carcinomas with spindle and/or giant cells
Small cell	Carcinosarcoma
Basaloid	Pulmonary blastoma
Small cell carcinoma	Carcinoid tumor
Combined small cell carcinoma	Typical carcinoid
Adenocarcinoma	Atypical carcinoid
Acinar	Carcinomas of salivary-gland type
Papillary	Mucoepidermoid carcinoma
Bronchioloalveolar carcinoma	Adenoid cystic carcinoma
Solid adenocarcinoma with mucin	Unclassified carcinoma
Adenocarcinoma with mixed subtypes	
Large cell carcinoma	
Large cell neuroendocrine carcinoma	
Basaloid carcinoma	
Lymphoepithelioma-like carcinoma	
Clear cell carcinoma	
Large cell carcinoma with rhabdoid phenotype	

Figure 19-8. The World Health Organization classification of malignant epithelial lung tumors [13].

CLINICAL PRESENTATION

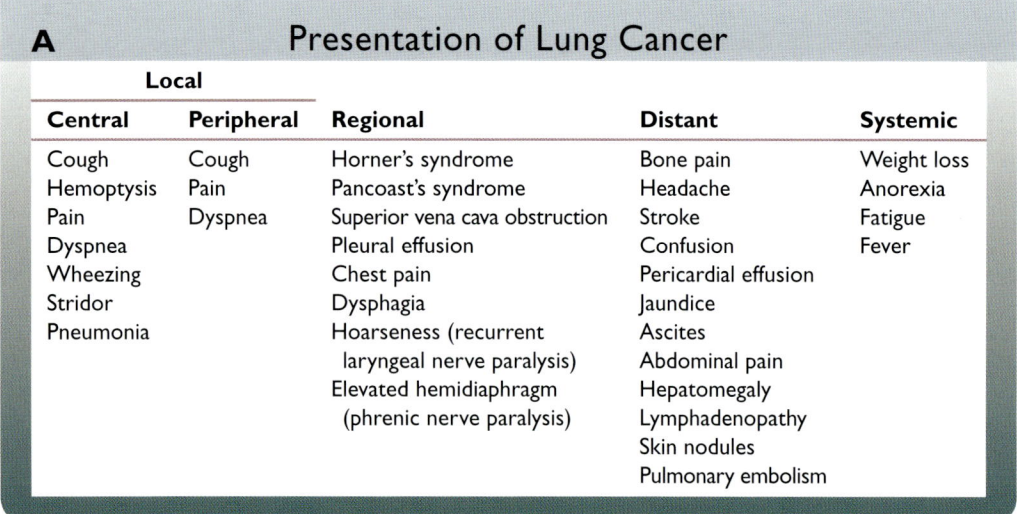

A   Presentation of Lung Cancer

Local				
Central	**Peripheral**	**Regional**	**Distant**	**Systemic**
Cough	Cough	Horner's syndrome	Bone pain	Weight loss
Hemoptysis	Pain	Pancoast's syndrome	Headache	Anorexia
Pain	Dyspnea	Superior vena cava obstruction	Stroke	Fatigue
Dyspnea		Pleural effusion	Confusion	Fever
Wheezing		Chest pain	Pericardial effusion	
Stridor		Dysphagia	Jaundice	
Pneumonia		Hoarseness (recurrent laryngeal nerve paralysis)	Ascites	
		Elevated hemidiaphragm (phrenic nerve paralysis)	Abdominal pain	
			Hepatomegaly	
			Lymphadenopathy	
			Skin nodules	
			Pulmonary embolism	

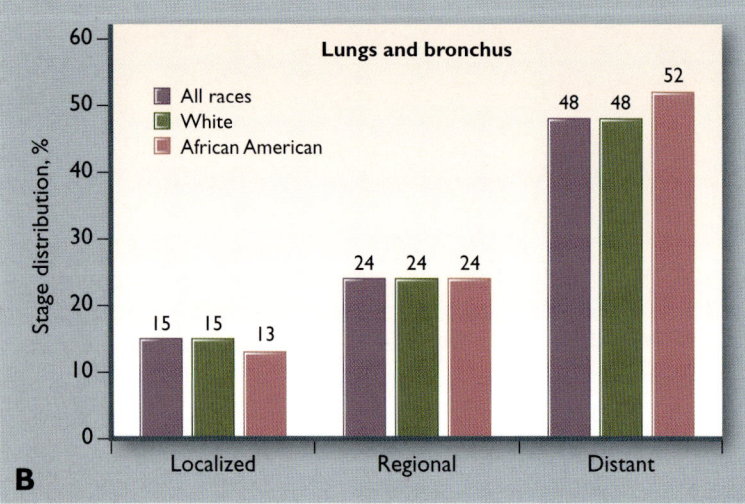

Figure 19-9. Clinical presentation of lung cancer. **A,** Patients with lung cancer may have local, regional, or metastatic disease at the time of presentation [12,14,15]. Symptoms are a late finding in the development of lung cancer. For instance, only 10% to 25% of patients who have a serendipitous, incidental diagnosis of lung cancer via chest radiography have symptoms attributable to lung cancer [16]. When looked at in a rigorous manner, seven symptoms (hemoptysis, weight loss, loss of appetite, dyspnea, thoracic pain, fatigue, and cough), one physical sign (finger clubbing), and two abnormal investigation results (thrombocytosis and abnormal spirometry) were associated with lung cancer in multivariable analyses. After excluding variables reported in the final 180 days before diagnosis, hemoptysis, dyspnea, and abnormal spirometry remained independently associated with cancer [17]. **B,** The lack of reliable early symptoms and an effective screening strategy are the likely reasons that 52% of lung cancer patients have distant metastases at the time of diagnosis [18].

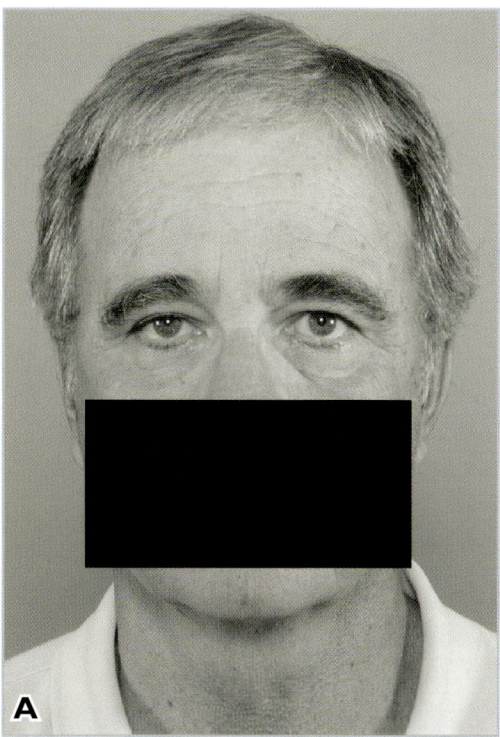
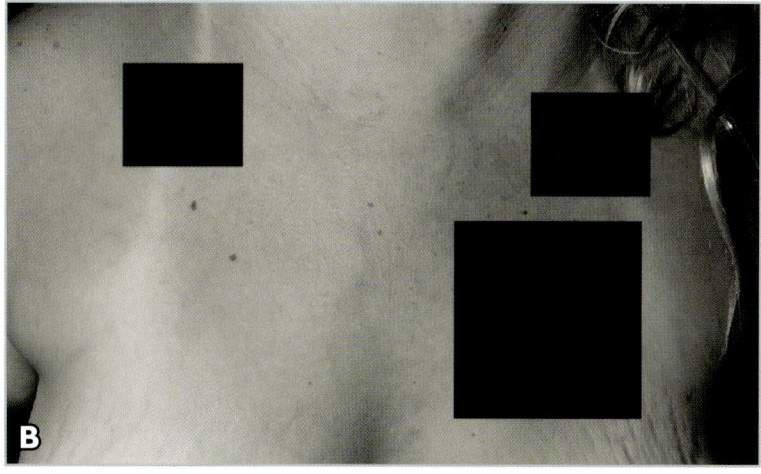

Figure 19-10. Local effects of lung cancer. Local mass effect and invasion result in regional signs and symptoms of lung cancer. Nerves, vessels, and airways are commonly compressed or invaded resulting in symptoms. **A,** Horner's Syndrome results from damage to sympathetic chain ganglia from a lung tumor in the upper thorax. This clinical syndrome consists of ipsilateral ptosis, miosis, and anhydrosis. This patient has a right-sided Horner's. **B,** Superior vena vava (SVC) syndrome results from obstruction of the SVC by the tumor. In this patient, dilated vessels are seen over the chest and breasts as well as massive supraclavicular and cervical adenopathy.

Paraneoplastic Syndromes in Lung Cancer

System	Syndrome	System	Syndrome
Endocrine and metabolic	Cushing's syndrome	Dermatologic	Dermatomyositis, polymyositis
	SIADH		Acanthosis nigricans
	Hypercalcemia/PTH-related peptide		Diffuse hyperpigmentation
	Gynecomastia		Erythema gyratum repens
	Galactorrhea		Erythema multiforme
	Acromegaly		Pruritus, urticaria
	Ectopic gonadotropic hormone		Tylosis
	Hyperthyroidism		Scleroderma
	Hypercalcitoninemia	Hematologic	Anemia
	Hypophosphatemia		Thrombocytosis
	Insulin-like activity		Nonspecific leukocytosis
	Hyperamylasemia		Leukoerythroblastic reaction
Neuromuscular	Peripheral neuropathy		Eosinophilia
	Corticocerebellar degeneration		Disseminated intravascular coagulation
	Eaton-Lambert syndrome		Polycythemia
	Cranial nerve abnormalities		Red cell aplasia
	Necrotizing myelopathy		Dysproteinemia
	Autonomic neuropathy	Cardiovascular	Migratory thrombophlebitis
	Encephalopathy		Nonbacterial verrucous (marantic) endocarditis
	Carcinomatous myopathy		Arterial thrombosis
Skeletal	Clubbing and pulmonary hypertrophic osteoarthropathy	Renal	Glomerulonephritis
			Proteinuria
			Nephrotic syndrome

Figure 19-11. Paraneoplastic syndromes. Paraneoplastic syndromes are reported in 2% to 20% of patients with lung cancer [19,20]. Extrapulmonary nonmetastatic manifestations of these syndromes may precede, coincide with, or follow the diagnosis of lung cancer. Their presence does not necessarily suggest that the lung cancer is unresectable. In some cases, the syndrome resolves immediately after resection of the primary tumor. In incurable cases, treatment of the associated symptoms or biochemical abnormalities (eg, hyperglycemia) may improve the patient's well being [21]. PTH—parathyroid hormone; SIADH—syndrome of inappropriate antidiuretic hormone secretion.

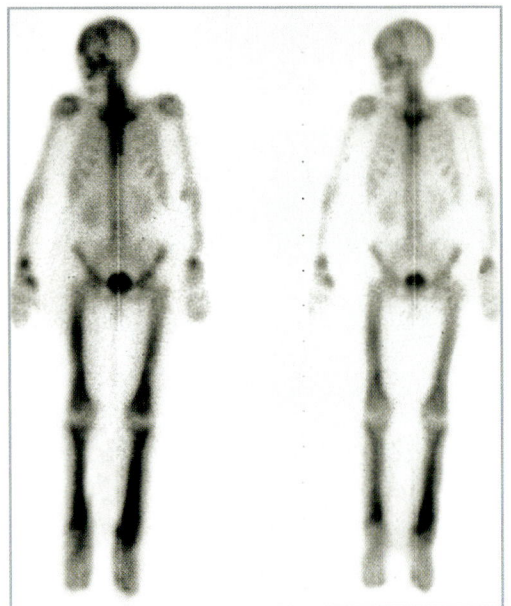

Figure 19-12. Bone scan showing hypertrophic pulmonary osteoarthropathy. New periosteal bone formation is highlighted in this bone scan of a patient with generalized hypertrophic pulmonary osteoarthropathy, a paraneoplastic disease reported to occur in 2% to 12% of patients with non–small cell lung cancer.

Lung Carcinomas and Associated Clinical Features			
Types of Carcinoma	Frequent Location	Initial Metastasis	Comments
Squamous cell	Central	Local invasion	Frequent cavitation and obstructive phenomena
			Hypercalcemia
			Cavitation rare
Small cell	Central	Lymphatics	Paraneoplastic syndromes
			Association with peripheral scars
Adenocarcinoma	Midlung, periphery	Lymphatics	Rapid growth with early metastases
Large cell	Periphery	Central nervous system, mediastinum	No correlation with cigarette smoking
Bronchioloalveolar	Periphery	Lymphatics, local invasion, hematogenous	Ground glass opacity

Figure 19-13. Clinical features of specific types of lung cancer. Although the initial presentations of lung cancer are diverse, each type of lung cancer is associated with a specific location, an initial pattern of metastasis, and other features. The specific clinical features may be helpful in the differential diagnosis and in selecting an appropriate work-up. (*Adapted from* Kiss [22].)

DIAGNOSIS AND STAGING

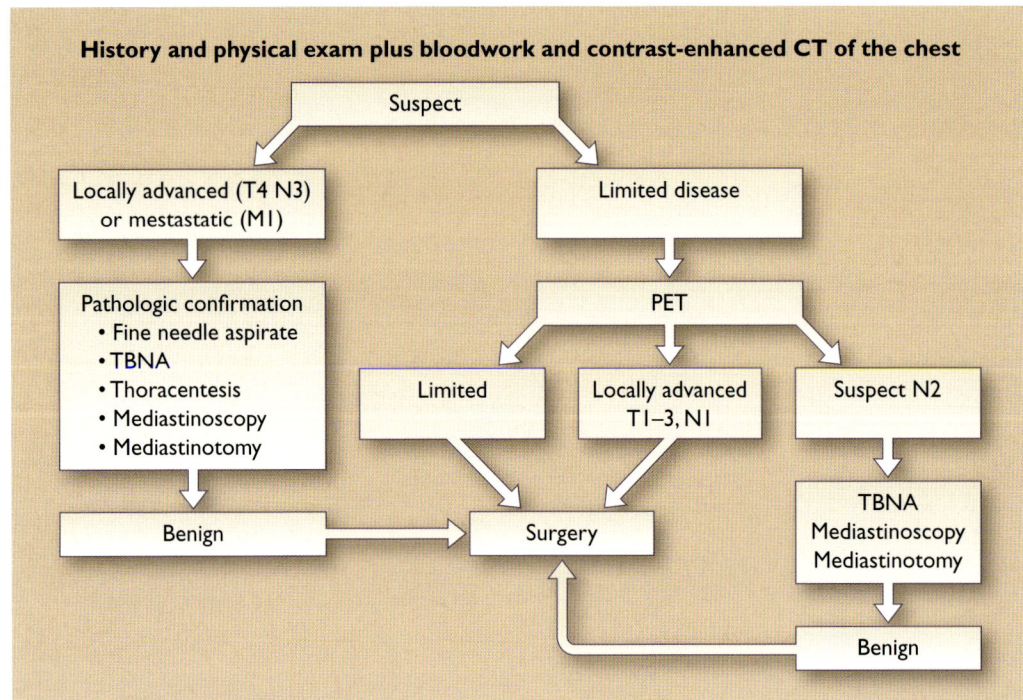

Figure 19-14. Approach to diagnosis and treatment. The acts of making a diagnosis and determining a stage should be given equal priority in the evaluation of suspected lung cancer. Tests that can do both simultaneously should be used preferentially. Diagnosis and staging require a methodical approach. Benign versus malignant status must be determined; the cell type must be identified; and information must be obtained regarding whether the problem is localized (resectable), regional, or metastatic. All patients suspected of having lung cancer should have a thorough history and physical exam. This should be accompanied by blood chemistry (including complete blood count, liver transaminases, and calcium) and by contrast-enhanced CT of the chest to include liver and adrenal glands. PET—positron emission tomography; TBNA—transbronchial needle aspiration.

Radiography

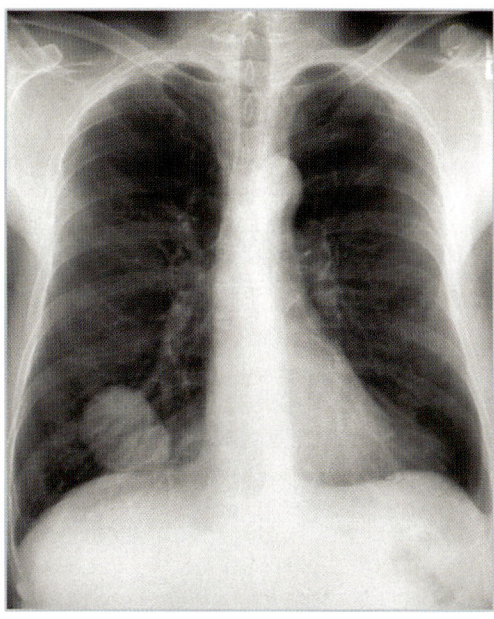

Figure 19-15. Conventional chest radiography. Standard posteroanterior and lateral chest radiographs comprise the primary method of detecting lung cancer. The accuracy of the chest radiograph in the detection of lung cancer is 70% to 88%; in the detection of hilar adenopathy, it is 61% to 71%, and in the detection of mediastinal adenopathy, it is 47% to 60% [16,23]. The detection of abnormalities can be helpful in the selection of subsequent evaluation techniques. The posteroanterior chest radiograph reveals a peripheral lobulated 4-cm mass in the right lower lobe, which is suggestive of adenocarcinoma.

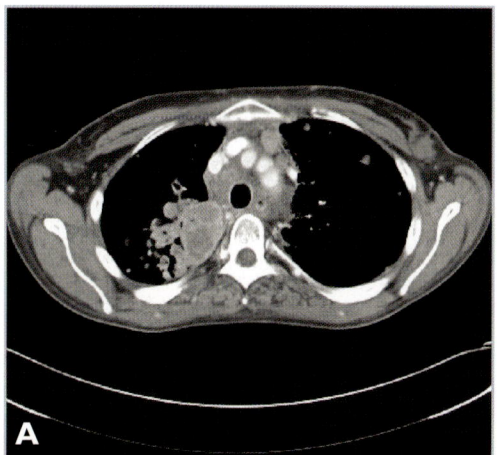 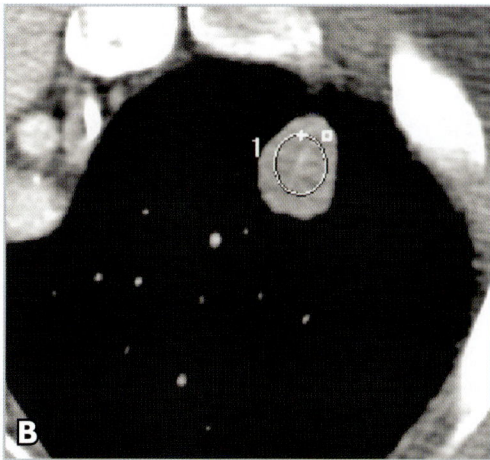 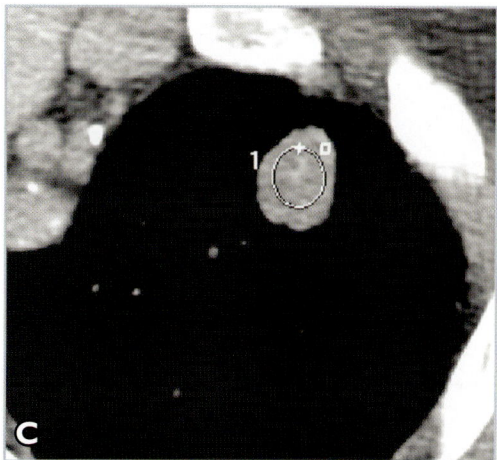

Figure 19-16. CT is the cornerstone imaging method for evaluation of lung cancer. In general, a chest CT is obtained in all patients with known or suspected lung cancer to help characterize nodules, determine the best biopsy or surgical approach, and assess the locoregional extent. CT has been the standard noninvasive method for mediastinal staging. It is generally accepted that the criterion for abnormality is a lymph node greater than 1 cm in short-axis diameter. In a recent review, the pooled sensitivity of CT was 0.51 (95% confidence interval [CI], 0.47 to 0.54), and the pooled specificity was 0.86 (95% CI, 0.84 to 0.88). The positive and negative likelihood ratios were 3.4 and 0.6, respectively [24]. Thus, other methods are needed to confidently prove or refute disease. **A,** CT of chest demonstrating dominant right suprahilar mass, mediastinal adenopathy, and contralateral metastasis in a patient with small cell lung carcinoma. Dynamic contrast-enhanced CT is a noninvasive method of evaluating lung nodules. If a nodule enhances less than 15 Hounsfield units after radiocontrast injection, it is strongly predictive of benignity (sensitivity 98%, specificity 58%) [25]. **B** and **C,** Negative CT enhancement study displaying the 1-minute and 4-minute images; the *circle* indicates the region of interest where the amount of enhancement is calculated.

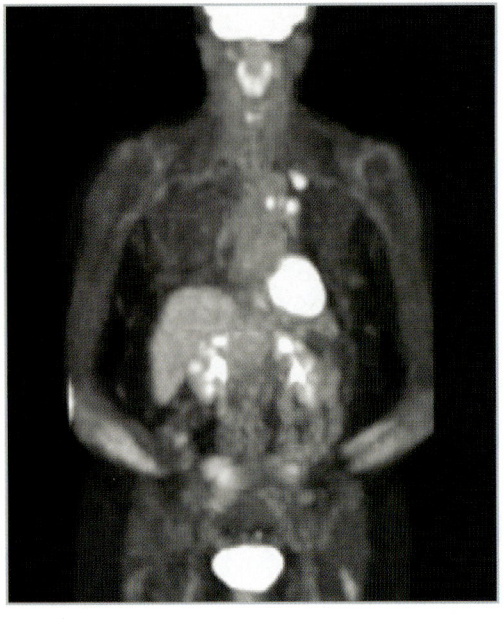

Figure 19-17. Positron emission tomography (PET). PET with 18F-fluoro-2-deoxy-D-glucose (FDG) is an emerging complementary tool in the diagnosis and staging of lung cancer. The overall sensitivity is 96%, the specificity is 79%, and the accuracy is 91% for diagnosis of indeterminate pulmonary nodules. The overall utility of PET for lymph node staging is sensitivity 89%, specificity 92%, and accuracy 90%. More importantly, PET can prevent a futile thoracotomy in 1 of 5 patients [26,27]. One caveat is that since the test is not 100% specific and the best chance for cure of lung cancer is with surgical resection, all positive results that would make a patient stage IIIB or IV (inoperable) should be confirmed by biopsy. This FDG-PET demonstrates enhancement in the left apex, hilum, and subcarinal area in a patient with non–small cell lung cancer.

Sputum Cytology

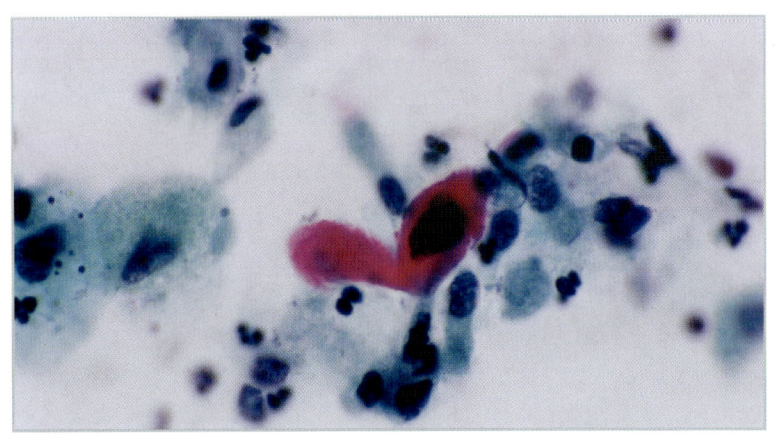

Figure 19-18. Color plate of a Papanicolaou smear showing squamous cell carcinoma. Sputum cytology is a noninvasive method to establish a diagnosis of carcinoma. The pooled sensitivity is 66% and the specificity is 99% in symptomatic patients suspected of having lung cancer, as opposed to a sensitivity of about 30% in a screening population [28]. A major limitation of sputum cytology is that it does not provide any staging information, which is often provided by other more invasive tests.

Bronchoscopy

Diagnostic Yield of Various Bronchoscopic Techniques

Procedure	Histologic Type	Average Diagnostic Yield, % (range)	Agreement with Definitive Diagnosis, % (range)
Bronchial washing	Squamous cell	79 (77–81)	93
	Adenocarcinoma	79 (75–83)	50
	Large cell	62 (50–73)	20
	Small cell	65 (64–66)	100
Bronchial brushing	Squamous cell	78 (52–93)	82 (78–87)
	Adenocarcinoma	69 (57–88)	82 (79–85)
	Large cell	62 (20–100)	58 (33–84)
	Small cell	66 (30–95)	80 (72–87)
Forceps biopsy	Squamous cell	75 (63–96)	88 (88–96)
	Adenocarcinoma	55 (50–67)	71 (46–82)
	Large cell	57 (23–80)	31 (20–38)
	Small cell	85 (69–100)	85 (70–100)

Figure 19-19. Diagnostic yield of various bronchoscopic techniques in lung cancer. The diagnostic yield in central tumors (squamous cell and small cell carcinoma) are acceptable, as demonstrated in the figure. The diagnostic yield in peripheral lesions is better using biplane (40%–80%) than conventional single-plane fluoroscopy (10%–30%). Tumor size also affects sensitivity, which is low (34%) in lesions less than 2 cm in diameter but rises to 63% when the lesion is greater than 2 cm in diameter [29]. This may be because tumors larger than 3 cm are supplied by three or more bronchi in 60% of cases, and lesions less than 3 cm are usually supplied by only one bronchus. When a bronchus is seen on CT leading directly to lesion ("Bronchus Sign") the yield is increased regardless of size. The overall sensitivity of bronchoscopy using all basic techniques (secretions, brushing, biopsy, and transbronchial needle aspiration) is 88% [29]. (*Adapted from* Arroliga and Matthay [30].)

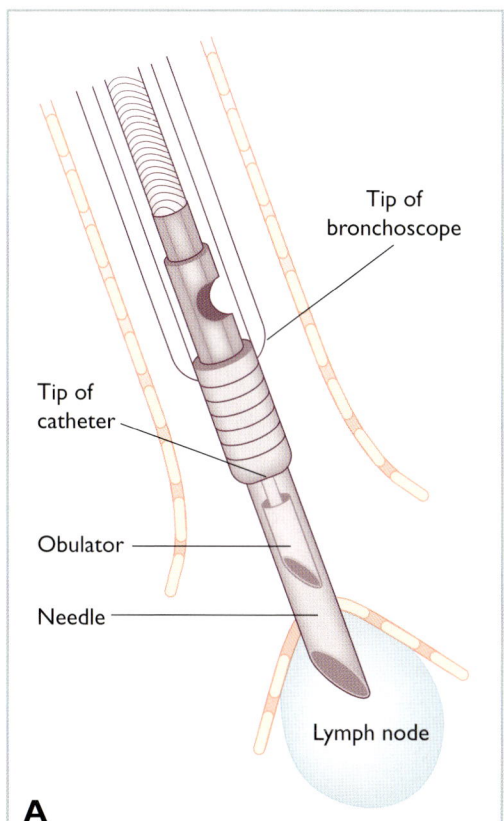 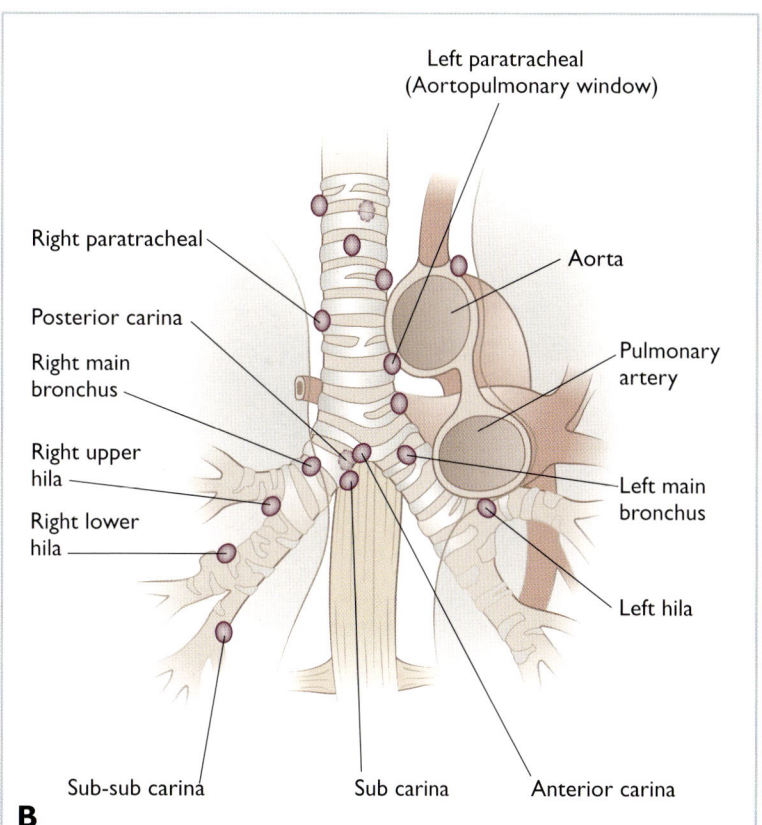

Figure 19-20. Transbronchial needle aspiration (TBNA). TBNA (**A**) is particularly useful in evaluating extrabronchial lesions or paratracheal, subcarinal, or hilar lymph nodes (**B**). The diagnostic yield of bronchial washing, brushing, and forceps biopsy for peripheral lung cancers is increased from 48% to 69% when TBNA is added. The diagnostic yield of TBNA when using the classic landmark technique to assess mediastinal lymphadenopathy is 93% with four passes and 100% with seven passes of the needle [31]. There are few complications with this technique. Nevertheless, TBNA has not been widely adopted by bronchoscopists.

Other Procedures

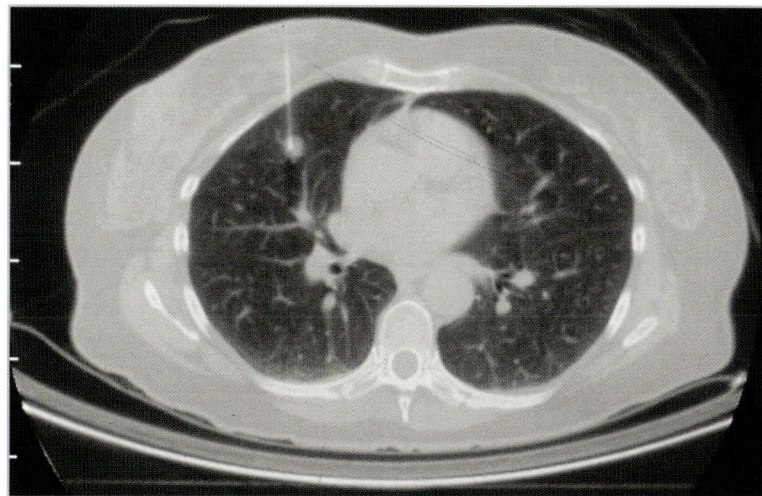 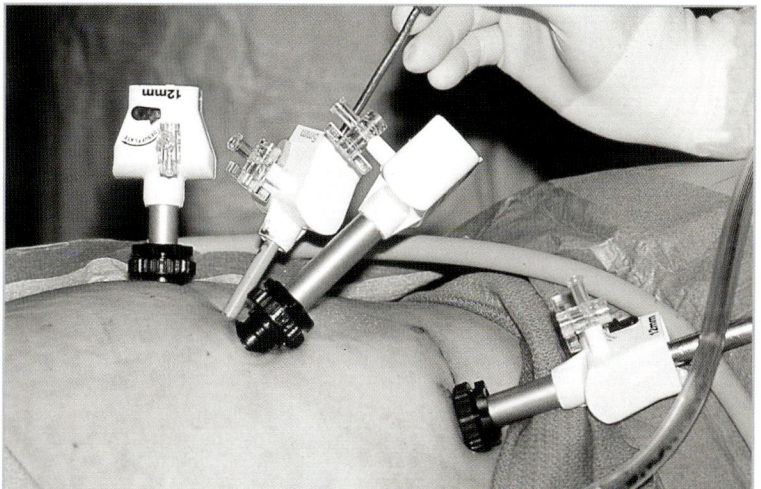

Figure 19-21. Percutaneous transthoracic needle aspiration (TTNA) using CT guidance. In peripheral lesions, percutaneous TTNA has a pooled sensitivity and specificity of 90% and 97%, respectively, independent of the size of the lesion [32]. Unfortunately, it is also associated with a higher incidence of adverse events. The incidence of pneumothorax with TTNA is 32% to 36% compared with less than 1% with bronchoscopy. The incidence of bleeding is also greater with TTNA (3.5%) than with bronchoscopy (< 1%).

Figure 19-22. Thoracoscopy. Biopsy using video-assisted thoracoscopic surgery of pleural lesions is particularly useful in the diagnosis of pleural metastatic lesions when pleural fluid cytology or "blind" percutaneous needle biopsy yields negative results. It also has a pivotal role in wedge resection of indeterminate nodules, whose status remains indeterminate despite noninvasive work-up in individuals with a high pretest probability for malignancy. In this scenario, if wedge were positive for malignancy, then definitive surgery could be done in patients with adequate pulmonary reserve and, conversely, if a benign diagnosis were to be obtained, then unneeded thoracotomy could be avoided [32].

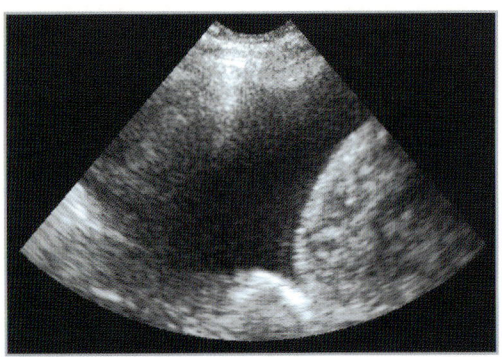

Figure 19-23. Thoracentesis. When a pleural effusion is found in a patient with suspected cancer, it is imperative that he/she undergo diagnostic thoracentesis. It is important to distinguish between malignant and benign effusion because malignant effusions upstage patients to T4, making them stage IIIB, and thus inoperable. There is a large variation in diagnostic yields of initial pleural fluid cytology, ranging from 62% to 90% [33]. Repeat thoracentesis will confirm malignancy in an additional 20% of malignant effusions. Closed pleural biopsy has a higher complication rate and adds little additional yield to thoracentesis. Between 10% and 20% of patients with malignant pleural effusions will still not have a diagnosis after serial thoracentesis. In such patients, thoracoscopy should be used. Although thoracoscopic biopsy requires local or general anesthesia, the diagnostic yield is greater than 95% [34].

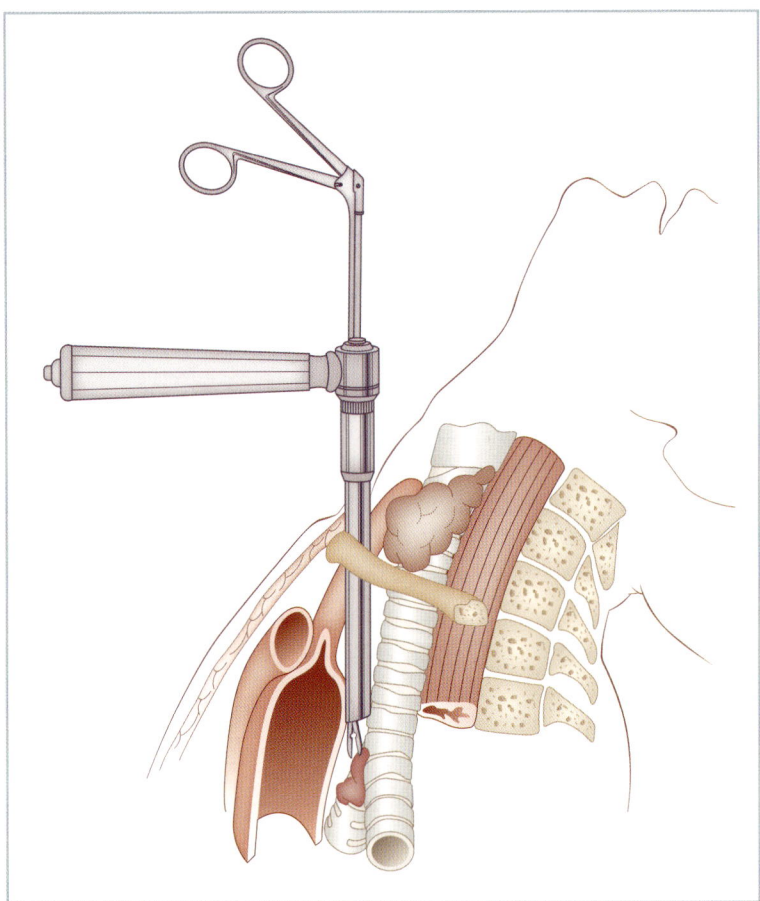

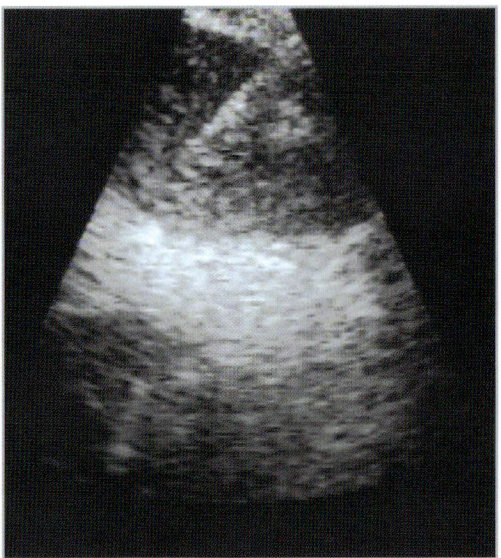

Figure 19-24. Mediastinoscopy and anterior mediastinotomy. Mediastinoscopy is an invasive, yet safe, procedure that can be used to identify malignant lymph nodes in the superior mediastinum [35]. The procedure involves an incision just above the suprasternal notch, insertion of a mediastinoscope alongside the trachea, and biopsy of the mediastinal nodes. Mediastinal lymph node metastasis usually denotes unresectability. The introduction of mediastinoscopy has reduced the frequency of staging thoracotomies from 30% to 50%, to 5% to 15% [36]. Anterior mediastinotomy is used to access aortopulmonic window lymph nodes that are not accessible via conventional mediastinoscopy.

Figure 19-25. Endobronchial ultrasound (EBUS)-guided transbronchial needle aspiration. EBUS-guided transbronchial needle aspiration (TBNA) is an emerging tool that has promise to establish itself as the definitive staging tool for the mediastinum. The diagnostic yield using EBUS-TBNA far exceeds that of conventional TBNA. In a recent study involving patients with CT-determined abnormal mediastinal nodes (> 1 cm), the sensitivity was 94%, the specificity was 100%, and the positive predictive value was 100% per patient for EBUS. There were no complications [37]. In another study of patients with CT-determined normal mediastinal lymph nodes, sensitivity was 92.3%, specificity was 100%, and negative predictive value was 96.3%. Again, no complications occurred. The authors also reported that EBUS-TBNA avoids unnecessary surgical exploration in 1 of 6 patients [38].

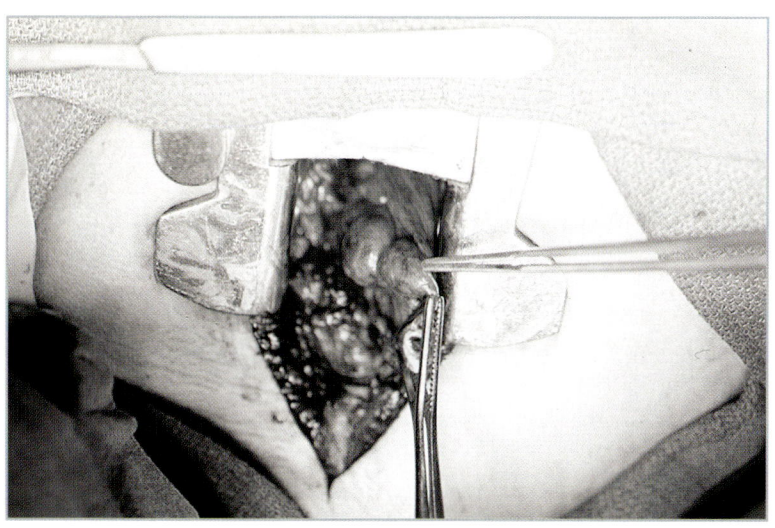

Figure 19-26. Thoracotomy. Thoracotomy should be considered for establishing a diagnosis in a highly suspicious lesion when the lesion is potentially resectable, the patient is sufficiently physiologically fit for resection, and there is no evidence of distant metastasis after a thorough and complete staging work-up [39].

Revised Internation Tumor, Node, and Metastasis Staging System for Lung Cancer

Primary tumor (T)		Regional lymph nodes (N)	
TX	Primary tumor cannot be assessed, or tumor is proven by the presence of malignant cells in sputum or bronchial washings but not visualized by imaging or bronchoscopy	NX	Regional lymph nodes cannot be assessed
T0	No evidence of primary tumor	N0	No regional lymph node metastasis
Tis	Carcinoma in situ	N1	Metastasis to ipsilateral peribronchial and/or ipsilateral hilar lymph nodes and intrapulmonary nodes involved by direct extension of the primary tumor
T1	Tumor < 3 cm in greatest dimension surrounded by lung or visceral pleura without bronchoscopic evidence of invasion more proximal than the lobar bronchus (*ie*, not in the main bronchus)	N2	Metastasis to ipsilateral mediastinal and/or subcarinal lymph nodes
T2	Tumor with any of the following features of size or extent: > 3 cm in greatest dimension; involves main bronchus; > 2 cm distal to the carina; invades the visceral pleura; associated with atelectasis or obstructive pneumonitis that extends to the hilar region but does not involve the entire lung	N3	Metastasis to contralateral mediastinal, contralateral, hilar ipsilateral, or contralateral scalene or supraclavicular lymph nodes
T3	Tumor of any size that directly invades any of the following: chest wall (including superior sulcus tumors), diaphragm, mediastinal pleura, parietal pericardium, or tumor in the main bronchus < 2 cm distal to the carina but without involvement of the carina or associated atelectasis or obstructive pneumonitis of the entire lung	**Distant metastasis (M)**	
T4	Tumor of any size that invades any of the following: mediastinum, heart, great vessels, trachea, esophagus, vertebral body, carina, or tumor with a malignant pleural or pericardial effusion or with satellite tumor nodules within the primary-tumor lobe of the lung	MX	Presence of distant metastasis cannot be assessed
		M0	No distant metastasis
		M1	Distant metastasis present

Figure 19-27. Staging of non–small cell lung cancer. Tumor, node, and metastasis staging is an inversely proportional prognosis in patients with non–small cell lung cancer. Five-year postoperative survival rates in patients with pathologic stage cancer are as follows: IA, 67%; IB, 57%; IIA, 55%; IIB, 39%; IIIA, 25%; IIIB, 5%; and IV, less than 1% [24,40–43].

Supraclavicular	Scalene (ipsi-/contralateral)	Mediastinal (Contralateral)	Mediastinal (Ipsilateral)	Subcarinal	Hilar (Contralateral)	Hilar (Ipsilateral)	Peribronchial (ipsilateral)	Lymph node (N)	T1	T2	T3	T4	Primary tumor (T)
+	/ +	/ +			/	+		N3	Stage IIIB				
-	-	-	+&/+	-				N2	Stage IIIA				
-	-	-	-	-	-	* +&/+		N1	Stage IIA	Stage IIB			
-	-	-	-	-	-	-	-	N0	Stage IA	Stage IB	Stage IIB		
Stage 0 (Tis, N0, M0)									T1	T2	T3	T4	Primary tumor (T)

(Stage IV M1 (any T, any N) spans top; M0 bracket on right side)

	T1	T2	T3	T4	Criteria
	a&b&c	Any of a,b,c,d	(a&c)/b/d	(a&c)/d	Criteria
	≤ 3 cm	> 3 cm	Any	Any	a. Size
	No invasion proximal to the lobar bronchus	Main bronchus (≥ 2 cm distal to the carina)	Main bronchus (< 2 cm distal to the carina)	–	b. Endobronchial location
	Surrounded by lung or visceral pleura	Visceral pleura	Chest wall **/ diaphragm/mediastinal pleura/ parietal pericardium	Mediastinum/trachea/ heart/great vessels/ esophagus/vertebral body/carina	c. Local invasion
	–	Atelectasis/ obstructive pneumonitis that extends to the hilar region but doesn't involve the entire lung	Atelectasis/ obstructive pneumonitis of the entire lung	Malignant pleural/ pericardial effusion or satellite tumor nodule(s) within the ipsilateral primary-tumor lobe of the lung	d. Other

Metastases (M)
M0: Absent
M1: Present
Separate metastatic tumor nodule(s) in the ipsilateral nonprimary-tumor lobe(s) of the lung also are classified M1

Tis: Carcinoma *in situ*

Staging is not relevant for occult carcinoma (Tx, N0, M0)

* Including direct extension to Intrapulmonary nodes
** Including superior sulcus tumor

(&: and) (/: or) (&/: and/or)

Figure 19-28. Tumor, node, and metastasis staging of non–small cell lung cancer. Accurate staging is central to choosing an appropriate treatment plan. There must be a careful and methodical search for disease that would exclude surgery (> N2 or M1).

Staging of Small Cell Lung Cancer

Limited disease (30%–40%)

Primary tumor confined to one hemithorax

Ipsilateral hilar supraclavicular, mediastinal lymph nodes

Extensive disease (60%–70%)

Metastatic lesions in the contralateral lung

Distant metastatic involvement (eg, brain, bone, liver)

Malignant pleural effusion

Figure 19-29. Staging of small cell lung cancer. Initial routine staging of small cell lung cancer (SCLC) should include a history, a physical exam, blood chemistries including liver transaminases and calcium, CT of the chest and abdomen, CT or MRI of the brain, and a bone scan. SCLC is divided into limited- and extensive-stage disease. Limited-stage disease is that which can be confined to a single radiation therapy port. Staging for SCLC is, therefore, designed to determine if there is limited or extensive disease. The extent of disease affects chemotherapy and radiation therapy options and is helpful when estimating survival time [44].

Approximate Frequencies of Metastatic Involvement by Lung Cancer		
	Frequency	
Metastatic Site	**All Lung Cancers, %**	**SCLC, %**
Central nervous system	20–50	10–30
Cervical lymph nodes	15–60	5 (extrathoracic)
Bone	25	29–35
Adrenal glands	—	20–40
Liver	1–35	25–28
Heart (including pericardium)	20	—
Bone marrow	—	19–50
Pleural effusion	8–15	—
Pulmonary embolism, infarction	10	—
Pancoast's syndrome	4–8	—
Superior vena cava syndrome	4	42.5

Figure 19-30. Frequency of metastasis to specific sites. Lung cancer may metastasize to a variety of sites. Because metastatic disease affects treatment options, a careful search for evidence of metastasis should be performed [12,14,15,45]. SCLC—small cell lung cancer.

TREATMENT

Contraindications for Pneumonectomy or Lobectomy
Predicted postoperative FEV_1 < 40%, or 0.8 L
$Paco_2$ > 45 mm Hg
Pao_2 < 50 mm Hg
Pulmonary hypertension (mean pulmonary artery pressure > 30 mm Hg)
Cor pulmonale
Maximum oxygen consumption < 10 mL/kg/min
Intractable congestive cardiac failure
Intractable ventricular arrhythmia
Recent myocardial infarction (< 3 mo)

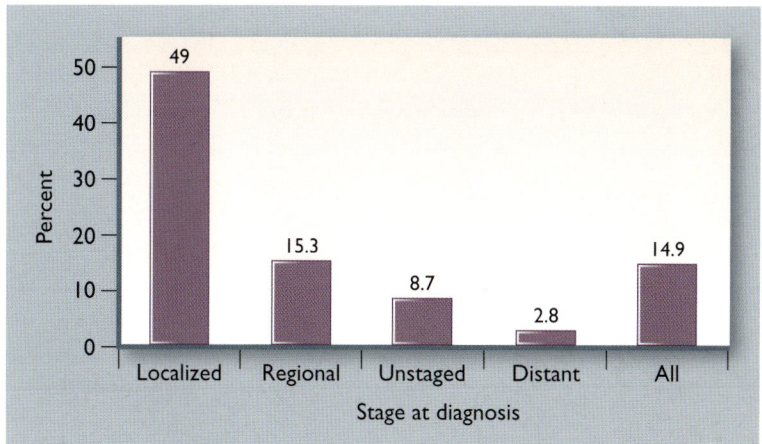

Figure 19-31. Treatment of non–small cell lung cancer. Thoracotomy with anatomic resection (lobectomy, pneumonectomy, segmentectomy) is the primary curative therapy for stage I and II operable patients with non–small cell lung cancer. Patients with stages IIIB and IV are generally considered to be incurable, and if functional status is good, they can be offered palliative chemotherapy or radiation if they have local effects or pain. Neoadjuvant chemotherapy and radiation are increasingly being used as a component of multimodality treatment for locally advanced disease (stage IIIA) [46]. However, routine use has not been justified by current trials. Contraindications for surgery are listed in the figure. Approximately two thirds of patients with surgically resected pathologic stage I disease will be cured. There is no role for adjuvant chemotherapy in stage I disease. Adjuvant chemotherapy has been established as an effective treatment in stage II patients and in stage IIIA patients who had unexpected N2 disease at the time of surgery [46,47]. Despite recent advances in therapy options, the survival rates among patients receiving treatment have remained essentially unchanged. The overall 5-year relative survival rate for lung cancer improved from 6.0% during the period of 1950 to 1954, to about 13.5% during the period of 1974 to 1988; from 2000 to 2004 there has been only a minimal increase in survival, to 14.9%. FEV_1—forced expiratory volume in 1 second.

Figure 19-32. Therapy in small cell lung cancer. Small cell lung cancer (SCLC) is extremely chemotherapy sensitive, with a 60% to 70% response rate. Unfortunately, most of these responses are not durable. Patients with limited stage disease should have combination radiation and platinum-based combination chemotherapy with curative intent. Only about 20% of patients will be cured. Those who achieve complete remission should be offered prophylactic cranial irradiation. Patients with extensive stage disease should receive platinum-based chemotherapy. The median survival time for limited-stage disease is about 20 months and is only about 10 months for extensive-stage disease. Patients who are found to have SCLC after having a pulmonary nodule resected, should have chemotherapy because early metastasis is quite common [44].

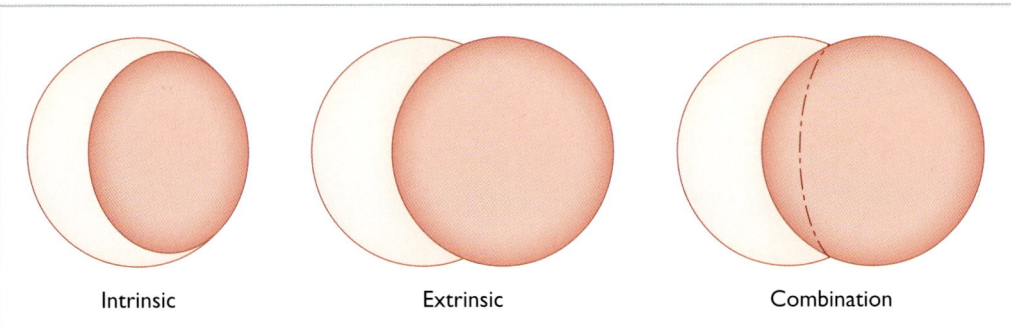

Figure 19-33. Classification of airway obstruction. Airway obstruction is classified as intrinsic, extrinsic, or a combination of the two. When cancer is entirely intraluminal without involvement of the airway wall, it is termed intrinsic. When an external mass exerts pressure on the extraluminal airway causing deformation, and when the wall and mucosa remain uninvolved, then it is purely extrinsic. When there are components of both types, it is termed combined. The type of lesion determines the palliative treatment modality used.

Classification of Endobronchial Therapy Modalities

Debulking	Cold	Hot
Rigid coring	Electrocautery	Cryotherapy
Cupped forceps	PDT	Argon plasma coagulation
Dilation	Brachytherapy	Laser (Nd:YAG, Nd:YAP, CO_2)
Rigid		
Balloon		

Figure 19-34. Endobronchial therapy options. PDT—photodynamic therapy.

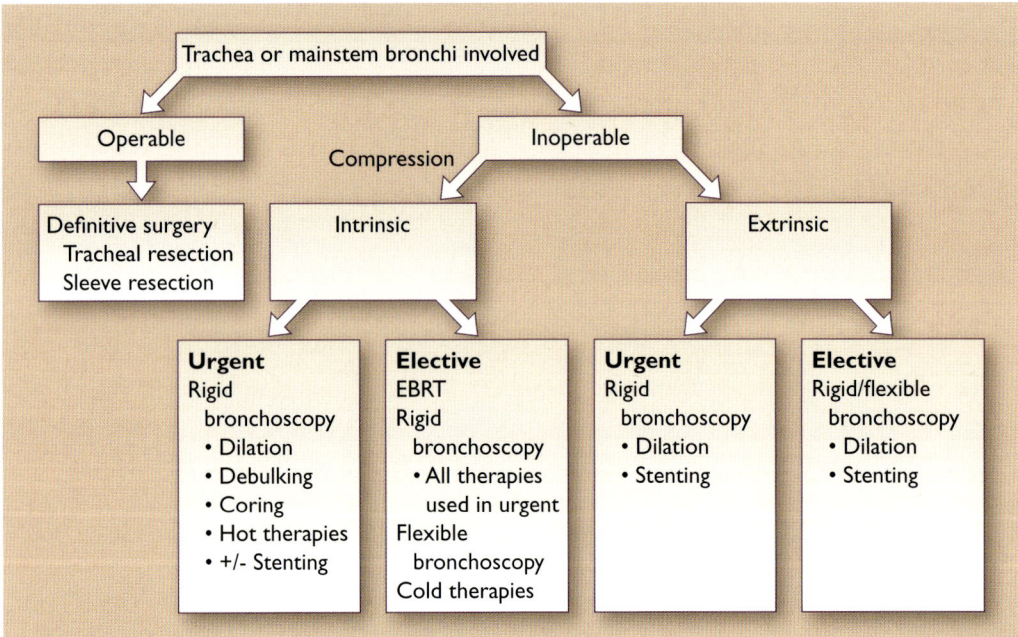

Figure 19-35. Algorithm for the palliative management of airway obstruction caused by malignancy. Approximately 40% of lung cancer deaths occur as a result of locoregional disease from either airway or vascular involvement. If the malignancy is not resectable, the patient is inoperable, or the disease is in the trachea or a main bronchi, then palliative endobronchial therapy may be indicated. To palliate inoperable disease of the airway, one can use external beam radiation therapy (EBRT), endobronchial therapies, or stenting. The choice of modality is determined by the urgency of the situation, the class of the obstruction, and/or the radiosensitivity of the lesion. For example, in many patients with bulky central disease secondary to small cell lung cancer, which is generally very chemotherapy and radiation sensitive, EBRT can result in rapid palliation. On the other hand, a patient with bulky central disease secondary to non–small cell lung cancer, which takes a while to respond to radiation, would be palliated faster with endobronchial therapy.

PROGNOSTIC FACTORS IN LUNG CANCER

Prognostic Markers in Stage I Non–Small Cell Lung Cancer

Variable	Favorable	Unfavorable
Anatomic and pathologic markers		
Tumor status	T1	T2
Histologic subtype*	Squamous	Large cell
Degree of tumor differentiation	Well differentiated	Poorly differentiated
Lymphatic vessel invasion	Absent	Present
Blood vessel invasion	Absent	Present
Mitotic index	Low	High
Degree of plasma cell infiltration	Present	Absent or minimal
Presence of tumor giant cells	Absent	Present
Adenocarcinoma subtype	Bronchioloalveolar, acinar, papillary	Solid tumor with mucus formation
Molecular genetic markers		
K-ras (oncogene) activation	No point mutation	Point mutation at codon 12
ras expression	Absent p21 staining	Strong p21 staining
C-erb B-2 expression	Normal	Increased
p53 (tumor-suppressor gene)	No mutation	Gene mutation present
p53 expression	Normal	Increased
Rb expression	Rb-positive	Rb-negative
bcl-2 expression	bcl-2–positive	bcl-2–negative
Differentiation markers		
Expression of blood group antigen on tumor cell	Conserved	Altered
Expression of H/Le^y/Le^b antigens	Negative staining with MIA-15-5	Positive staining with MIA-15-5
Proliferation markers		
DNA content (flow cytometry)	Diploid	Aneuploid
S-phase fraction (flow cytometry)	Low	High
Mitotic index	< 13 mitoses/10 high-powered fields	≥ 13 mitoses/10 high-powered fields
Proliferation index using Ki-67 nuclear antigen	< 3.5	> 3.5
Thymidine labeling index	< 2.9	> 2.9
Nucleolar organizing regions (mean), n	< 3.8/cell	> 3.8/cell
PCNA	< 5% of tumor cells stained with PCNA	> 5% of tumor cells stained with PCNA
Markers of metastatic propensity		
Intensity of angiogenesis	Low	High
Basement membrane deposition (squamous cell carcinoma)	Extensive	Limited
Soluble interleukin-2 receptor value	Postoperative < preoperative	Postoperative > preoperative
Ability to establish in vitro cell lines	No	Yes

*Adenocarcinoma is intermediate in prognostic value.

Figure 19-36. Prognostic factors in stage I non–small cell lung cancer. The three major prognostic factors in non–small cell lung cancer (NSCLC) are stage of the disease, Karnofsky performance status, and weight loss. About 50% of patients with clinical stage I and 30% to 40% with pathologic stage I disease experience recurrence and die after curative resection [48]. Other anatomic, pathologic, and molecular markers reported to be highly predictive of outcome in stage I NSCLC are shown in the figure. PCNA–proliferating cell nuclear antigen. (*Adapted from* Strauss *et al.* [48].)

Indicators of a Poor Prognosis in Small Cell Lung Cancer

Biochemical			
Low	Elevated	Clinical	Therapeutic
Hemoglobin	Leukocytes	Race nonwhite	Slow response rate
Platelets	LDH	Age > 60 y	Failure to achieve complete response
Na, Cl	CEA	Male gender	Unable to be resected
Albumin	Gamma-glutamyl transpeptidase	Weight loss	Low-dose density
Uric acid		Extensive disease	No radiotherapy (limited disease)
Bicarbonate		Liver, central nervous system, marrow sites/increasing number of sites	

CEA–carcinoembryonic antigen; LDH–lactate dehydrogenase.

Figure 19-37. Prognostic markers in small cell lung cancer. Although the median survival time among patients with limited disease is 20 months and that of patients with extensive disease is 10 months [45], use of prognostic factors may help in selecting patients for more specific, intensive treatment to prolong survival and achieve a cure. (*Adapted from* Skarin [49].)

SCREENING

Screening Pitfalls

Lack of proof of effectiveness

Survival statistics may be misleading in the absence of prospective, randomized controlled data; mortality may be unchanged because of the following:

Lead time bias: survival appears longer because of earlier diagnosis, but the ultimate course and outcome of the disease are unchanged (age-adjusted disease-specific mortality unchanged)

Length time bias: less aggressive tumors are detected more often than their true population distribution because there is a longer potential asymptomatic period during which screening may occur; outcome thereby appears improved in the screened population

Overdiagnosis bias: lesions with no effect on mortality are detected (either the lesions are very indolent or the patient expires from other causes before appearance of tumor symptoms)

Cost

Poor specificity

Figure 19-38. Lung cancer screening. Theoretically, earlier detection and intervention should lead to enhanced resectability and decreased age-adjusted lung cancer mortality. Randomized, controlled trials determined that serial chest radiography and sputum cytology are ineffective screens for lung cancer [50–52]. Low-dose spiral CT (LDCT) has been studied in several prospective cohort studies and has shown no convincing stage shift. A high number of false positive nodules and ancillary findings were noted [53–57]. The American Cancer Society, the National Cancer Institute, and the US Public Health Service do not recommend for or against using LDCT to screen for lung caner. The American College of Chest Physicians does not recommend LDCT except in the context of a well-designed clinical trial [56]. It remains to be determined in a randomized, controlled trial whether CT screening will result in reduced lung cancer mortality. No single specific tumor marker is available for screening asymptomatic patients; however, some are being evaluated for their potential prognostic value when used alone or in combination with other clinical, histopathologic, or biochemical variables. Potential new markers are tumor suppressor genes, loss of heterozygosity, methylation, expression of telomerase, gene expression arrays, and proteomics [58]. Other potential strategies include immunocytology, automated sputum cytometry, and autofluorescence bronchoscopic surveillance [10,59,60]. Although promising, further clinical validation as well as subsequent cost-effectiveness evaluation needs to be done before any formal recommendation can be made for or against these techniques.

REFERENCES

1. Jemal A, Siegel R, Ward E, et al.: Cancer statistics, 2007. *CA Cancer J Clin* 2007, 57(1): 43–66.

2. Surveillance, Epidemiology, and End Results (SEER) Program: *SEER*Stat Database: Mortality—All COD, Public-Use With State, Total U.S. (1969–2004)*, National Cancer Institute, DCCPS, Surveillance Research Program, Cancer Statistics Branch, April 2007. Accessible online at www.seer.cancer.gov. Underlying mortality data provided by NCHS, accessible online at www.cdc.gov/nchs.

3. Surveillance, Epidemiology, and End Results (SEER) Program: *SEER*Stat Database: Incidence—SEER 9 Regs Limited-Use, Nov 2006 Sub (1973–2004)*, National Cancer Institute, DCCPS, Surveillance Research Program, Cancer Statistics Branch, April 2007, based on the November 2006 submission. Accessible online at www.seer.cancer.gov.

4. Surveillance, Epidemiology, and End Results (SEER) Program: *SEER*Stat Database: Incidence—SEER 9 Regs Public-Use, Nov 2002 Sub (1973–2000)*, National Cancer Institute, DCCPS, Surveillance Research Program, Cancer Statistics Branch, April 2003, based on the November 2002 submission. Accessible online at www.seer.cancer.gov.

5. Surveillance, Epidemiology, and End Results (SEER) Program: *SEER*Stat Database: Mortality—All COD, Public-Use With State, Total U.S. (1969–2000)*, National Cancer Institute, DCCPS, Surveillance Research Program, Cancer Statistics Branch, April 2003. Accessible online at www.seer.cancer.gov. Underlying mortality data provided by NCHS, accessible online at www.cdc.gov/nchs.

6. Ries LAG, Eisner MP, Kosary CL, et al., eds: *SEER Cancer Statistics Review, 1975–2000*. Bethesda, MD: National Cancer Institute; 2003. Accessible online at http://seer.cancer.gov/csr/1975_2000.

7. Alberg AJ, Ford JG, Samet JM: Epidemiology of lung cancer: ACCP evidence-based clinical practice guidelines, edn 2. *Chest* 2007, 132(Suppl 3):29S–55S.

8. Kabat GC: Recent developments in the epidemiology of lung cancer. *Semin Surg Oncol* 1993, 9(2):73–79.

9. Shopland DR, Eyre HJ, Pechacek TF: Smoking-attributable cancer mortality in 1991: is lung cancer now the leading cause of death among smokers in the United States? *J Natl Cancer Inst* 1991, 83(16):1142–1148.

10. Hirsch FR: Early detection of lung cancer: clinical perspectives of recent advances in biology and radiology. *Clin Cancer Res* 2001, 7(1):5–22.

11. Ferguson MK: Synchronous primary lung cancers. *Chest* 1993, 103(Suppl 4):398S–400S.

12. Vaporciyan AA, et al.: Cancer of the lung, In *Cancer Medicine*. Edited by Bast RC. Hamilton, ON: BC Decker Inc.; 2000.

13. Brambilla E, Travis WD, Colby TV, et al.: The new World Health Organization classification of lung tumours. *Eur Respir J* 2001, 18(6):1059–1068.

14. Patel AM, Peters SG: Clinical manifestations of lung cancer. *Mayo Clin Proc* 1993, 68(3):273–277.

15. Prager D.: Bronchogenic carcinoma. In *Textbook of Respiratory Medicine*. Edited by Murray JF, Nadel JA. Philadelphia: WB Saunders; 2000:415–1451.

16. Karsell PR, McDougall JC: Diagnostic tests for lung cancer. *Mayo Clin Proc* 1993, 68(3):288–296.

17. Hamilton W, Peters TJ, Round A, Sharp D: What are the clinical features of lung cancer before the diagnosis is made? a population based case-control study. *Thorax* 2005, 60(12):1059–1065.

18. Jemal A, Murray T, Samuels A, et al.: Cancer statistics, 2003. *CA Cancer J Clin* 2003, 53(1):5–26.

19. Gerber RB, Mazzone P, Arroliga AC: Paraneoplastic syndromes associated with bronchogenic carcinoma. *Clin Chest Med* 2002, 23(1):257–264.

20. Patel AM, Davila DG, Peters SG: Paraneoplastic syndromes associated with lung cancer. *Mayo Clin Proc* 1993, 68(3):278–287.

21. Thomas L, Kwok Y, Edelman MG: Management of paraneoplastic syndromes in lung cancer. *Curr Treat Options Oncol* 2004, 5(1):51–62.

22. Kiss GT: Pulmonary diseases: carcinoma of the lung. In *Practical Guide to the Care of the Medical Patient*. Edited by Ferri F. St. Louis: Mosby Year Book; 1991:519–524.

23. Swensen SJ, Brown LR: Conventional radiography of the hilum and mediastinum in bronchogenic carcinoma. *Radiol Clin North Am* 1990, 28(3):521–538.

24. Silvestri GA, Gould MK, Margolis ML, et al.: Noninvasive staging of non–small cell lung cancer: ACCP evidenced-based clinical practice guidelines, edn 2. *Chest* 2007, 132(Suppl 3):178S–201S.

25. Swensen SJ, Jett JR, Hartman TE, et al.: Lung cancer screening with CT: Mayo Clinic experience. *Radiology* 2003, 226(3):756–761.

26. van Tinteren H, Hoekstra OS, Smit EF, et al.: Effectiveness of positron emission tomography in the preoperative assessment of patients with suspected non–small cell lung cancer: the PLUS multicentre randomised trial. *Lancet* 2002, 359(9315):1388–1393.

27. Vansteenkiste JF, Stroobants SG: The role of positron emission tomography with 18F-fluoro-2-deoxy-D-glucose in respiratory oncology. *Eur Respir J* 2001, 17(4):802–820.

28. Schreiber G, McCrory DC: Performance characteristics of different modalities for diagnosis of suspected lung cancer: summary of published evidence. *Chest* 2003, 123(Suppl 1):115S–128S.

29. Rivera MP, Mehta AC: Initial diagnosis of lung cancer: ACCP evidence-based clinical practice guidelines, edn 2. *Chest* 2007, 132(Suppl 3):131S–148S.

30. Arroliga AC, Matthay RA: The role of bronchoscopy in lung cancer. *Clin Chest Med* 1993, 14(1):87–98.

31. Chin R Jr, McCain TW, Lucia MA, et al.: Transbronchial needle aspiration in diagnosing and staging lung cancer: how many aspirates are needed? *Am J Respir Crit Care Med* 2002, 166(3):377–381.

32. Rivera MP, Detterbeck F, Mehta AC: Diagnosis of lung cancer: the guidelines. *Chest* 2003, 123(Suppl 1):129S–136S.

33. Neragi-Miandoab S: Malignant pleural effusion: current and evolving approaches for its diagnosis and management. *Lung Cancer* 2006, 54(1):1–9.

34. Fenton KN, Richardson JD: Diagnosis and management of malignant pleural effusions. *Am J Surg* 1995, 170(1):69–74.

35. Mentzer S.: Mediastinoscopy, thoracoscopy, and video-assisted thoracic surgery in the diagnosis and staging of lung cancer. *Chest* 1997, 112(4):239S–241S.

36. Pearson FG: Staging of the mediastinum: role of mediastinoscopy and computed tomography. *Chest* 1993, 103(Suppl 4):346S–348S.

37. Herth FJ, Eberhardt R, Vilmann P, et al.: Real-time endobronchial ultrasound guided transbronchial needle aspiration for sampling mediastinal lymph nodes. *Thorax* 2006, 61(9):795–798.

38. Herth FJ, Ernst A, Eberhardt R, et al.: Endobronchial ultrasound-guided transbronchial needle aspiration of lymph nodes in the radiologically normal mediastinum. *Eur Respir J* 2006, 28(5):910–914.

39. Moffatt SD, Mitchell JD, Whyte RI: Role of video-assisted thoracoscopic surgery and classic thoracotomy in lung cancer management. *Curr Opin Pulm Med* 2002, 8(4):281–286.

40. Lababede O, Meziane MA, Rice TW: TNM staging of lung cancer: a quick reference chart. *Chest* 1999, 115(1):233–235.

41. Mountain CF: A new international staging system for lung cancer. *Chest* 1986, 89(Suppl 4):225S–233S.

42. Mountain CF: Revisions in the international system for staging lung cancer. *Chest* 1997, 111(6):1710–1717.

43. Mountain CF: The international system for staging lung cancer. *Semin Surg Oncol* 2000, 18(2):106–15.

44. Simon GR, Turrisi A: Management of small cell lung cancer: ACCP evidence-based clinical practice guidelines, edn 2. *Chest* 2007, 132(Suppl 3):324S–339S.

45. Simon GR, Wagner H: Small cell lung cancer. *Chest* 2003, 123(90010):259S–271S.

46. Robinson LA, Ruckdeschel JC, Wagner H, et al.: Treatment of non–small cell lung cancer—stage IIIa: ACCP evidence-based clinical practice guidelines, edn 2. *Chest* 2007, 132(Suppl 3):243S–265S.

47. Scott WJ, Howington J, Feigenberg S, et al.: Treatment of non–small cell lung cancer stage I and stage II: ACCP evidence-based clinical practice guidelines, edn 2. *Chest* 2007, 132(Suppl 3):234S–242S.

48. Strauss GM, Kwiatkowski DJ, Harpole DH, et al.: Molecular and pathologic markers in stage I non–small cell carcinoma of the lung. *J Clin Oncol* 1995, 13(5):1265–1379.

49. Skarin AT: Analysis of long-term survivors with small-cell lung cancer. *Chest* 1993, 103(Suppl 4):440S–444S.

50. Fontana RS: Lung cancer screening: the Mayo program. *J Occup Med* 1986, 28(8):746–50.

51. Melamed MR: Screening for early lung cancer: results of the Memorial Sloan-Kettering study in New York. *Chest* 1984, 86(1):44–53.

52. Tockman MS: Survival and mortality form lung cancer in a screened population: the Johns Hopkins study. *Chest* 1986, 89(4):324S–26S.

53. Kaneko M, Kusumoto M, Kobayashi T, et al.: Computed tomography screening for lung carcinoma in Japan. *Cancer* 2000, 89(Suppl 11):2485–2488.

54. MacRedmond R, Logan PM, Lee M, et al.: Screening for lung cancer using low dose CT scanning. *Thorax* 2004, 59(3):237–241.

55. Swensen SJ, Jett JR, Hartman TE, et al.: CT screening for lung cancer: five-year prospective experience. *Radiology* 2005, 235(1):259–265.

56. Bach PB, Silvestri GA, Hanger M, et al.: Screening for lung cancer: ACCP evidence-based clinical practice guidelines, edn 2. *Chest* 2007, 132(Suppl 3):69S–77S.

57. Henschke CI, Yankelevitz DF, Libby DM, et al.: Survival of patients with stage I lung cancer detected on CT screening. *N Engl J Med* 2006, 355(17):1763–1771.

58. Bunn PA Jr: Molecular biology and early diagnosis in lung cancer. *Lung Cancer* 2002, 38(1):S5–8.

59. Kennedy TC, Lam S, Hirsch FR: Review of recent advances in fluorescence bronchoscopy in early localization of central airway lung cancer. *Oncologist* 2001, 6(3):257–262.

60. Palcic B, Garner DM, Beveridge J, et al.: Increase of sensitivity of sputum cytology using high-resolution image cytometry: field study results. *Cytometry* 2002, 50(3):168–176.

PULMONARY NEOPLASMS OTHER THAN LUNG CANCER

Peter Mazzone, Carol Farver, Peter B. O'Donovan, and Raed A. Dweik

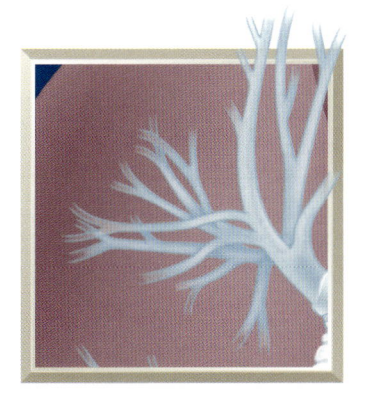
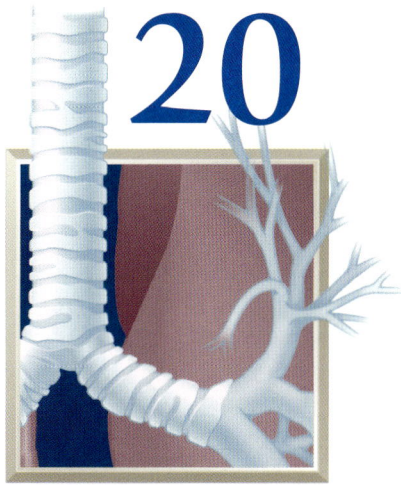
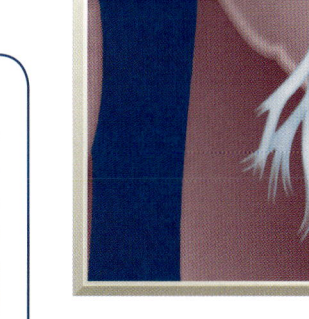

Pulmonary neoplasms other than the four major primary bronchogenic carcinomas include typical and atypical carcinoids, hamartomas, mucous gland tumors, papillomas, juvenile laryngotracheal papillomatosis, mesenchymal tumors, sclerosing hemangiomas, intravascular bronchioloalveolar tumors (epithelioid hemangioendotheliomas), teratomas, blastomas, and inflammatory pseudotumors. Although many of these tumors are rare, they need to be considered in the differential diagnosis when a patient presents with a lung nodule or a mass. This chapter reviews the clinical presentation and the radiographic and histologic features of these tumors.

CARCINOID TUMORS

Typical Carcinoid Tumors

Distinguishing Features of Typical and Atypical Carcinoid Tumors		
Feature	**Typical Carcinoid**	**Atypical Carcinoid**
Histologic pattern	Neuroendocrine	Neuroendocrine
Mitoses	Absent or rare	2–10 per 10 HPFs
Necrosis	Rare	Characteristic
Lymph node metastases, %	5–15	40–57
Distant metastases, %	2	20
5-year survival, %	87–93	44–75

Figure 20-1. Histologic and prognostic differences between typical and atypical carcinoids. Carcinoid tumors of the lung are neuroendocrine tumors. They account for 20% to 32% of all carcinoid tumors. Annual incidences had been reported in the 2 to 5 per 1 million range, but recently the incidence has increased to 11 to 17 per 1 million. They are divided into low-grade, typical carcinoids and intermediate-grade, atypical carcinoids. Approximately four out of five carcinoids are typical. They are distinguished from atypical carcinoids by their histologic features. Atypical carcinoids are more aggressive tumors. They more often involve the lymph nodes, and they have a poorer prognosis than do typical carcinoids [1–8]. HPFs—high-power fields. (*Adapted from* Arroliga *et al.* [9].)

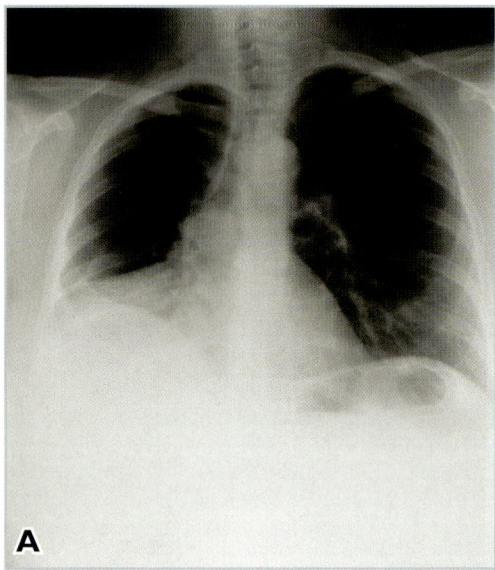 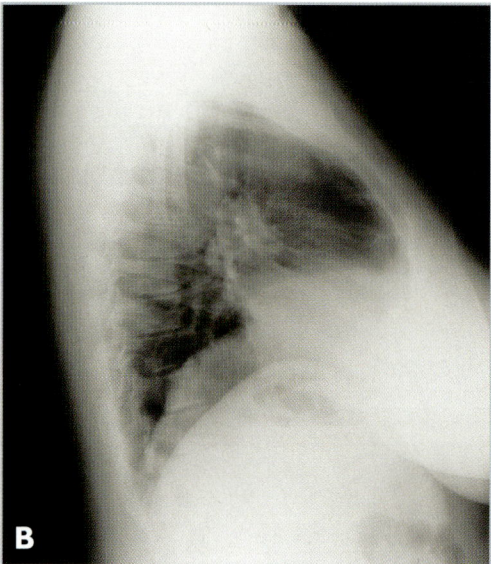 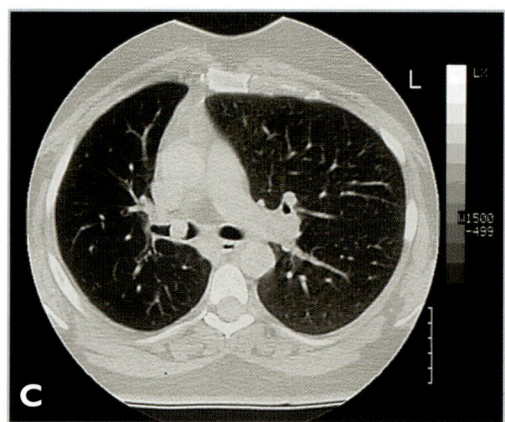

Figure 20-2. Typical carcinoid tumors: posteroanterior (**A**) and lateral (**B**) chest radiographs of a patient with a carcinoid tumor of the bronchus intermedius. The tumor resulted in right middle lobe collapse. A CT of the same patient (**C**) demonstrates a well-circumscribed lesion in the bronchus intermedius. Notice the loss of volume in the right lung. In up to 80% of cases, typical carcinoids are located in the mainstem or lobar bronchi. They may obstruct the airway, with 40% or more having radiographic evidence of segmental or lobar atelectasis, with or without postobstructive pneumonia [1,10–12]. Given the carcinoids' central location, the most common presenting symptoms are cough, hemoptysis, dyspnea, and wheezing. Between 30% and 50% of the time, the individual is asymptomatic [1,12,13]. Carcinoid tumors may rarely lead to ectopic Cushing's syndrome (ECS). The classic Cushingoid appearance is present in most cases, hypertension is prominent, and hypokalemia is found in approximately 50% of cases [14]. It has been suggested that typical bronchial carcinoids producing ECS are a more aggressive subtype, being locally more invasive with more lymph node metastases [15], but others have not found this to be the case [16,17]. Bronchopulmonary carcinoids have been reported in patients with MEN 1 [18], and have been reported to secrete growth hormone-releasing hormone as well [19]. Lesions in the periphery are usually well demarcated, round, and radiopaque, with sharp and often notched margins [11]. Hilar adenopathy is uncommon in either presentation and, if present, is probably due to inflammation [11]. Cavitation is uncommon, although it may occur in atypical carcinoids. Other uncommon radiologic features of typical carcinoids include calcification and satellite nodules [10,11]. Typical carcinoids are four times more likely than atypical carcinoids to be central in location (see Fig. 20-3) [12].

Continued on the next page

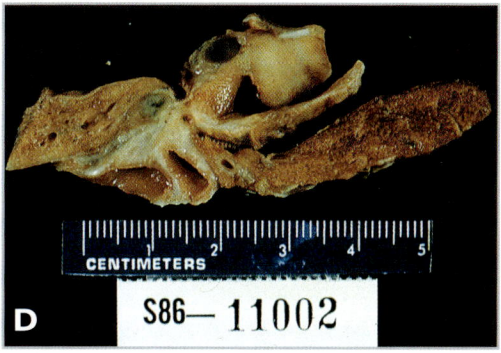
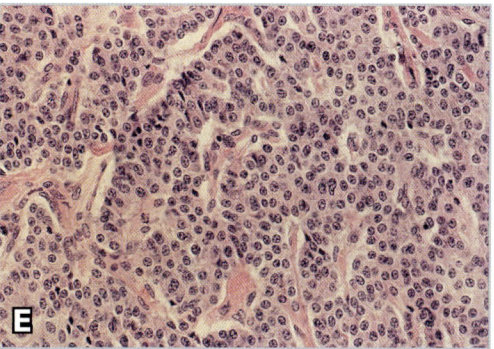

Figure 20-2. (Continued) (**D**) Gross specimen of a carcinoid tumor, obtained from a different patient. Notice the well-encapsulated, yellow, homogenous, endobronchial mass protruding into the lumen of the airway. (**E**) Microscopic specimen of a typical carcinoid tumor. The tumor is composed of nests of cells with slightly spindled nuclei, finely stippled chromatin, and a "salt-and-pepper" pattern. The cells have a moderate amount of pink cytoplasm that lack distinct borders. The cell nests are highlighted by intervening congested vessels. The degree of nuclear pleomorphism is mild to moderate, and mitotic figures are rare. The histologic pattern in central tumors may be different from that in peripheral tumors [20]. Although both usually have medium-sized, uniform epithelial cells with limited nuclear pleomorphism and limited mitoses, the pattern of cell growth in peripheral lesions may be less organized, more crowded, and without orientation. A spindle pattern is also more common in peripheral carcinoid tumors [20,21]. When the tumor is less than 5 mm in diameter a label of carcinoid tumorlet is applied. A potentially premalignant lesion, diffuse idiopathic pulmonary neuroendocrine cell hyperplasia, has been reported in some carcinoid resection specimens. When imaged with positron emission tomography–CT scanning the uptake tends to be less than other neuroendocrine tumors of the lung [22] but still yields positive findings in many patients [23,24]. Diagnosis is usually made by bronchoscopy. Bronchoscopic resection and treatment with cryotherapy have been reported to be successful in selected groups [25,26]. Surgical resection, often with parenchyma-sparing procedures, remains the treatment of choice [27]. The presence of typical histology and lack of nodal metastases portend a better prognosis.

ATYPICAL CARCINOID TUMORS

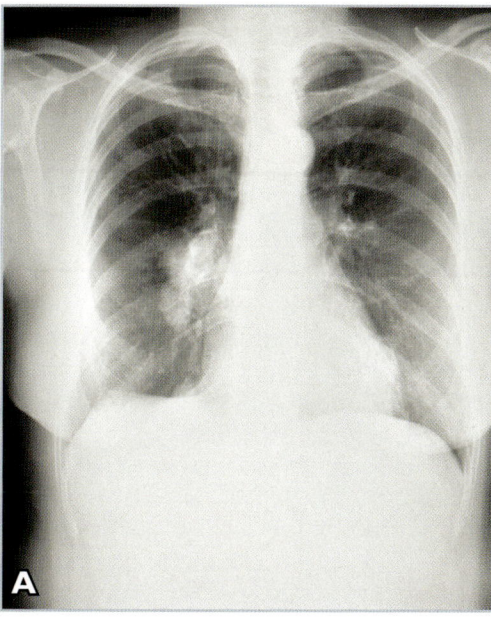
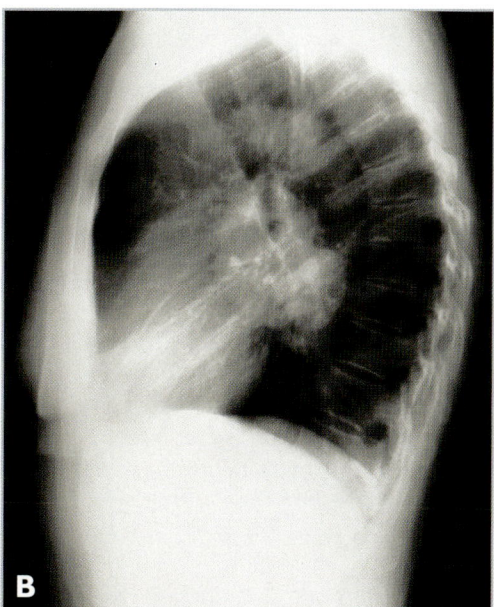
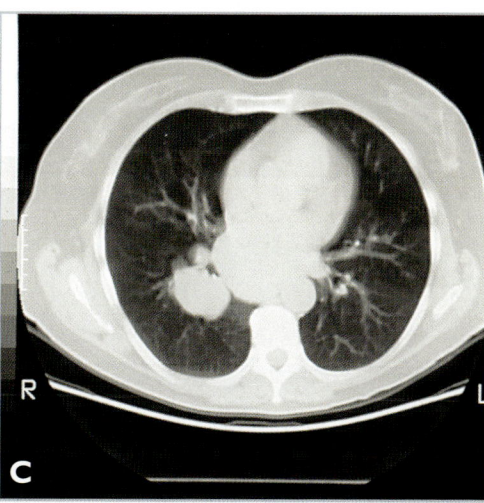

Figure 20-3. Atypical carcinoid tumors. Posteroanterior (**A**) and lateral (**B**) chest radiographs of a patient with an atypical carcinoid presenting as a right-middle lobe infiltrative mass. Chest radiographs of patients with atypical carcinoids usually show a round or ovoid mass, 1.5 to 10 cm in diameter. The mass may be lobulated or spiculated, or it may have smooth borders. Atypical carcinoids are more common peripherally than typical carcinoids. Thus, they are less likely to lead to endobronchial obstruction [28]. A CT of the chest (**C**) shows atypical carcinoids significantly larger than typical carcinoids, and lymph node involvement may be seen in as many as 40% of cases [28].

Continued on the next page

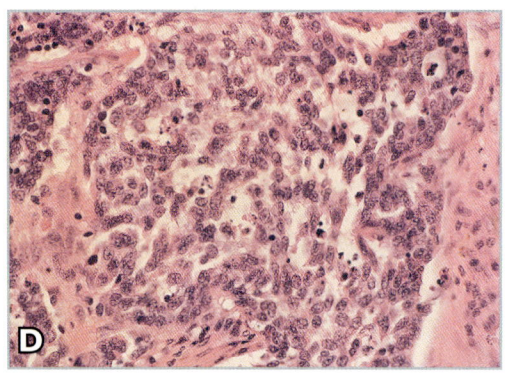
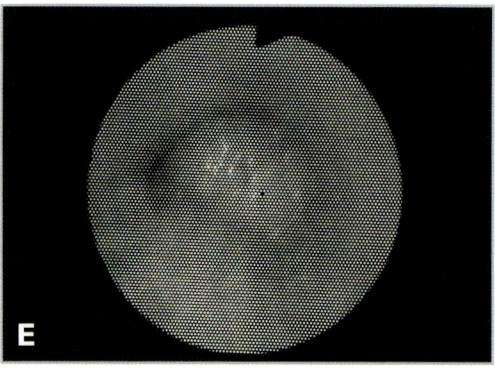

Figure 20-3. *(Continued)* Microscopic studies (**D**) demonstrate that, unlike typical carcinoids, atypical carcinoid tumors are necrotic and have an increased number of mitotic figures [9,20,21,29]. Histologically, atypical carcinoids are defined as a neuroendocrine tumor with 2 to 10 mitotic counts per 10 high-power fields, or with coagulative necrosis [2]. These tumors show patterns of discrete nests of cells separated by a fibrovascular stroma. Architectural features are more varied in atypical carcinoids. The cells have a fine granular eosinophilic cytoplasm, and their borders tend to be indistinct. The nuclei are predominantly ovoid and hyperchromatic. They are also anaplastic and have larger and more numerous nucleoli than the nuclei of typical carcinoids [9,20,21,28,29]. They can be overdiagnosed as small cell carcinoma on small crushed bronchial biopsies [30]. Again, diagnosis is usually made by bronchoscopy (**E**). On bronchoscopic examination, typical and atypical carcinoid lesions are described as having a polypoid, shiny, glistening, vascular appearance [11]. Contrary to the earlier belief that bronchoscopic biopsy may put patients at risk of significant bleeding, several recent reports show that significant hemorrhage is not a major problem [2,11,31,32]. Atypical carcinoids are more aggressive than typical carcinoids. They have a survival between that of typical carcinoids and high-grade neuroendocrine tumors (large cell neuroendocrine carcinoma and small cell carcinoma). Higher mitotic rate, a tumor size of 3.5 cm or greater, and female gender are negative prognostic factors, whereas the presence of rosettes on histology is a positive prognostic factor. Resection is the treatment of choice. There is a poor response to chemotherapy and radiation therapy [5,33] *(Panel E courtesy of A.C. Mehta, MD.)*

HAMARTOMA

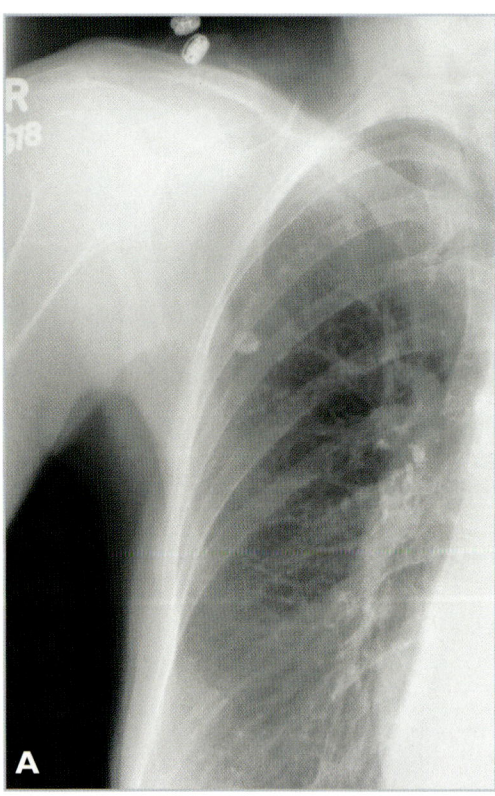
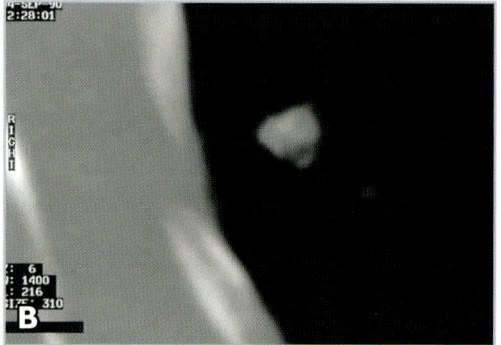
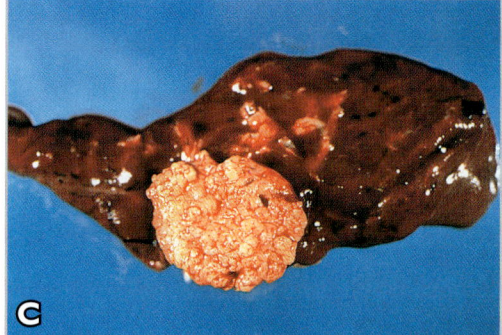
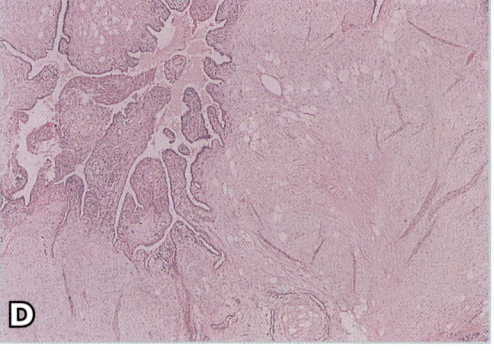

Figure 20-4. Hamartoma. Hamartoma is the most common benign pulmonary tumor. It accounts for 6% to 8% of solitary pulmonary nodules (SPN). Most patients with hamartomas are asymptomatic. The most common presentation is an SPN that is usually detected incidentally on a chest radiograph. Approximately 10% of hamartomas grow endobronchially and may present with cough, dyspnea, wheezing, or hemoptysis [34–36,37]. Multiple hamartomas have been reported as part of uncommon syndromes (*eg*, Cowden syndrome, Carney triad) [38]. **A**, Posteroanterior chest radiograph of a patient with a hamartoma presenting incidentally as a right upper lobe solitary nodule. The chest radiograph in patients with hamartoma is rarely diagnostic. It usually shows a round, homogenous, occasionally lobulated peripheral opacity. Calcification is seen in 10% of cases, but the classically described "popcorn" calcification is rare. Although most hamartomas are 2 to 3 cm in size, their size may range from 1 to 8.5 cm, and tumors involving a whole lobe have been reported [34,35]. **B**, CT of a patient with a solitary nodule suggestive of a hamartoma. CT of the chest may be helpful in determining whether an SPN is a hamartoma. Nodules less than 2.5 cm in diameter and containing fat or having a typical benign calcification pattern (as demonstrated in this scan) suggest the diagnosis of hamartoma [36,39]. **C**, Gross specimen showing a hamartoma as a well-circumscribed, smooth mass that "shells out" of the surrounding lung. On gross examination, hamartomas are usually gray-pink, well circumscribed, uniform, and rubber-hard but not encapsulated [40]. **D**, Microscopic specimen, with benign lobules of cartilage entrapping adjacent air spaces. Other mesenchymal elements, including fat and smooth muscle, can be seen. Histologically, a hamartoma may contain cartilage, fat, or both. It may also contain entrapped epithelium that is not an intrinsic part of the tumor. Chronic inflammation and fibrosis may also be evident in lung tissue adjacent to the lesion [40]. Fine needle aspiration has been reported to be useful in diagnosing hamartomas. The potential for a false positive diagnosis of primary lung cancer exists [41,42].

MUCOUS GLAND TUMORS

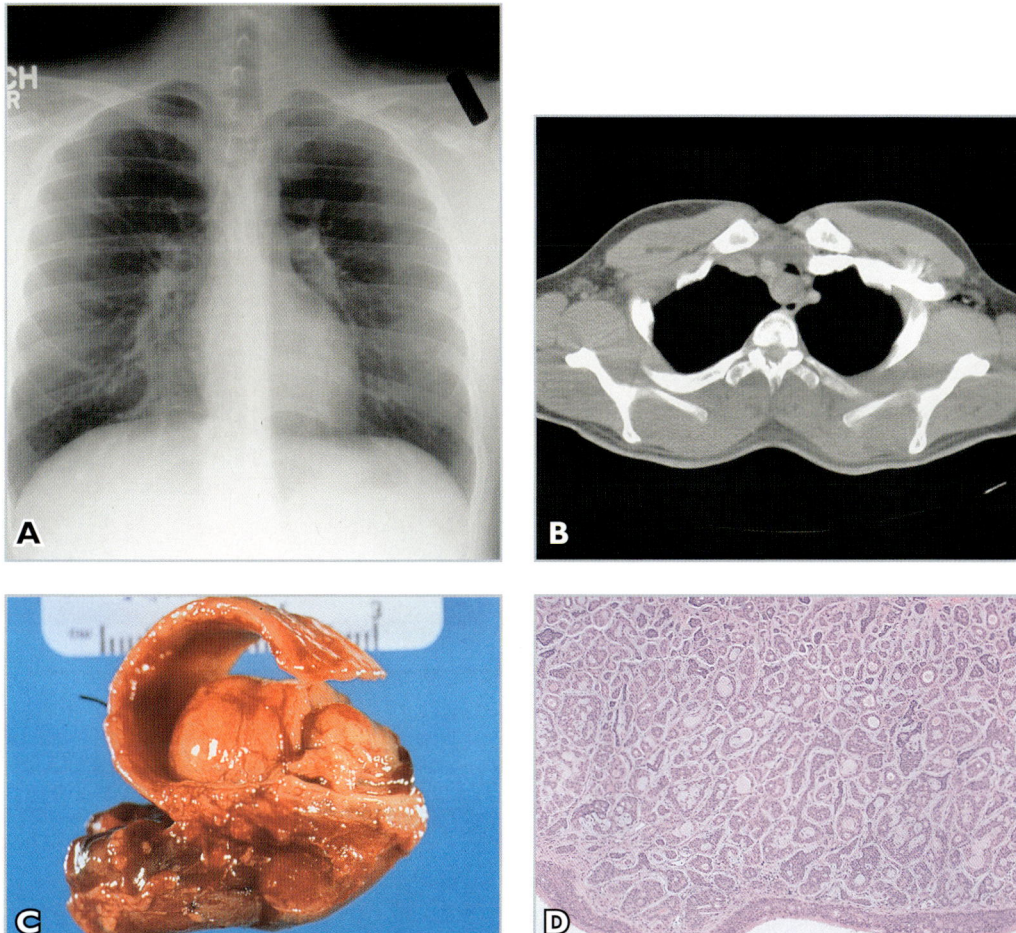

Tumors Arising from the Tracheobronchial Mucous Glands and Their Ducts

- Adenoid cystic carcinomas (cylindromas)
- Mucoepidermoid carcinomas
- Mixed (pleomorphic) adenomas
- Cystadenomas
- Oxyphilic bronchial gland adenomas

Figure 20-5. Mucous gland tumors. These rare tumors arise from the exocrine cells of the mucous glands and their ducts in the trachea and bronchi. Patients with mucous gland tumors usually present with symptoms of bronchial obstruction. Histologically, these tumors have features similar to those of salivary gland tumors.

Figure 20-6. Adenoid cystic carcinoma. **A,** Posteroanterior chest radiograph of a patient who had dry cough and dyspnea on exertion, which progressed in the past 3 months to dyspnea at rest. On physical examination, he was found to have stridor. The large mass in the trachea turned out to be an adenoid cystic carcinoma. The etiology of adenoid cystic carcinoma is unknown, and smoking does not seem to be a predisposing factor. The tumor can present in individuals in their 30s and 40s, with a median age at presentation of 54. A cough is present in 70% of individuals at the time of diagnosis. Dyspnea, wheezing, obstructive pneumonias, and hemoptysis are not uncommon. Approximately 80% of these tumors arise from the trachea, main carina, and mainstem bronchi, and the rest arise from lobar bronchi. Lymph node involvement has been reported in 30% of the cases, and distant metastases in 40% [43–45]. **B,** CT of the chest of the same patient, showing a mass obstructing the trachea. **C,** Gross specimen, obtained from another patient, demonstrating a firm, polypoid, tan-pink mass infiltrating the bronchial wall. Adenoid cystic carcinomas grow slowly and are locally invasive [43,44]. **D,** The histologic features of adenoid cystic carcinomas are similar to those of salivary gland tumors [46]. Malignant glands infiltrate the underlying bronchial epithelium. These glands have a microcystic, cribriform, and trabecular pattern. The cystic spaces contain acidic mucin. A thickened basement membrane surrounds the glands. Cytologic features—small, uniform cells with dark nuclei, scant cytoplasm, and acellular balls of basement membrane material—may be diagnostic [47]. Surgical resection by lobectomy or pneumonectomy is the treatment of choice. Recurrence is not uncommon, and multiple procedures may be needed [46]. Adenoid cystic carcinomas show poor response to chemotherapy and some response to radiotherapy. Survival rates are reported to be 57% at 5 years and 45% at 10 years for those who undergo resection [44–46].

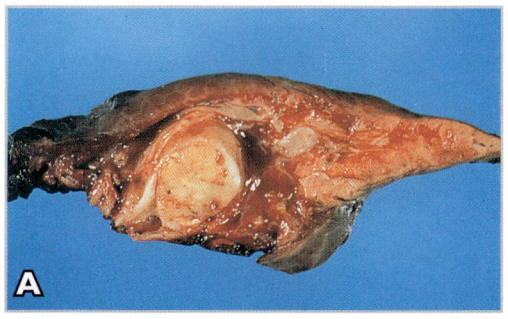
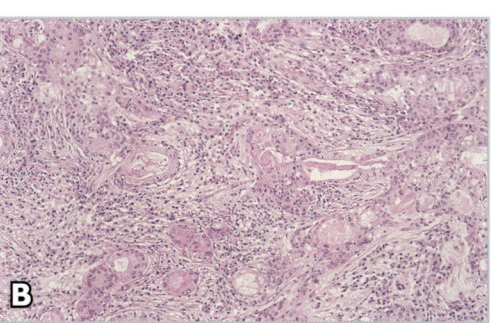

Figure 20-7. Mucoepidermoid carcinoma. **A,** Gross pathology of a low-grade mucoepidermoid carcinoma appearing as a spherical, tan-white mass occluding the bronchus. Based on microscopic histopathology and clinical behavior, mucoepidermoid tumors can be divided into low- and high-grade tumors. Low-grade tumors are grossly well-circumscribed, exophytic, endobronchial lesions.

Continued on the next page

Figure 20-7. *(Continued)* **B**, Microscopic specimen showing a low-grade tumor that contains a mixture of solid and cystic components. The glandular component predominates, and cellular atypia is absent [48,49]. Notice the malignant glands with abundant mucinous cystic spaces filled with a weakly acidic mucous substance invading the bronchial epithelium. More solid areas of transitional cells or nonkeratinizing squamous cells are seen adjacent to these cystic areas. Some cells appear to be between glandular and squamous. Mitoses are rare or absent. High-grade tumors are larger than low-grade tumors. They also have a predominantly solid component and marked atypia and mitotic activity [49]. Cytology features—the presence of mucinous, squamous, and intermediate cells, at times associated with extracellular mucin—are suggestive of the diagnosis [47]. They are difficult to distinguish from adenosquamous carcinomas. Clinically, patients with more aggressive high-grade tumors have a worse prognosis. The tumors most commonly arise in a segmental bronchus, with around 40% involving the mainstem bronchi, main carina, or trachea [45]. Only 10% have metastases at presentation [45]. On CT they appear as smoothly oval or lobulated airway masses that adapt to the branching features of the airways. Heterogeneous contrast enhancement is frequently seen [50]. Punctate calcifications can be seen within the tumor [51]. Surgical resection is the treatment of choice. Survival rates of 87% at 5 and 10 years have been reported [45]. Survival is better in central tumors than in those arising in the periphery [52].

PAPILLOMA

Classification of Benign Papillomas of the Tracheobronchial Tree

Tumor	Cell Type	Clinical Presentation
Multiple papillomas	Squamous	Young children; larynx
Juvenile		
Adult		
Solitary papilloma	Squamous	Adults; lobar and segmental bronchi
Solitary papilloma	Columnar or cuboidal with or without squamous metaplasia	Adults; may undergo malignant transformation
Inflammatory polyps	Columnar	Patients with chronic respiratory infections

Figure 20-8. Papilloma. Squamous papillomas of the upper and lower respiratory tract are exophytic tumors derived from the surface epithelium and bronchial mucous glands [53]. A classification schema for these tumors appears in the figure [54]. The most common type of papilloma is juvenile papillomatosis, which occurs primarily in children and most commonly in the larynx [54,55]. Extension to the trachea, proximal bronchi, or both occurs in 5% to 12% of cases, and the lung parenchyma is involved in 1% to 7% of cases [55,56]. The symptoms are those of an obstructive airway lesion, that is, wheezing, dyspnea, cough, and hemoptysis [55,57]. (*Adapted from* Maxwell et al. [54].)

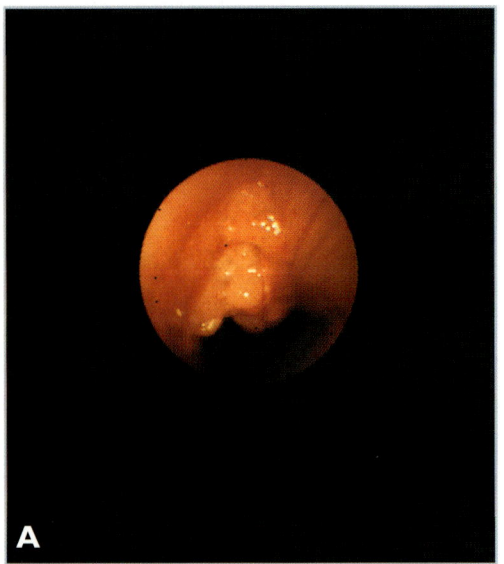 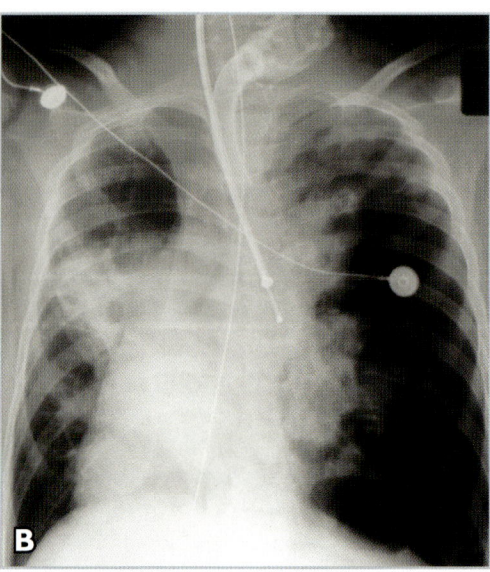

Figure 20-9. Juvenile papillomatosis. (**A**) Bronchoscopy of a patient with juvenile papillomatosis, demonstrating typical pink, polypoid, exophytic lesions with a "bunch-of-grapes" appearance [55]. Juvenile papillomas are benign tumors caused by the human papilloma virus (HPV), especially types 6 and 11 [55,58]. Mothers of individuals with respiratory papillomatosis have evidence of HPV infection in the genital tract [59]. Patients who have HPV-11, and those who are diagnosed when younger than 3 years of age are prone to develop more aggressive disease [60]. Malignant transformation can occur, typically 25 years after the initial diagnosis and 15 years after pulmonary spread [61]. The risk of malignant transformation is greater in adults, in parenchymal lesions, after radiation therapy, and in those infected with HPV-11 [61–64]. (**B**) Radiograph of a patient with pulmonary parenchymal extension of tracheobronchial papillomas. These parenchymal lesions occur in 1% to 7% of cases and are at risk of undergoing a transformation into squamous cell carcinoma [55,56,62].

Continued on the next page

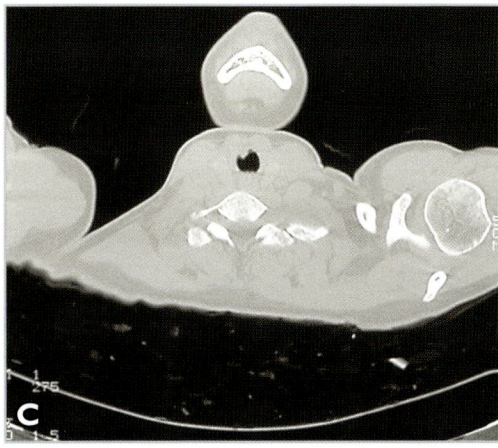 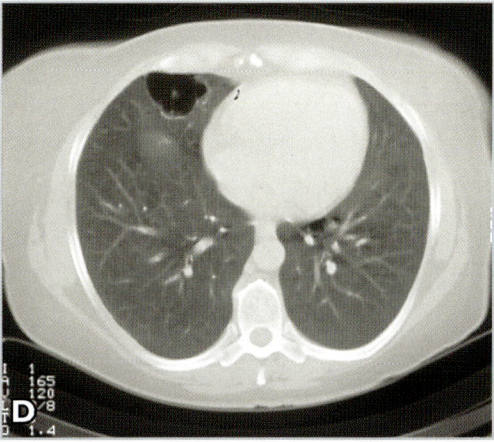

Figure 20-9. *(Continued)* CTs of a patient with a tracheal lesion (**C**) and cavitary parenchymal involvement (**D**). Histologically, these papillomas consist of a core of fibrous connective tissue covered by squamous epithelium [53–55]. There is no curative therapy for these tumors. They tend to recur, leading to the name recurrent respiratory papillomatosis. Standard management consists of laser excision of the lesions [55]. Other palliative approaches include the use of lymphoblastoid interferon-alpha [55,65] and photodynamic therapy [55,66,67]. Acyclovir, leukocyte interferon, isotretinoin, and methotrexate have not clearly proven useful [55,68]. (*Panel A courtesy of A.C. Mehta, MD.*)

MESENCHYMAL TUMORS OF THE LUNG

Mesenchymal Pulmonary Neoplasms

Benign	Malignant*
Leiomyoma*	Fibrosarcoma
Fibroma	Leiomyosarcoma
Bronchial lipoma	Malignant fibrous histiocytoma
Cavernous hemangioma	Liposarcoma
Endobronchial schwannoma	Extraosseous osteosarcoma
Granular cell tumor	Chondrosarcoma
Neurofibroma	Rhabdomyosarcoma
	Hemangiopericytoma
	Carcinosarcoma

*Need to exclude metastasis from extrapulmonary sites.

Figure 20-10. Mesenchymal tumors of the lung. Patients with benign mesenchymal tumors of the lung usually present with bronchial obstruction and atelectasis or with a solitary pulmonary nodule on a chest radiograph. Leiomyomas are the most common soft-tissue tumors of the lung and resemble uterine leiomyomas histologically. Although primary pulmonary leiomyomas and leiomyosarcomas have been reported [69], most smooth muscle tumors of the lung are well-differentiated metastases from extrathoracic (usually uterine) leiomyosarcomas. Several other mesenchymal tumors can be found in the lung and are listed here [69].

OTHER PULMONARY NEOPLASMS

Other Pulmonary Neoplasms

Tumor	Age, y (range)	Male-to-Female Ratio	Clinical Presentation	Cells of Origin	Diagnosis/ Therapy	Prognosis	Notes
Sclerosing hemangioma [70,71]	30s (15–69)	1:4	60%–80% asymptomatic nodule; hemoptysis, cough, chest pain	Pulmonary epithelial cells	Surgical resection	Excellent	Four histologic patterns: solid, hemorrhagic, papillary, sclerotic
Intravascular bronchoalveolar tumor–epithelioid hemangioendothelioma [72–74]	30s (12–61)	1:4	45% asymptomatic; pleuritic pain, cough, progressive dyspnea, weight loss, clubbing	Endothelial	Surgical resection	Poor	Multiple resections may be necessary
Teratoma [75–76]	Young adults (10–30)	1:1	Mainly asymptomatic; chest pain, hemoptysis, cough	Multiple: endodermal, mesodermal, ectodermal	Surgical resection	Benign (mature), malignant (immature)	Metastatic germ cell tumors need to be excluded
Blastoma [77–80]	40s (10–60)	2.6:1	Mainly asymptomatic nodule; hemoptysis, chest pain, cough, dyspnea, fever	Epithelial, mesenchymal, (histology resembles fetal lung)	Surgical resection	Poor (similar to adenocarcinoma): 2 of 3 recur	May herald other dysplastic and neoplastic diseases in patient and family
Primary melanoma [81–82]	Adults (29–80)	1:1	Cough, sputum, hemoptysis, dyspnea, weight loss	Epithelial	Surgical resection	11-y survival reported	Exclude metastasis
Inflammatory pseudotumor–plasma cell granuloma [83–85]	Children*, young adults, adults (11–64)	1:1	Cough, chest pain, hemoptysis (if endobronchial)	Plasma cells	Surgical resection	Recurs in 10%–20% of cases if incompletely excised	May represent pulmonary reaction to previous (infectious?) insult

*Most common pulmonary neoplasm in children.

Figure 20-11. Clinical and pathologic characteristics of additional pulmonary neoplasms [70–85].

NOVEL DIAGNOSTICS

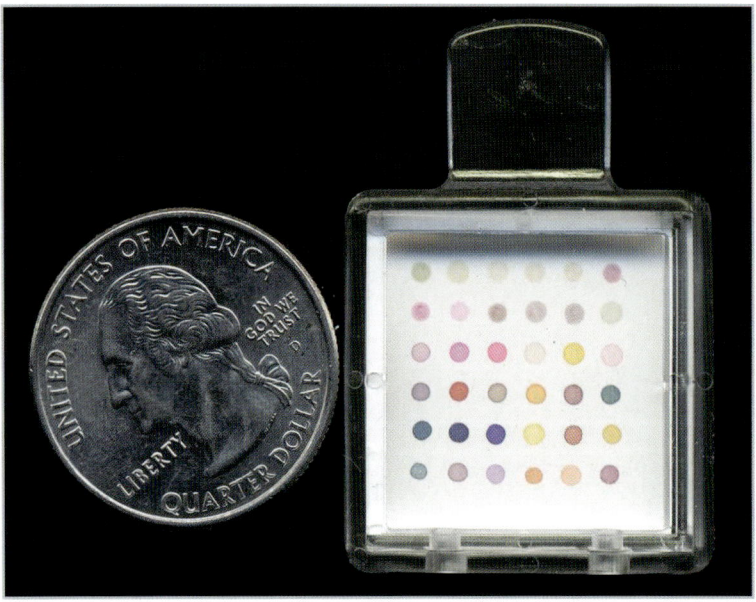

Figure 20-12. Colorimetric sensor. Several novel methods are being developed to diagnose cancers of the lung. These have included proteomic analysis of microscopic tissue samples, genomic profiling of normal airway epithelial cells, protein microarrays of blood specimens, and breath testing [86–89]. The signature of a colorimetric sensor exposed to a patient's breath may one day be able to accurately diagnose cancers of the lung. The sensor's color pattern changes after being exposed to breath. A unique pattern may identify cancer.

REFERENCES

1. Fink G, Krelbaum T, Yellin A, et al.: Pulmonary carcinoid: presentation, diagnosis, and outcome in 142 cases in Israel and review of 640 cases from the literature. Chest 2001, 119:1647–1651.

2. Travis WD, Rush W, Flieder DB, et al.: Survival analysis of 200 pulmonary neuroendocrine tumors with clarification of criteria for atypical carcinoid and its separation from typical carcinoid. Am J Surg Pathol 1998, 22:934–944.

3. Skuladottir H, Hirsch FR, Hansen HH, Olsen JH: Pulmonary neuroendocrine tumors: incidence and prognosis of histological subtypes: a population-based study in Denmark. Lung Cancer 2002, 37:127–135.

4. Soga J, Yakuwa Y: Bronchopulmonary carcinoids: an analysis of 1875 reported cases with special reference to a comparison between typical and atypical varieties. Ann Thorac Cardiovasc Surg 1999, 5:211–219.

5. Beasley MB, Thunnissen FBJM, Brambilla E, et al.: Pulmonary atypical carcinoid: predictors of survival in 106 cases. Human Pathol 2000, 31:1255–1265.

6. Maggard MA, O'Connell JB, Ko CY: Updated population-based review of carcinoid tumors. Ann Surg 2004, 240:117–122.

7. Perez EA, Koniaris LG, Snell SE, et al.: 7201 carcinoids: increasing incidence overall and disproportionate mortality in the elderly. World J Surg 2007, 31:1022–1030.

8. Li AF, Hsu CY, Li A, et al.: A 35-year retrospective study of carcinoid tumors in Taiwan: differences in distribution with a high probability of associated second primary malignancies. Cancer 2007, doi: 10.1002/cncr.23159.

9. Arroliga AC, Carter D, Matthay RA: Other primary neoplasms of the lung. In Pulmonary and Critical Care Medicine. Edited by Bone RC, et al. St. Louis: Mosby Yearbook; 1993:1–16.

10. Davila DG, Dunn WF, Tazelaar HD, et al.: Bronchial carcinoid tumors. Mayo Clinic Proc 1993, 68:795–803.

11. Nessi R, Basso Ricci P, Vasso Ricci S, et al.: Bronchial carcinoid tumors: radiologic observations in 49 cases. J Thorac Imaging 1991, 6:47–53.

12. Warren WH, Faber LP, Could VE: Neuroendocrine neoplasm of the lung: a clinicopathologic update. J Thorac Cardiovasc Surg 1989, 98:321–332.

13. Wilkens EW, Grillo HC, Moncure AC, et al.: Changing times in surgical management of bronchopulmonary carcinoid tumor. Ann Thorac Surg 1984, 38:339–342.

14. Amer KMA, Ibrahim NBN, Forrester-Wood CP, et al.: Lung carcinoid related Cushing's syndrome: report of three cases and review of the literature. Postgrad Med J 2001, 77:464–467.

15. Shrager JB, Wright CD, Wain JC, et al.: Bronchopulmonary carcinoid tumors associated with Cushing's syndrome: a more aggressive variant of typical carcinoid. J Thorac Cardiovasc Surg 1997, 114:367–375.

16. Deb SJ, Nichols FC, Allen MS, et al.: Pulmonary carcinoid tumors with Cushing's syndrome: an aggressive variant or not? Ann Thorac Surg 2005, 79:1132–1136.

17. Scanagatta P, Montresor E, Pergher S, et al.: Cushing's syndrome induced by bronchopulmonary carcinoid tumours: a review of 98 cases and our experience of two cases. Chir Ital 2004, 56:63–70.

18. Sachithanandan N, Harle RA, Burgess JR: Bronchopulmonary carcinoid in multiple endocrine neoplasia type 1. Cancer 2005, 103:509–515.

19. de Jager CM, de Heide LJ, van den Berg G, et al.: Acromegaly caused by a growth hormone-releasing hormone secreting carcinoid tumour of the lung: the effect of octreotide treatment. Neth J Med 2007, 65:263–266.

20. Froudarakis M, Fournel P, Burgard G, et al.: Bronchial carcinoids: a review of 22 cases. Oncology 1996, 53:153–158.

21. DeCaro LF, Paladugu R, Benfield JR, et al.: Typical and atypical carcinoids within the pulmonary APUD tumor spectrum. J Thorac Cardiovasc Surg 1983, 86:528–536.

22. Chong S, Lee KS, Kim BT, et al.: Integrated PET/CT of pulmonary neuroendocrine tumors: diagnostic and prognostic implications. Am J Roentgenol 2007, 188:1223–1231.

23. Daniels CE, Lowe VJ, Aubry MC, et al.: The utility of fluorodeoxyglucose positron emission tomography in the evaluation of carcinoid tumors presenting as pulmonary nodules. Chest 2007, 131:255–260.

24. Kruger S, Buck AK, Blumstein NM, et al.: Use of integrated PET/CT imaging in pulmonary carcinoid tumours. J Intern Med 2006, 260:545–550.

25. Luckraz H, Amer K, Thomas L, et al.: Long-term outcome of bronchoscopically resected endobronchial typical carcinoid tumors. J Thorac Cardiovasc Surg 2006, 132:113–115.

26. Bertoletti L, Elleuch R, Kaczmarek D, et al.: Bronchoscopic cryotherapy treatment of isolated endoluminal typical carcinoid tumor. Chest 2006, 130:1405–1411.

27. Rea F, Rizzardi G, Zuin A, et al.: Outcome and surgical strategy in bronchial carcinoid tumors: single institution experience with 252 patients. Eur J Cardiothorac Surg 2007, 31:186–191.

28. Foster BB, Mueller NL, Miller RR, et al.: Neuroendocrine carcinomas of the lung: clinical, radiologic, and pathologic correlation. Radiology 1989, 170:441–445.

29. Paladugu RR, Benfield JR, Pak HY, et al.: Bronchopulmonary Kulchitzky cell carcinomas: a new classification scheme for typical and atypical carcinoma. Cancer 1985, 55:1303–1311.

30. Pelosi G, Rodriguez J, Viale G, Rosai J. Typical and atypical pulmonary carcinoid tumor overdiagnosed as small-cell carcinoma on biopsy specimens: a major pitfall in the management of lung cancer patients. Am J Surg Pathol 2005, 29:179–187.

31. Hurt R, Bates M: Carcinoid tumors of the bronchus: a 33-year experience. Thorax 1984, 39:617–623.

32. Rozenman J, Pausner R, Lieberman Y, et al.: Bronchial adenoma. Chest 1987, 92:145–147.

33. Wirth LJ, Carter MR, Janne PA, Johnson BE. Outcome of patients with pulmonary carcinoid tumors receiving chemotherapy or chemoradiotherapy. Lung Cancer 2004, 44:213–220.

34. Gjevre JG, Meyers JL, Prakash UBS: Pulmonary hamartomas. Mayo Clin Proc 1996, 71:14–20.

35. Van den Bosh JMM, Wagenaar SS, Corrin B, et al.: Mesenchymoma of the lung (so called hamartoma): a review of 154 parenchymal and endobronchial cases. Thorax 1987, 42:790–793.

36. Caskey CJ, Templeton PA, Zerhouni EA: Current evaluation of the solitary pulmonary nodule. Radiol Clin North Am 1990, 28:511–520.

37. Lien YC, Hsu HS, Li WY, et al.: Pulmonary hamartoma. J Chin Med Assoc 2004, 67:21–26.

38. Bini A, Grazia M, Petrella F, Chittolini M. Multiple chondromatous hamartomas of the lung. Interact Cardiovasc Thorac Surg 2002, 1:78–80.

39. Siegelman SS, Khouri NF, Scott WW, et al.: Pulmonary hamartoma: CT findings. Radiology 1986, 160:313–317.

40. Perez-Atayde AR, Seiler MW: Pulmonary hamartoma: an ultrastructural study. Cancer 1984, 53:485–492.

41. Saqi A, Shaham D, Scognamiglio T, et al.: Incidence and cytological features of pulmonary hamartomas indeterminate on CT scan. Cytopathology 2007, doi 10.1111/j.1365-2303.2007.00439.x.

42. Hughes JH, Young NA, Wilbur DC, et al.: Fine-needle aspiration of pulmonary hamartoma: a common source of false-positive diagnoses in the College of American Pathologists Interlaboratory Comparison Program in Nongynecologic Cytology. Arch Pathol Lab Med 2005, 129:19–22.

43. Li W, Ellerbrolk NA, Libshitz HI: Primary malignant tumors of the trachea: a radiological and clinical study. Cancer 1990, 66:894–899.

44. Kanematsu T, Yohena T, Uehara T, et al.: Treatment outcome of resected and nonresected primary adenoid cystic carcinoma of the lung. Ann Thorac Cardovasc Surg 2002, 8:74–77.

45. Molina JR, Aubry MC, Lewis JE, et al.: Primary salivary gland-type lung cancer: spectrum of clinical presentation, histopathologic and prognostic factors. Cancer 2007, 110:2253–2259.

46. Spencer H: Bronchial mucous gland tumor. Virchows Arch [A] 1979, 383:101–115.

47. Segletes LA, Steffee CH, Geisinger KR: Cytology of primary pulmonary mucoepidermoid and adenoid cystic carcinoma: a report of four cases. Act Cytol 1999, 43:1091–1097.

48. Klacsman PG, Olson JL, Eggleston JC: Mucoepidermoid carcinomas of the bronchus: an electron microscopic study of the low grade and the high grade variants. Cancer 1979, 43:1720–1733.

49. Yousem SA, Hochholzer L: Malignant fibrous histiocytoma of the lung. Cancer 1987, 60:2532–2541.

50. Ishizumi T, Tateishi U, Watanabe SI, Matsuno Y. Mucoepidermoid carcinoma of the lung: high-resolution CT and histopathologic findings in five cases. Lung Cancer 2007, 10.1016/j.lungcan.2007.08.022.

51. Kim TS, Lee KS, Han J, et al.: Mucoepidermoid carcinoma of the tracheobronchial tree: radiographic and CT findings in 12 patients. Radiology 1999, 212:643–648.

52. Shimizu J, Watanabe Y, Oda M, et al.: Clinicopathologic study of mucoepidermoid carcinoma of the lung. Int Surg 1998, 83:1–3.

53. Spencer H, Dail DH, Arneaud J: Non-invasive bronchial epithelial papillary tumors. Cancer 1980, 45:1486–1497.

54. Maxwell RJ, Gibbons JR, O'Hara MD: Solitary squamous papilloma of the bronchus. Thorax 1985, 40:68–71.

55. Dweik RA, Patel SR, Mehta AC: Tracheal papillomatosis. J Bronchology 1994, 1:226–227.

56. Silver RD, Rimell FL, Adams GL, et al.: Diagnosis and management of pulmonary metastasis from recurrent respiratory papillomatosis. Otolaryn Head Neck Surg 2003, 129:622–629.

57. Kramer SS, Wehaunt WD, Stocker JT, Kashima H: Pulmonary manifestations of juvenile laryngotracheal papillomatosis. AJR Am J Roentgenol 1985, 144:687–694.

58. Quiney RE, Wells M, Lewis FA, et al.: Laryngeal papillomatosis: correlation between severity of the disease and presence of HPV6 and 11 detected by in situ DNA hybridization. J Clin Pathol 1989, 42:694–698.

59. Gerein V, Schmandt S, Babkina N, et al.: Human papilloma virus (HPV)–associated gynecological alteration in mothers of children with recurrent respiratory papillomatosis during long-term observation. Cancer Detect Prev 2007, 31:276–281.

60. Wiatrak BJ, Wiatrak DW, Broker TR, Lewis L. Recurrent respiratory papillomatosis: a longitudinal study comparing severity associated with human papilloma viral types 6 and 11 and other risk factors in a large pediatric population. Laryngoscope 2004, 114:1–23.

61. Gerein V, Rastorguev E, Gerein J, et al.: Incidence, age at onset, and potential reasons of malignant transformation in recurrent respiratory papillomatosis patients: 20 years experience. Otolaryngol Head Neck Surg 2005, 132:392–394.

62. Lie ES, Engh V, Boysen M, et al.: Squamous cell carcinoma of the respiratory tract following laryngeal papillomatosis. Acta Otolaryngol (Stockh) 1994, 114:209–212.

63. Cook JR, Hill A, Humphrey PA, et al.: Squamous cell carcinoma arising in recurrent respiratory papillomatosis with pulmonary involvement: emerging common pattern of clinical features and human papillomavirus serotype association. Mod Pathol 2000, 13:914–918.

64. Lele SM, Pou AM, Ventura K, et al.: Molecular events in the progression of recurrent respiratory papillomatosis to carcinoma. Arch Pathol Lab Med 2002, 126:1184–1188.

65. Leventhal BG, Kashima HK, Mounts P, et al.: Long-term response of recurrent respiratory papillomatosis to treatment with lymphatoid interferon a-n1. N Engl J Med 1991, 325:613–617.

66. Dweik RA, Mehta AC: Bronchoscopic management of malignant airway disease. Clin Pulm Med 1996, 3:43–51.

67. Kavuru MS, Mehta AC, Eliachar I: Effect of photodynamic therapy and external beam radiation therapy on juvenile laryngotracheal papillomatosis. Am Rev Resp Dis 1990, 141:509–510.

68. Morrison GAJ, Evans JNG: Juvenile respiratory papillomatosis: acyclovir reassessed. Int J Paediatr Otorhinolaryngol 1993, 26:193–197.

69. Tench WD, Dail D, Gmelich JT, et al.: Benign metastasizing leiomyomas: a review of 21 cases [abstract]. Lab Invest 1978, 38: 367–368.

70. Katzenstein AA, Gmelich JT, Carrinton CB: Sclerosing hemangioma of the lung: a clinicopathologic study of 51 cases. Am J Surg Pathol 1980, 4:343–356.

71. Yousem SA, Wick MR, Singh G, et al.: So-called sclerosing hemangiomas of the lung: an immunohistochemical analysis with comparison with fetal lung in its pseudoglandular stage. Am J Clin Pathol 1990, 93:167–175.

72. Van Kasteren ME, Van der Wurff AA, Palmen FM, et al.: Epithelioid haemangioendothelioma of the lung: clinical and pathological pitfalls. European Respir J 1995, 8:1616–1619.

73. Weiss SW, Ishak KG, Dail DH, et al.: Epithelioid hemangioendothelioma and related lesions. Semin Diag Pathol 1986, 3:259–287.

74. Miettinen M, Collan Y, Halttunen P, et al.: Intravascular bronchoalveolar tumor. Cancer 1987, 60:2471–2475.

75. Ashley DJB: Origin of teratomas. Cancer 1973, 32:390–394.

76. Collier FC, Dowling EA, Plott D, et al.: Teratoma of the lung. Arch Pathol 1959, 68:138–142.

77. Yousem SA, Hochholzer L: Primary pulmonary hemangiopericytoma. Cancer 1987, 59:549–555.

78. Priest JR, Watterson J, Strong L, et al.: Pleuropulmonary blastoma: a marker for familial disease. J Pediatr 1996, 128:220–224.

79. Koss MN, Hochholzer L, O'Leary T: Pulmonary blastomas. Cancer 1991, 67:2368–2381.

80. Novotny JE, Huiras CM: Resection and adjuvant chemotherapy of pulmonary blastoma: a case report. Cancer 1995, 76:1537–1539.

81. Bagwell SP, Flynn SD, Cox PM, et al.: Primary malignant melanoma of the lung. Am Rev Respir Dis 1989, 139:1543–1547.

82. Jennings TA, Axiotis CA, Kress Y, et al.: Primary malignant melanoma of the lower respiratory tract. Am J Clin Pathol 1990, 94:649–655.

83. Dweik RA, Goldfarb J, Alexander F, Stillwell PC: Actinomycosis and plasma cell granuloma, coincidence or coexistence: patient report and review of the literature. Clin Pediatr 1997, 36:229–233.

84. Biselli R, Ferlini C, Fattorossi A, et al.: Inflammatory myofibroblastic tumor (inflammatory pseudotumor). Cancer 1996, 77:778–784.

85. Hancock BJ, Di Lorenzo M, Youssef S, et al.: Childhood primary pulmonary neoplasms. J Pediatr Surg 1993, 28:1133–1136.

86. Yanagisawa K, Shyr Y, Xu BJ, et al.: Proteomic patterns of tumor subsets in non–small cell lung cancer. Lancet 2003, 362:433–439.

87. Spira A, Beane JE, Shah V, et al.: Airway epithelial gene expression in the diagnostic evaluation of smokers with suspect lung cancer. Nature Med 2007, 13:361–366.

88. Zhong L, Hidalgo EG, Stromberg AJ, et al.: Using protein microarray as a diagnostic assay for non–small cell lung cancer. Am J Respir Crit Care Med 2005, 172:1308–1314.

89. Mazzone PJ, Hammel J, Dweik R, et al.: Diagnosis of lung cancer by the analysis of exhaled breath with a colorimetric sensor array. Thorax 2007, 62:565–568.

SOLITARY PULMONARY NODULE

Hina Sahi, Elif Kupeli, and Atul C. Mehta

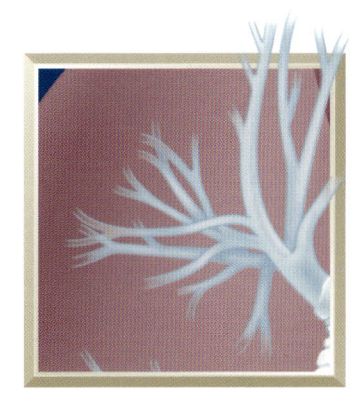
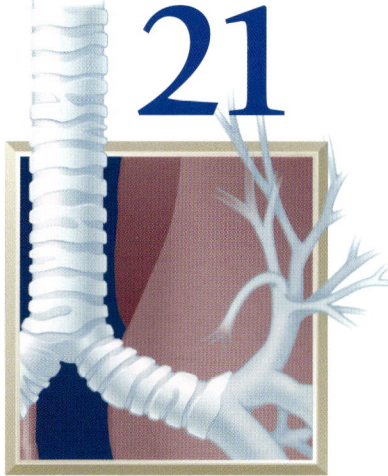
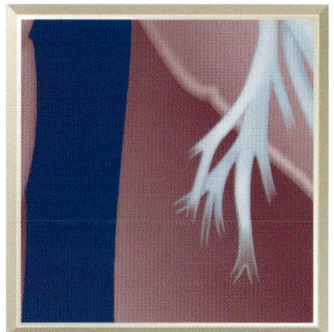

The finding of a solitary pulmonary nodule (SPN) on a chest radiograph is a common problem in pulmonary medicine. SPNs are seen in approximately 1 in 500 chest radiographs and are caused by a variety of conditions ranging from infectious granulomas to lung cancer. An estimated 150,000 new benign or malignant SPNs are discovered each year in the United States [1], of which 10% to 70% are malignant [2–3]. Because asymptomatic bronchogenic carcinomas commonly present as SPNs, and because surgical resection within one month of diagnosis results in a 10-year survival rate of 92% [4], it is important to identify them promptly to ensure optimal treatment. Similarly, it is important to avoid the morbidity and mortality associated with thoracotomy in patients with benign disease. Thus, the workup for SPN focuses on distinguishing benign from malignant nodules, considering the size of the lesion and the clinical probability of cancer. This chapter focuses on lesions less than or equal to 8 mm in size and describes how clinicians can distinguish benign from malignant nodules in a practical manner.

DEFINITION

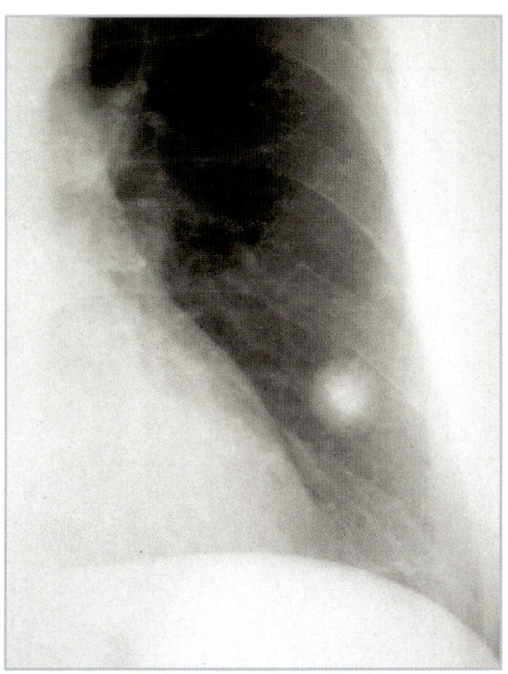

Figure 21-1. Chest radiograph of a solitary pulmonary nodule. A solitary pulmonary nodule is defined as a single spherical lesion less than or equal to 3 cm in diameter, surrounded by aerated lung and not associated with mediastinal adenopathy, atelectasis, pneumonitis, or satellite lesions [5–6]. Lesions greater than 3 cm in diameter are referred to as masses; 80% to 90% of these masses are malignant [7].

DIFFERENTIAL DIAGNOSIS

Differential Diagnosis of Solitary Pulmonary Nodules

Neoplasm	Benign	Hamartoma
		Lipoma
		Fibroma
		Inflammatory pseudotumor
	Malignant	Bronchogenic carcinoma
		Carcinoid tumor
		Lymphoma (non-Hodgkin's)
	Metastasis	Breast, renal, colon, head and neck, sarcoma, germ cell, thyroid
Infection	Granuloma	Mycobacteria
		Fungi (histoplasma, coccidioidomycosis)
	Infected bulla	
	Septic embolus	Bacteria (anaerobes, *Staphylococcus*, gram negative)
	Abscess	Nocardia
	Round pneumonia	Pneumooccus
	Parasitic	Eichinococcus, Ascariasis, Pneumocystis
		Dirofilaria (dog heartworm)
Inflammatory	Connective tissue	Wegener's granulomatosis
		Rheumatoid (necrobiotic) nodule
	Sarcoidosis	
Vascular	AV malformation	
	Hematoma	
	Pulmonary infarct	
	Pulmonary artery aneurysm	
	Pulmonary venous varix	
Airway	Congenital lesion	Bronchogenic cyst
		Bronchial atresia
	Mucocele	

Figure 21-2. Common causes of solitary pulmonary nodules. Infectious granulomas, bronchogenic carcinomas, and metastatic disease are the most common causes of solitary pulmonary nodules. AV—arteriovenous.

Prevalence of Malignancy in Solitary Pulmonary Nodules in Studies of Lung Cancer Screening

Study	Subjects, n	Prevalence of SPNs With Nodule < 3 cm, % (n/total)	Prevalence of Cancer in Patients With Nodules, % (n/total)	Prevalence of Cancer in all Patients, % (n/total)
Veronesi et al. [11]	5109	NR (10% recall rate)	Approx 10 (54/520)	1 (54/5189)
Henschke et al. [12]	2897	21.3% (616 of 2897)	13 (81/616)	2.8 (81/2897)
	1660	8% (26/1660)	3.8 (1/26)	
Li et al. [13] Li et al. [14] Takashima et al. [15] Hasegawa et al. [16] Sone et al. [17]	7847	NR	10.1 (76/747)	1% of the nodules receiving follow-up scans (76/7847)
Swensen et al. [18]	1520	51% (782/1520)	1.1% of 2244 nodules measured in serial CT; 3.5 (36/1038) of participants with nodules ≤ 20 mm; 3.8 (40/1049) of participants with nodules of any size;	
Swensen et al. [19]			1.4 (40/2832) of nodules of any size	
Nawa et al. [20]	7956	26.3% (2099/7956)	1.7 (20/2099)	0.44 (35/7956)
Henschke et al. [21]	1000	23% (233/1000)	12 (27/233)	2.7 (27/1000)
Diederich et al. [22]	> 700	20% for SPNs		1.1 (8/700)

Figure 21-3. Causes of solitary pulmonary nodules. Benign processes are the most common causes of solitary pulmonary nodules (SPNs), although their incidence has decreased over time. The most common causes of benign SPNs in positron emission tomography

Continued on the next page

Figure 21-3. *(Continued)* studies were healed or nonspecific granulomas, accounting for 25% of all benign causes. Another 15% of benign nodules are active granulomatous infections, including tuberculosis [8]. Although malignant nodules are most commonly primary bronchogenic carcinomas (35%), metastases and bronchial carcinoids account for 23% and 1%, respectively [9]. Adenocarcinoma and squamous cell carcinoma are the most common histologic subtypes [10]. The prevalence of SPNs (8%–51%) and the prevalence of malignancy in patients with SPNs (1.1%–12%) vary significantly across lung cancer screening studies. This variation stems from the inconsistency among studies in terms of method, enrolled population, and result reporting. *(Adapted from* Wahidi et al. [23].)

DIAGNOSIS

Stage	Patients, n	Survival at 1 y, %	Survival at 5 y, %
Clinical TNM*			
cIA	687	91	61
cIB	1189	72	38
cIIA	29	79	34
cIIB	357	59	24
cIIIA	511	50	13
cIIIB	1030	34	5
cIV	1427	19	1
Pathologic TNM†			
pIA	511	94	67
pIB	549	87	57
pIIA	76	89	55
pIIB	375	73	39
pIIIA	399	64	23

*Staging based on all diagnostic and evaluative information obtained before the institution of treatment or decision for no treatment.
†Staging based on pathologic examination of resected specimens.

Figure 21-4. Cumulative proportion of patients with bronchogenic carcinoma surviving 5 years, by clinical stage of disease. Bronchogenic carcinomas presenting as solitary pulmonary nodules that are resected early usually correspond to TNM (tumor, node, metastasis) stage I. Recent data from the International Early Lung Cancer Action program (I-ELCAP) study found that survival at 10 years in patients with stage I cancer was 92% if they underwent surgical resection within 1 month of diagnosis, leading the authors to conclude that CT can detect lung cancer that is "curable" [4]. However, the validity of their recommendations needs to be substantiated by further studies. Although it may be possible for the clinician to distinguish between benign and malignant nodules based on clinical and radiographic features made visible through modern imaging techniques such as spiral CT and positron emission tomography, most nodules cannot be differentiated by these tests alone. Tissue specimens are required for a final diagnosis. *(Adapted from* Mountain [24].)

HISTORY

Important Features To Be Investigated in Patients with Solitary Pulmonary Nodules

- Age
- Gender
- Area of residence
- History of smoking
- History of chest trauma
- History of intra- or extrathoracic malignancy
- Occupational history
- History of emphysema

Figure 21-5. Factors suggesting the nature of solitary pulmonary nodules. A detailed medical history can help the clinician identify patients who are more likely to have malignant solitary pulmonary nodules (SPNs). Among the many risk factors studied, age, smoking, and history of malignancy have been shown to be the most useful. A benign process is the causative factor in most SPNs found in patients younger than 35 years of age and in two thirds of patients younger than 50 years [25]. Smoking and prior cancer increase the likelihood of malignancy. Incidence of lung cancer correlates directly with the pack-years of cigarettes smoked [26]. It has been reported that more than 80% of SPNs found in patients with previous extrathoracic cancer are malignant at thoracotomy [27]. Area of residence and travel to areas with high prevalence rates for tuberculosis, coccidioidomycosis, or histoplasmosis are important considerations because they may suggest that the nodule is benign [28]. Occupational exposures to compounds such as asbestos, uranium, nickel, cadmium, and radon gas increase the probability of cancer [29]. After controlling for the number of cigarettes smoked, patients with obstructive pulmonary function tests have a higher risk of acquiring lung cancer, especially in the larger airways [30].

Imaging Studies

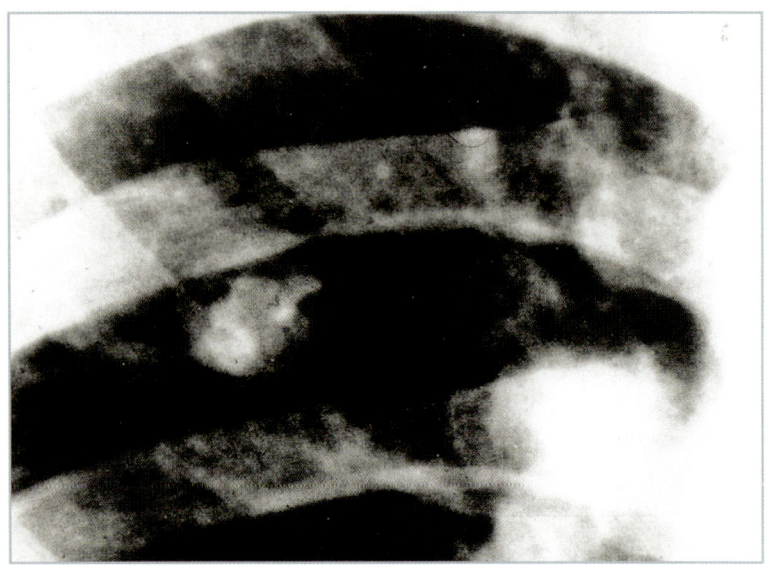

Figure 21-6. Chest radiograph of hamartoma presenting as a solitary pulmonary nodule. A solitary pulmonary nodule (SPN) can be detected on chest radiograph when it is 8 to 10 mm in diameter [31]. It is usually seen in frontal and lateral views. If it is visualized in only one view, an extrapulmonary cause should be ruled out. Approximately 20% of patients with extrathoracic malignancy have multiple lesions at thoracotomy, even when they appear as SPNs on chest radiographs [27]. Growth rate, calcification, nodule size, and appearance of nodule edges are helpful characteristics in differentiating malignant from benign SPNs on chest radiographs. Other features such as cavitation and satellite lesions are less reliable. Previous chest radiographs are invaluable for determining the growth rate and doubling time (dT) of the nodule and should be obtained for comparison even if they are reportedly negative. Growth rate is the time necessary for the nodule to double in volume; approximately 30 doublings are required to produce a lesion that is 1 cm in diameter. A dT of 30 to 360 days is consistent with a malignant process [32]. A dT of more than 500 days strongly suggests that the nodule is benign; no growth for more than 2 years is considered one of the features of benignity. However, bronchoalveolar cell carcinomas and carcinoid tumors occasionally appear stable for 2 or more years [33].

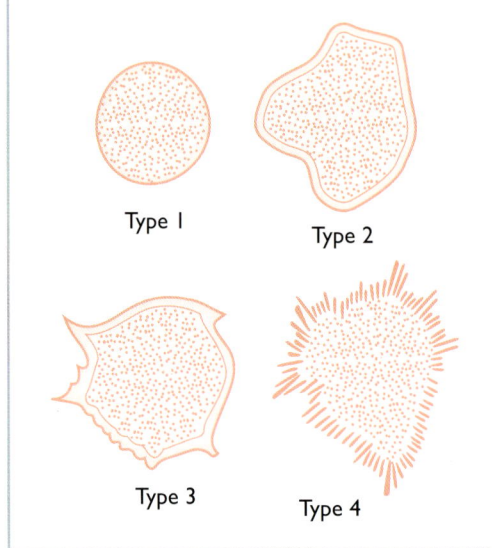

Figure 21-7. Classification of nodular margins. Nodule margins are divided into four categories, with types 3 and 4 (scalloped or spiculated margins [7,34]) suggesting malignancy, and types 1 and 2 suggesting benignity [3]. Nodule margins are better appreciated with CT (see Fig. 21-9) than with plain film. (*Adapted from* Siegelman *et al.* [3].)

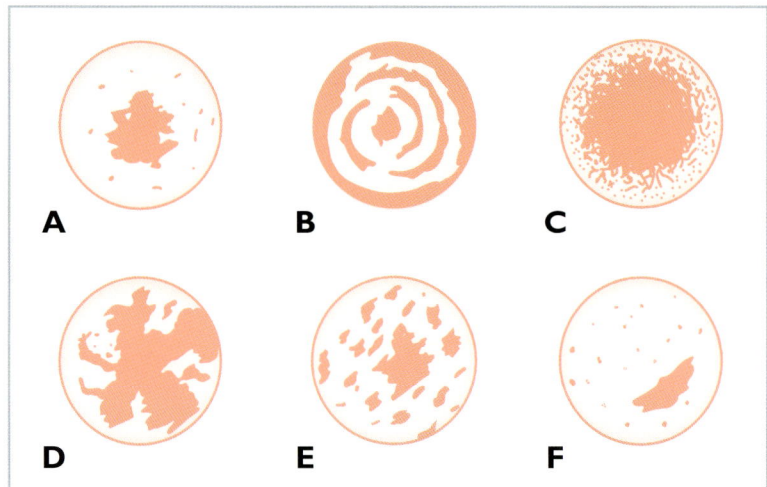

Figure 21-8. Calcification patterns in solitary pulmonary nodules. Calcification often suggests a benign process [6]. Patterns of calcification that may be present in a solitary pulmonary nodule include central (**A**), laminated (**B**), diffuse (**C**), popcorn (**D**), stippled (**E**), and eccentric (**F**). A solitary pulmonary nodule with a stippled or eccentric pattern of calcification must be considered indeterminate and requires further work-up [28]. Central, laminated, or diffuse calcification patterns suggest benignity. The presence of popcorn calcification is characteristic of hamartoma, but this is rare, occurring in approximately 5% to 10% of cases. CT is also more sensitive than the plain film for the detection of calcification: in one study, 7% of nodules that were believed to be definitely calcified by chest radiography lacked calcium on CT (see Fig. 21-9). (*Adapted from* Siegelman *et al.* [3].)

A. Prevalence of Malignancy in Nodules with Varying Edge Characteristics

Study	Participants, n	Nodules, n	Overall Prevalence of Malignancy, %	Nodule Characteristic	Prevalence of Malignancy, %
Tozaki et al. [35]	45	45	64	Smooth	22
				Lobulated	58
				Irregular	83
Takashima et al. [15]	13,786	80	39	Spiculated	35
				Lobulated	50
Swenson et al. [36]	163	163	68	Inflitrating	76
				Lobulated	100
				Smooth infiltrating	58
				Lobulated	78
				Smooth	69

B. Prevalance of Malignancy in Nodules of Varying Size

Study	Participants, n	Nodules, n	Overall Prevalence of Malignancy, %	Nodule Size	Prevalence of Malignancy, %
Henschke et al. [12]	2897	616	2.8	< 5 mm	0
				5–9 mm	6
Takashima et al. [15]	13,786	80	39	< 10 mm	31
				10–15 mm	64
				> 20 mm	67
Henschke et al. [37]	233	233	12	2–5 mm	0.7
				6–10 mm	20
				11–20 mm	45
				21–45 mm	80
Henschke et al. [38]	1000	233	12	2–5 mm	1
				6–10 mm	24
				11–20 mm	33
				21–45 mm	80
Suzuki et al. [39]	92	92	39	< 5 mm	100
				5–10 mm	21
				10–20 mm	41
				> 20 mm	64
Zerhouni et al. [7]	369	384	60	0–1 cm	55
				1–2 cm	51
				2–3 cm	82

Figure 21-9. **A** and **B**, Prevalence of malignancy with varying nodule characteristics. The prevalence of malignancy in nodules measuring less than 5 mm is exceedingly low (range 0%–1%). The risk of malignancy is higher in nodules measuring between 5 and 10 mm (range 6%–28%) and is very high in nodules in which the diameter is less than 2 cm (range 64%–82%). Solitary pulmonary nodule morphology may be classified as solid, partly solid, or exhibiting ground glass opacities (GGO). The prevalence of malignancy in solid nodules is generally lower (7%–9%), whereas pure GGOs tend to be predominantly malignant (59%–73%) [13,15].

Studies of patients with incidental or screening-detected nodules show that the risk for malignancy is approximately 20% to 30% in nodules with smooth edges and varies from 33% to 100% in nodules with irregular, lobulated, or spiculated borders. (*Panel A adapted from* Wahidi et al. [23]; *Panel B adapted from* Wahidi et al. [23].)

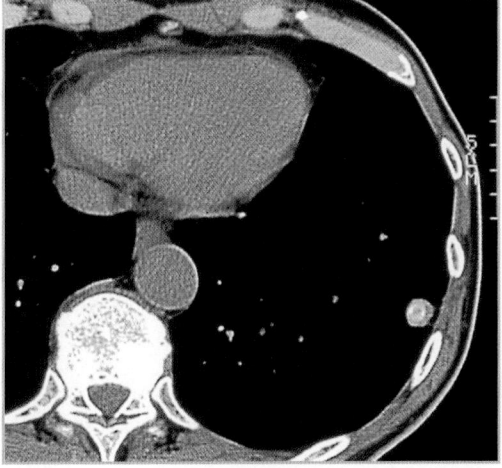

Figure 21-10. CT of a patient with solitary pulmonary nodule. CT provides better representation of nodule margins and calcification patterns than do plain film radiographs. CT also provides better definition of other characteristics, such as fat and vascular connections. For example, the diagnostic feature of hamartoma on a CT consists of focal high attenuation due to calcium and low attenuation due to fat. In fact, a nodule containing a fat density can be classified as a hamartoma with high confidence. The degree of enhancement seen on a CT after injection of nonionic contrast dye can be helpful in distinguishing malignant nodules from benign nodules because the blood supply of malignant lesions is qualitatively and quantitatively different from that of benign lesions. Using an attenuation of 20 Hounsfield Units as the threshold for a positive test result, the sensitivity and specificity for malignancy are 98% and 73%, respectively [40]. Other advantages of CT include staging of the tumor, detecting multiple lesions, and guiding transthoracic needle aspiration and bronchoscopic biopsies. In recent years, there has been renewed interest in lung cancer screening using low-dose CT.

Continued on the next page

Figure 21-10. *(Continued)* Results of the Early Lung Cancer Action Program (ELCAP), showed that low-dose CT, when compared with chest radiography, detected noncalcified nodules three times more commonly (23% vs 7%), malignancy four times more commonly (2.7% vs 0.7%), and stage I malignancies six times more commonly (2.3% vs 0.4%). Moreover, the sizes of the malignancies detected on low-dose CTs were smaller than those detected on chest radiographs: 96% of the CT-detected tumors were resectable and 85% were stage I [38]. Also, high-resolution CT is more sensitive than CT in delineating tumor–bronchus relationships. An air bronchogram leading to a solitary pulmonary nodule increases the likelihood of malignancy [41]. However, helical CT is useful in detecting nodules smaller than 5 mm in diameter and in evaluating areas of the lung that are difficult to examine because of respiratory motion (*eg*, the lung bases adjacent to the diaphragm).

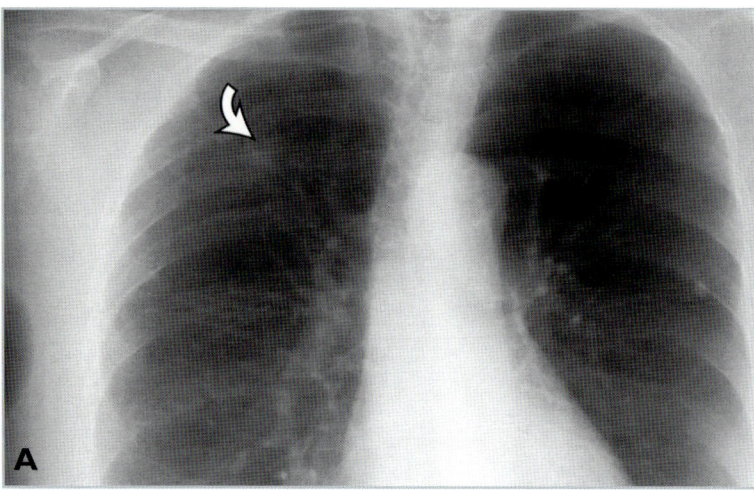 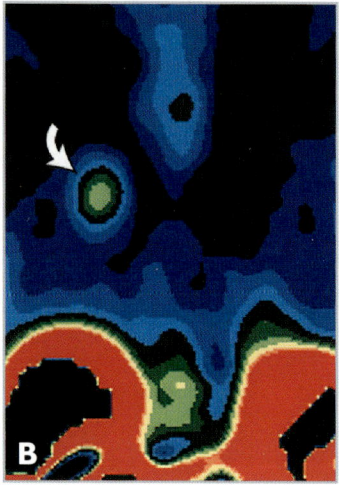

Figure 21-11. A, Chest radiograph demonstrating a solitary pulmonary nodule (*arrow*). **B,** Positron emission tomograph of the same lesion shown with greater uptake of F-18 fluorodeoxyglucose than surrounding normal tissue (*arrow*). In one study, positron emission tomographic–F-18 fluorodeoxyglucose (PET-FDG) correctly classified 27 of 30 nodules less than 3 cm in diameter with a specificity of 80% and a sensitivity of 95% [42]. PET-FDG was shown to be superior to the traditional Bayesian approach in classifying lesions as benign or malignant [43]. A decision-analysis model used to assess its cost effectiveness demonstrated that a CT-plus-PET strategy decreased surgical procedures by 15% and produced a total estimated cost savings of $91 to $2200 per patient [44]. Another potential benefit of PET-FDG is the detection of occult metastases and improved staging. False-negative results can occur for scar adenocarcinomas, carcinoids, bronchioloalveolar carcinomas, and tumors smaller than 10 mm in diameter [42,45,46]. False-positive results can occur in hyperglycemia, caseating granulomas with active inflammation, and histoplasma organisms [47]. Integration of both anatomical and functional images via a new generation of hybrid PET-CT scanners represents a more efficient and accurate approach to identifying and staging lung nodules, compared to PET-FDG alone [48]. This should also permit localization of the best biopsy site.

BIOPSY PROCEDURES

Success Rate of Flexible Bronchoscopy

Study	Patients, n	Overall, %	Transbronchial Biopsy, %	Cytology Brush, %	Cytology Wash, %	Size of Lesion < 2 cm, %	Size of Lesion > 2 cm, %
Stringfield *et al.* [49]	27	48	28	31	24	33	50
Cortese and McDougall [50]	48	60	46	40	43	0	66
Radke *et al.* [51]	97	56	52	33	—	29	64
Fletcher and Levin* [52]	101	36	27	16	4	13	46
Wallace and Deutsch* [53]	133	20	20	12	9	5	34
Shiner *et al.*[54]	71	68	65	37	10	—	68
Chechani *et al.* [55]	49	73	57	52	35	54	75
Baaklini *et al.* [56]	177	60	52	41	40	23	67

*Some patients did not undergo all the procedures (brushings, washings, transbronchial biopsies).

Figure 21-12. Flexible bronchoscopy. In most cases, a solitary pulmonary nodule (SPN) cannot be classified as benign or malignant on the basis of clinical and radiographic characteristics alone. Other options available for making a tissue diagnosis include flexible bronchoscopy, percutaneous needle aspiration, video-assisted thoracotomy, and open thoracotomy. The success rate of flexible bronchoscopy in diagnosing SPNs is summarized in the figure. Although brush biopsy and bronchial washing (lavage) play important complementary roles, bronchoscopic lung biopsy is the most sensitive sampling method, with an overall success rate of 36% to 68% [57]. Nodule size and location affect the diagnostic yield with flexible bronchoscopy. Lesions less than or equal to 2 cm in size have a diagnostic yield of 14% when located in the peripheral third of the lung, as compared to 31% when located in the inner two thirds of the lung. If the CT reveals a bronchus leading to the lesion, the yield is 60% [58]. New techniques that may increase the diagnostic yield of fiberoptic bronchoscopy include electromagnetic navigation bronchoscopy [59], bronchoscopy with ultrasound [60–61], and CT- guided bronchoscopy [62]. (*Adapted from* Mehta *et al.* [57].)

Diagnostic Yield of Bronchoalveolar Lavage

Study	Patients, n	Bronchoalveolar Lavage Yield
Shiner et al. [54]	71	9/38 (24%)
Pirozynski [63]	145	52/145 (40%)
		94/145 (65%)*
de Garcia et al. [64]	35	10/35 (28%)
Total	251	71/218 (33%)

*Includes patients in whom malignant cells were present, but correct cell type could not be identified.

Figure 21-13. Diagnostic yield of bronchoalveolar lavage in patients with solitary pulmonary nodules. Bronchoalveolar lavage complements the bronchoscopic brush biopsy. However, with a diagnostic yield of only 28% to 65%, it is a less reliable diagnostic method than bronchoscopic lung biopsy (see Fig. 21-11). (*Adapted from* Mehta et al. [57].)

Factors Suggesting a Higher Diagnostic Yield with Flexible Bronchoscopy

- Solitary pulmonary nodule > 2 cm
- Positive "bronchus sign" on high-resolution CT
- Strong clinical suspicion of malignancy
- Location in the middle or inner third on chest radiography (≤ 2 cm from the hilum)
- Location in right-middle or lingular lobes

Figure 21-14. Factors that increase the diagnostic yield of flexible bronchoscopy. In addition to nodule size and location, the diagnostic yield with flexible bronchoscopy is increased by a positive "bronchus sign" on CT. (*Adapted from* Mehta et al. [57].)

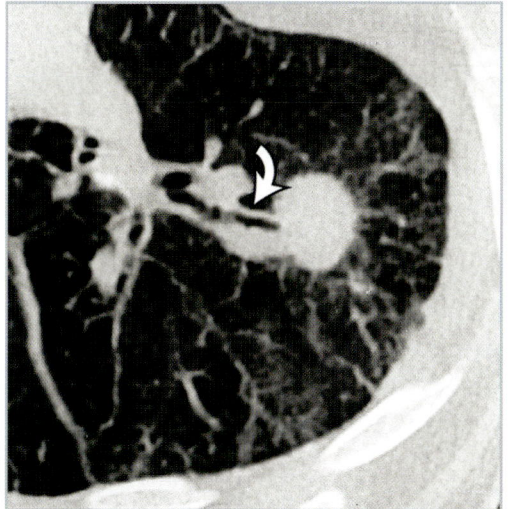

Figure 21-15. "Bronchus sign" on CT. The term *bronchus sign* was used to describe the CT finding of a bronchus (*arrow*) leading directly to or contained within a nodule or mass. The presence of a bronchus sign indicates a higher diagnostic yield (60%) with flexible bronchoscopy than if the sign were absent (14%) [65].

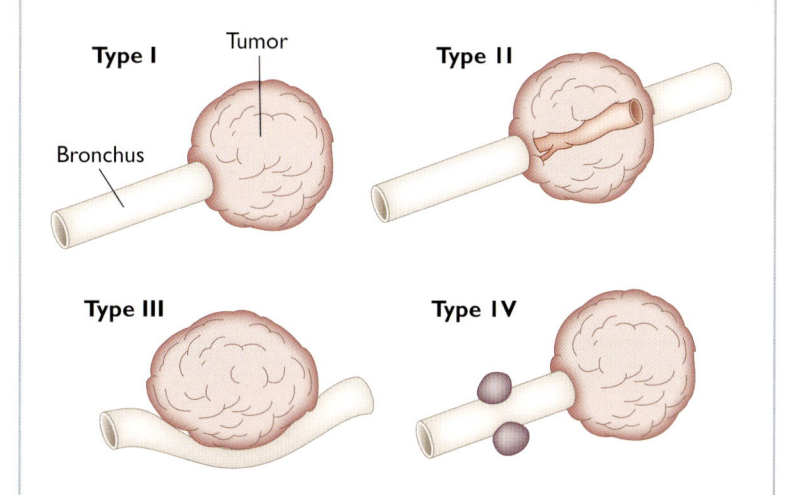

Figure 21-16. Classification of nodule–bronchus relationships. Based on its anatomic relationship with the bronchus, the solitary pulmonary nodule (SPN) is classified as one of four types: type 1, in which the bronchial lumen is patent up to the tumor; type 2, in which the bronchus is contained in the tumor mass; type 3, in which the tumor compresses and narrows the bronchus, but the bronchial mucosa is intact; or type 4, in which the proximal bronchial tree is narrowed by peribronchial or submucosal spread of the tumor or by enlarged lymph nodes [66]. When high-resolution CT indicates that the SPN is a type-1 or type-2 lesion, conventional sampling methods (transbronchial biopsy with brushing and washing) will be adequate to obtain a tissue diagnosis. However, if the SPN is a type-3 or type-4 lesion, transbronchial needle aspiration may be the diagnostic procedure of choice. Complications of flexible bronchoscopy methods include pneumothorax (1.0%–3.8%) [67] and significant bleeding (< 2%) [68]. (*Adapted from* Tsuboi et al. [66].)

Indications for Percutaneous Needle Aspiration

- Small nodules < 2 cm
- Peripheral location of the solitary pulmonary nodule (outer third of the lung)
- Negative flexible bronchoscopy in an indeterminate lesion accessible to percutaneous needle aspiration

*These patients should have no contraindication to percutaneous needle aspiration, such as inability to hold breath, severe pulmonary hypertension, or bleeding diathesis.

Figure 21-17. Percutaneous needle aspiration. Percutaneous needle aspiration (PCNA) is preferred for tissue diagnosis of small (< 2 cm) and peripheral nodules (outer third of the lung), for which the diagnostic yield of flexible bronchoscopy is very low. The choice of fluoroscopy, ultrasound, or CT guidance for PCNA is based on lesion characteristics (size and location) and on the experience of the radiologist. CT is better for the biopsy of nodules adjacent to vascular structures or nerves, and for nodules that are not seen on fluoroscopy. Fluoroscopy allows real-time monitoring of the needle course and is often easier in patients who are less cooperative with breath holding. Transthoracic ultrasonography can be used only to guide biopsy of peripheral lung lesions and not to direct biopsy of most lung nodules because air in the lung parenchyma blocks ultrasound. The diagnostic yield of PCNA varies between studies, ranging from 43% to 97% [69–70]. PCNA is successful in obtaining a diagnosis in 65% of nodules larger than 1 cm in diameter, and in more than 80% of nodules larger than 2 cm.

Continued on the next page

Figure 21-17. *(Continued)* PCNA can be used to identify 95% of malignant nodules [71] and, therefore, has a significant negative predictive value. However, it yields a specific diagnosis in 70% of benign nodules [70]; thus, a nonspecific diagnosis of so-called benign nodules on PCNA does not rule out malignancy [72], and a repeat PCNA or removal of a solitary pulmonary nodule is advisable if clinical suspicion for malignancy is high. Some new technical advances, such as the addition of core biopsy to routine fine-needle aspiration (FNA), may enhance the accuracy of benign diagnoses. In a study of 50 patients, the accuracy of benign diagnoses increased from 31% with FNA alone to 69% with core biopsy. The addition of core samples did not increase the accuracy of malignant diagnoses [73]. The utility of on-site cytologic examination could also increase the success rate of PCNA and minimize complication risks and discomfort to patients. Complications of the procedure include pneumothorax (30%) and bleeding.

Indications for Video-Assisted Thoracoscopic Surgery

Indeterminate nodule that is peripheral (outer one third of lung) and inaccessible to flexible bronchoscopy or CT–guided needle aspiration (small lesion, located under ribs or scapula or near area of emphysema or bullous disease)

Wedge resection of indeterminate or malignant solitary pulmonary nodule in a patient with limited pulmonary reserve who cannot tolerate thoracotomy and wedge resection

Figure 21-18. Indications for video-assisted thoracoscopic surgery. Video-assisted thoracoscopic surgery may be a less invasive option than open thoracotomy when an indeterminate nodule cannot be classified as benign by flexible bronchoscopy or percutaneous needle aspiration. Open lung resection, lobectomy, or pneumonectomy, if required, can be performed during the same procedure if the solitary pulmonary nodule is malignant [74]. (*Adapted from* Fein *et al.* [75].)

Indications for Open Thoracotomy

Solitary pulmonary nodule diagnosed as malignant by flexible bronchoscopy or CT–guided needle aspiration in a patient with adequate pulmonary reserve

Indeterminate nodule of > 3 cm with negative metastatic work-up in a patient with adequate pulmonary reserve

Figure 21-19. Indications for open thoracotomy. Open thoracotomy is the procedure of choice for malignant solitary pulmonary nodules. The mortality rate varies from 1.4% for segmentectomy to 6.2% for pneumonectomy [76]. (*Adapted from* Fein *et al.* [75].)

MANAGEMENT

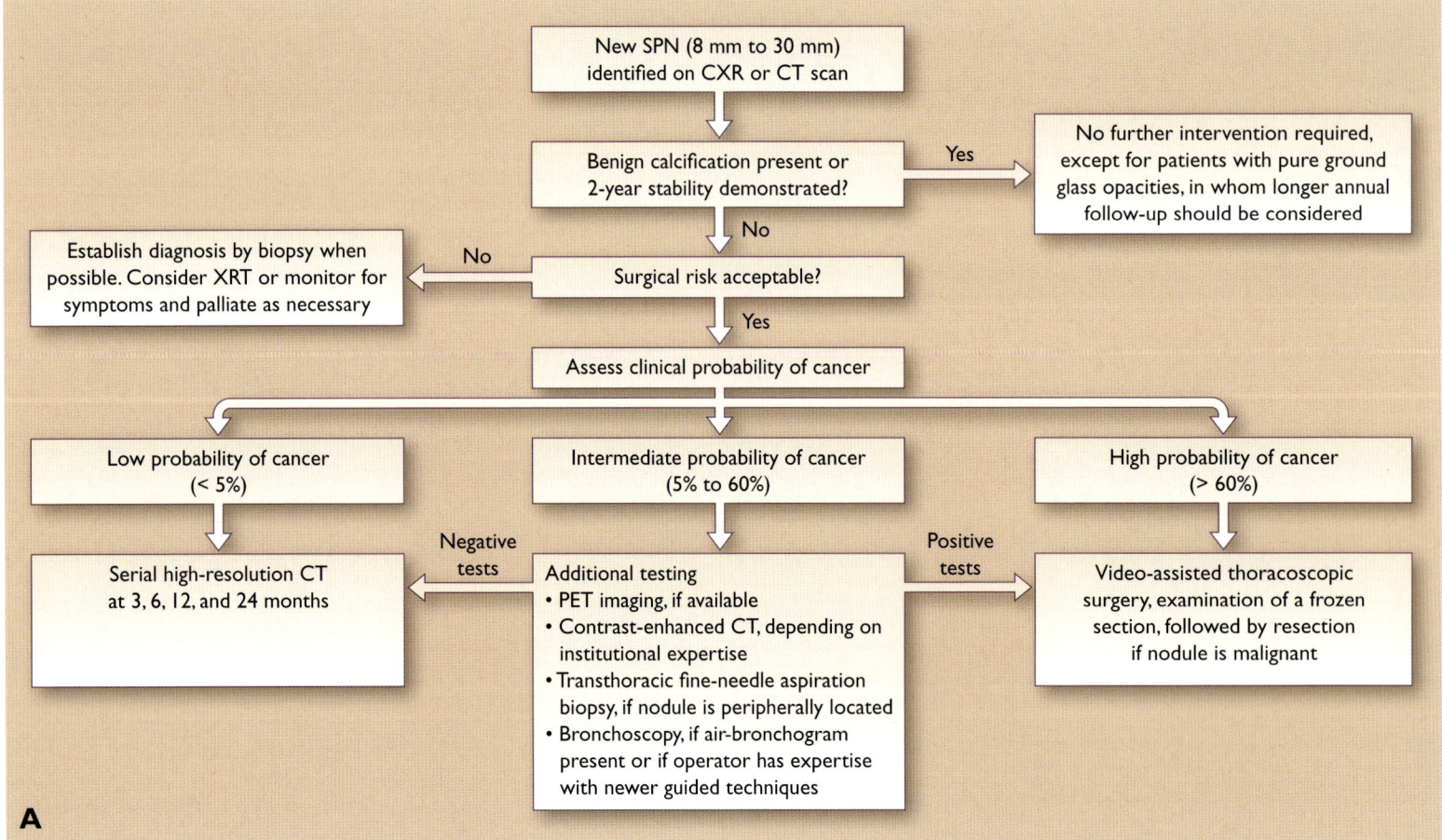

Figure 21-20. A, Algorithm for management of the solitary pulmonary nodule. Based on a detailed history and physical examination, a clinical probability of malignancy can be calculated, and with the results of noninvasive studies such as chest radiographs and CT, a solitary pulmonary nodule (SPN), based on nodule characteristics, can be categorized as benign, indeterminate, or malignant.

Continued on the next page

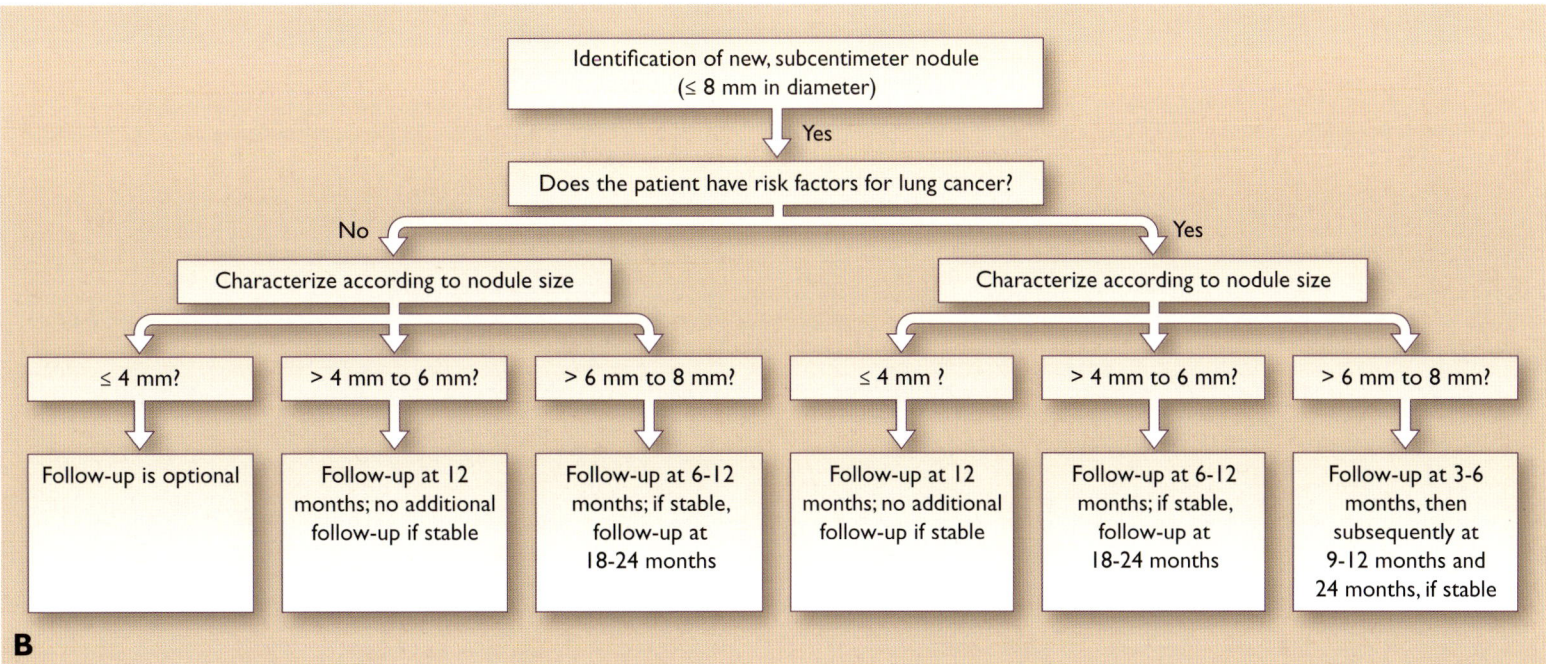

Figure 21-20. *(Continued)* "Watchful waiting," an active process that involves close monitoring and serial chest radiographs, may be used for patients with SPNs that are probably benign (eg, a nodule in a patient younger than 35 years of age who has no additional risk factors, or a nodule that becomes smaller or remains stable for a 2-year period). For malignant SPNs, thoracotomy and resection of the nodule is advocated. For indeterminate nodules, variables such as nodule characteristics, patient's age, history of smoking, and prior malignancy must be considered. Based on the literature and on cost-effectiveness analyses, the approach to patients with indeterminate nodules favors positron emission tomography (PET) because it allows more precise risk stratification. This is important particularly in older patients with concurrent medical illnesses in whom the surgical risk is high, and avoiding unnecessary surgery is essential. If the PET is negative, serial chest radiograph or CT follow-up is justified. Similarly, a positive PET justifies the risk associated with surgery because malignancy is likely. For patients without co-morbidities who have a relatively high risk for cancer, early thoracotomy is an option. However, in clinical situations in which potential differences between choice strategies are small, patient preference may play an important role in decision making. **B,** Recommended management algorithm for patients with subcentimeter pulmonary nodules that measure less than 8 mm in diameter. CXR—chest x-ray; XRT—x-ray therapy. *(Panel A adapted from Ost et al. [33]; Panel B adapted from Gould et al. [8].)*

REFERENCES

1. Leef JL III, Klein JS: The solitary pulmonary nodule. *Radiol Clin North Am* 2002, 40:123–143, ix.

2. Khouri NF, Meziane MA, Zerhouni EA, *et al.*: The solitary pulmonary nodule: assessment, diagnosis, and management. *Chest* 1987, 91:128–133.

3. Siegelman SS, Khouri NF, Leo FP, *et al.*: Solitary pulmonary nodules: CT assessment. *Radiology* 1986, 160:307–312.

4. International Early Lung Cancer Action Program Investigators, Henschke CI, Yankelevitz DF, *et al.*: Survival of patients with stage I lung cancer detected on CT screening. *N Engl J Med* 2006, 355:1763–1771.

5. Good CA, Wilson TW: The solitary circumscribed pulmonary nodule: study of seven hundred five cases encountered roentgenologically in a period of three and one-half years. *JAMA* 1958, 166:210–215.

6. Lillington GA: Management of solitary pulmonary nodules. *Dis Mon* 1991, 37:271–318.

7. Zerhouni EA, Stitik FP, Siegelman SS, *et al.*: CT of the pulmonary nodule: a cooperative study. *Radiology* 1986; 160:319-327.

8. Gould MK, Fletcher J, Iannettoni MD, *et al.*: Evaluation of patients with pulmonary nodules: when is it lung cancer? [ACCP evidence-based clinical practice guidelines, edn 2] *Chest* 2007, 132:108S–130S.

9. Tan BB, Flaherty KR, Kazerooni EA, *et al.*: The solitary pulmonary nodule. *Chest* 2003, 123:89S–96S.

10. Bandoh S, Fujita J, Tojo Y, *et al.*: Diagnostic accuracy and safety of flexible bronchoscopy with multiplanar reconstruction images and ultrafast Papanicolaou stain: evaluating solitary pulmonary nodules. *Chest* 2003; 124:1985–1992.

11. Veronesi G, Bellomi M, Spaggiari L, *et al.*: Low dose spiral computed tomography for early diagnosis of lung cancer: results of baseline screening in 5,000 high-risk volunteers [ASCO Annual Meeting Proceedings Part 1]. *J Clin Oncol* 2006, 24(Suppl):7029.

12. Henschke CI, Yankelevitz DF, Naidich DP, *et al.*: CT screening for lung cancer: suspiciousness of nodules according to size on baseline scans. *Radiology* 2004, 231:164–168.

13. Li F, Sone S, Abe H, *et al.*: Malignant versus benign nodules at CT screening for lung cancer: comparison of thin-section CT findings. *Radiology* 2004, 233:793–798.

14. Li F, Sone S, Abe H, *et al.*: Lung cancers missed at low-dose helical CT screening in a general population: comparison of clinical, histopathologic, and imaging findings. *Radiology* 2002, 225:673–683.

15. Takashima S, Sone S, Li F, *et al.*: Small solitary pulmonary nodules (< or = 1 cm) detected at population-based CT screening for lung cancer: reliable high-resolution CT features of benign lesions. *AJR Am J Roentgenol* 2003, 180:955–964.

16. Hasegawa M, Sone S, Takashima S, *et al.*: Growth rate of small lung cancers detected on mass CT screening. *Br J Radiol* 2000, 73:1252–1259.

17. Sone S, Li F, Yang ZG, *et al.*: Results of three-year mass screening programme for lung cancer using mobile low-dose spiral computed tomography scanner. *Br J Cancer* 2001, 84:25–32.

18. Swensen SJ, Jett JR, Hartman TE, *et al.*: Lung cancer screening with CT: Mayo Clinic experience. *Radiology* 2003, 226:756–761.

19. Swensen SJ, Jett JR, Sloan JA, et al.: Screening for lung cancer with low-dose spiral computed tomography. *Am J Respir Crit Care Med* 2002, 165:508–513.

20. Nawa T, Nakagawa T, Kusano S, et al.: Lung cancer screening using low-dose spiral CT: results of baseline and 1-year follow-up studies. *Chest* 2002, 122:15–20.

21. Henschke CI, Yankelevitz DF, Libby DM, et al.: Early lung cancer action project: annual screening using single-slice helical CT. *Ann N Y Acad Sci* 2001, 952:124–134.

22. Diederich S, Wormanns D, Lenzen H, et al.: Screening for asymptomatic early bronchogenic carcinoma with low dose CT of the chest. *Cancer* 2000, 89:2483–2484.

23. Wahidi MM, Govert JA, Goudar RK, et al.: Evidence for the treatment of patients with pulmonary nodules: when is it lung cancer? [ACCP evidence-based clinical practice guidelines, edn 2] *Chest* 2007, 132:94S–107S.

24. Mountain CF: Revisions in the International System for Staging Lung Cancer. *Chest* 1997, 111:1710–1717.

25. Cummings SR, Lillington GA, Richard RJ: Estimating the probability of malignancy in solitary pulmonary nodules: a Bayesian approach. *Am Rev Respir Dis* 1986, 134:449–452.

26. Wynder, EL, Graham, EA: Tobacco smoking as a possible etiologic factor in bronchiogenic carcinoma: a study of 684 proved cases. *JAMA* 1950, 143:329–336.

27. Neifeld JP, Michaelis LL, Doppman JL: Suspected pulmonary metastases: correlation of chest x-ray, whole lung tomograms, and operative findings. *Cancer* 1977, 39:383–387.

28. Swensen SJ, Jett JR, Payne WS, et al.: An integrated approach to evaluation of the solitary pulmonary nodule. *Mayo Clin Proc* 1990, 65:173–186.

29. Libby DM, Smith JP, Altorki NK, et al.: Managing the small pulmonary nodule discovered by CT. *Chest* 2004,125:1522–1529.

30. Tockman MS: Epidemiology of lung cancer. In *Other Host Factors and Lung Cancer Susceptibility*. Edited by JM Samet. New York: Marcel Dekker; 1994:397–412.

31. Goldmeier, E. Limits of visibility of bronchogenic carcinoma. *Am Rev Respir Dis* 1965, 91:232–239.

32. Yankelevitz DF, Reeves AP, Kostis WJ, et al.: Small pulmonary nodules: volumetrically determined growth rates based on CT evaluation. *Radiology* 2000, 217:251–256.

33. Ost D, Fein AM, Feinsilver, SH: Clinical practice: the solitary pulmonary nodule. *N Engl J Med* 2003, 348:2535–2542.

34. Zwirewich CV, Vedal S, Miller RR, et al.: Solitary pulmonary nodule: high-resolution CT and radiologic-pathologic correlation. *Radiology* 1991, 179:469–476.

35. Tozaki M, Ichiba N, Fukuda K: Dynamic magnetic resonance imaging of solitary pulmonary nodules: utility of kinetic patterns in differential diagnosis. *J Comput Assist Tomogr* 2005, 29:13–19.

36. Swensen SJ, Brown LR, Colby TV, et al.: Pulmonary nodules: CT evaluation of enhancement with iodinated contrast material. *Radiology* 1995, 194:393–398.

37. Henschke CI, Yankelevitz DF, Mirtcheva R, et al.: CT screening for lung cancer: frequency and significance of part-solid and nonsolid nodules. *AJR Am J Roentgenol* 2002, 178:1053–1057.

38. Henschke CI, McCauley DI, Yankelevitz DF, et al.: Early Lung Cancer Action Project: overall design and findings from baseline screening. *Lancet* 1999, 354:99–105.

39. Suzuki K, Nagai K, Yoshida J, et al.: Video-assisted thoracoscopic surgery for small indeterminate pulmonary nodules: indications for preoperative marking. *Chest* 1999, 115:563–568.

40. Swensen SJ, Brown LR, Colby TV, et al.: Lung nodule enhancement at CT: prospective findings. *Radiology* 1996, 201:447–455.

41. Naidich DP, Harkin TJ: Airways and lung: correlation of CT with fiberoptic bronchoscopy. *Radiology* 1995, 197:1–12.

42. Dewan NA, Gupta NC, Redepenning LS, et al.: Diagnostic efficacy of PET-FDG imaging in solitary pulmonary nodules. Potential role in evaluation and management. *Chest* 1993, 104:997–1002.

43. Dewan NA, Shehan CJ, Reeb SD, et al.: Likelihood of malignancy in a solitary pulmonary nodule: comparison of Bayesian analysis and results of FDG-PET scan. *Chest* 1997, 112:416–422.

44. Gambhir SS, Shepherd JE, Shah BD, et al.: Analytical decision model for the cost-effective management of solitary pulmonary nodules. *J Clin Oncol* 1998, 16:2113–2125.

45. Erasmus JJ, McAdams HP, Patz EF Jr, et al.: Evaluation of primary pulmonary carcinoid tumors using FDG PET. *AJR Am J Roentgenol* 1998, 170:1369–1373.

46. Higashi K, Ueda Y, Seki H, et al.: Fluorine-18-FDG PET imaging is negative in bronchioloalveolar lung carcinoma. *J Nucl Med* 1998, 39:1016–1020.

47. Gupta NC, Frank AR, Dewan NA, et al.: Solitary pulmonary nodules: detection of malignancy with PET with 2-[F-18]-fluoro-2-deoxy-D-glucose. *Radiology* 1992, 184:441–444.

48. Freudenberg LS, Rosenbaum SJ, Beyer T, et al.: PET Versus PET/CT dual-modality imaging in evaluation of lung cancer. *Radiol Clin North Am* 2007, 45:639–644.

49. Stringfield JT, Markowitz DJ, Bentz RR, et al.: The effect of tumor size and location on diagnosis by fiberoptic bronchoscopy. *Chest* 1977, 72:474–476.

50. Cortese DA, McDougall JC: Biopsy and brushing of peripheral lung cancer with fluoroscopic guidance. *Chest* 1979, 75:141–145.

51. Radke JR, Conway WA, Eyler WR, et al.: Diagnostic accuracy in peripheral lung lesions: factors predicting success with flexible fiberoptic bronchoscopy. *Chest* 1979, 76:176–179.

52. Fletcher EC, Levin DC: Flexible fiberoptic bronchoscopy and fluoroscopically guided transbronchial biopsy in the management of solitary pulmonary nodules. *West J Med* 1982, 136:477–483.

53. Wallace JM, Deutsch AL: Flexible fiberoptic bronchoscopy and percutaneous needle lung aspiration for evaluating the solitary pulmonary nodule. *Chest* 1982, 81:665–671.

54. Shiner RJ, Rosenman J, Katz I, et al.: Bronchoscopic evaluation of peripheral lung tumours. *Thorax* 1988, 43:887–889.

55. Chechani V: Bronchoscopic diagnosis of solitary pulmonary nodules and lung masses in the absence of endobronchial abnormality. *Chest* 1996, 109:620–625.

56. Baaklini WA, Reinoso MA, Gorin AB, et al.: Diagnostic yield of fiberoptic bronchoscopy in evaluating solitary pulmonary nodules. *Chest* 2000, 117:1049–1054.

57. Mehta AC, Kathawalla SA, Chan CC, et al.: Role of bronchoscopy in the evaluation of SPN. *J Bronchol* 1995, 4:315–322.

58. Naidich DP, Sussman R, Kutcher WL, et al.: Solitary pulmonary nodules: CT-bronchoscopic correlation. *Chest* 1988; 93:595–598.

59. Gildea TR, Mazzone PJ, Karnak D, et al.: Electromagnetic navigation diagnostic bronchoscopy: a prospective study. *Am J Respir Crit Care Med* 2006, 174:982–989.

60. Herth FJ, Ernst A, Becker HD: Endobronchial ultrasound-guided transbronchial lung biopsy in solitary pulmonary nodules and peripheral lesions. *Eur Respir J* 2002, 20:972–974.

61. Herth FJ, Eberhardt R, Becker HD, et al.: Endobronchial ultrasound-guided transbronchial lung biopsy in fluoroscopically invisible solitary pulmonary nodules: a prospective trial. *Chest* 2006, 129:147–150.

62. Tsushima K, Sone S, Hanaoka T, et al.: Comparison of bronchoscopic diagnosis for peripheral pulmonary nodule under fluoroscopic guidance with CT guidance. *Respir Med* 2006, 100:737–745.

63. Pirozynski M: Bronchoalveolar lavage in the diagnosis of peripheral, primary lung cancer. *Chest* 1992, 102:372–374.

64. Garcia J, Bravo C, Miravitlles M, et al.: Diagnostic value of bronchoalveolar lavage in peripheral lung cancer. *Am Rev Respir Dis* 1993, 147:649–652.

65. Gaeta M, Pandolfo I, Volta S, et al.: Bronchus sign on CT in peripheral carcinoma of the lung: value in predicting results of transbronchial biopsy. *AJR Am J Roentgenol* 1991, 157:1181–1185.

66. Tsuboi E, Ikeda S, Tajima M, *et al.*: Transbronchial biopsy smear for diagnosis of peripheral pulmonary carcinomas. *Cancer* 1967, 20:687–698.

67. Blasco SH, Sanchez Hernandez IM, Villena G, *et al.*: Safety of transbronchial biopsy in outpatients. *Chest* 1991, 99:562–565.

68. Cordasco EM Jr, Mehta AC, Ahmad M: Bronchoscopically induced bleeding: a summary of nine years' Cleveland clinic experience and review of the literature. *Chest* 1991, 100:1141–1147.

69. Khouri NF, Stitik FP, Erozan YS, *et al.*: Transthoracic needle aspiration biopsy of benign and malignant lung lesions. *AJR Am J Roentgenol* 1985, 144:281–288.

70. Levine MS, Weiss JM, Harrell JH, *et al.*: Transthoracic needle aspiration biopsy following negative fiberoptic bronchoscopy in solitary pulmonary nodules. *Chest* 1988, 93:1152–1155.

71. Westcott JL: Percutaneous transthoracic needle biopsy. *Radiology* 1988, 169:593–601.

72. Calhoun P, Feldman PS, Armstrong P, *et al.*: The clinical outcome of needle aspirations of the lung when cancer is not diagnosed. *Ann Thorac Surg* 1986, 41:592–596.

73. Boiselle PM, Shepard JA, Mark EJ, *et al.*: Routine addition of an automated biopsy device to fine-needle aspiration of the lung: a prospective assessment. *AJR Am J Roentgenol* 1997, 169:661–666.

74. Ginsberg RJ: Thoracoscopy: a cautionary note. *Ann Thorac Surg* 1993, 56:801–803.

75. Fein AM, Feinsilver SH, Ares CA: Fishman's pulmonary diseases and disorders. In *The Solitary Pulmonary Nodule: A Systemic Approach*. Edited by AP Fishman. New York: Mc Graw Hill; 1998:1727–1737.

76. Ginsberg RJ, Hill LD, Eagan RT, *et al.*: Modern thirty-day operative mortality for surgical resections in lung cancer. *J Thorac Cardiovasc Surg* 1983, 86:654–658.

PRIMARY PLEURAL AND CHEST WALL TUMORS

Aneil Mujoomdar, Jasleen Kukreja, and David J. Sugarbaker

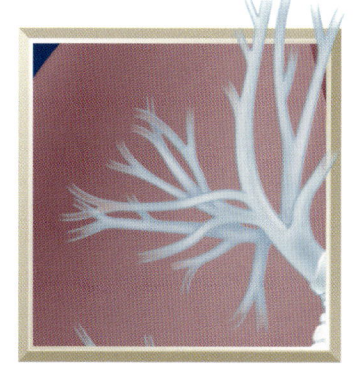
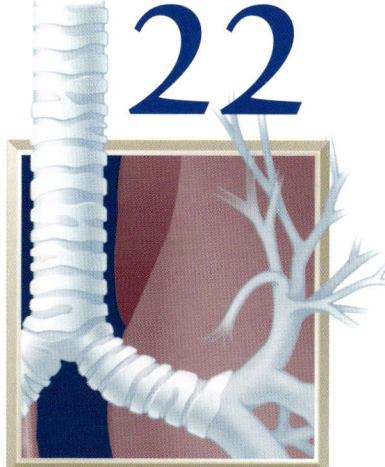
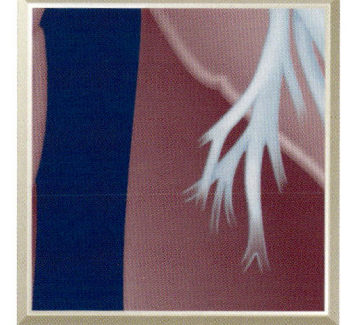

Compared with neoplasms of the lung parenchyma, pleural and chest wall tumors are uncommon. Furthermore, primary pleural and chest wall tumors must be distinguished from the more common metastatic as well as benign and reactive processes that affect the pleural space. This chapter considers various aspects of pleural and chest wall tumors, with an emphasis on pathology and diagnostic radiology. Tumors metastatic to the pleural space are not considered.

The most common primary tumor of the pleura is malignant pleural mesothelioma (MPM). The diagnosis of MPM is usually conducted on the basis of a spectrum of clinical findings such as dyspnea and pleural effusion, as well as typical CT or MRI results verified against pathologic findings on electron microscopy and immunohistochemical stains [1]. None of these findings is pathognomonic, however, and the differential diagnosis usually involves mesothelioma versus adenocarcinoma or sarcoma. Typical early CT indications of malignant mesothelioma include a unilateral pleural effusion and multiple, discrete pleural-based masses. As the disease progresses, diffuse pleural involvement with encasement of the lung and obliteration of the pleural space are seen. In locally advanced MPM, direct extension into the adjacent mediastinum, pericardium, diaphragm, and chest wall can be appreciated on CT. A CT is essential for the initial diagnosis and staging of mesothelioma [2]. MRI does not appear to offer an advantage over CT in the management of patients with mesothelioma [3], although MRI may be more accurate in detecting transdiaphragmatic invasion. Positron emission tomography (PET) and integrated CT-PET may have a role in staging, by identifying mediastinal nodes and extrathoracic disease, as well as in assessing treatment response [4,5].

Pleural fluid cytology and closed pleural biopsy are usually inadequate for pathologic diagnosis [6]. As a consequence of the widespread use of thoracoscopy, thoracoscopic pleural biopsy has now replaced open surgical biopsy as the preferred means for diagnosis [7]. Much has been published about the pathology of mesothelioma, but the challenge for the pathologist to distinguish MPM from other metastatic carcinomas of the pleura, especially adenocarcinoma, remains. Centers experienced in MPM routinely use immunohistochemistry and electron microscopy to differentiate MPM from other tumors. A strong positivity of MPM for cytokeratin distinguishes it from sarcomas, whereas weak reactivity with carcinoembryonic antigen (CEA) and positive staining with calretinin argue against adenocarcinoma [8,9]. On electron microscopy, MPMs have long, sinuous microvilli. In contrast, adenocarcinomas have short, glycocalyx-covered, straight microvilli [10,11].

Overall, the prognosis for patients with MPM remains grim. Single-modality therapy in the form of chemotherapy, surgery, or radiotherapy has generally been ineffective. However, newer chemotherapeutic agents—in particular, gemcitabine and pemetrexed in combination with cisplatin—have shown improved rates for survival [12,13]. Similarly, surgical procedures (pleurectomy with decortication or extrapleural pneumonectomy) alone rarely offer a cure. Radiation as a single-modality therapy is generally reserved for palliative control. Multimodality therapy, including surgery followed by adjuvant chemoradiation, has shown promise in a select cohort [14].

Another, far more rare tumor that deserves mention is the solitary fibrous tumor of the pleura (SFTP). This tumor was initially thought to represent a localized form of mesothelioma, but subsequent work with immunohistochemistry and electron microscopy led to a unique classification independent of MPM. Most patients with SFTP present with symptoms of cough, chest pain, or dyspnea, and there is a well-established association between SFTP and clubbing, hypertrophic pulmonary osteoarthropathy, and hypoglycemia[15].

Primary chest wall tumors account for 2% of all primary tumors [16]. Usually, they are of soft tissue, bone, cartilage, or hematologic origin. Most bony chest wall tumors are located in the ribs (85%), with the remainder found around the scapula, sternum, or clavicle [17]. Sixty percent of primary chest wall tumors that may manifest as painless chest masses or painful ulcerating lesions are malignant [18]. Their evaluation usually includes a chest radiograph with rib tomograms, a CT of the chest, and a bone scan to evaluate the extent of the mass as well as to assess for metastasis. MRI is useful when vascular, spinal cord, or mediastinal invasion is in question.

Chest wall tumors generally have a nonspecific imaging appearance. Therefore, the histologic diagnosis is essential for distinguishing benign from malignant tumors. In addition, a preoperative diagnosis may also be used to identify patients with Ewing's sarcoma, plasmacytoma, or embryonal rhabdomyosarcoma, for which the primary therapy consists of combination chemotherapy. Because needle biopsy has poor specificity and is subject to sampling error, open surgical biopsy remains the procedure of choice for histologic diagnosis. Excisional rather than incisional biopsy is preferred, although the latter may occasionally be appropriate for a large tumor. Frequently, surgical resection, which requires a multidisciplinary team approach, is the treatment of choice.

PLEURAL TUMORS

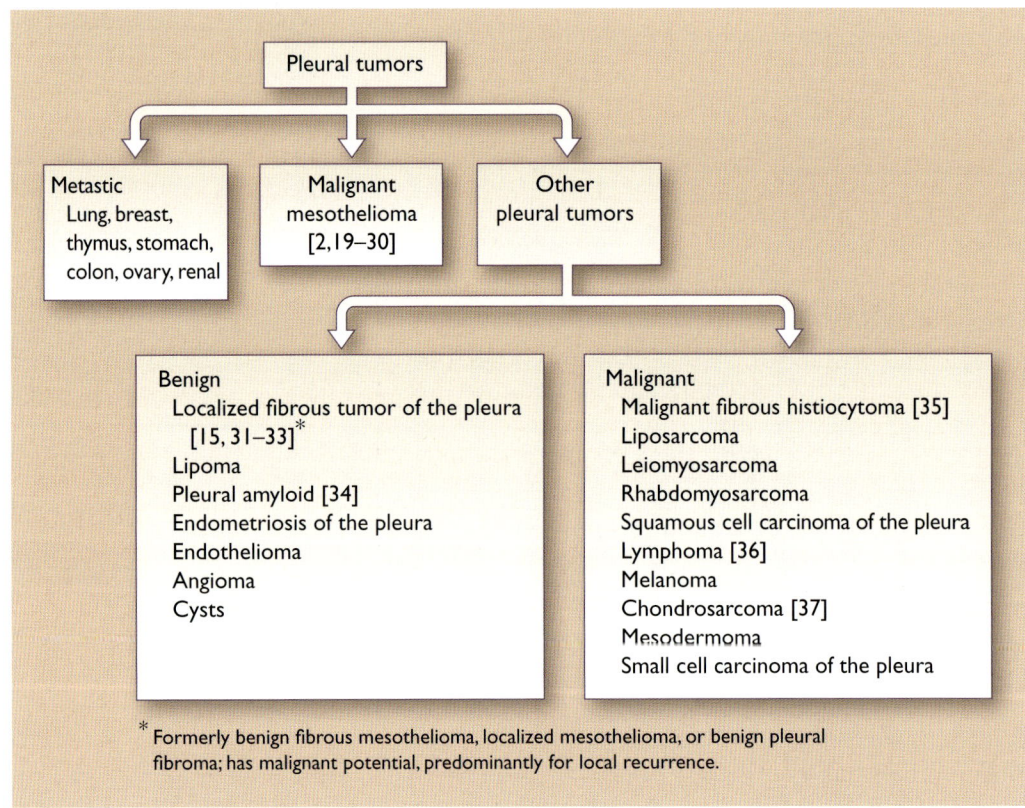

Figure 22-1. Chest wall tumors: overview of the differential diagnosis for pleural tumors. Malignant mesothelioma is the most common primary pleural tumor.

Clinical Features of Malignant Mesothelioma

Age	40–70 y
Male-to-female ratio	5:1
Risk factors	Asbestos exposure (eg, shipyard workers, miners)
	Spouse of asbestos worker
	Irradiation
	Beryllium exposure
Latency period after asbestos exposure	30–45 y
Type of asbestos fiber	Crocidolite ≥ amosite > tremolite > chrysotile
Incidence	Nonasbestos exposure—1:1,000,000
	Asbestos exposure—0.2–2:100
History of asbestos exposure	13%–76%
Smoking history	36%–71%
Symptoms to diagnosis	
< 6 mo	70%
> 6 mo	28%
Survival without treatment (after diagnosis)	6.8–15 mo

Figure 22-2. Epidemiologic and clinical features of malignant mesothelioma [14,24,25].

The Revised* Brigham/DFCI Staging System for Malignant Pleural Mesothelioma

Stage	Description
I	Disease completely resected within the capsule of the parietal pleura without adenopathy; ipsilateral pleura, lung, pericardium, diaphragm, or chest wall disease limited to previous biopsy sites
II	All of stage I with positive resection margins and/or intrapleural adenopathy
III	Local extension of disease into the chest wall or mediastinum, into the heart or through the diaphragm, into the peritoneum, or with extrapleural lymph node involvement
IV	Distant metastatic disease

*Patients with Butchart stage II or III disease are combined into stage III; stage I represents patients with resectable disease and negative nodes; stage II indicates resectable disease but positive nodes.

Figure 22-3. Brigham/Dana Farber Cancer Institute staging system. Accurate staging of malignant pleural mesothelioma is essential to determining survival, predicting prognosis, and guiding treatment. Several staging systems have been proposed, including Butchart's staging system, the International Mesothelioma Interest Group's staging system, and the Brigham/Dana Farber Cancer Institute (DFCI) modified staging system. The Brigham/DFCI staging system, which is based on the largest clinical series published to date as well as on prognostic indicators of resectability, nodal status, and tumor histology, is the most clinically relevant system [2,14,38]. (Adapted from Sugarbaker et al. [39]; with permission.)

Results of Extrapleural Pneumonectomy and Pleurectomy

	Therapeutic Options	
	EPP	**Pleurectomy**
Mortality, %	3.8–31.0	1.5–11.0
Median survival, mo	4.5–19.0	9.0–21.0
2-y survival, %	10.0–38.0	8.9–32.0
5-y survival, mo	3.5–28.5	—

Figure 22-4. Results of extrapleural pneumonectomy and pleurectomy. Extrapleural pneumonectomy (EPP) as a single-modality therapy offers no added advantage over pleurectomy and carries a higher mortality rate [14,29,40,41].

Treatment Options for Malignant Mesothelioma

Single-modality therapy:
  Debulking surgery
    Extrapleural pneumonectomy
    Pleurectomy
  Radiation [28]
    External beam irradiation
    Implantation of radioactive isotopes
  Chemotherapy [12, 13, 24]
    Doxorubicin, cyclophosphamide, *cis*-platinum, gemcitabine, pemetrexed
Multimodality therapy:
  Surgery and adjuvant radiation
  Surgery and adjuvant chemotherapy
  Surgery and adjuvant chemoradiation

Figure 22-5. Treatment options for malignant mesothelioma. The surgical options for patients with malignant mesothelioma include 1) extrapleural pneumonectomy, which involves removal of the parietal and mediastinal pleura, lung, pericardium, and ipsilateral diaphragm; and 2) pleurectomy, which entails removal of the parietal and visceral pleura with or without resection of the pericardium and ipsilateral hemidiaphragm. Surgery as a single-modality therapy is rarely curative. Multimodality therapy offers a survival advantage over single-modality therapy [12,13,24,28].

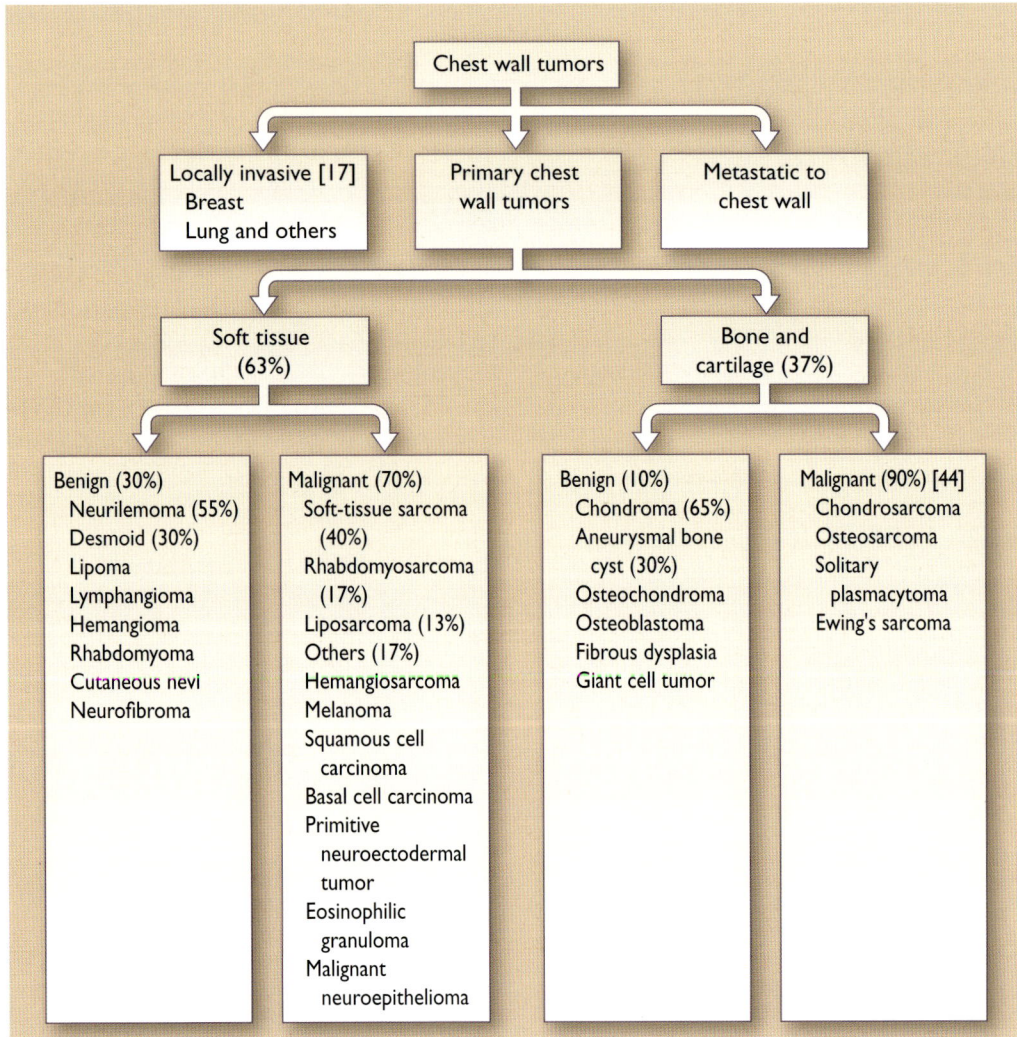

Figure 22-6. Chest wall tumors: overview of the differential diagnosis for chest wall tumors. These tumors are usually of soft tissue, bone, cartilage, or hematologic origin [17,42–49].

Clinical Features of Common Malignant Chest Wall Tumors

	Soft Tissue Sarcoma	Chondrosarcoma	Ewing's Sarcoma	Osteosarcoma	Plasmacytoma
Incidence in chest wall, %	6	20	5–10	15	< 10
Male-to-female ratio	2:1	1.3:1	1.6:1	1.5:1	2.4:1
Age, y (mean)	< 1–86 (38)	5–86 (49)	2–39 (16)	11–78 (42)	35–75 (59)
Site					
Rib, %	—	43	55	34	62
Scapula, %	—	36	34	32	4
Sternum, %	—	16	3	26	12
Clavicle, %	—	5	8	8	21
Symptoms					
Mass only, %	73	43	3	16	21
Mass and pain, %	13	37	8	68	17
Pain only, %	1	12	6	10	54
Others, %	2	7	2	5	8
Radiographic appearance	—	Ill-defined (cortical bone destruction)	Onion peel	Sunburst pattern	Diffuse osteolytic
Incidence, %	35	18	75	68	40–60
Site of metastasis	Lung, pleura, brain, liver, spleen	Lung, liver, bone	Lung, bone, brain, lymph nodes	Lung, bone, colon	—

Figure 22-7. Clinical features of common malignant chest wall tumors. Overall, these tumors are relatively uncommon. Most patients are symptomatic with a mass involving the soft tissues or rib and scapula [17,42–52].

Treatment and Prognosis for Common Malignant Chest Wall Tumors

	Soft Tissue Sarcoma	Chondrosarcoma	Ewing's Sarcoma	Osteosarcoma	Plasmacytoma
Treatment	Complete resection ± radiotherapy; chemotherapy	Complete resection	Combination chemotherapy followed by radiotherapy; limited role for resection	Resection followed by postoperative chemotherapy protocol	Radiotherapy/resection for local control
Local recurrence rate after resection, %	27	39	—	10	5
5-y survival, %	49–90	27–64	50	15	30
Indicators of poor prognosis	Metastasis	Metastasis	Metastasis	Metastasis	Multiple myeloma
	High-grade histology	Age > 50 y		Sternal tumor	
	Pain	Local recurrence		Incomplete resection	

Figure 22-8. Treatment and prognosis for chest wall tumors. Treatment depends on the histology of the primary malignant tumor. Resection is the primary therapy in all cases except Ewing's sarcoma and plasmacytoma [17,42–52].

PATHOLOGY OF PLEURAL TUMORS

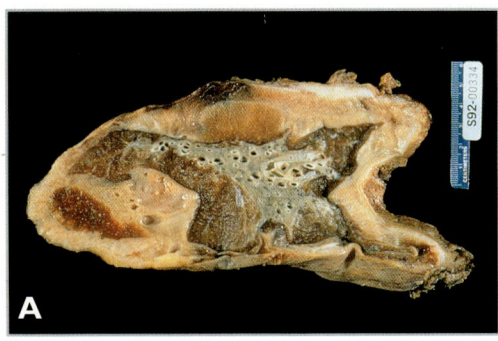
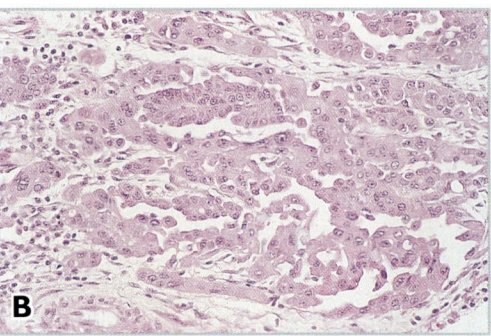
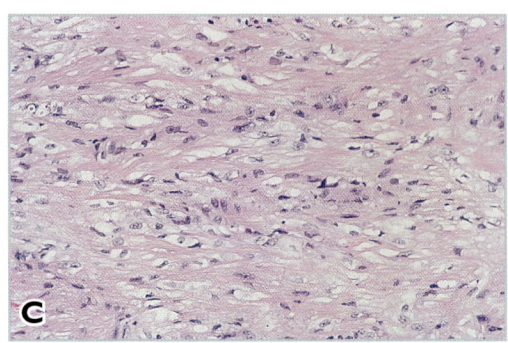

Figure 22-9. Malignant mesothelioma. **A,** Gross specimen of malignant mesothelioma, demonstrating typical dense thickening of the pleura by firm gray-white tissue, which may show areas of cystic degeneration and mucinous material containing hyaluronic acid. The tumor usually arises in the parietal pleura but quickly involves the visceral pleura, causing these two layers to fuse into a dense, white encasement of the lung. The tumor extends into the lung via the major and minor fissures and interlobular septae; it generally also extends into, and through, the diaphragm. The underlying lung is characteristically atelectatic, but otherwise unremarkable, and pleural effusions are common. **B,** Microscopic specimen of malignant mesothelioma. Malignant mesotheliomas are classified histologically as belonging to one of three groups: epithelial, sarcomatous, or mixed. **B** is an example of epithelial mesothelioma, which has a tubopapillary architecture with cuboidal tumor cells containing one eccentric nucleolus and ample eosinophilic cytoplasm. **C,** Example of sarcomatous mesothelioma, composed of atypical spindle-like cells with hyperchromatic nuclei of varying nuclear pleomorphism and mitotic activity. The cells are surrounded by varying amounts of collagen.

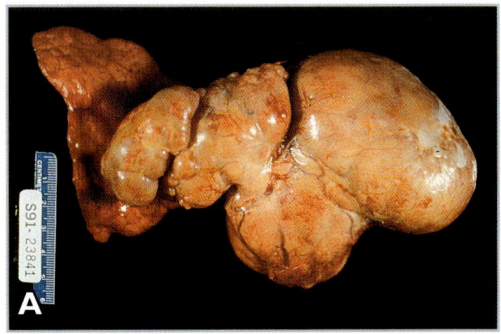
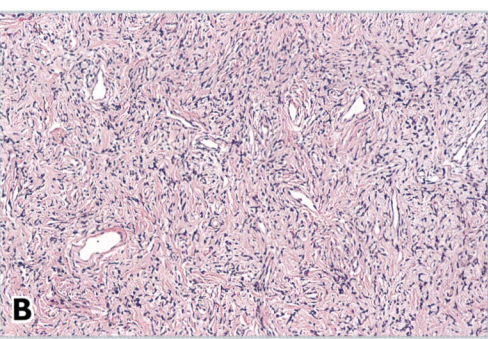

Figure 22-10. Localized fibrous tumor of the pleura. **A,** Gross specimen of a pleural tumor. Most tumors are nodular, whorled, or lobulated. On cut section, they are composed of firm, gray-white tissue with focal cystic degeneration. They are attached to the pleura by a single pedicle, which contains vessels, or are broad-based with a sessile attachment. **B,** Microscopic specimen of a pleural tumor. The tumor is composed of spindle-like cells with collagen arranged in a variety of patterns, which include a storiform pattern, a hemangiopericytoma-like pattern, and a disorderly or random pattern of fibroblast-like cells. Dense, wirelike bands of collagen can be seen, and small vessels with hyalinized walls are common.

PATHOLOGY OF CHEST WALL TUMORS

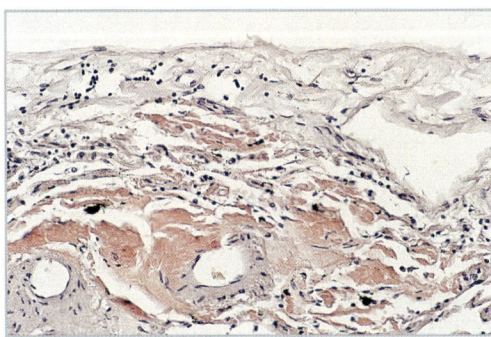
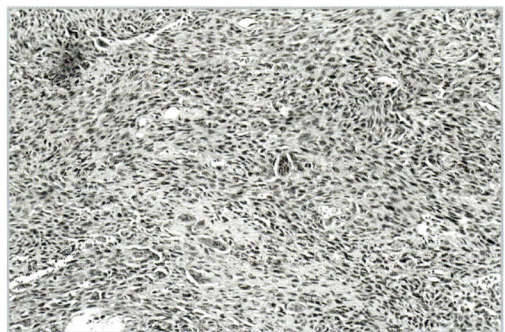

Figure 22-11. Microscopic specimen demonstrating amyloid of the pleura. This Congo red stain reveals congophilic deposits of amyloid within the visceral pleura. The amyloid has a characteristic acellular eosinophilic appearance that reveals apple-green birefringence.

Figure 22-12. Microscopic specimen demonstrating malignant fibrous histiocytoma. This neoplasm contains a polymorphous population of spindled cells arranged in a storiform and fascicular pattern. The tumor cells include fibroblasts and myofibroblasts, histiocytic-like cells, and multinucleated giant cells. A variable number of chronic inflammatory cells, including lymphocytes and plasma cells, are usually present. Increased mitotic activity and necrosis indicate a poor prognosis.

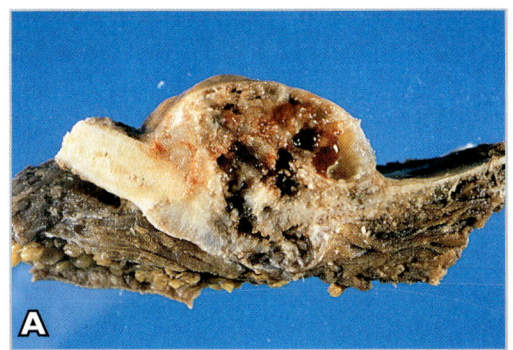
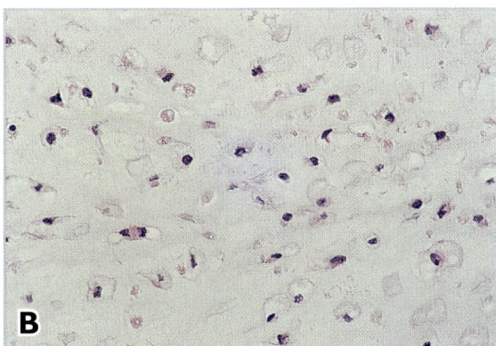

Figure 22-13. Chondrosarcoma. **A,** Gross specimen of chondrosarcoma, which usually presents as a soft-to-firm lobulated mass that is well circumscribed, often with a distinct fibrous capsule. On cut section, it is gelatinous and gray to brown with varying amounts of hemorrhage. The tumor size varies from 1 to 15 cm.
B, Microscopic specimen, demonstrating that the tumor consists of chondrocytes and intervening cartilage. The cells contain small, dark nuclei with varying degrees of cellularity and pleomorphism, which distinguish these lesions from benign cartilage.

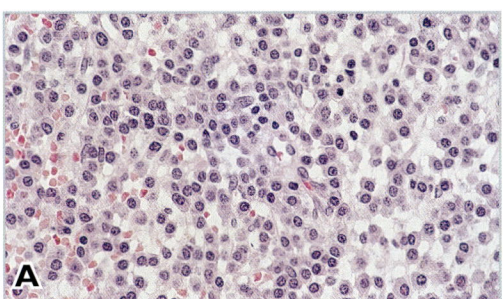
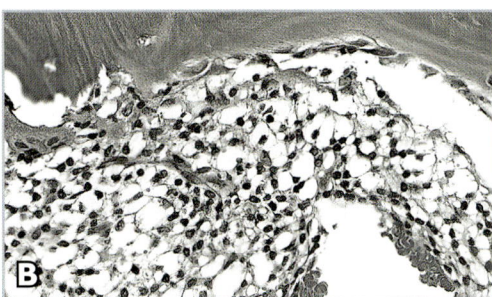

Figure 22-14. Plasmacytoma. **A,** Microscopic specimen, demonstrating that the tumor is composed of a homogeneous population of plasma cells with varying degrees of cytologic atypia and little or no intervening stroma. Occasionally, amyloid deposition is present. **B,** The tumor cells erode adjacent bone, resulting in a reparative lining of osteoblasts along with an osseous border.

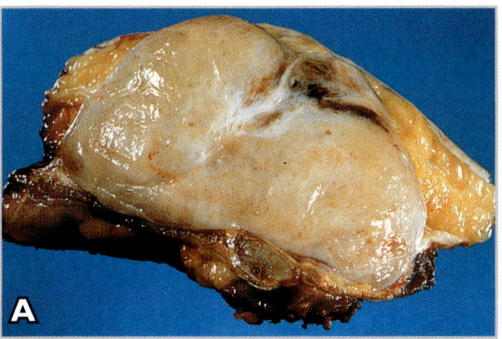
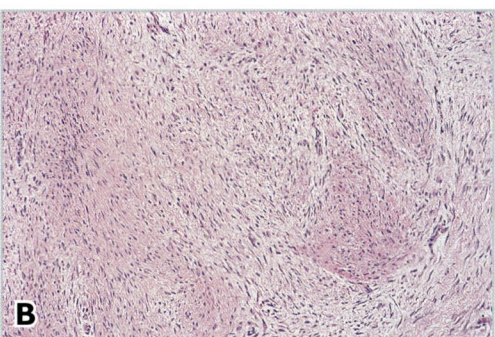

Figure 22-15. Desmoid. **A,** Gross specimen, demonstrating that the tumor consists of a firm, glistening white mass with a trabeculated surface resembling scar tissue. Desmoids commonly reach a maximum dimension of 5 to 10 cm, and tumors as large as 20 cm may be found. **B,** Microscopic specimen of a tumor consisting of spindle-shaped cells with a relatively uniform appearance and interspersed collagen. Cellular atypia or hyperchromasia is rare. The cells and collagen are arranged in long, rather ill-defined bundles with a poorly circumscribed and infiltrative border.

Figure 22-16. Microscopic specimen of osteochondroma showing a lesion with a thick proliferating cartilage cap overlying poorly organized cancellous bone. Irregular endochondral ossification at the base of the cartilage cap can be seen.

RADIOLOGY OF PLEURAL TUMORS

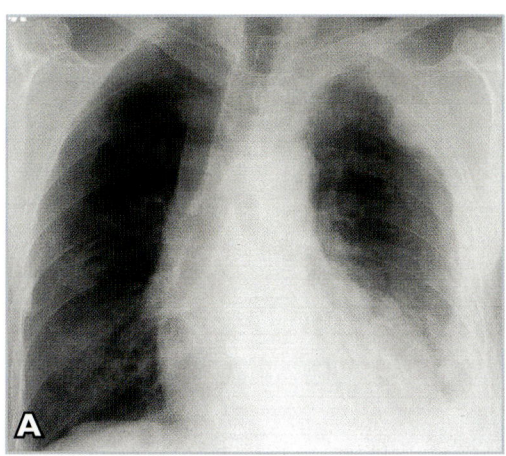
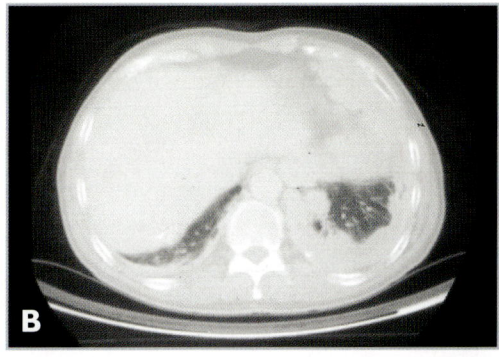

Figure 22-17. Radiographic findings of malignant mesothelioma. **A,** Posteroanterior chest radiograph of a 70-year-old white man with a 7-month history of cough and exertional dyspnea. Recently, the patient, who had worked as a railroad worker and pipe fitter for 40 years, experienced chest discomfort on the left side.

Continued on the next page

Figure 22-17. *(Continued)* Posteroanterior and lateral views of his chest radiograph demonstrate extensive left pleural nodular thickening encasing the left lung, a pattern compatible with malignant pleural mesothelioma. There are also bilateral calcified pleural plaques indicative of pleural changes related to prior asbestos exposure. **B,** A CT of the chest demonstrates extensive pleural disease involving the entire left hemithorax with involvement of the medial and lateral aspects of the pleura compatible with malignant mesothelioma. The bulkiest portion of the tumor is seen in the anterior left-middle and lower pleural space, best observed near the origin of the left hemidiaphragm. There is no definite extension through the diaphragm, but there is evidence of extension into the left major fissure. There are multiple bilateral calcified pleural plaques indicative of prior asbestos exposure.

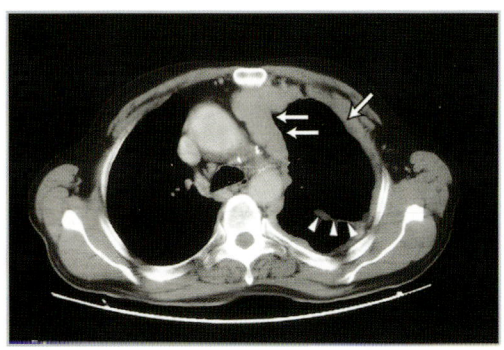

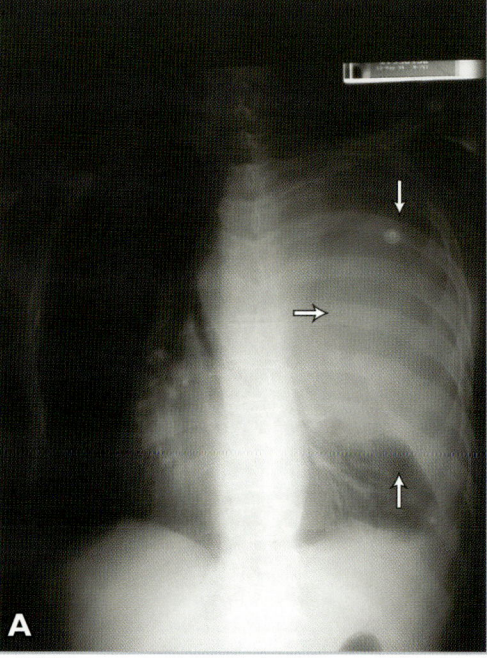

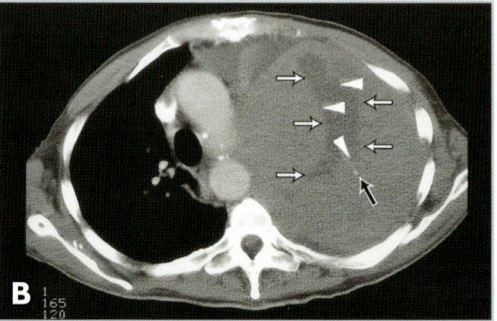

Figure 22-18. Malignant mesothelioma. Axial CT through the upper chest of a 62-year-old man demonstrates diffuse nodular thickening of the left pleura (*arrows*) extending into the major fissure (*arrowheads*) due to malignant mesothelioma.

Figure 22-19. Localized fibrous tumor of the pleura. **A,** Posteroanterior chest radiograph of a 78-year-old man with progressive shortness of breath and large, slowly growing density in the left side of the chest (*arrows*). **B,** CT of the midthorax demonstrates a large, well-defined soft-tissue pleural mass (*white arrows*) with a central cleft (*arrowheads*) and calcification (*black arrow*) compatible with a localized fibrous tumor of the pleura.

RADIOLOGY OF CHEST WALL TUMORS

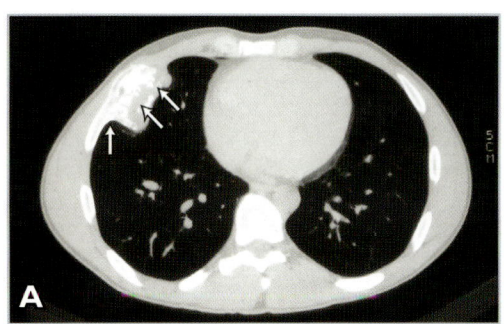

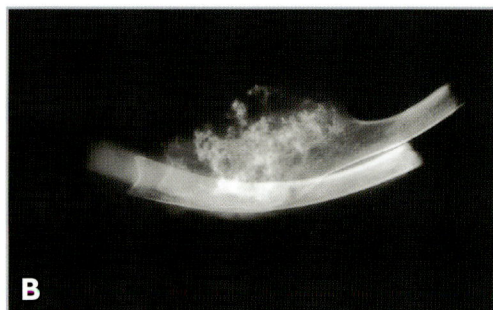

Figure 22-20. Costal chondrosarcoma. **A,** A 27-year-old man's slowly enlarging right lower chest wall mass. An axial CT through the lower chest demonstrates an expansile lesion involving the posterior aspect of the right sixth rib at the costochondral junction (*arrows*). **B,** Resected specimen confirms the presence of a low-grade chondrosarcoma of the rib.

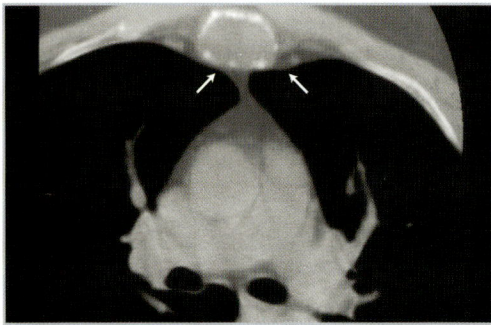

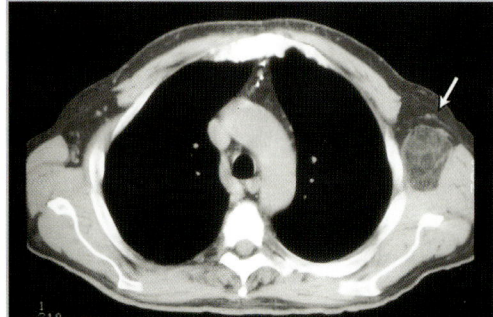

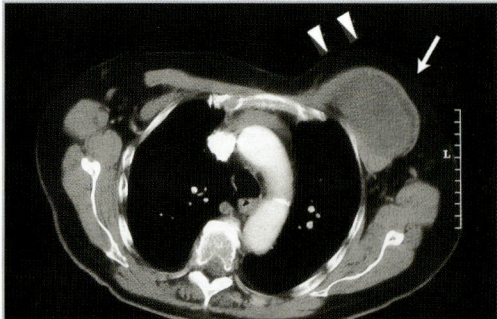

Figure 22-21. Plasmacytoma in a 48-year-old man with sternal pain. Axial scans through the body of the sternum demonstrate a soft-tissue mass (*arrows*) infiltrating and expanding the sternum. Biopsy specimens confirmed the presence of a plasmacytoma.

Figure 22-22. Liposarcoma in an 82-year-old man with a palpable left axillary mass. Axial CT obtained at the level of the aortic arch demonstrates a well-defined fatty lesion in the left axilla (*arrow*) with multiple septae through the lesion, compatible with a liposarcoma.

Figure 22-23. Soft-tissue sarcoma in an 80-year-old man with left chest wall swelling. Axial CT obtained at the level of the aortic arch demonstrates a large soft-tissue mass (*arrow*) seen in the left chest wall below the left pectoralis major muscle (*arrowheads*) due to a soft-tissue sarcoma.

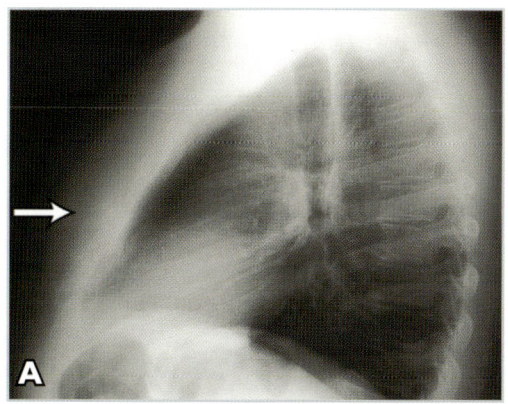
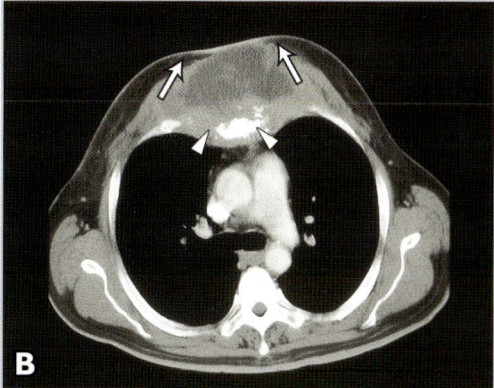

Figure 22-24. Chest wall lymphoma. **A,** Lateral view of the chest in a 48-year-old man presenting with non-Hodgkin's lymphoma and chest wall swelling, demonstrating marked soft-tissue thickening in the presternal region (*arrow*). **B,** Axial CT at the level of the carina demonstrates a large necrotic chest wall mass (*arrows*) with involvement of the sternum (*arrowheads*).

REFERENCES

1. Zellos LS, Sugarbaker DJ: Multimodality treatment of diffuse malignant mesothelioma. *Semin Oncol* 2002, 29:41–50.

2. IMIG, International Mesothelioma Interest Group: A proposed new international TNM staging system for malignant pleural mesothelioma. *Chest* 1995, 108:1122–1128.

3. Patz EF Jr, Shaffer K, Piwnica-Worms DR, et al.: Malignant pleural mesothelioma: value of CT and MR imaging in predicting resectability. *AJR Am J Roentgenol* 1992, 159:961–966.

4. Gerbaudo VH, Britz-Cummingham S, Sugarbaker DJ, Treves ST: Metabolic significance of the pattern, intensity and kinetics of 18F-FDG uptake in malignant pleural mesothelioma. *Thorax* 2003, 58:1077–1082.

5. Steinert HC, Santos Dellea MM, Burger C, Stahel R: Therapy response evaluation in malignant pleural mesothelioma with integrated PET-CT imaging. *Lung Cancer* 2005, 49(suppl 1):S33–35.

6. Renshaw AA, Dean BR, Antman KH, et al.: The role of cytologic evaluation of pleural fluid in the diagnosis of malignant mesothelioma. *Chest* 1997, 111:106–109.

7. Harris RJ, Kavuru MS, Rice TW, Kirby TJ: The diagnostic and therapeutic utility of thoracoscopy: a review. *Chest* 1995, 108:828–841.

8. Ordonez NG: In search of a positive immunohistochemical marker for mesothelioma: an update. *Adv Anatom Pathol* 1998, 1:53–60.

9. Wirth PR, Legier J, Wright GLJ: Immunohistochemical evaluation of seven monoclonal antibodies for differentiation of pleural mesothelioma from lung adenocarcinoma. *Cancer* 1991, 76:655–662.

10. Burns TR, Greenberg SD, Mace ML, Johnson EH: Ultrastructural diagnosis of epithelial malignant mesothelioma. *Cancer* 1985, 56:2036–2040.

11. Hammar SP, Bolen JW: Pleural neoplasms. In *Pulmonary Pathology*. Edited by Dail DH. New York: Springer-Verlag; 1988:973–1028.

12. Tomek S, Emri S, Krejcy K, Manegold C: Chemotherapy for malignant pleural mesothelioma: past results and recent developments. *Br J Cancer* 2003, 88:167–174.

13. Vogelzang NJ, Rusthoven JJ, Symanowski J, et al.: Phase III study of pemetrexed in combination with cisplatin versus cisplatin alone in patients with malignant pleural mesotheliomas. *J Clin Oncol* 2003, 21:2636–2644.

14. Sugarbaker DJ, Flores RM, Jaklitsch MT, et al.: Resection margins, extrapleural nodal status, and cell type determine postoperative long-term survival in trimodality therapy of malignant pleural mesothelioma: results in 183 patients. *J Thorac Cardiovasc Surg* 1999, 117:54–63.

15. Briselli M, Mark EJ, Dickersin GR: Solitary fibrous tumors of the pleura: eight new cases and review of 360 cases in the literature. *Cancer* 1981, 47:2678–2689.

16. Okumura T, Asamura H, Kondo H, et al.: Hemangioma of the rib: a case report. *Jpn J Clin Oncol* 2000, 30:354–357.

17. Anderson BO, Burt ME: Chest wall neoplasms and their management. *Ann Thorac Surg* 1994, 58:1774–1781.

18. Athanassiadi K, Kalavrouziotis G, Rondogianni D, et al.: Primary chest wall tumors: early and long term results of surgical treatment. *Eur J Cardiothorac Surg* 2001, 19:589–593.

19. Pisani RJ, Colby TV, William DE: Malignant mesothelioma of the pleura. *Mayo Clin Proc* 1988, 63:1234–1244.

20. Antman KH: Natural history and epidemiology of malignant mesothelioma. *Chest* 1993, 103:373–376.

21. Vogelzang NJ: Malignant mesothelioma: diagnostic and management strategies for 1992. *Semin Oncol* 1992, 19:64–71.

22. Hammar SP: The pathology of benign and malignant pleural disease. *Chest Surg Clin North Am* 1994, 4:405–431.

23. Roggli VL, Pratt PC, Brody AR: Asbestos fiber type in malignant mesothelioma: an analytical scanning electron microscopic study of 94 cases. *Am J Ind Med* 1993, 23:605–614.

24. Alberts AS, Falkson G, Goedhals L, et al.: Malignant pleural mesothelioma: a disease unaffected by current therapeutic maneuvers. *J Clin Oncol* 1988, 6:527–535.

25. Antman KH, Shemin R, Ryan L, et al.: Malignant mesothelioma: prognostic variables in a registry of 180 patients, the Dana-Farber Cancer Institute and Brigham and Women's Hospital experience over two decades, 1965–1985. *J Clin Oncol* 1988, 6:147–153.

26. Chailleux E, Dabouis G, Pioche D, et al.: Prognostic factors in diffuse malignant pleural mesothelioma: a study of 167 patients. *Chest* 1988, 93:159–162.

27. Carbone M, Kratzke RA, Testa JR: The pathogenesis of mesothelioma. *Semin Oncol* 2002, 29:2–17.

28. Ball DL, Cruickshank DG: The treatment of malignant mesothelioma of the pleura: review of five-year experience, with special reference to radiotherapy. *Am J Clin Oncol* 1990, 13:4–9.

29. Allen KB, Faber LP, Warren WH: Malignant pleural mesothelioma: extrapleural pneumonectomy and pleurectomy. *Chest Surg Clin North Am* 1994, 4:113–126.

30. Sugarbaker DJ, Heher EC, Lee TH, et al.: Extrapleural pneumonectomy, chemotherapy, and radiotherapy in the treatment of diffuse malignant pleural mesothelioma. *J Thorac Cardiovasc Surg* 1991, 101:10–15.

31. England DM, Hochholzer L, McCarthy MT: Localized benign and malignant fibrous tumors of the pleura: a clinicopathological review of 223 cases. *Am J Surg Pathol* 1989, 13:640–658.

32. Saifuddin A, Da Costa P, Chalmers AG, et al.: Primary malignant localized fibrous tumors of the pleura: clinical, radiological and pathological features. *Clin Radiol* 1992, 45:13–17.

33. Hartmann CA, Schutze H: Mesothelioma-like tumors of the pleura: a review of 72 autopsy cases. *J Cancer Res Clin Oncol* 1994, 120:331–347.

34. Kavuru MS, Adamo JP, Ahmad M, et al.: Amyloidosis and pleural disease. *Chest* 1990, 98:20–23.

35. Rizkalla K, Ahmad D, Garcia B, *et al.*: Primary malignant fibrous histiocytoma of the pleura: a case report and review of the literature. *Respir Med* 1994, 88:711–714.

36. Kavuru MS, Tubbs R, Miller ML, Wiedemann HP: Immunocytometry and gene rearrangement analysis in the diagnosis of lymphoma in an idiopathic pleural effusion. *Am Rev Respir Dis* 1992, 145:209–211.

37. Bailey SC, Head HD: Pleural chondrosarcoma. *Ann Thorac Surg* 1990, 49:996–997.

38. Butchart EG, Ashcroft T, Barnsley WC, Holden MP: Pleuropneumonectomy in the management of diffuse malignant mesothelioma of the pleura. Experience with 29 patients. *Thorax* 1976, 31:15–24.

39. Sugarbaker DJ, Strauss GM, Lynch TJ, *et al.*: Node status has prognostic significance in the multimodality therapy of diffuse, malignant mesothelioma. *J Clin Oncol* 1993, 11:1172–1178.

40. Jaklitsch MT, Grondin SC, Sugarbaker DJ: Treatment of malignant mesothelioma. *World J Surg* 2001, 25:210–217.

41. Singhal S, Kaiser L: Malignant mesothelioma: options for management. *Surg Clin North Am* 2002, 82:797–831.

42. Eng J, Sabanathan S, Pradhan GN, Mearns AJ: Primary bony chest wall tumors. *J R Coll Surg Edinb* 1990, 35:44–47.

43. Burt M, Fulton M, Wessner-Dunlap S, *et al.*: Primary bony and cartilaginous sarcomas of chest wall: results of therapy. *Ann Thorac Surg* 1992, 54:226–232.

44. Burt ME: Primary malignant tumors of the chest wall: the Memorial Sloan-Kettering Cancer Center Experience. *Chest Surg Clin North Am* 1994, 4:137–153.

45. King RM, Pairolero PC, Trastek VF, *et al.*: Primary chest wall tumors: factors affecting survival. *Ann Thorac Surg* 1986, 41:597–601.

46. Burt M, Karpeh M, Ukoha O, *et al.*: Medical tumors of the chest wall: solitary plasmacytoma and Ewing's sarcoma. *J Thorac Cardiovasc Surg* 1993, 105:89–96.

47. Grosfeld JL: Primary tumors of the chest wall and mediastinum in children. *Semin Thorac Cardiovasc Surg* 1994, 6:235–239.

48. Pezzella AT, Fall SM, Pauling FW, Sadler TR: Solitary plasmacytoma of the sternum: surgical resection with long-term follow-up. *Ann Thorac Surg* 1989, 48:859–862.

49. Incarbone M, Pastorino U: Surgical treatment of chest wall tumors. *World J Surg* 2001, 25:218–230.

50. Miser JS, Kinsella TJ, Triche TJ, *et al.*: Preliminary results of treatment of Ewing's sarcoma in children and young adults: six months of intensive combined modality therapy without maintenance. *J Clin Oncol* 1988, 6:484–490.

51. Faber LB, Somers J, Templeton AC: Chest wall tumors. *Curr Probl Surg* 1995, 32:661–747.

52. Liptay MJ, Fry WA: Malignant bone tumors of the chest wall. *Semin Thorac Cardiovasc Surg* 1999, 11:278–284.

MEDIASTINAL MASSES

23

*M. Yesim Ersoy,
Carlos A. Jimenez,
and Rodolfo C. Morice*

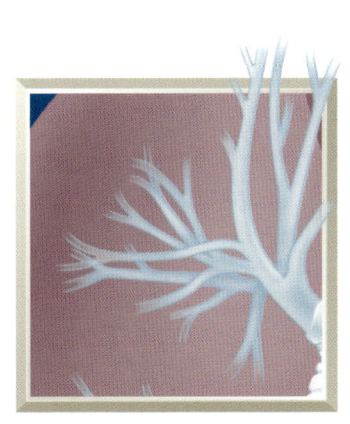
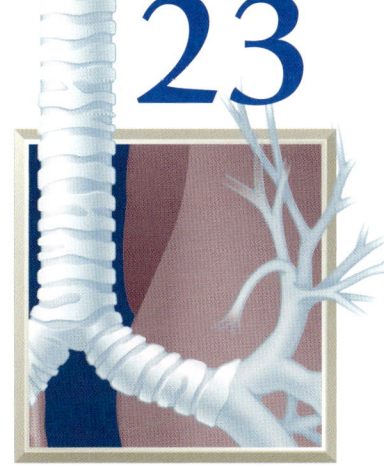
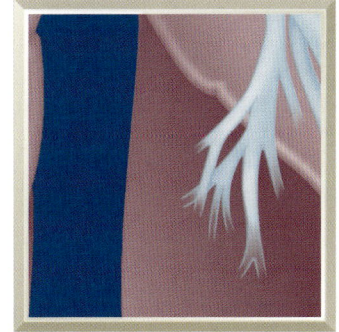

The mediastinum is the region of the chest bounded laterally by the mediastinal pleural reflections of both lungs, anteriorly by the undersurface of the sternum, and posteriorly by the vertebral bodies of the thoracic vertebrae. Longitudinally, it extends from the thoracic inlet to the diaphragm. Because of the variety of tissues it contains, tumors that originate in the mediastinum are numerous and diverse.

Clinical manifestations of these tumors range from vague or asymptomatic to a multiplicity of endocrine or systemic syndromes. The tumors can invade or compress airways and vital cardiovascular structures. In such cases, dramatic, life-threatening clinical presentations can occur [1].

ANATOMIC CONSIDERATIONS

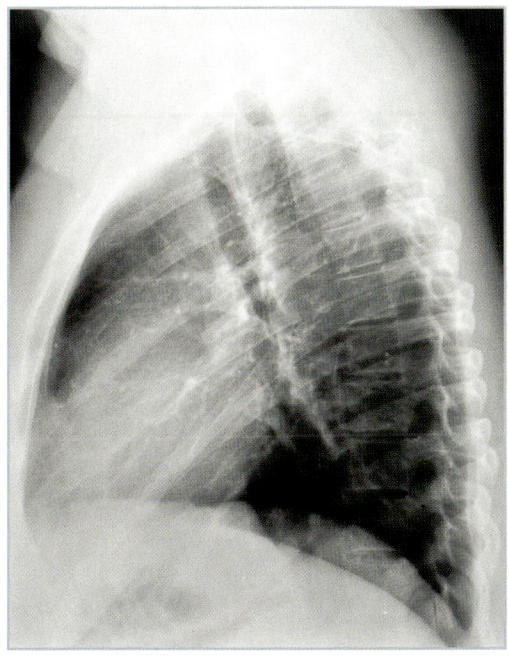
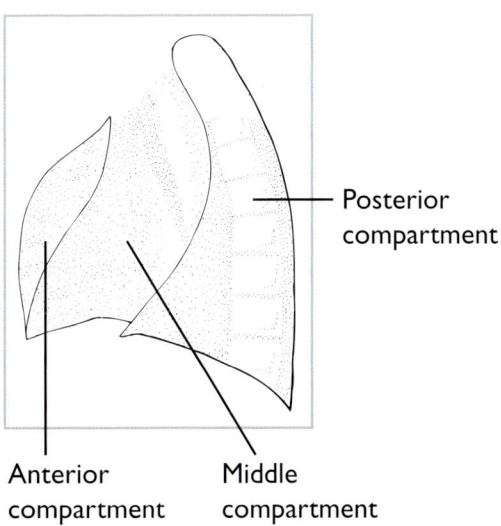

Figure 23-1. Radiograph showing mediastinal compartments. The mediastinum is divided into anterior, middle, and posterior compartments. The anterior compartment is bounded anteriorly by the sternum and posteriorly by the anterior surface of the pericardium, aorta, and brachiocephalic vessels. This compartment contains the thymus gland, lymph nodes, connective tissue, internal mammary arteries and veins, and ectopic parathyroid glands or thyroid tissue. The middle compartment contains the heart and pericardium, the ascending and transverse sections of the aorta, the brachiocephalic vessels, and the superior and inferior vena cava. It also contains the thoracic portion of the trachea and proximal main stem bronchi, and the pulmonary arteries and veins. The phrenic and upper portion of the vagus nerves, as well as numerous lymphatics and connective tissue, are also located within this compartment. The posterior compartment is bounded anteriorly by the dorsal surface of the pericardium, caudally by the diaphragm, laterally by the mediastinal pleural reflections, and posteriorly by the vertebral bodies of the thoracic spine. The paravertebral or costovertebral regions, although not truly within the mediastinum, are generally considered part of the posterior mediastinal compartment. The latter contains the esophagus, the descending aorta, azygos and hemiazygos veins, the thoracic duct, autonomic nerves, adipose and connective tissue, and lymph nodes.

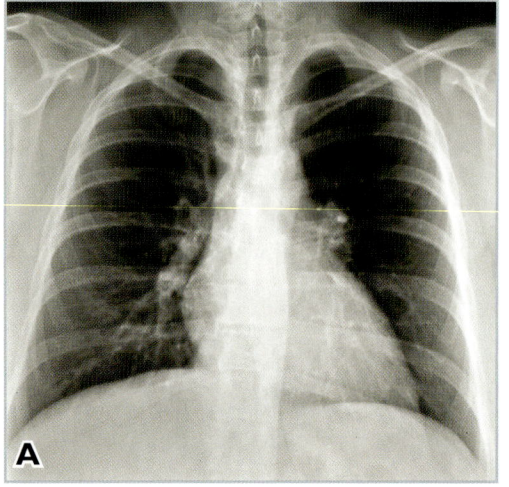
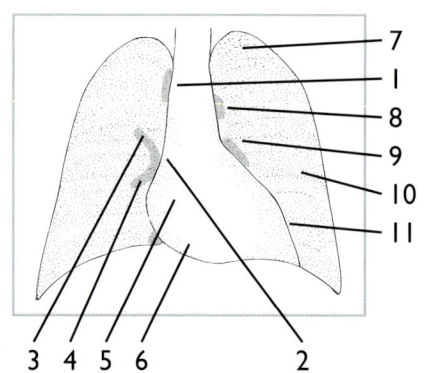
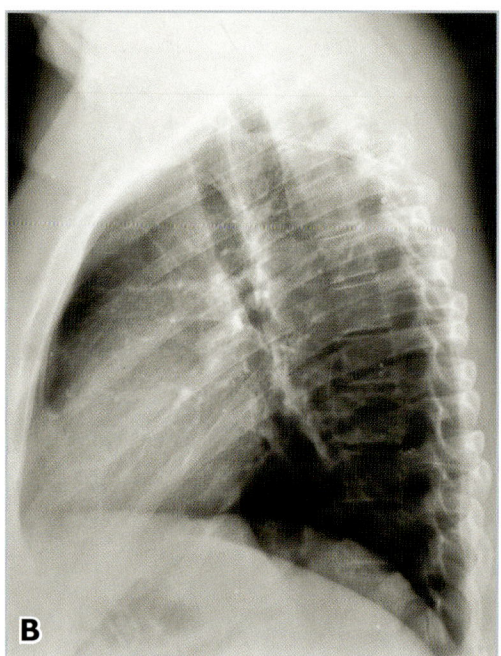
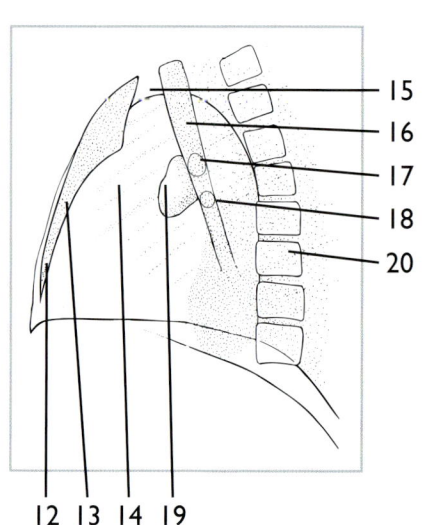

Figure 23-2. Radiographs showing normal mediastinal borders and lines. Recognition of the normal structures that make up the mediastinal contours and lines on a posteroanterior and lateral chest radiograph remains the fundamental method for detecting mediastinal abnormalities. **A,** On the posteroanterior chest radiograph, the right mediastinal border is defined by the superior vena cava (*1*); azygos vein (*2*); right hilum, formed by the juxtaposed shadows of the right upper lobe pulmonary vein (*3*) and right interlobar pulmonary artery (*4*); the right atrium (*5*); and the pericardial fat pad (*6*) at the diaphragmatic-pericardial junction. On the left side, the upper mediastinal contour is formed by the left subclavian artery (*7*); the aortic arch (*8*); and the aortopulmonary window (*9*), a space occupied largely by mediastinal fat between the aortic arch and the left pulmonary artery (*10*). The shadow of the left ventricle (*11*) forms the remainder of the left infrahilar mediastinal border. Normally, the left atrium is rarely visualized. **B,** On a lateral chest radiograph, the anterior mediastinal space is well demarcated by the undersurface of the sternum (*12*), the ventral border of the pericardium (*13*), the ascending portion of the aortic arch (*14*), and the brachiocephalic vessels (*15*). In the middle compartment, the air column of the trachea (*16*), as well as the openings of the right upper lobe bronchi (*17*) and left upper lobe bronchi (*18*), are visualized. The more dense shadows located anteriorly and posteriorly to the bronchial openings correspond to the right interlobar artery (*19*) and the confluence of pulmonary veins (*20*), respectively.

DIAGNOSTIC TECHNIQUES

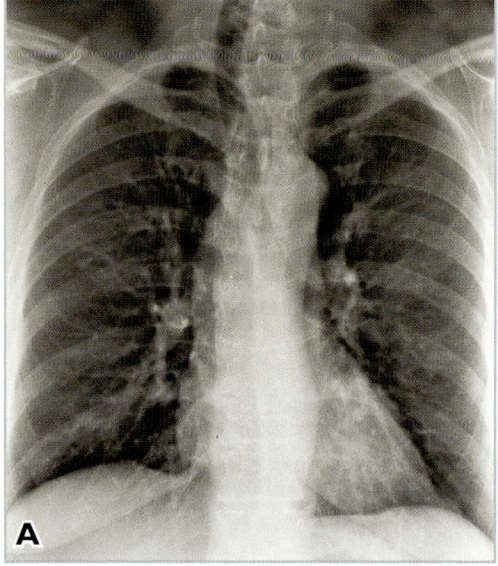
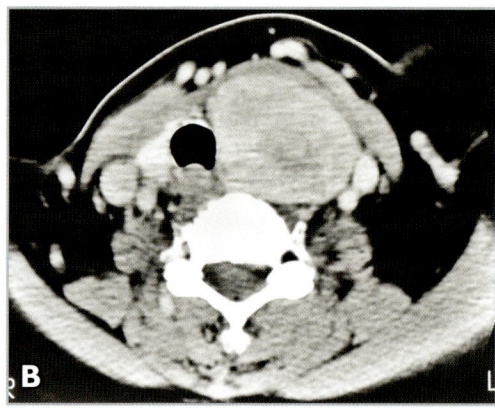

Figure 23-3. A, Frontal chest radiograph showing displacement of the trachea from left to right in the lower neck and upper mediastinal area, caused by an intrathoracic goiter. On a standard chest radiograph, the distortion or obliteration of normal mediastinal lines is key to the initial identification of mediastinal disease. The correlation of the radiographic findings with presence or absence of symptoms and clinical examination is sufficient in some cases to establish a diagnosis. In most cases, however, further evaluation is necessary [2]. **B,** CT of the chest shows lateral tracheal displacement and outward displacement of brachiocephalic vessels. It defines the mass as solid and contained anteriorly by the pretracheal fascia with no invasion of adjacent tissues. A CT of the chest has a much higher sensitivity for smaller lesions than does a conventional radiograph, and it allows for better definition of superimposed structures. It also clarifies the association of adjacent tissues and the presence or absence of invasion, and it differentiates between tissue densities.

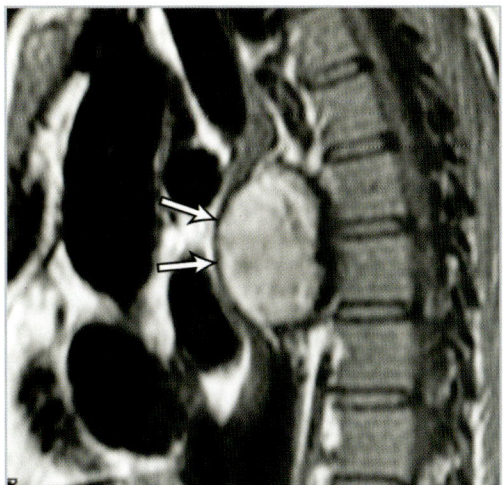

Figure 23-4. MRI of the mediastinum. An advantage of MRI over CT is its ability to visualize vascular structures without requiring intravenous contrast enhancement. MRI is also helpful for confirming the cystic nature of mediastinal lesions that appear solid on CTs. Because of its multiplanar capability, MRI is the preferred method for imaging neurogenic tumors. In this role, it also displays sagittal and coronal planes of mediastinal structures without requiring cumbersome patient repositioning or reformatting of transverse sections, as is the case with CT. In spite of recent advances in MRI, this technique is at present largely used as an adjunct to CT in the evaluation of mediastinal abnormalities [3]. This image of a patient with a primary mediastinal pleomorphic sarcoma shows the location of the mass, and anterior displacement of the esophagus (*arrows*) is well-visualized from the perspective of the sagittal view. Blood flowing within cardiovascular structures is perceived as a radiolucency. No known significant biologic risks are associated with the use of the magnetic field at current imaging levels. However, magnetic field interference prevents the use of MRI in patients who have internal metallic devices, such as pacemakers or prostheses. Contrast enhanced MRI has been associated with nephrogenic systemic fibrosis in patients with renal dysfunction [4].

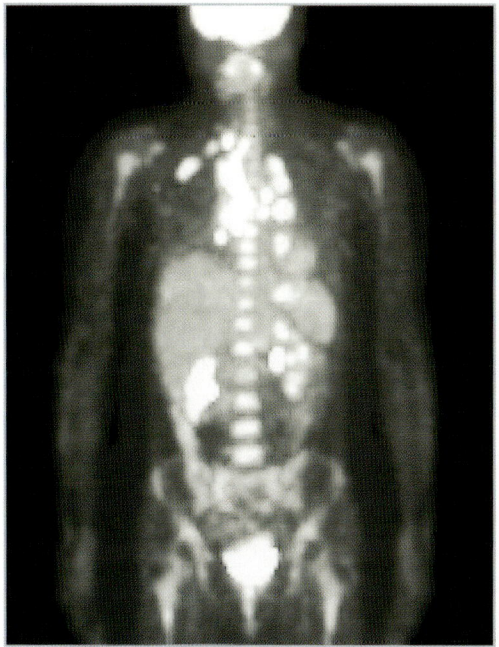

Figure 23-5. Positron emission tomography image of a patient with a history of nodular sclerosis Hodgkin's disease who was referred for initial staging evaluation. There is multicompartmental disease, with multiple lymph nodes identified in the mediastinum along the paratracheal, both of the hilar, and the prevascular regions, as well as extension to the right supraclavicular and right axillary nodal regions. Positron emission tomography (PET) is based on identifying the increased glycolytic activity in malignant cells. It uses the radionuclide fluorine-18 fluorodeoxyglucose (FDG). Because of an increase in membrane glucose transporters and phosphorylation, FDG is preferentially concentrated within malignant cells. FDG PET has gained acceptance for the initial staging of cancer, for diagnosis of recurrent malignancy, and for monitoring response to therapy. Its specificity is hampered by the fact that inflammatory conditions may also exhibit increased radioactive glucose uptake [5].

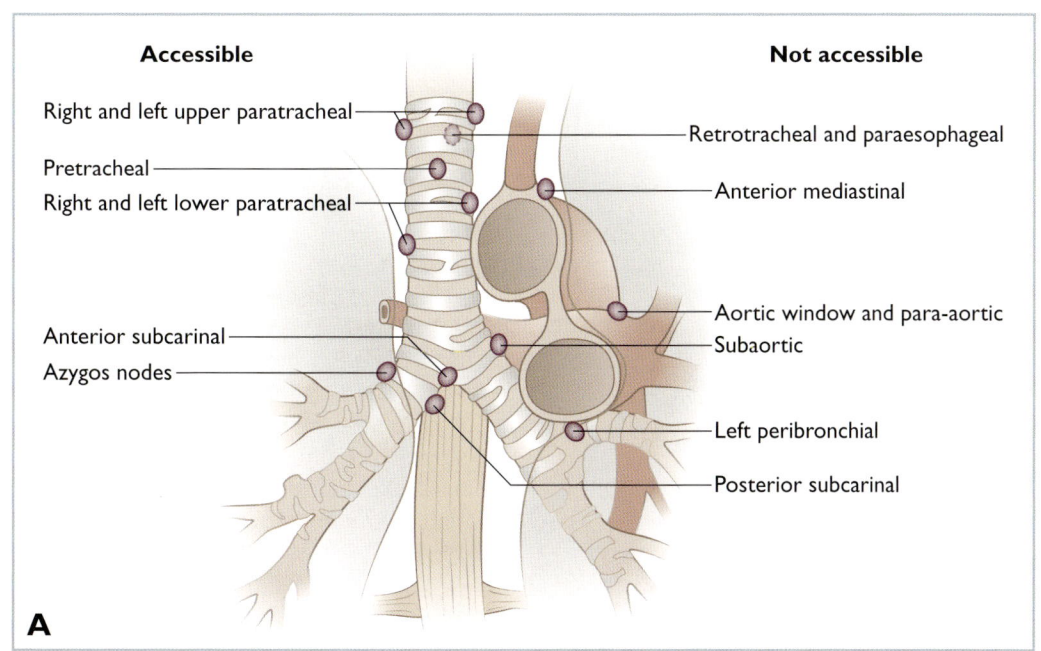

Figure 23-6. A, Accessibility of lymph nodes for biopsy with standard mediastinoscopy. Most of the paratracheal, pretracheal, and anterior subcarinal lymph nodes are accessible through standard cervical mediastinoscopy. Nodes in the anterior or posterior compartments, as well as the hilar, para-aortic, subaortic, and lower left paratracheal regions are not accessible through this procedure. Extended cervical mediastinoscopy or anterior mediastinotomy would be required for tissue biopsy of these areas [6].

Continued on the next page

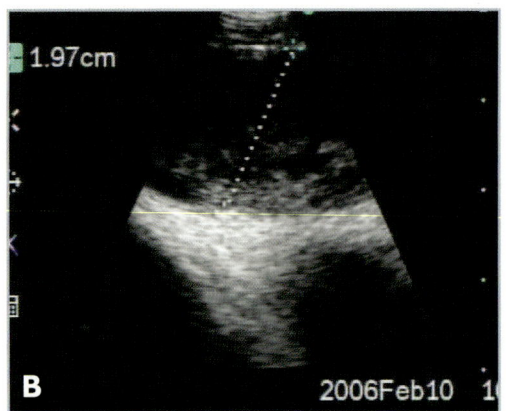

Figure 23-6. *(Continued)* B, Mediastinal lymph nodes can also be aspirated with a transbronchial biopsy needle during bronchoscopy or percutaneously with CT guidance. Endobronchial ultrasound guided transbronchial needle aspiration (EBUS-TBNA) is a recently introduced real-time bronchoscopic biopsy technique that is rapidly gaining widespread acceptance as the minimally invasive procedure of choice for mediastinal lymph node sampling. Lymph node stations that can be accessed by EBUS-TBNA include the highest mediastinal, the upper and lower paratracheal, the subcarinal, the hilar, and the interlobar nodes [7]. A right lower paratracheal lymph node visualized and sampled bronchoscopically with ultrasound guidance is visible in the figure. Endoscopic ultrasound-guided fine-needle aspiration (EUS-FNA) is also a useful adjunct in endoscopy for the diagnosis of mediastinal diseases. EUS imaging is performed from the esophagus, and FNA sampling is performed in real time. The mediastinal lymph node stations that can be accessed by EUS include the subcarinal, the subaortic, the paraesophageal, and the inferior pulmonary ligament [8].

FREQUENCY AND DISTRIBUTION OF MEDIASTINAL MASSES

Compartmental Distribution of Mediastinal Masses

Anterior Compartment	Middle Compartment	Posterior Compartment
Thymic tumors	Metastasis to lymph nodes	Neurogenic tumors
Germ cell tumors	Benign lymphadenopathy	Meningoceles
Thyroid masses	Lymphomas	Thoracic spine neoplasms
Lymphomas	Bronchogenic cysts	Hiatal hernia
Parathyroid masses	Pleuropericardial cysts	Bochdalek hernia
Mesenchymal tumors	Vascular masses	Neurenteric cysts
	Morgagni hernia	Gastroenteric cysts
		Thoracic duct cysts

Figure 23-7. Compartmental distribution of mediastinal masses. A practical classification of mediastinal masses based on the usual location of the mass within a mediastinal compartment is useful. However, tumors may extend across compartmental boundaries or have a wide distribution throughout several compartments, such as is the case with lymphoma. Tumors arising from the heart or esophagus are usually not categorized as mediastinal tumors.

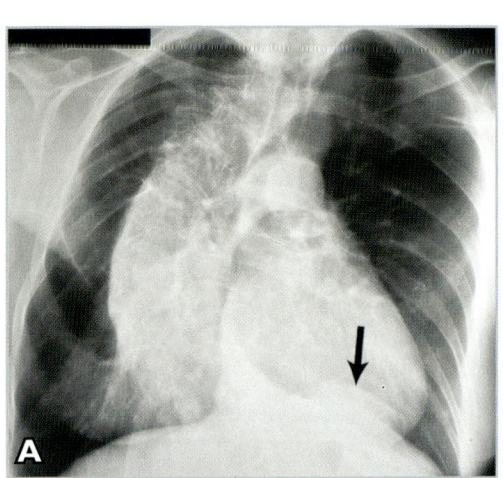
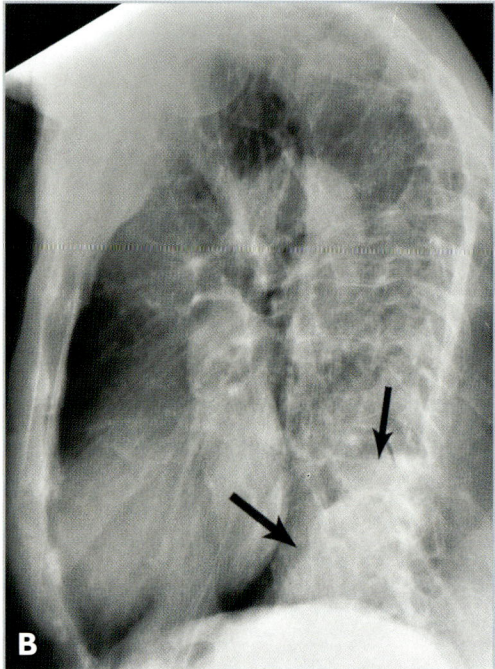

Figure 23-8. Radiographs showing lesions extending into the mediastinum similar to mediastinal tumors. A, Frontal view shows severe scoliosis of the thoracic spine and a retrocardiac density over the left hemidiaphragm (*arrow*). B, On the lateral view, the smooth density that overlies the lower thoracic spine represents a hernia (*arrows*) through the foramen of Bochdalek. Foramen of Morgagni hernias present as a mass on the right side of the cardiophrenic angle [9].

ANTERIOR MEDIASTINAL MASSES

Thymic Tumors

Benign	Malignant
Benign thymoma (encapsulated)	Malignant thymoma (invasive)
Thymic hyperplasia	Thymic carcinoma
Thymolipoma	Thymic carcinoid
Thymic cysts	Small cell carcinoma of the thymus
Benign germ cell tumors of the thymus	Lymphoma of the thymus
	Malignant germ cell tumors of the thymus
	Metastatic neoplasms

Figure 23-9. Thymic tumors. Thymic neoplasms constitute approximately 50% of tumors found in the anterior mediastinal compartment in adults but are rare in children. The primary forms of these tumors originate from normal thymic tissue components: epithelial cells, lymphoid tissue, germ cells, neuroendocrine cells, and adipose tissue. Although atypia is occasionally found in some of the epithelial cells, cytologic characteristics do not differentiate between benign or malignant thymomas. Their classification as malignant or benign depends on the presence or absence of encapsulation and of invasion to adjacent tissue [10]. Most often, malignant thymomas invade locally, but widespread intrathoracic and sometimes transdiaphragmatic invasion can occur.

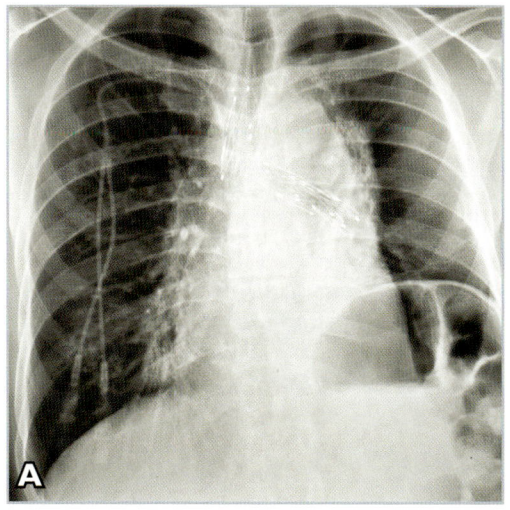
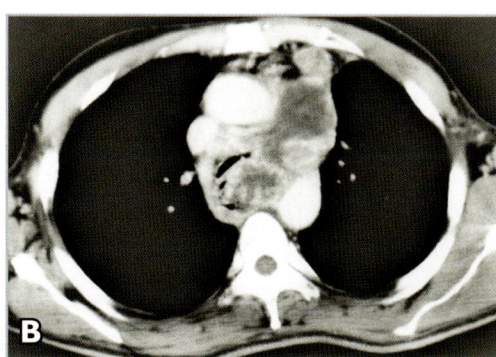

Figure 23-10. Radiographs of thymic carcinoma. **A,** Frontal chest radiograph shows obliteration of the right mediastinal contour and right upper chest by confluent and multilobulated masses. **B,** CT at the level of the aortic arch shows neoplastic invasion of the anterior mediastinal compartment with extension into the chest wall. Histologic examination revealed a thymic carcinoma (lymphoepithelioma-like variant). These rare tumors of the thymus are radiologically and macroscopically indistinguishable from invasive thymomas. They spread locally across lymph nodes of various mediastinal compartments, the pleura, and the pericardium. Extrathoracic metastases are also common. Two main histologic varieties exist: squamous cell and lymphoepithelioma-like carcinomas.

Classification of Germ Cell Tumors

Benign
  Benign teratoma (dermoid cyst)
Malignant
  Seminoma
  Nonseminomatous tumors
    Malignant teratoma
    Choriocarcinoma
    Teratocarcinoma
    Endodermal sinus tumor
    Embryonal carcinoma
    Mixed histologic types

Figure 23-11. Classification of germ cell tumors [11]. Primary mediastinal germ cell tumors account for approximately 10% of all mediastinal tumors. In adult patients, approximately 80% of these tumors are benign. Benign teratomas are slow-growing tumors that are equally distributed among men and women and usually do not produce symptoms. Rarely, they may rupture into the pleural or pericardial space or form bronchial fistulae. Primary malignant mediastinal germ cell tumors occur most frequently in men from 20 to 35 years of age. Pure seminomas are slow growing and are often asymptomatic. Nonseminomatous varieties are more aggressive; most patients have symptoms caused by compression, invasion, or metastatic disease. In addition, several hematologic malignancies are associated with nonseminomatous germ cell tumors [12]. Tissue and serologic markers present in malignant germ cell neoplasms are helpful in differentially diagnosing them from benign teratomas [13].

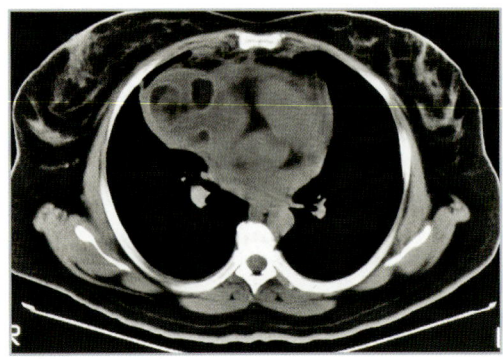

Figure 23-12. CT of a benign teratoma. This CT reveals a well-circumscribed tumor with a partial calcific rim and with heterogenous density contents. Numerous cysts are seen within the mass. These contain various adipose and soft-tissue densities that are characteristic of benign teratoma. Multicystic spaces were lined with various fully differentiated epithelia. Hair, fat, and cartilaginous tissue were present within the cysts. These tumors, also known as dermoids or epidermoid cysts, have an excellent prognosis after complete surgical removal [14].

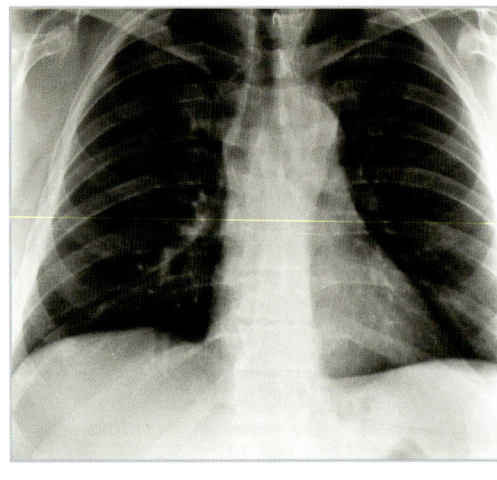

Figure 23-13. Posteroanterior radiograph of the chest of a young man showing widening of the mediastinal borders as a result of seminoma. Although relatively slow growing, seminomas invade adjacent tissues and most often present with symptoms. Unless metastases have occurred, systemic manifestations are rare. Serum human chorionic gonadotropin is elevated in approximately 10% of patients who have primary mediastinal seminomas. Surgical removal is rarely indicated because most seminomas are locally invasive and metastases are present in more than 50% of patients at time of diagnosis. (*From* Morice [15]; with permission.)

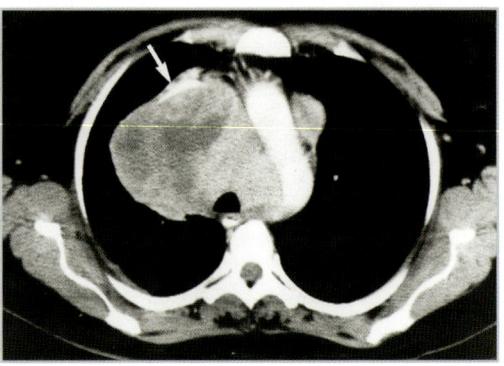

Figure 23-14. CT of a nonseminomatous mediastinal tumor (choriocarcinoma). This image shows a large mass on the right side of the upper thorax. It is located predominantly in the anterior mediastinum, but it encroaches into the middle mediastinum. The mass is partially necrotic and invades the perivascular structures. The superior vena cava (*arrow*) appears distorted and compressed. In comparison to other mediastinal tumors, choriocarcinomas grow very rapidly. These tumors present almost invariably with signs and symptoms of local invasion. More than two thirds of patients present with gynecomastia associated with elevated serum levels of human chorionic gonadotropin [16].

Primary Mediastinal Masses of Mesenchymal Origin

Adipose tissue	Fibrous tissue
Lipoma	Fibroma
Liposarcoma	Fibrosarcoma
Mediastinal lipomatosis	Benign fibrous histiocytoma
Vascular tissue	Malignant fibrous histiocytoma
Hemangioma	Mesodermal tissue
Angiosarcoma	Benign mesenchymoma
Hemangiopericytoma	Malignant mesenchymoma
Lymphangioma	Miscellaneous
Muscle tissue	Osteosarcoma
Leiomyoma	Granulocytic sarcoma
Leiomyosarcoma	Synovial sarcoma
Rhabdomyoma	Pleomorphic adenoma
Rhabdomyosarcoma	

Figure 23-15. Primary mediastinal masses of mesenchymal origin. Such masses are rare—they account for approximately 6% of all mediastinal masses in adults and 10% in children [17]. Because of mesenchymal tissue's broad distribution, tumors derived from it can occur in all mediastinal compartments. Lipomas are the most common of all mesenchymal tumors in the mediastinum and are easily identifiable by their characteristic density on CTs. Primary mediastinal liposarcomas are extremely rare and almost always present with symptoms caused by compression or invasion of neural or bronchovascular structures [18]. Mesenchymal tumors of vascular origin are very rare. Hemangiomas are the most common and comprise less than 0.5% of all mediastinal masses [19]. Rather than being true neoplasms, hemangiomas are developmental vascular proliferations. They present as rounded or lobulated, well-defined densities. Occasionally, phleboliths can be seen within the mass. These can be isolated or multifocal, as in patients with Rendu-Osler-Weber syndrome. Hemangiosarcomas are rare, aggressive tumors with dismal prognosis. Mediastinal lymphangiomas, most often seen in children, represent developmental abnormalities and are sometimes associated with chylothorax [20]. Mediastinal tumors of muscular origin, other than those arising from esophageal smooth muscle, are infrequent. They arise from vascular muscle components or, in cases of rhabdomyosarcomas, can originate from teratomas that undergo single-tissue differentiation. Mediastinal fibrous tumors are most often primaries of pleura and of neural structures with secondary extension into the mediastinum. Few cases of primary mediastinal benign and malignant fibrous histiocytomas have been reported. Tumors of pluripotential mesodermal tissue that occur in the mediastinum are thought to arise from teratomatous differentiation. Other tumors, such as pleomorphic adenoma, originate from the ectopic glandular bronchial epithelium within mediastinal lymph nodes.

MIDDLE MEDIASTINAL MASSES

Mediastinal Lymph Node Enlargement

Benign, Infectious

Granulomatous
  Tuberculosis
  Fungi
Mononucleosis
Reactive lymphadenitis

Benign, Noninfectious

Granulomatous
  Sarcoidosis
  Silicosis
  Hypersensitivity pneumonitis
  Wegener's granulomatosis
  Associated with neoplasms
Angioimmunoblastic lymphadenopathy
Amyloidosis
Drug induced (eg, diphenylhydantoin)
Lymphoid hamartoma
Angiofollicular hyperplasia (eg, Castelman's disease)

Malignant

Primary large cell lymphoma of the mediastinum
Hodgkin's and lymphoblastic lymphomas
Metastasis to mediastinal lymph nodes

Figure 23-16. Mediastinal lymph node enlargement. Lymph node enlargement, which is usually caused by systemic infections, noninfectious inflammatory conditions, and extramediastinal malignancy, is the most common cause of mediastinal abnormality. Although most mediastinal lymph nodes are located in the middle compartment, numerous nodal chains exist throughout the mediastinum. Therefore, conditions that cause lymph node enlargement most often affect several mediastinal compartments simultaneously. Specific diagnosis of mediastinal lymph node abnormalities usually requires tissue or bacteriologic confirmation. However, various patterns in the distribution of the lymphadenopathy may provide clues to help guide the patient work-up based on possible causes. Symmetrical, bilateral hilar lymphadenopathy is a feature of sarcoidosis. Asymmetric hilar distribution with involvement of substernal and cervical nodes is often seen in lymphomas. Granulomatous infections tend to cause a more focal and unilateral distribution.

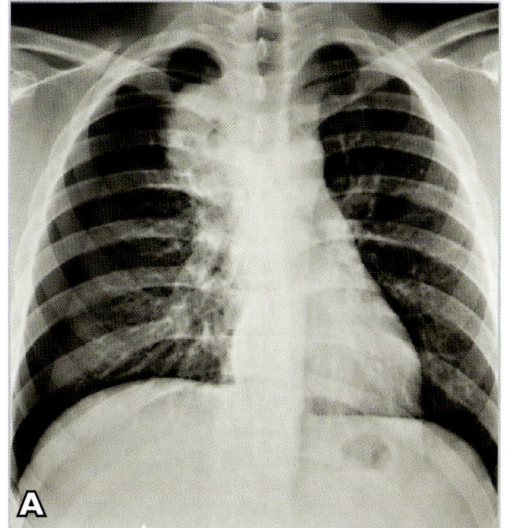

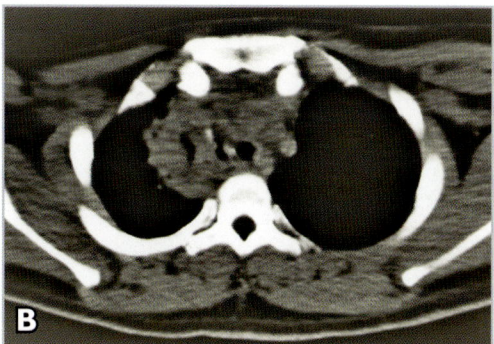

Figure 23-17. Wegener's granulomatosis presenting as a mediastinal mass. **A,** Frontal chest radiograph shows widening of upper mediastinal profile by a right paratracheal mass that extends down to the azygous area. The trachea appears compressed and deviated to the left. There is a right pneumothorax after needle biopsy of the mass. **B,** CT confirms the presence of a solid mass with obliteration of soft-tissue planes of trachea and vascular structures. The main diagnostic categories considered in this case of a man 21 years of age, who had a history of fever, weight loss, and mild hemoptysis, included lymphoma and granulomatous infections. Bronchoscopic examination in this patient showed extensive tracheal and right main-stem bronchial narrowing with mucosal infiltration and partial necrosis. The diagnosis of "limited" Wegener's granulomatosis was made by tissue analysis obtained via mediastinoscopy and corroborated by the presence of positive serology tests for antineutrophil cytoplasmic autoantibodies [21].

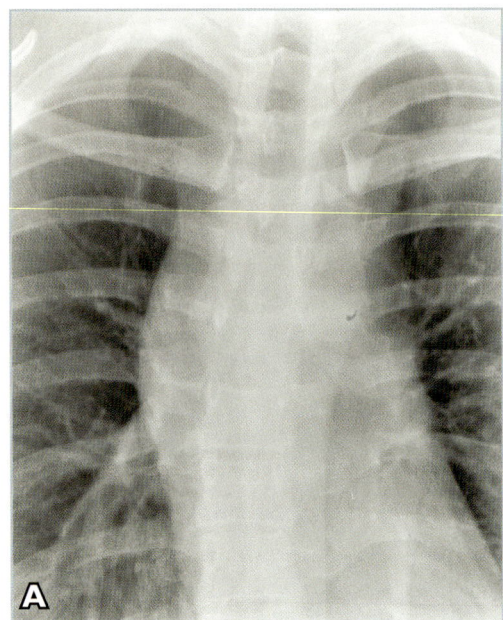 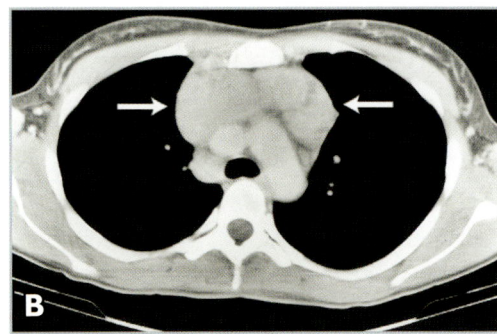

Figure 23-18. Nodular sclerosing Hodgkin's lymphoma. **A,** Frontal radiograph shows a large mediastinal mass protruding on both sides of the mediastinal borders. **B,** CT reveals several confluent, lobulated, solid masses that fill the anterior mediastinal space entirely and wrap around the middle mediastinal vascular structures (*arrows*). Lymphomas constitute approximately 20% of all mediastinal neoplasms in adults [22]. Most lymphomas that occur in the mediastinum also appear in extra-thoracic sites. However, three lymphoma types are known for their preferential mediastinal location: Hodgkin's disease, lymphoblastic lymphoma [23], and large cell lymphoma [24]. Of these, the nodular sclerosing form of Hodgkin's disease is by far the most common of the mediastinal lymphomas. Constitutional symptoms, rather than local compressive manifestations, are usually observed with mediastinal Hodgkin's disease. The other two non-Hodgkin's varieties—lymphoblastic lymphoma and large cell lymphoma—are more aggressive, usually cause compressive symptoms, and have a worse prognosis [25].

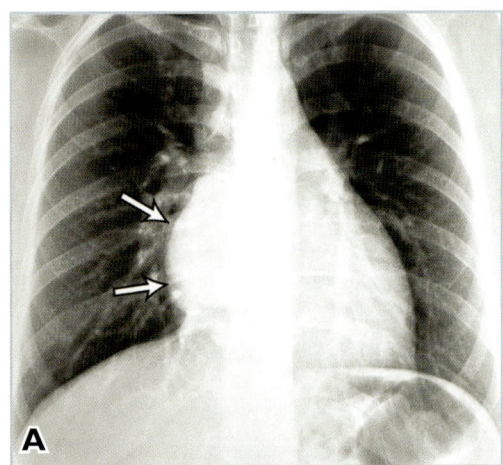 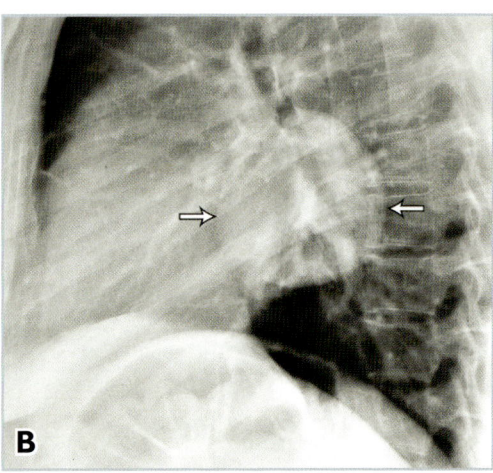

Figure 23-19. Mediastinal bronchogenic cyst. **A,** Posteroanterior chest radiograph discloses a homogeneous, infracarinal, soft-tissue mass superimposed on the cardiac shadow (*arrows*). **B,** The lateral radiograph identifies a round, sharply defined mass in the retrocardiac area (*arrows*). These radiologic features are characteristic of bronchogenic cysts. These cysts are congenital and are often detected during childhood or adolescence. Compressive airway manifestations occur particularly in infants: more than 50% of them are asymptomatic. Some may remain undiagnosed into adulthood. Occasionally, fistula formation and drainage of the cystic contents into the bronchial tree can occur. Development of fever, pain, and change in the size of the cyst are indications of infection or intracystic bleeding. Nearly two thirds of bronchogenic cysts are located near the main carina. Less often, they may be associated with a lobar or segmental bronchus and have an intrapulmonary rather than mediastinal location [26].

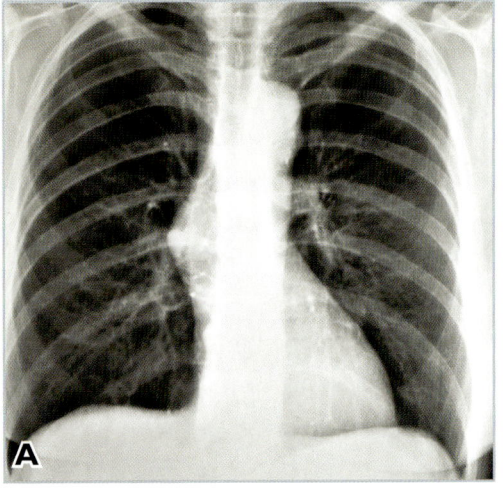 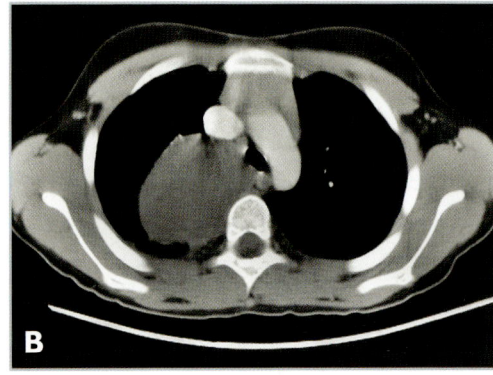

Figure 23-20. Aneurysm of the ascending aorta. **A,** Posteroanterior radiograph of an asymptomatic woman aged 63 years shows a smooth, abnormal density that overlaps the right hilar area. **B,** CT confirms a fusiform aneurysm of the ascending aorta with dense calcification of its wall. Aortic aneurysms are the most common cause of mediastinal vascular masses. They can have multiple causes, but most are atherosclerotic. Among various other causes, aortic aneurysms can be related to Marfan syndrome, trauma, mycotic infection, rheumatic aortitis, and syphilis. Sixty percent of thoracic aortic aneurysms affect the descending aorta; the rest affect the ascending portion and transverse arch.

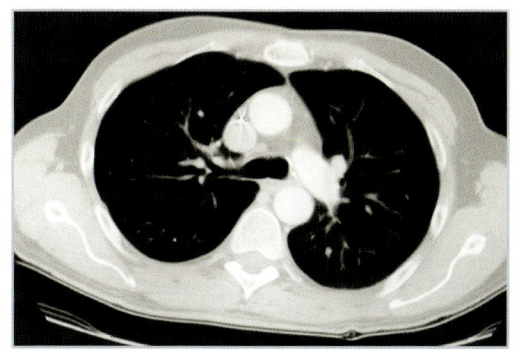

Figure 23-21. CT showing the presence of two aortic arches surrounding the trachea. In most cases, this form of congenital malformation becomes evident in childhood [27]. Dyspnea, occasionally confused with asthma, can occur when the trachea is significantly compressed. Other forms of congenital abnormalities of the thoracic aorta include right aortic arch, aortic diverticula, cervical aortic arch, and pseudocoarctation of the aorta.

POSTERIOR MEDIASTINAL MASSES

Classification of Neurogenic Mediastinal Tumors

Nerve Sheath Origin	Autonomic Ganglia Origin	Paraganglionic Origin
Benign	**Benign**	**Benign**
Neurofibroma	Ganglioneuroma	Pheochromocytoma
Neurilemoma	**Malignant**	Benign paraganglioma
(benign schwannoma)	Ganglioneuroblastoma	(chemodectoma)
Granular cell tumor	Neuroblastoma	**Malignant**
Melanotic schwannoma		Malignant pheochromocytoma
Malignant		Malignant paraganglioma
Malignant schwannoma		(chemodectoma)
(neurogenic sarcoma)		

Figure 23-22. Classification of neurogenic mediastinal tumors. Neurogenic tumors of the mediastinum account for approximately 20% of all mediastinal tumors in adults and 40% in children. The clinical presentation and prognosis of these tumors varies with the age of the population. In children, most derive from autonomic ganglia, more than 50% are malignant, and most cause compressive or invasive manifestations. In adults, most are of nerve sheath origin and are benign and asymptomatic. Tumors of nerve sheath origin present as paraspinal masses [28]. Of these, neurilemomas present as solitary and well-encapsulated tumors. Occasionally, they can degenerate into malignant schwannomas [29]. Neurofibromas are most often multiple and are typically seen in patients with von Recklinghausen's disease. Neoplasms derived from autonomic ganglia represent a continuum of various levels of differentiation. These range from the benign and mature ganglioneuroma to the malignant and most anaplastic neuroblastoma. In addition to local compressive or invasive manifestations, these tumors can secrete a variety of hormones that result in gastrointestinal and vasoactive systemic syndromes. Paraganglionic tumors can occur in all mediastinal compartments. They can be catecholamine-secreting pheochromocytomas or nonfunctioning paragangliomas. In addition to catecholamines, some paraganglionic tumors can secrete a variety of substances, such as vasoactive intestinal peptide and parathyroid-like and corticotrophin hormones [30].

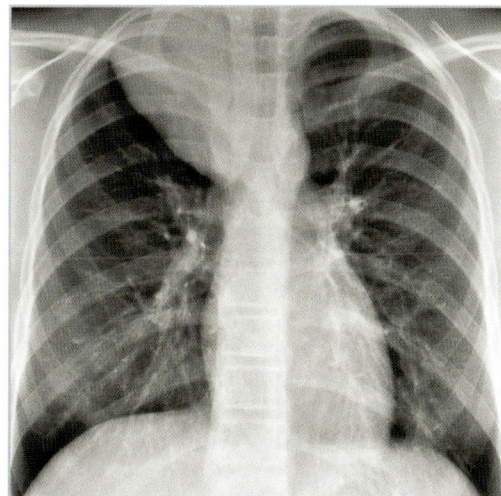

Figure 23-23. Radiograph of a ganglioneuroma. This frontal radiograph shows a well-demarcated opacity that occupies the right upper paramediastinal area and the apical lung field. These tumors are primarily found in young children. They are most often large and of paravertebral location. In contrast to tumors of nerve sheath origin, foraminal intraspinal extension is rare.

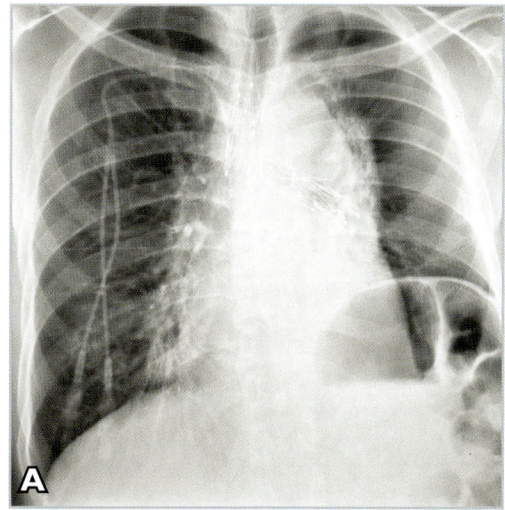
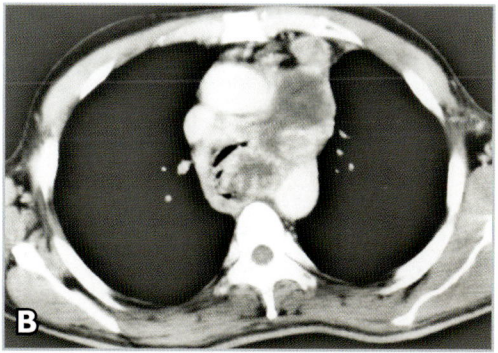

Figure 23-24. Malignant paraganglioma. Paragangliomas or chemodectomas originate from chemoreceptor-autonomic tissue. Thus, most arise from and are located in the ascending or transverse portion of the aortic arch, where normal chemoreceptor aortic bodies are usually found [31]. **A,** Frontal radiograph shows an ill-defined mass that obliterates the aortopulmonary window and left hilum. The left hemidiaphragm is elevated because of paralysis, which indicates neoplastic phrenic nerve invasion. Endoluminal stents have been placed in the trachea and right main stem bronchus. **B,** CT shows an extensive, necrotic mass at the level of the aortic arch with extension throughout all mediastinal spaces at this level. The tracheal lumen is severely reduced and displaced.

REFERENCES

1. Williams HJ, Alton HM: Imaging of pediatric mediastinal abnormalities. *Paediatr Respir Rev* 2003, 4:55–66.

2. Laurent F, Latrabe V, Lecesne R, *et al.*: Mediastinal masses: diagnostic approach. *Eur Radiol* 1998, 8:1148–1159.

3. Erasmus JJ, McAdams HP, Donnelly LF, *et al.*: MR imaging of mediastinal masses. *Magn Reson Imaging Clin N Am* 2000, 8:59–89.

4. Marckmann P, Skov L, Rossen K, *et al.*: Nephrogenic systemic fibrosis: suspected causative role of gadodiamide used for contrast-enhanced magnetic resonance imaging. *J Am Soc Nephrol* 2006, 17(9):2359–2362.

5. Kostakoglu L, Agress H, Goldsmith SJ: Clinical role of FDG PET in evaluation of cancer patients. *Radiographics* 2003, 23:315–340.

6. LeBlanc JK, Espada R, Ergun G: Non-small-cell lung cancer staging techniques and endoscopic ultrasound. *Chest* 2003, 123:1718–1725.

7. Yasufuku K, Chiyo M, Koh E, *et al.*: Endobronchial ultrasound guided transbronchial needle aspiration for staging of lung cancer. *Lung Cancer* 2005, 50(3):347–354.

8. Fritscher-Ravens A, Soehendra N, Schirrow L, *et al.*: Role of transesophageal endosonography-guided fine-needle aspiration in the diagnosis of lung cancer. *Chest* 2000, 117:339–345.

9. Mouroux J, Venissac N, Alifano M, Padovani B: Morgagni hernia and thoracic deformities. *Thorac Cardiovasc Surg* 2003, 51:44–45.

10. Truong MT, Sabloff BS, Gladish GW, *et al.*: Invasive thymoma. *Am J Roentgenol* 2003, 181:1504.

11. International Germ Cell Cancer Collaborative Group: International Germ Cell Consensus Classification: a prognostic factor-based staging system for metastatic germ cell cancers. *J Clin Oncol* 1997, 15:594–603.

12. Wood DE: Mediastinal germ cell tumors. *Semin Thorac Cardiovasc Surg* 2000, 12:278–289.

13. Collins KA, Geisinger KR, Wakely PR Jr, *et al.*: Extragonadal germ cell tumors: a fine needle aspiration biopsy study. *Diagn Cytopathol* 1995, 12:223–229.

14. Moran CA, Suster S: Primary germ cell tumors of the mediastinum: I. Analysis of 322 cases with special emphasis on teratomatous lesions and a proposal for histopathologic classification and clinical staging. *Cancer* 1997, 80:681–690.

15. Morice RC: Mediastinal disease. In *Pulmonary and Critical Care Medicine*, edn 3 (vol II). Edited by Bone RC. St Louis: Mosby-Year Book; 1995:1–25.

16. Schwabe J, Calaminus G, Varhoff W: Sexual precocity and recurrent beta-human chorionic gonadotropin upsurges preceding the diagnosis of a malignant mediastinal germ-cell tumor in a 9-year-old boy. *Ann Oncol* 2002, 13:973–977.

17. Strollo DC, Rosado de Christenson ML, Jett JR: Primary mediastinal tumors: part 1, tumors of the anterior mediastinum. *Chest* 1997, 112:511–522.

18. Gladish G, Sabloff BM, Munden RF, *et al.*: Primary thoracic sarcomas. *Radiographics* 2002, 22:631–637.

19. Moran CA, Suster S: Mediastinal hemangiomas: a study of 18 cases with emphasis on the spectrum of morphological features. *Hum Pathol* 1995, 26:416–421.

20. Lee KH, Song KS, Kwon Y, *et al.*: Mesenchymal tumours of the thorax: CT findings and pathological features. *Clin Radiol* 2003, 58:934–944.

21. Jennette JC, Falk RJ: Small-vessel vasculitis. *N Engl J Med* 1997, 337:1512–1523.

22. Grosfeld JL, Skinner MA, Rescorla FJ, *et al.*: Mediastinal tumors in children: experience with 196 cases. *Ann Surg Oncol* 1994, 1:121–127.

23. Shepherd SF, A'Hern RP, Pinkerton CR: Childhood T-cell lymphoblastic lymphoma: does early resolution of mediastinal mass predict for final outcome? The United Kingdom Children's Cancer Study Group (UKCCSG). *Br J Cancer* 1995, 72:752–756.

24. Aisenberg AC: Primary large cell lymphoma of the mediastinum. *Semin Oncol* 1999, 26:251–258.

25. Rodriguez J, Pugh WC, Romaguera JE, Cabanillas F: Primary mediastinal large cell lymphoma. *Hematol Oncol* 1994, 12:175–184.

26. Jeung M, Gasser B, Gangi A, *et al.*: Imaging of cystic masses of the mediastinum. *Radiographics* 2002, 22:S79–S93.

27. Goo HW, Park IS, Ko JK, *et al.*: CT of congenital heart disease: normal anatomy and typical pathologic conditions. *Radiographics* 2003, 23:S147–S165.

28. Marchevsky AM: Mediastinal tumors of peripheral nervous system origin. *Semin Diagn Pathol* 1999, 16:65–78.

29. Fukai I, Masaoka A, Yamakawa Y, *et al.*: Mediastinal malignant epithelioid schwannoma. *Chest* 1995, 108:574–575.

30. Trump DL, Livingston JL, Baylin SB: Watery diarrhea syndrome in an adult with ganglioneuroma-pheochromocytoma. *Cancer* 1977, 40:1526–1532.

31. Nwose P, Galbis JM, Okafor O, Torre W: Mediastinal paraganglioma: a case report. *Thorac Cardiovasc Surg* 1998, 46:376–379.

METASTASES TO THE LUNGS

Carlos A. Jimenez, Georgie A. Eapen, and Rodolfo C. Morice

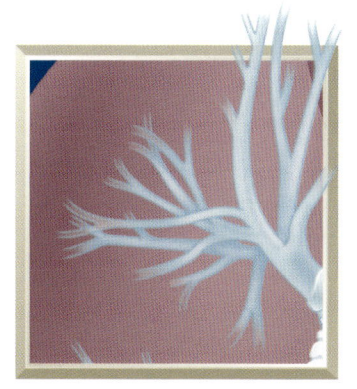
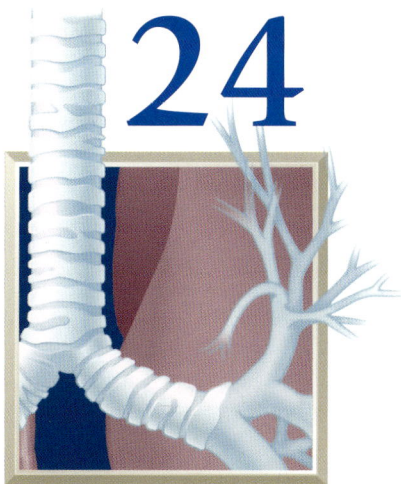
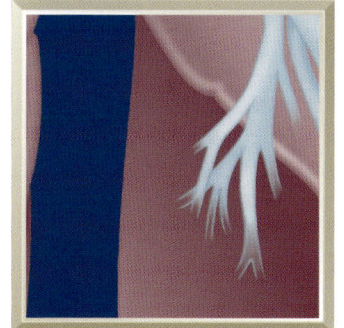

It has been suggested that there are six essential acquired capabilities in cell physiology that collectively dictate malignant growth in most, if not all, human tumors: self-sufficiency in growth signals, insensitivity to growth-inhibitory signals, evasion of program cell death, limitless replicative potential, sustained angiogenesis, and tissue invasion and metastasis [1]. Secondary neoplastic involvement of the lungs is clinically important because of its prognostic implications and common occurrence. As a group, pulmonary metastases represent the most common form of pulmonary malignancies. Lung metastases are diagnosed in 30% to 40% of all patients with cancer [2]. Most patients lack significant respiratory symptoms at the time of initial presentation; the diagnosis is often made by abnormal findings on radiologic studies of the chest. The primary site is often clinically apparent before symptoms of pulmonary involvement develop. Clinical manifestations such as dyspnea and cough are ominous signs of advanced disease. Wheezing, hemoptysis, hoarseness, and respiratory distress may also occur because of malignant invasion of the tracheobronchial tree, mediastinal structures, or pleura. Despite the overall grave prognosis, surgical resection of pulmonary metastases and newer chemotherapy regimens have led to improved outcomes in selected patients.

Extrapulmonary tumors may reach the lungs by several routes: hematogenous, lymphogenous, direct invasion, and endobronchial dissemination. Of these, metastatic spread through the pulmonary or bronchial arteries is the most common. Retrograde extension into lymphatic channels from pulmonary and hilar lymph nodes can occur, but this presentation is most commonly the result of lymphatic penetration from hematogenous peripheral tumor implants. A combination of several mechanisms of tumor spread may also occur in a patient. The location of the primary tumor, access to the vascular system, and tumor and local tissue factors are important determinants for the development and progression of pulmonary metastases.

PATTERNS OF METASTASES

Common Patterns of Pulmonary Metastases					
Micronodular	**Coarse Nodules**	**Cannonball**	**Lymphatic–Interstitial**	**Tumor Emboli**	**Tracheobronchial**
Thyroid	Head and neck	Sarcomas	Breast	Hepatoma	Renal
Renal	Gastric	Germ cell	Stomach	Renal	Thyroid
Choriocarcinoma	Gynecological	Renal	Pancreas	Choriocarcinoma	Melanoma
Breast	Lymphoma	Colorectal	Prostate	Gastric	Colorectal
Bone sarcomas	Choriocarcinoma	Melanoma	Lymphoma	Atrial myxoma	Breast

Figure 24-1. Common patterns of pulmonary metastases. Any neoplasm can invade the lungs, but some tumors have a particular predilection for pulmonary dissemination. Various appearances of pulmonary metastases on the chest radiograph may offer clues as to the origin of the primary neoplasm [3]. The primary neoplasms listed in this table are ranked based on their likelihood to produce a particular configuration of pulmonary metastases.

PULMONARY NODULES

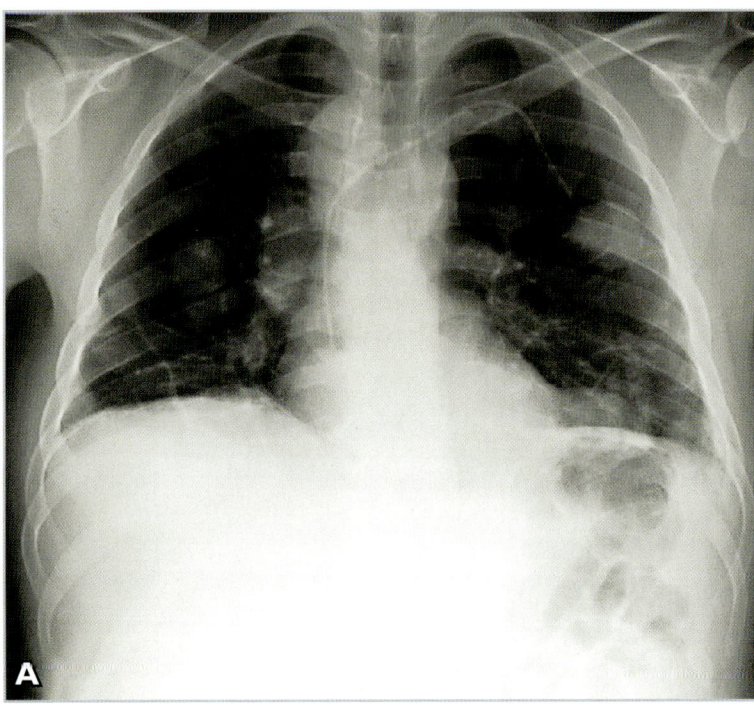
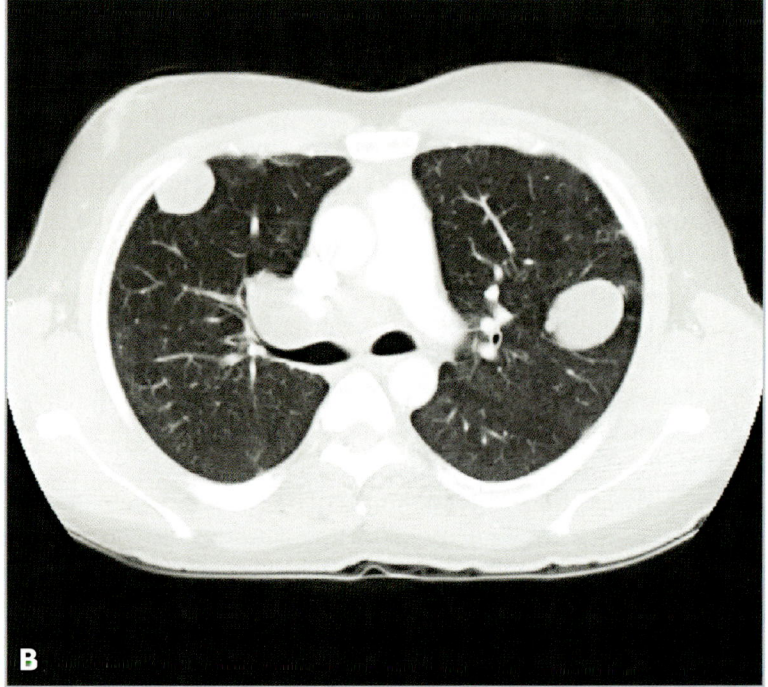

Figure 24-2. Pulmonary nodules. Most commonly, pulmonary metastases present as multiple pulmonary nodules. The pattern of nodules ranges from diffuse micronodular (miliary) to large, well-defined single or multiple masses ("cannonballs"). The uniformity and small size of the pulmonary nodules suggest a simultaneous dissemination from a highly vascular tumor. Irregular size of nodular metastases indicates sequential embolic inoculations and different growth patterns. Nodules are preferentially located in the periphery and lower lung regions corresponding to zones of higher pulmonary blood flow. Characteristically, these nodules are smooth and well circumscribed. Both hemorrhage in the periphery of the nodule and posttreatment changes may induce irregular margins. Calcification within the nodules can occur and should not be misinterpreted as a manifestation of benign disease. This calcification can be found after chemotherapy or irradiation of tumors and in metastases from sarcomas of bone, cartilage, and synovial tissues. Calcium deposits can also occur in adenocarcinomas from the ovaries, thyroid, breasts, and gastrointestinal tract. CT is the preferred method for evaluation of pulmonary metastases. High-resolution scanners are sensitive and can detect nodules as small as 1 to 2 mm in diameter. Posteroanterior (**A**) and CT roentgenograms (**B**) of a patient with a metastatic germ cell tumor reveal multiple nodules of homogenous density ranging in size from 5 mm to 3 cm, distributed throughout both lungs. These lesions predominate in the bases and mid-lung zones. Hilar and mediastinal lymphadenopathy are also present.

Continued on the next page

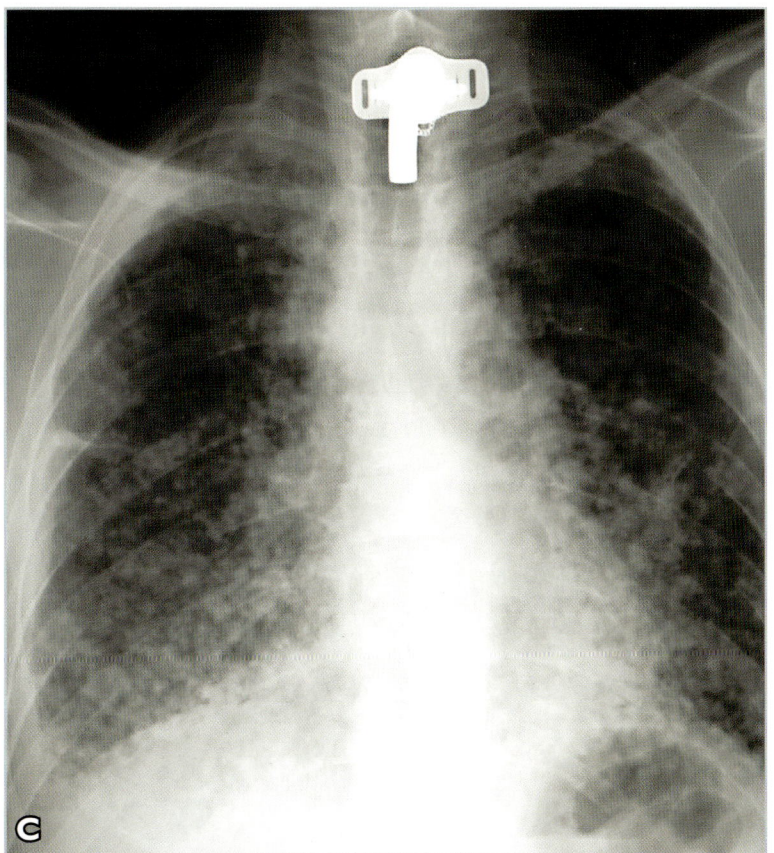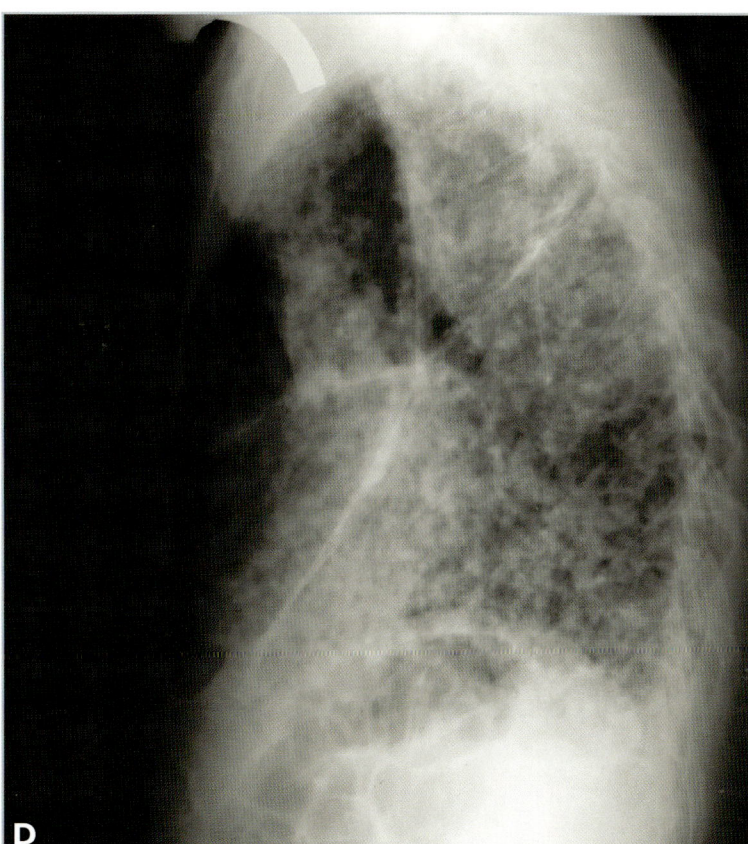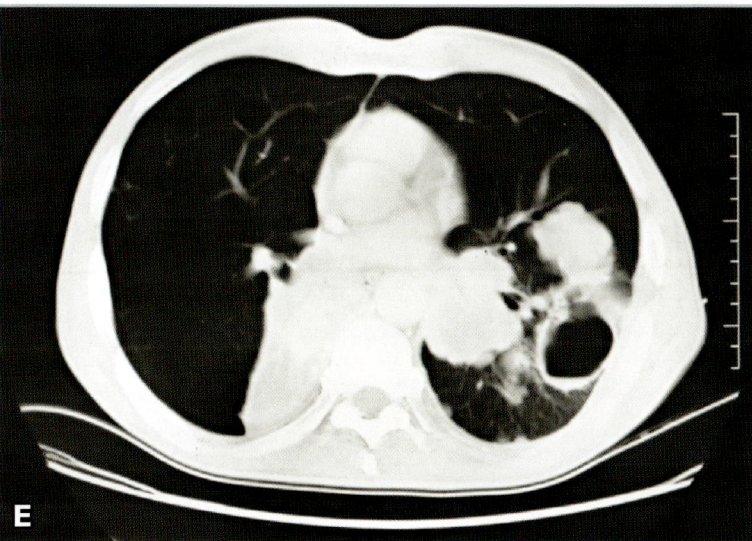

Figure 24-2. *(Continued)* Posteroanterior (**C**) and lateral roentgenogram (**D**) of a 42-year-old man reveal widespread micronodular metastases from a papillary thyroid carcinoma. In some areas, the small nodules are well circumscribed. In other areas, they become coalescent and less defined. This pattern has been described as "snowstorm." Note the presence of a metal tracheostomy cannula after radical neck surgery and a right pleural effusion. A CT through the upper thorax (**E**) shows large nodules from a metastatic adenoid cystic carcinoma of the parotid gland. One of the nodules is cavitated. Intranodular cavitation is most common in metastatic sarcomas and squamous cell carcinomas of the head and neck.

LYMPHATIC/INTERSTITIAL INFILTRATES

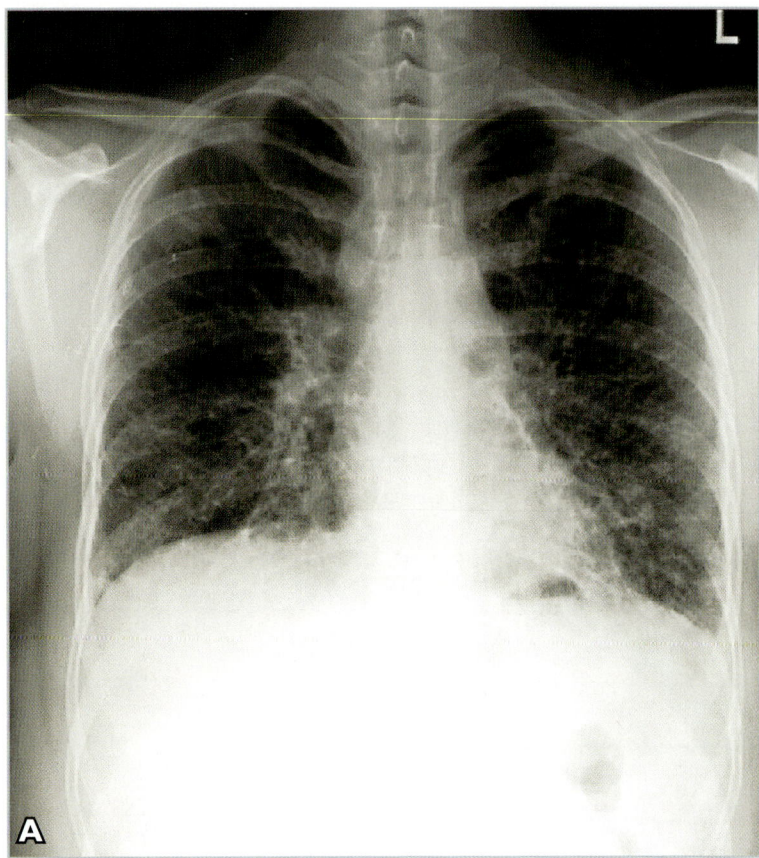
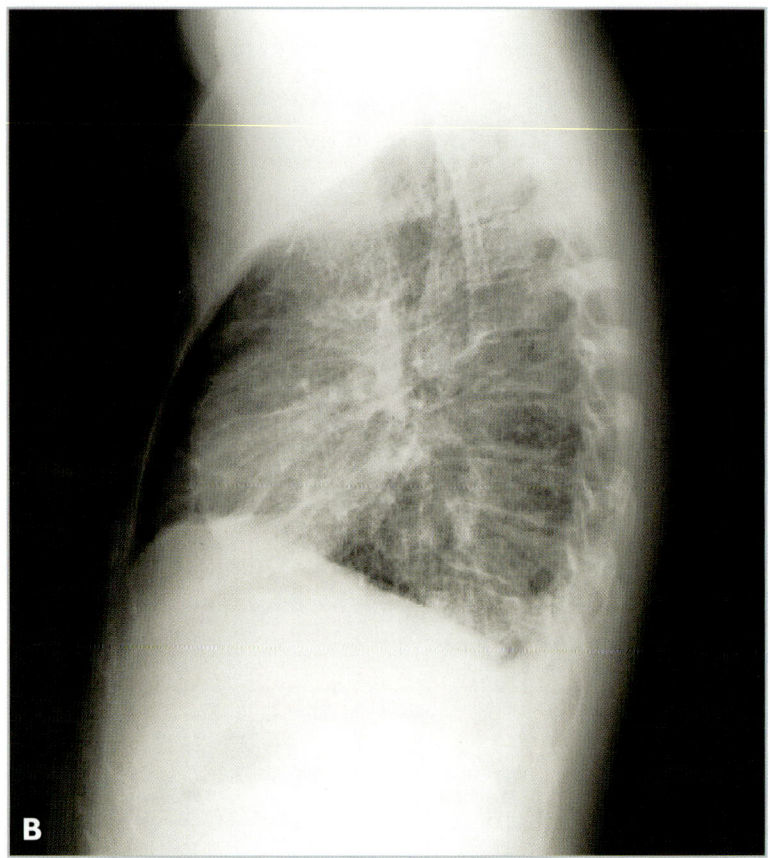

Figure 24-3. Lymphatic or interstitial patterns. Lymphatic or interstitial patterns are rarely caused by pure lymphatic invasion. Instead, they are mostly caused by fibroblastic reactions to the tumor in the perivascular and interlobular interstitium. Roentgenographically, a lymphatic or interstitial pattern presents as an accentuation of interstitial markings, an appearance of peripheral septal lines (Kerley B lines), and a thickening of interlobar fissures. These findings are more pronounced at the lung bases. Micronodular tumor extension can coexist with lymphatic infiltration. This combination results in a reticulonodular pattern on the chest radiograph. Loss of pulmonary compliance associated with malignant interstitial infiltration is evident by a generalized reduction in lung volumes. Pleural effusion and mediastinal adenopathy are frequently present in association with a lymphatic pattern of pulmonary metastases. The most common clinical manifestation of lymphangitic metastases is dyspnea of gradual onset. In some cases, cough and wheezing suggestive of airway disease may be the prominent symptoms. Posteroanterior (**A**) and lateral (**B**) chest roentgenograms reveal a bilateral, coarse linear, and reticular interstitial pattern. Well-formed Kerley B lines are also evident. There is bilateral enlargement of hilar lymph nodes. This 27-year-old woman with invasive ductal carcinoma of the breast had been treated with a modified radical right mastectomy and a prophylactic simple left mastectomy. She had also received combined chemoradiation therapy. At the time the chest roentgenograms were obtained, the patient complained of a 1-month history of progressive dyspnea. Lymphatic spread of adenocarcinoma was confirmed by transbronchial lung biopsies.

TRACHEOBRONCHIAL METASTASES

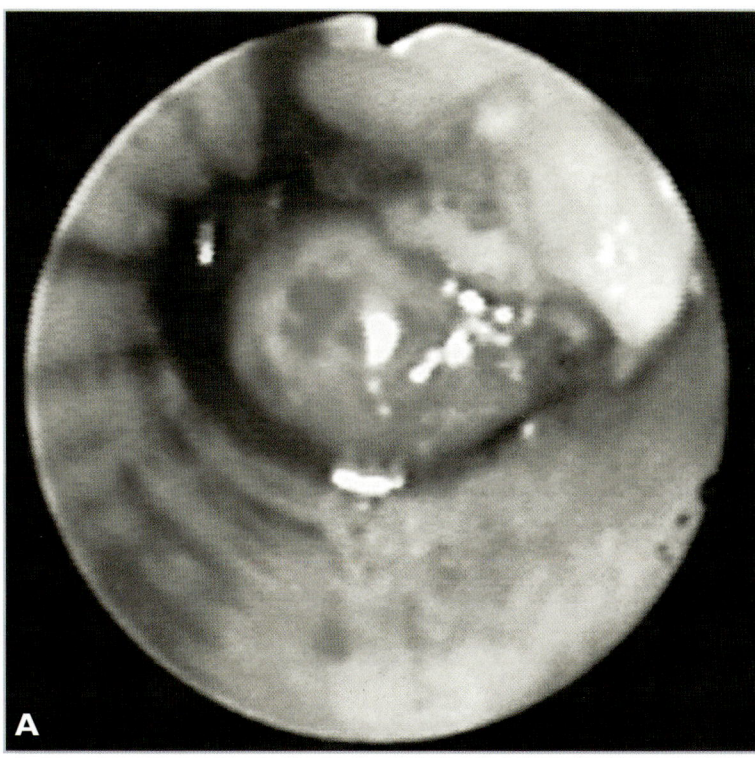

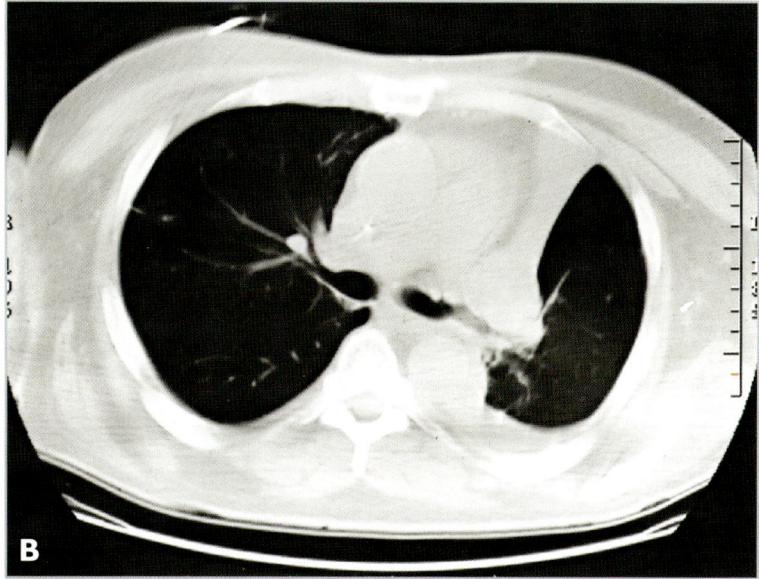

Figure 24-4. Endobronchial malignant invasion. Metastatic malignant invasion of the tracheal or bronchial wall is often the result of contiguous penetration from adjacent metastases to mediastinal lymph nodes or from submucosal lymphatic infiltration. Occasionally, tracheobronchial metastases can occur as isolated forms of endoluminal airway invasion in the absence of demonstrable pulmonary or mediastinal involvement. **A,** Bronchoscopic image of the left mainstem bronchus. This shows a friable, fungating mass that originates from the left upper lobe and extends into the left mainstem bronchus. This 59-year-old man with metastatic renal adenocarcinoma presented with dyspnea and hemoptysis. **B,** CT of the left hilar area shows a very large mass with endobronchial extension, causing left upper lobe atelectasis.

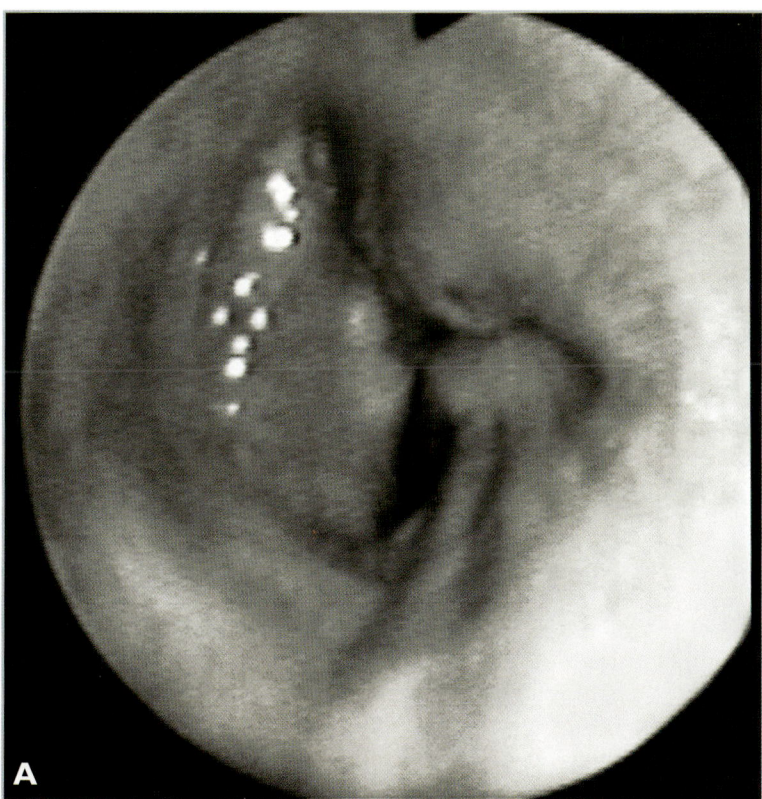

Figure 24-5. A, Endobronchial photograph of the right bronchus intermedius of a 64-year-old woman with metastatic choriocarcinoma. Bronchoscopic findings indicate concentric submucosal and endobronchial malignant infiltration of the right bronchus intermedius and right middle lobe.

Continued on the next page

| *Metastases to the Lungs* |
315

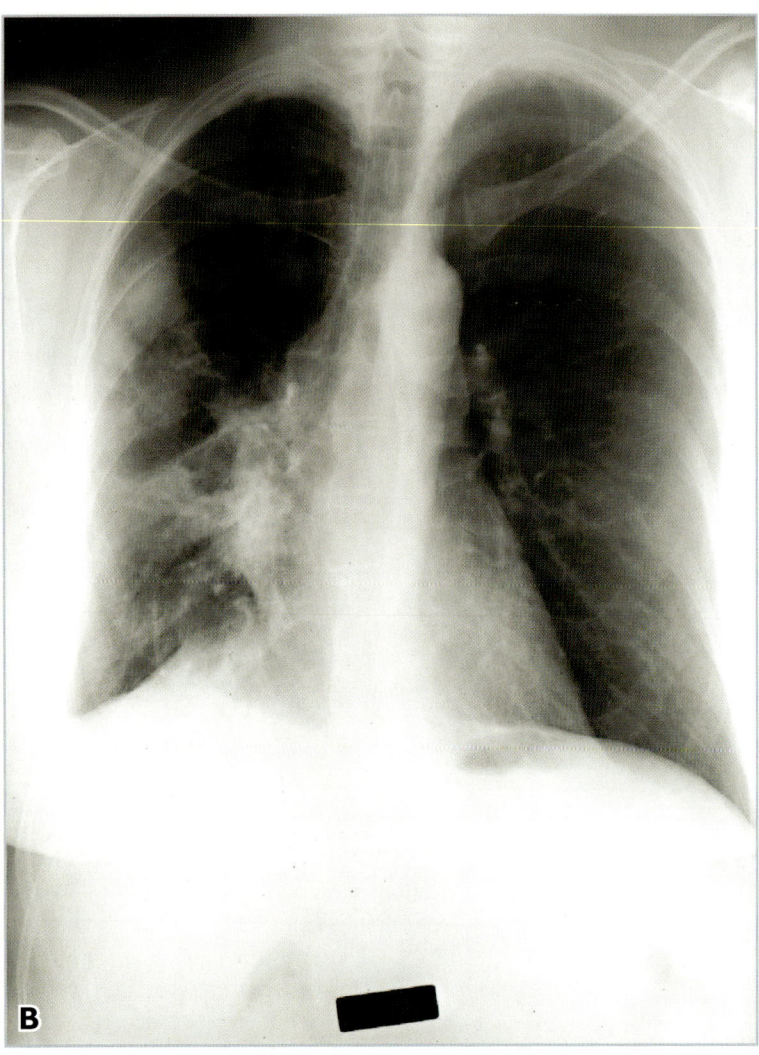

Figure 24-5. *(Continued)* **B,** Posteroanterior roentgenogram reveals middle lobe collapse and a right hilar mass. There are also adjacent parenchymal nodular densities caused by focal pulmonary metastases.

TUMOR EMBOLI

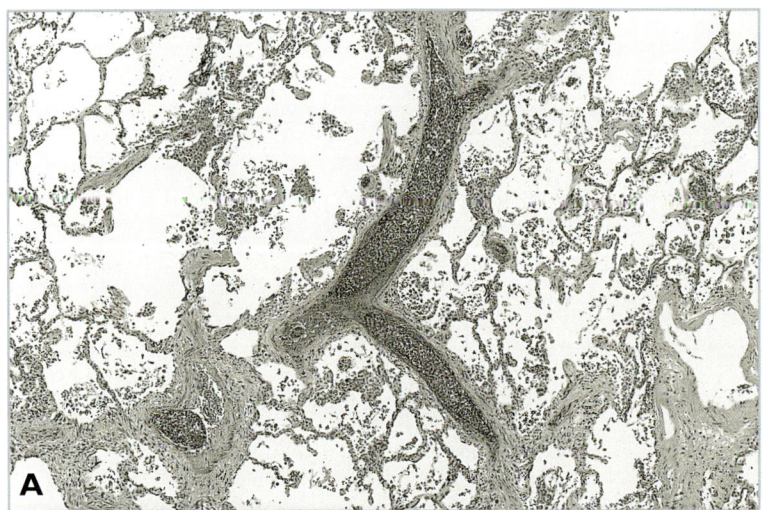
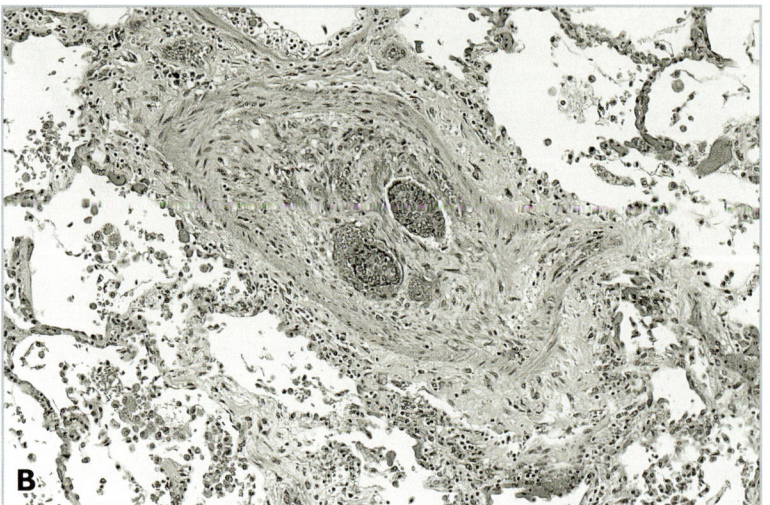

Figure 24-6. Tumor emboli. Tumor emboli are common autopsy findings in patients with malignancies. Symptoms from this form of dissemination are usually absent. When present, clinical manifestations are similar to other forms of pulmonary thromboembolism: acute onset of dyspnea, hypoxemia, and cor pulmonale. In most cases, these tumors affect arterioles and small arteries. Tumor cells usually do not invade the vessel walls, but intimal fibrosis is often present. Occasionally, tumor emboli originating from primary neoplasms that invade the inferior vena cava, such as renal carcinomas and hepatomas, may be large. These can cause occlusion of the main pulmonary artery or its segmental branches, resulting in sudden death. **A,** Low-power photomicrograph of an autopsy specimen from a patient with salivary gland carcinoma. Small arterial branches contain aggregates of metastatic carcinoma. **B,** Higher-power microscopy of the same specimen. There is a complete occlusion of a small artery caused by plugs of carcinoma surrounded by organizing thrombus and intimal proliferation.

TREATMENT AND PROGNOSIS OF PULMONARY METASTASES

Selection of Patients for Resection of Pulmonary Metastases

- Primary tumor is under control
- Metastases can be completely resected
- Absence of extrapulmonary metastases, or if present, ability to also be completely resected
- Adequate pulmonary function to allow resection
- Effective systemic therapy is not available or has already been given prior to resection

Figure 24-7. Selection of patients for resection of pulmonary metastases. Most pulmonary metastases in adults cannot be cured. With appropriate selection, surgical resection of lung metastases can lead to prolonged survival and quality of life [4]. Metastasectomy with curative intent is an option in some types of cancers, such as germ cell tumors, neuroblastoma, and gestational trophoblastic neoplasms. Surgical resection is indicated when residual disease is present in the lung after systemic chemotherapy.

Factors Associated with Improved Outcome after Pulmonary Metastasectomy

- Complete resection
- Unilateral involvement
- Single metastasis
- Smaller size of metastasis
- Longer disease-free interval
- Longer tumor doubling time
- Absence of lymph node involvement
- Asymptomatic
- Type of tumor
- No recurrence after metastasectomy

Figure 24-8. Factors associated with improved outcome after pulmonary metastasectomy. Complete resection of the entire tumor is the most important factor associated with long-term survival after metastasectomy. Other factors, listed in this figure, have shown variable significance as prognostic indicators. Patients with germ cell tumors have the best overall survival rate: 68% at 5 years and 63% at 10 years [5]. Disease-free interval refers to the time from the resection of the primary tumor to the time of diagnosis of lung metastases. Patients without mediastinal nodal involvement at the time of pulmonary metastasectomy have longer median survival [6]. Surgical approaches attempt to remove all disease with maximal preservation of viable lung parenchyma. Metastases are most often located in the periphery and can be excised with mechanical stapling, laser, or electrocautery. Bilateral metastases can be approached by median sternotomy, staged thoracotomies, or bilateral thoracosternotomy ("clamshell" incision). The role of video-assisted thoracoscopy (VATS) for treatment of metastatic disease has not been fully defined. Inability to palpate the lung during VATS may result in incomplete resection [7].

Management of Tracheobronchial Metastases

Indications	Therapies
Dyspnea related to tracheobronchial malignancy, not to systemic disease	Laser
Tracheobronchial obstruction with functional lung distal to obstruction or postobstructive pneumonia	Argon plasma coagulation
Hemoptysis	Electrocautery
Intractable cough	Stents
	Brachytherapy
	Balloon or mechanical dilation
	Photodynamic therapy
	Cryotherapy
	Gene therapy

Figure 24-9. Management of tracheobronchial metastases. Neoplastic airway invasion is common among patients with metastatic malignancies. These patients may have symptoms related to tracheobronchial tumor extension, such as dyspnea, bleeding, intractable cough, and postobstructive pneumonia. In selected cases, bronchoscopic interventions can prevent imminent death, offer clinical stability that will allow additional cancer treatment, or palliate symptoms. Proper patient selection for endobronchial therapy is crucial. For patients with hemoptysis, the bleeding source must be endobronchial and within the reach of the bronchoscope. Arterial embolization may be considered when the source of bleeding is beyond the reach of the bronchoscope. Obstructive airway lesions should be ablated to regain significant lung function or relieve postobstructive pneumonia. In the absence of postobstructive pneumonia, there will be no benefit from endobronchial therapy if the lung distal to the obstruction is nonfunctional. Patients selected for endobronchial therapies should have respiratory rather than systemic symptoms of widespread malignancy. Argon plasma coagulation is a form of noncontact electrocoagulation [8]. It offers the simplicity and low cost of an electrocoagulator with the noncontact approach of an Nd:YAG laser. Patients with diffuse, concentric malignant infiltration and with significant distortion of anatomic landmarks are best treated with endobronchial brachytherapy [9]. Similarly, obstructions caused by lesions that extrinsically compress the airway are best palliated with endoluminal stents and dilation [10].

Prognostic Grouping of Patients with Lung Metastases

Group	Resectable	Disease-free Interval, mo	Number of Metastases	Median Survival, mo
I	Yes	≥ 36	Single	61
II	Yes	≥ 36	Multiple	34
III	Yes	< 36	Single	34
IV	Yes	< 36	Multiple	24
V	No	—	—	14

Figure 24-10. Prognostic grouping of patients with lung metastases. Three parameters of prognostic significance were included by the International Registry of Lung Metastasis: resectability, disease-free interval (DFI), and number of metastases. DFI and number of metastases were independent risk factors in patients with resectable disease. Patients with germ cell and Wilms' tumors, which have the best prognosis, were not included in these groups. The median survival rate for all others was 33 months, with a 5-year survival of 34% and a 10-year survival of 23%. According to the major tumor types, epithelial tumors (37% survival at 5 years and 21% at 10 years; median 40 months) and sarcomas (31% survival at 5 years and 26% at 10 years; median 29 months) behaved similarly. Melanomas had the worst prognosis (21% survival at 5 years and 14% at 10 years; median 19 months). Other studies have reported 5-year survival for single histologies of 27% to 49% for breast carcinoma, 39% to 53% for colorectal carcinoma, 43% for head and neck malignancies [11], 75.7% for endometrial adenocarcinoma, and 86.5% for choriocarcinoma [12]. (*Adapted from* Pastorino *et al.* [5].)

REFERENCES

1. Hanahan D, Weinberg RA: The hallmarks of cancer. *Cell* 2000, 100:57–70.

2. Burt M: Pulmonary metastases. In *Fishman's Pulmonary Diseases and Disorders,* edn 3. Edited by Fishman AP, Elias JA, Fishman JA, *et al.* New York: McGraw-Hill; 1998:1851–1860.

3. Fraser RS, Muller NL, Colman N, Pare PD: Neoplastic secondary neoplasms. In Fraser and Pare's *Diagnosis of Diseases of the Chest,* edn 4. Edited by Fraser RS, Muller NL, Colman N, Pare PD. Philadelphia: WB Saunders Company; 1999:1381–1417.

4. Robert JH, Vala D, Sayegh Y, Spiliopoulos A: The surgical treatment of lung metastases: an update. *Crit Rev Oncol Hematol* 1998, 28:91–96.

5. Pastorino U, Buyse M, Friedel G, *et al.,* the International Registry of Lung Metastases: Long-term results of lung metastasectomy: prognostic analysis based on 5206 cases. *J Thorac Cardiovasc Surg* 1997, 113:37–49.

6. Pfannschmidt J, Klode J, Muley T, *et al.*: Nodal involvement at the time of pulmonary metastasectomy: experiences in 245 patients. *Ann Thorac Surg* 2006, 81:448–454.

7. Ferson P, Keenan RJ, Luketich JD: The role of video-assisted thoracic surgery in pulmonary metastases. *Chest Surg Clin N Am* 1998, 8:59–76.

8. Morice RC, Ece T, Ece F, Keus F: Endobronchial argon plasma coagulation for treatment of hemoptysis and neoplastic airway obstruction. *Chest* 2001, 119:781–787.

9. Kelly JF, Delclos ME, Morice RC, *et al.*: High-dose-rate endobronchial brachytherapy effectively palliates symptoms due to airway tumors: the 10-year M.D. Anderson Cancer Center experience. *Int J Radiat Oncol Biol Phys* 2000, 48:697–702.

10. Saad CP, Murthy S, Krizmanich G, Mehta A: Self-expandable metallic airway stents and flexible bronchoscopy. *Chest* 2003, 124:1993–1999.

11. Downey RJ: Surgical treatment of pulmonary metastases. *Surg Oncol Clin N Am* 1999, 8:341–354.

12. Anraku M, Yokoi K, Nakagawa K, *et al.*: Pulmonary metastases from uterine malignancies: results of surgical resection in 133 patients. *J Thorac Cardiovasc Surg* 2004, 127:1107–1112.

PLEURAL DISEASE

*Steven A. Sahn,
John T. Huggins,
and Peter Doelken*

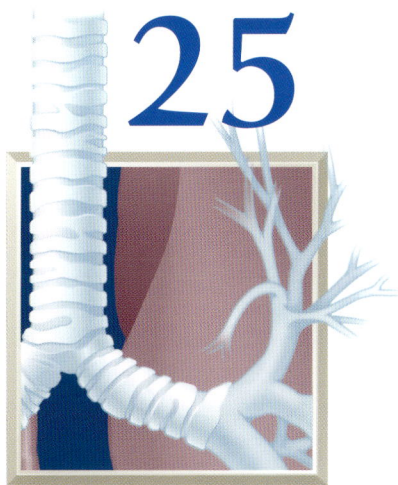
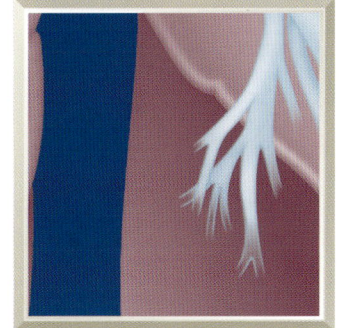

The normal pleural space is approximately 10 to 20 μm wide and is separated by a single-cell lining of mesothelial cells that form the parietal and visceral pleura. Diseases affecting any organ and systemic illnesses may cause pleural effusions, pleural thickening, pneumothorax, and pleural tumors.

Pleural effusion represents an abnormal accumulation of fluid in the pleural space and is the result of dysequilibrium between fluid formation and removal. There are eight plausible mechanisms responsible for pleural effusion development: (1) an increase in microvascular pressure (congestive heart failure), (2) a decrease in perimicrovascular pressure (atelectasis and trapped lung), (3) a decrease in oncotic pressure (nephrotic syndrome), (4) an increase in capillary permeability (parapneumonic effusion), (5) a decrease in lymphatic drainage (malignancy), (6) thoracic duct rupture (chylothorax), (7) trauma (hemothorax), and (8) movement of extravascular fluid to the pleural space (urinothorax and duropleural fistula).

A specific diagnosis can be established definitively by pleural fluid analysis; however, the majority of cases require careful attention to medical history and radiographic findings in conjunction with thoughtful interpretation of pleural fluid characteristics to establish a presumptive diagnosis. The identification of pleural fluid acidosis (pH < 7.30) and low pleural fluid glucose (PF/S < 0.5), pleural fluid eosinophilia (eosinophils/total nucleated cell count > 10%), or pleural fluid lymphocytosis (lymphocytes/total nucleated cell count > 80%) helps narrow the differential diagnosis of the exudative effusion.

Pneumothorax represents extra-alveolar air in the pleural space. The diagnosis of pneumothorax on an upright chest radiograph relies on identification of the 1 mm visceral pleural line; however, in critically ill patients, radiographs are typically imaged in a supine or semi-erect position. Supine, the typical radiographic findings for pneumothorax are not seen, and clinicians must rely on indirect signs to identify patients having pneumothorax. These signs include hyperlucency in anteromedial and subpulmonic recesses, deep sulcus sign, and depression of the hemidiaphragm.

The incidence of spontaneous pneumothorax is increased in all patients who have pre-existing lung disease, in comparison with the general population. The incidence and recurrence rates for pneumothorax are highly variable among pulmonary disorders; lymphangioleiomyomatosis has both the highest incidence and the highest recurrence rate. Smoking is an independent risk factor for the development of spontaneous pneumothorax. The spontaneous development of pneumothorax in a nonsmoking, premenopausal woman has a limited differential that includes thoracic endometriosis, lymphangioleiomyomatosis, and connective tissue disorders such as Marfan and Ehlers-Danlos syndromes.

The most common primary pleural tumor is malignant mesothelioma, which is the signal neoplasm for asbestos exposure. The diagnosis of malignant mesothelioma is based on a spectrum of clinical findings, typical CT findings, and histologic features. Differentiating adenocarcinoma from mesothelioma may be problematic, and an accurate diagnosis depends heavily on immunohistochemical analysis.

Mechanisms of Pleural Fluid Formation in Disease

Mechanism	Clinical Example	Classification
↑ Microvascular pressure	Congestive heart failure	Transudate
↓ Perimicrovascular pressure	Atelectasis	Transudate
↓ Oncotic pressure	Hypoalbuminemia	Transudate
↑ Capillary permeability	Pneumonia	Exudate
↓ Lymphatic drainage	Malignancy	Exudate
Peritoneal–pleural communication	Hypatic hydrothorax	Transudate
Thoracic duct rupture	Chylothorax	Exudate
Iatrogenic	Extravascular central venous catheter migration with saline infusion	Transudate

Figure 25-1. Mechanisms of pleural fluid formation in disease. ↑—increase in; ↓—decrease in. (*Adapted from* Sahn [1].)

Pleural Fluid Analysis

Disease	Diagnostic Pleural Fluid Tests
Empyema	Observation (pus, putrid odor)
Malignancy	Positive cytology
Lupus pleuritis	Presence of lupus erythematosus cells
Tuberculous pleurisy	Positive AFB stain, culture
Esophageal rupture	High amylase (salivary); low PF pH; presence of food particles and squamous epithelial cells
Fungal pleurisy	Positive KOH stain, culture
Chylothorax	Triglycerides (> 110 mg/dL); presence of chylomicrons on lipoprotein electrophoresis
Hemothorax	Hematocrit (PF/blood > 0.5)
Urinothorax	Creatinine (PF/serum > 1.0)
Peritoneal dialysis	Protein (< 1 g/dL) and glucose (300–400 mg/dL)
Rheumatoid pleurisy	Characteristic cytology
Glycinothorax	Glycine in PF (complication of transurethral surgery with glycine bladder infection)

Figure 25-2. Pleural fluid analysis. The figure lists diagnoses that can be established definitely by pleural fluid analysis. AFB—acid-fast bacilli; KOH—potassium hydroxide; PF—pleural fluid. (*Adapted from* Sahn [1].)

Pleural Fluid Lymphocyte-Predominant Exudates (≥ 80%)

Disease	Comments
Tuberculous effusion	Most common cause of lymphocyte-predominant exudates; usually 90%–95% lymphocytes
Chylothorax	2000–20,000 lymphocytes/μL; lymphoma most common cause
Lymphoma	Often 100% of nucleated cells are lymphocytes; diagnostic yield on cytology or pleural biopsy higher with non-Hodgkin's lymphoma
Yellow nail syndrome	A cause of a persistent exudate
Rheumatoid pleurisy	Usually associated with trapped lung (chronic)
Sarcoidosis	Usually > 90% lymphocytes; stage II or III
Acute lung rejection	Pleural fluid may be first manifestation of rejection

Figure 25-3. Pleural fluid lymphocyte-predominant exudates (≥ 80%). (*Adapted from* Sahn [1].)

Pleural Fluid Eosinophilia

Disease	Comments
Pneumothorax	The most common cause
Hemothorax	May take 1–2 wk to develop after blood enters pleural space
Benign asbestosis	25%–30% incidence; up to 50% eosinophils
Pulmonary embolism	Associated with infarction and hemorrhagic effusion
Parasitic disease	Paragonimiasis, hydatid disease, amebiasis, ascariasis
Fungal disease	Histoplasmosis, coccidioiodomycosis
Drug induced	Dantrolene, bromocriptine, nitrofurantoin, valproic acid
Carcinoma	5%–8% with PFE*
Churg-Strauss syndrome	High PF eosinophil counts; associated with blood eosinophilia
Tuberculous pleurisy	Rare
Sarcoid pleurisy	Rare
Lymphoma	Hodgkin's disease (rare)

*PFE/total nucleated PF cells > 10%.

Figure 25-4. Pleural fluid eosinophilia. PF—pleural fluid; PFE—pleural fluid eosinophils. (*Adapted from* Sahn [1].)

Diagnoses Associated with Pleural Fluid Acidosis and Low Glucose Concentration

Diagnosis	Usual pH (Incidence)	Usual Glucose Concentration, mg/dL
CPE, empyema	5.50–7.29 (~100%)	< 40 (may be 0)
Esophageal rupture	5.50–7.00 (~100%)	< 60 (may be 0)
Chronic rheumatoid pleurisy	7.00 (80%)	0–30
Malignancy	6.95–7.29 (suggests chronicity)	30–59
Tuberculous effusion	7.00–7.29 (20%)	30–59
Lupus pleuritis	7.00–7.29 (20%)	30–59

Figure 25-5. Diagnoses associated with pleural fluid acidosis (pH < 7.30) and low glucose concentration (pleural fluid/serum < 0.5). CPE—complicated parapneumonic effusion. (*Adapted from* Sahn [1].)

Causes of Transudative Pleural Effusions

Disease	Comments
Congestive heart failure	Acute diuresis may result in high PF/serum protein ratio
Hepatic hydrothorax	Rare without clinical ascites
Nephrotic syndrome	Small, subpulmonic, and bilateral
Peritoneal dialysis	Large right effusion may develop acutely within 48–72 h of initiating dialysis
Hypoalbuminemia	Anasarca usually present; serum albumin < 1.5 g/dL
Urinothorax	Caused by ipsilateral obstructive uropathy
Atelectasis	Small effusion caused by increased intrapleural negative pressure
Constrictive pericarditis	Bilateral effusions due to pulmonary and systemic venous hypertension
Trapped lung	A result of remote inflammation
Superior vena cava obstruction	May be a result of acute systemic venous hypertension or acute blockage of thoracic lymph flow
Subarachnoid-pleural fistula	Cerebrospinal fluid leaks into pleural space after trauma
EV drainage of CVC	Associated with left-sided catheters; saline infusion

Figure 25-6. Causes of transudative pleural effusions. PF—pleural fluid; EV—extravascular; CVC—central venous catheter. (*Adapted from* Sahn [1].)

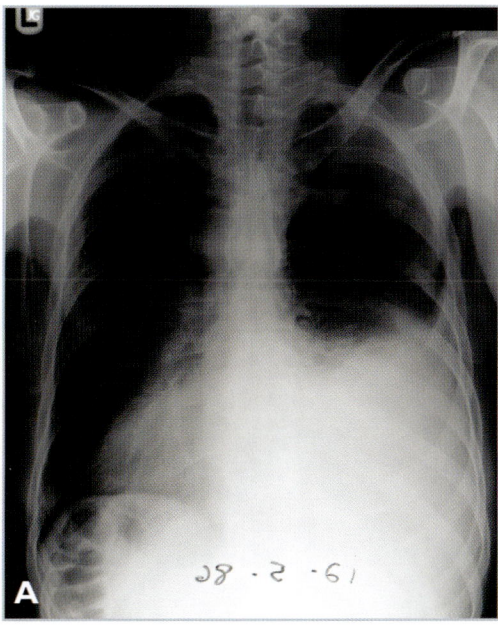
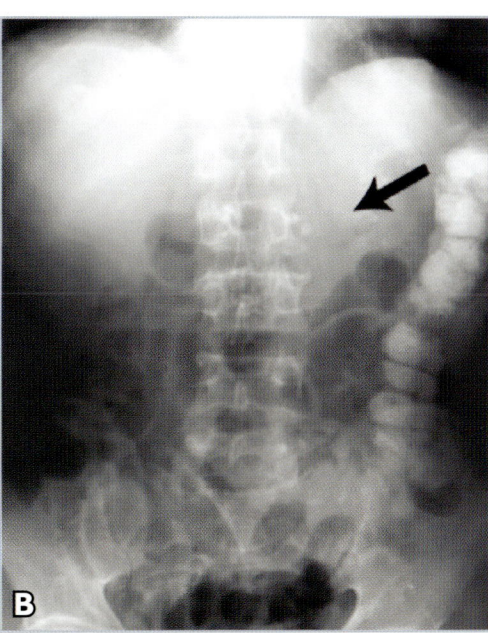

Figure 25-7. Pancreatic pleural fistula. **A,** Posteroanterior chest radiograph showing a large left-sided pleural effusion. **B,** Abdominal radiograph obtained prior to the development of the pleural effusion revealing extensive pancreatic calcification (*arrow*) consistent with the diagnosis of chronic pancreatitis. The pathogenesis of pleural fluid formation in chronic pancreatitis involves pancreatic duct disruption with fistula formation and movement of fluid into the pleural space. Chronic pancreatic effusions are large-to-massive unilateral left-sided effusions that recur rapidly after thoracentesis. The pleural effusion in chronic pancreatitis is typically a serous or hemorrhagic exudate with amylase levels exceeding 100,000 IU/L [2–4].

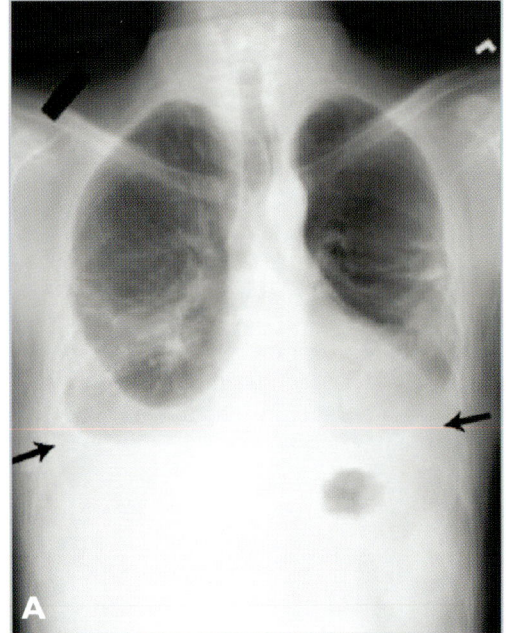
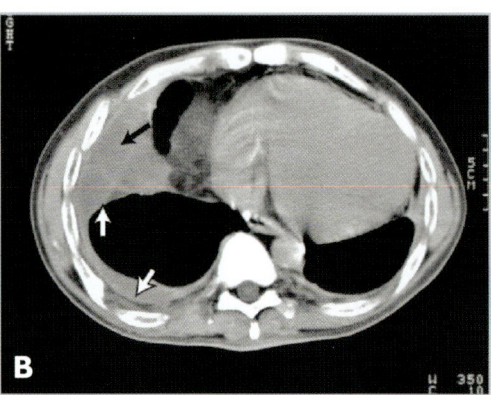

Figure 25-8. Fibrosing uremic pleuritis. **A,** Posteroanterior chest radiograph of a 55-year-old man with end-stage renal disease showing significant pleural disease that could represent pleural thickening or pleural effusions (*arrows*). **B,** CT revealing parietal and visceral pleural thickening (*white arrows*) and a loculated pleural effusion (*black arrow*). Uremic pleural effusions have been reported in 3% to 5% of patients receiving chronic dialysis [5]. In a study of 100 hospitalized patients on long-term hemodialysis with pleural effusions, uremic pleurisy was thought to be the cause in 16% of the cases [6]. Uremic pleurisy typically presents with fever, cough, dyspnea, chest pain, and pleural friction rub. The chest radiograph usually shows a moderate unilateral pleural effusion, although massive and bilateral effusions have been reported [6,7]. The pleural fluid is a serosanguineous or bloody exudate having less than 1500 nucleated cells/μL and a predominance of lymphocytes. Although the pleural fluid creatinine concentration is high, the pleural fluid–serum creatinine ratio is less than unity, compared with a urinothorax, in which the pleural fluid–serum creatinine ratio is greater than 1 and is a transudate. The effusion generally resolves over several weeks with continued dialysis. A late pleural sequela of uremic pleuritis is the development of a trapped lung [8,9].

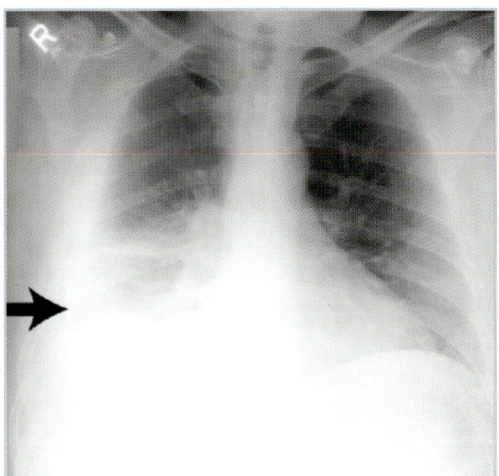
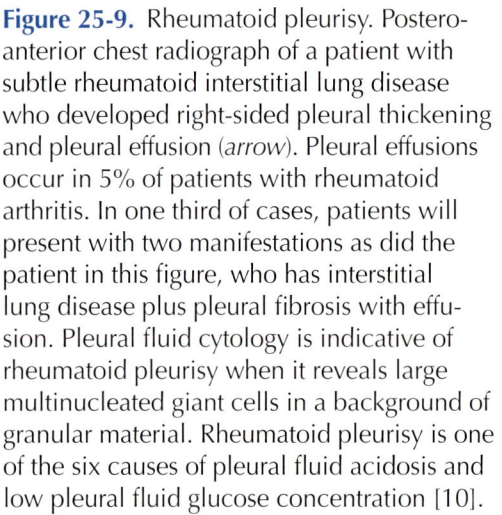

Figure 25-9. Rheumatoid pleurisy. Posteroanterior chest radiograph of a patient with subtle rheumatoid interstitial lung disease who developed right-sided pleural thickening and pleural effusion (*arrow*). Pleural effusions occur in 5% of patients with rheumatoid arthritis. In one third of cases, patients will present with two manifestations as did the patient in this figure, who has interstitial lung disease plus pleural fibrosis with effusion. Pleural fluid cytology is indicative of rheumatoid pleurisy when it reveals large multinucleated giant cells in a background of granular material. Rheumatoid pleurisy is one of the six causes of pleural fluid acidosis and low pleural fluid glucose concentration [10].

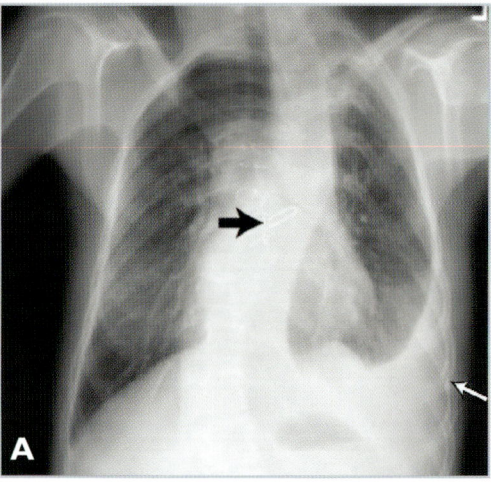
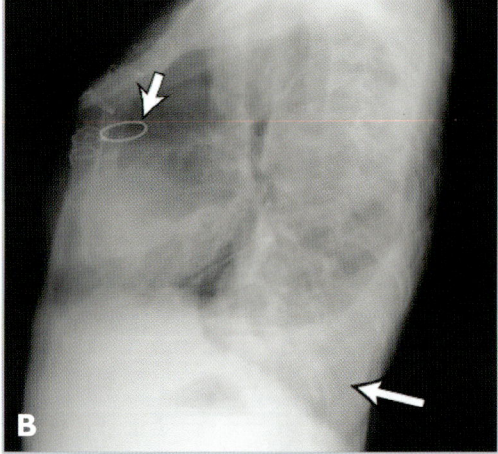

Figure 25-10. Chylothorax associated with Noonan's syndrome. **A,** Posteroanterior chest radiograph of a 30-year-old woman with Noonan's syndrome who developed mild dyspnea on exertion. The chest radiograph shows sternal wires, pulmonic valve replacement (*black arrow*), scoliosis, and a left pleural effusion (*white arrow*). **B,** Lateral chest radiograph confirms that the previous valve replacement was of the pulmonic valve (*top arrow*) and also confirms the presence of the pleural effusion (*bottom arrow*). Diagnostic thoracentesis confirmed the presence of a chylous effusion. Noonan's syndrome is a hereditary syndrome in which affected patients have a phenotype of short stature, webbed neck, and pectus excavatum. Congenital heart defects occur frequently and include pulmonary valve stenosis due to a dysplastic valve, atrial septal defect, and ventricular septal defect [11,12]. The development of chylothorax has been reported in this syndrome and is most likely related to underlying lymphangiectasis [13–15].

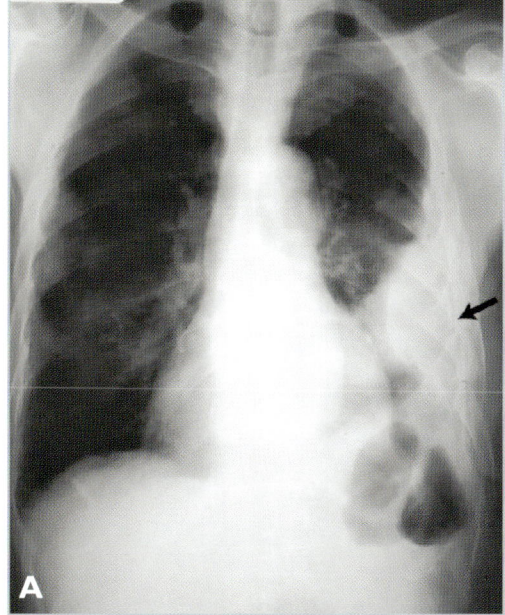
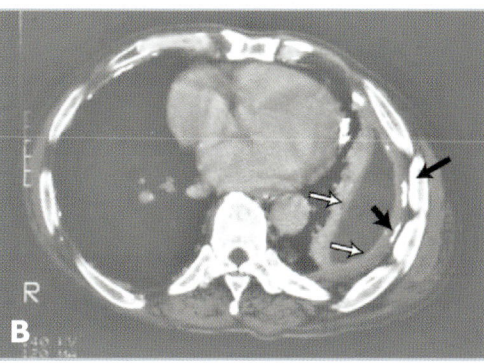

Figure 25-11. Tuberculous empyema. **A,** Posteroanterior chest radiograph of a 68-year-old man who was diagnosed with a tuberculous empyema when he presented with an abnormal chest radiograph. The radiograph shows a left loculated pleural effusion (*arrow*). **B,** CT of a tuberculous empyema shows a thick pleural rind (*white arrows*) and rib thickening (*top black arrow*) that surrounds a loculated pleural effusion. Pericardial and pleural calcification (*bottom black arrow*) can be seen. Much less common than tuberculous pleural effusion, tuberculous empyema represents chronic, active infection of the pleural space, although the patient may be asymptomatic for years [16]. Pleural fluid analysis reveals purulent fluid that is smear-positive for acid-fast bacilli. Chest CTs are virtually diagnostic for tuberculous empyema if a thick, calcific pleural rind and periosteal rib thickening surrounding the loculated pleural fluid are both evident [17]. Problems associated with treatment include both the inability to re-expand the entrapped lung and the inability to achieve therapeutic drug levels in the pleural space [18,19].

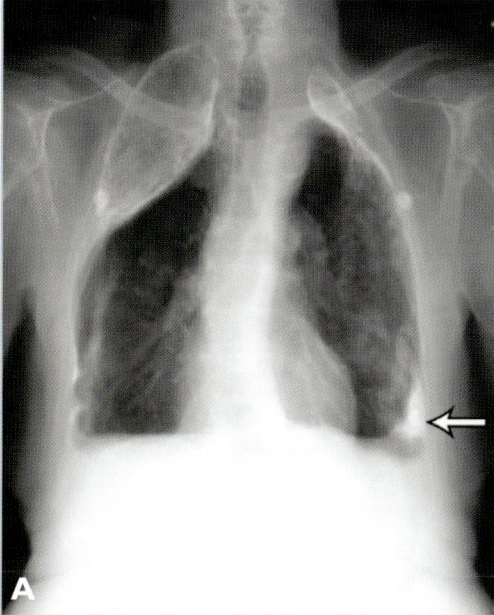
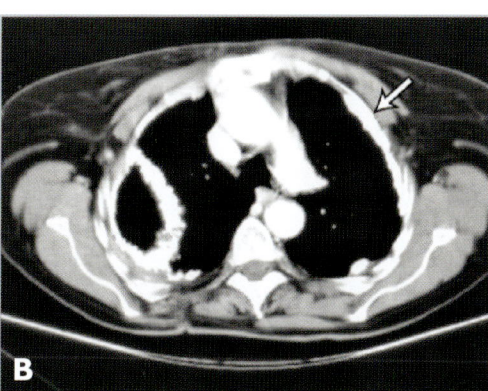

Figure 25-12. Oleothorax. Oleothoraces in a 68-year-old woman who had been treated for tuberculosis at age 20. **A,** A posteroanterior chest radiograph demonstrates bilateral, calcified extrapleural opacities in the apices. The calcification process is the end result of prior oleothoraces. Blunting of both costophrenic angles secondary to pleural thickening is also seen. An area of pleural calcification is noted in the left costophrenic angle (*arrow*). **B,** A chest CT taken at the level of the lung apex shows a heavily calcified lenticular shape of the oleothoraces. Pleural calcification can also be seen on the left (*arrow*). Prior to the introduction of antituberculosis chemotherapy and surgical techniques for lung resection, the mainstay for pulmonary tuberculosis treatment involved the placement of various extrapleural materials to occupy space and maintain lung collapse. Collapsing the lung in the area of active infection was thought to limit the spread of tuberculous infection to an uninvolved lung and to prevent the spread of infection by producing a low-oxygen environment. Successful treatment resulted in fibrosis and encapsulation of the diseased portion of the lung. One of the methods used to achieve and maintain collapse involved extrapleural plombage. Plombage centered around the creation of an extrapleural space by dissecting periosteum and intercostal muscles off the ribs and filling the space with various materials, including vegetable and mineral oil, to produce an oleothorax [20,21].

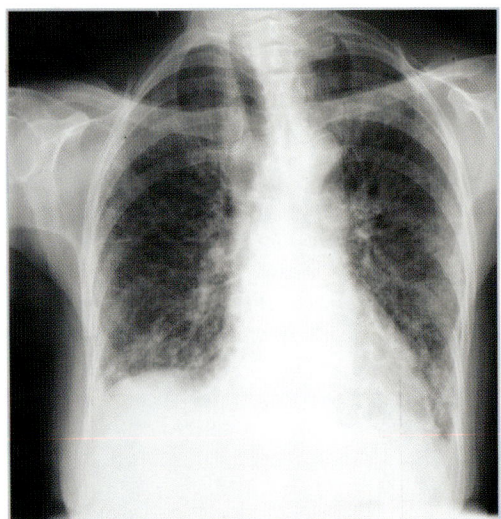

Figure 25-13. Nitrofurantoin pulmonary toxicity. Posteroanterior chest radiograph of an 84-year-old woman who presented with acute dyspnea following treatment for urinary tract infection with nitrofurantoin. The radiograph demonstrates coarse bibasilar reticulonodular infiltrates and small bilateral pleural effusions. After cessation of nitrofurantoin, radiographic abnormalities and symptoms resolved. Nitrofurantoin causes acute pleuropulmonary effects in 5% to 25% of patients. The acute effects may present within hours of starting drug therapy. Patients present with fever, dyspnea, and cough. Radiographic abnormalities include bibasilar alveolar and interstitial infiltrates. Pleural effusions are observed in up to one third of cases and rarely occur in the absence of parenchymal abnormalities (see Fig. 25-3) [22–24]. Holmberg and Boman [23] reported that of 447 patients noted as having pulmonary reactions to nitrofurantoin, 232 (52%) had infiltrates alone, 68 (15%) had infiltrates and effusions, 14 (3%) had only an effusion, and 70 (21%) had normal chest radiographs. Peripheral blood eosinophilia—as high as 83%—is a frequent finding with nitrofurantoin toxicity, and pleural fluid eosinophilia has been described [23]. Nitrofurantoin-induced pleural effusions are typically bilateral. Treatment consists of prompt drug withdrawal. Adjunctive corticosteroids may hasten resolution of symptoms if they are severe at presentation.

The chronic disease, in contrast, presents with insidiously progressive dyspnea, nonproductive cough, interstitial pneumonitis, and fibrosis [22]. Pleural effusions are rarely associated with chronic nitrofurantoin use [23]. Pleural thickening has been described with chronic nitrofurantoin-induced pleuropulmonary disease [22,23]. The severity of the chronic pulmonary reaction with nitrofurantoin appears to be related to both the dosage and the duration of therapy. Unfortunately, when fibrosis develops, pulmonary function is usually permanently impaired and may continue to deteriorate despite discontinuation of the drug [25].

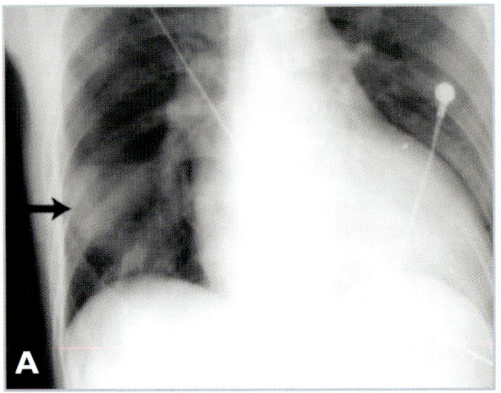 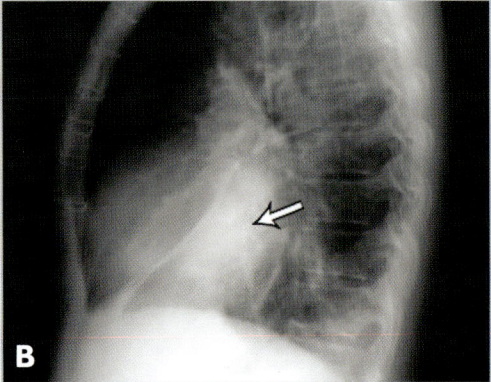 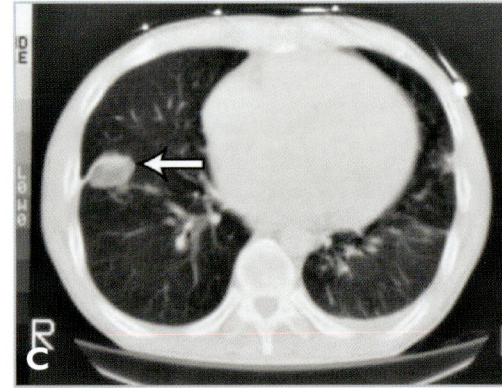

Figure 25-14. Pulmonary pseudotumor. Pulmonary pseudotumor in a 68-year-old man with a history of congestive heart failure. **A,** Posteroanterior chest radiograph showing a prior sternotomy, a large cardiac silhouette, and a well-circumscribed opacity in the right lower lung field (arrow). **B,** Lateral chest radiograph showing fluid in the right major fissure and a large opacity overlying the cardiac silhouette (arrow). **C,** Chest CT showing a lenticular-shaped opacity (arrow) confined to the right major fissure. These findings are highly suggestive of a pulmonary pseudotumor. Chest radiograph 1 week after diuretic therapy showed complete resolution of the "tumor" (not shown).

A loculated interlobar pleural effusion often mimics a pulmonary tumor if viewed in only one projection. A careful roentgenographic evaluation using multiple views makes it possible to distinguish between a primary lung mass and a pseudotumor caused by a loculated interlobar pleural effusion. The radiographic findings, which suggest the presence of a pseudotumor, are of a lenticular configuration and are confined to an interlobar fissure [26].

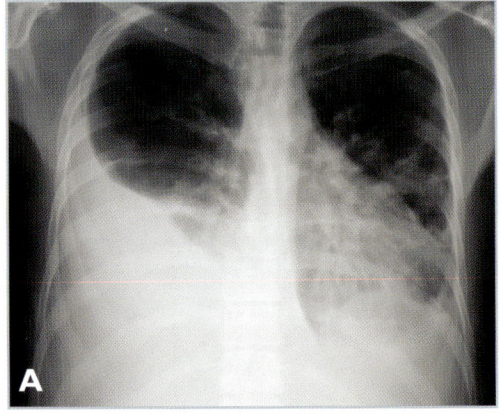 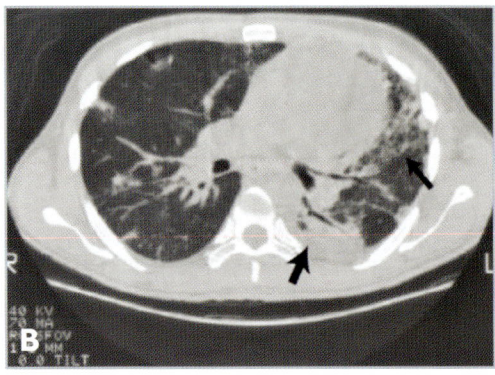

Figure 25-15. Kaposi sarcoma. **A,** Posteroanterior chest radiograph of an AIDS patient with Kaposi sarcoma reveals a large right-sided pleural effusion with contralateral mediastinal shift and patchy, ill-defined nodules in the left mid-lung zone. **B,** A prior CT better defines the nodular infiltrates along the bronchovascular bundle (arrows). Kaposi sarcoma is an AIDS-defining malignancy, closely associated with the presence of human herpesvirus-8 [27–29]. Pleural effusions caused by Kaposi sarcoma are cytologically negative exudates that are serosanguineous or hemorrhagic [27]. The pleural effusions usually occur in the presence of bilateral pulmonary parenchymal infiltrates [28].

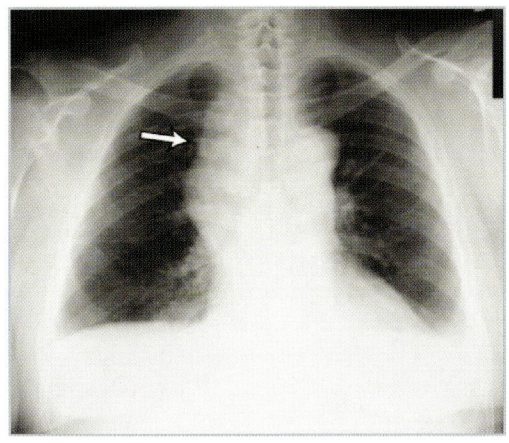

Figure 25-16. Pleural effusions in association with non-Hodgkin's lymphoma. This posteroanterior chest radiograph shows an AIDS patient with bilateral pleural effusion secondary to non-Hodgkin's lymphoma (NHL). The radiograph demonstrates bulky right paratracheal (*arrow*) and hilar lymphadenopathy and blunting of both costophrenic angles. Flow cytometry on the pleural fluid was consistent with B-cell NHL. Intrathoracic involvement with NHL is less common than in Hodgkin's disease [30,31]. In HIV disease, NHL is typically an aggressive B-cell tumor and is frequently associated with pleural effusions. In a review of 38 patients with AIDS and pleuropulmonary manifestations of NHL, pleural effusions were detected in 44% of patients by means of chest radiography and in 68% by means of CT [32]. The pleural fluid is an exudate and may be chylous.

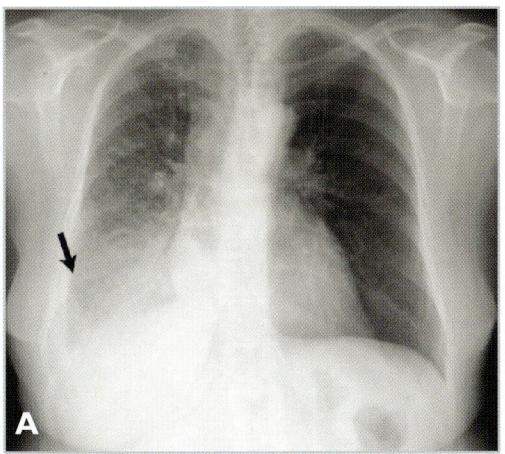 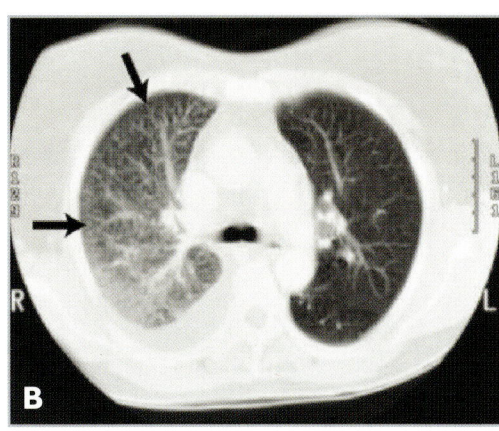

Figure 25-17. Lymphangitic carcinomatosis. Posteroanterior chest radiograph and CT of a 60-year-old man with gastric adenocarcinoma and unilateral lymphangitic carcinomatosis.

A, Posteroanterior chest radiograph revealing a diffuse reticular infiltrate, Kerley's B lines (*arrow*), and a small pleural effusion on the right. **B,** CT showing the peripheral septal lines arranged in a polygonal configuration (*arrows*) associated with small nodules and pleural effusion. The tumors commonly causing lymphangitic carcinomatosis are adenocarcinomas of lung, breast, stomach, pancreas, or prostate origin. Progressive dyspnea is the most common symptom. The presence of mediastinal/hilar lymphadenopathy, unilateral or bilateral pleural effusions, and Kerley's B lines are highly suggestive of this metastatic process.

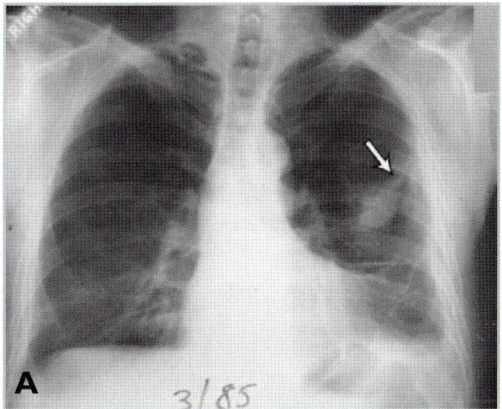 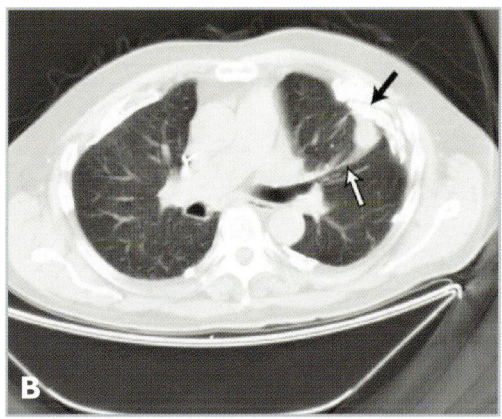

Figure 25-18. Rounded atelectasis. **A,** Posteroanterior chest radiograph showing a peripheral mass in the left upper lung field. There is a curvilinear density (*arrow*) radiating from the mass, with associated pleural thickening. **B,** On conventional CT, a swirling of vessels and bronchi (*white arrow*) from the pleural-based mass ("comet tail" sign) is seen in association with calcified pleural thickening (*black arrow*). These radiographic findings are consistent with the diagnosis of rounded atelectasis of asbestos origin. Rounded atelectasis represents peripheral atelectatic lung induced by a fibrotic process along the pleural surface. The lung is "tacked down" and twisted on itself, pulling blood vessels and bronchi into the atelectatic region, resulting in the appearance of a "comet tail" artifact [33]. Rounded atelectasis usually occurs in the region of greatest pleural fibrosis. When these radiographic features are present, the diagnosis of rounded atelectasis can be made confidently, avoiding the need for transthoracic needle biopsy [34].

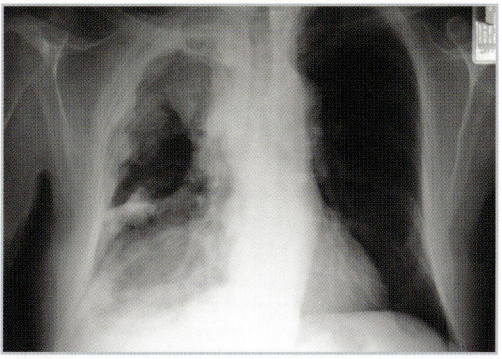

Figure 25-19. Malignant mesothelioma. This posteroanterior chest radiograph is of a former shipyard worker who presented with pleuritic, progressive chest pain. There is pleural thickening with nodular masses on the parietal pleura. Asbestos acts as a carcinogen of mesothelioma, with a latency period of 30 to 45 years [35–37]. Virtually all patients with mesothelioma are symptomatic at presentation, with chest pain and dyspnea being the most common complaints.

Radiographically, mesothelioma most often presents with diffuse, confluent pleural thickening with nodularity along the pleural surface. Between 40% and 95% of patients will have pleural effusions at presentation. Differentiating adenocarcinoma from mesothelioma is technically challenging because no monoclonal antibody specific for mesothelioma has been identified.

Continued on the next page

Figure 25-19. *(Continued)* With an immunohistochemical approach in which four different antibodies, including anticarcinoembryonic antigen (CEA), Leu M1 (CD 15), Ber-EP4, and B72.3, are applied to the tumor, the vast majority of adenocarcinomas will stain to at least one of these markers, whereas mesotheliomas will be nonreactive [38].

Median survival without treatment is 6.8 to 15 months. Surgical procedures (pleurectomy with decortication or extrapleural pneumonectomy) rarely offer a cure. Combination chemotherapy with or without radiation does not appear to have any advantage over single-agent chemotherapy [39–42].

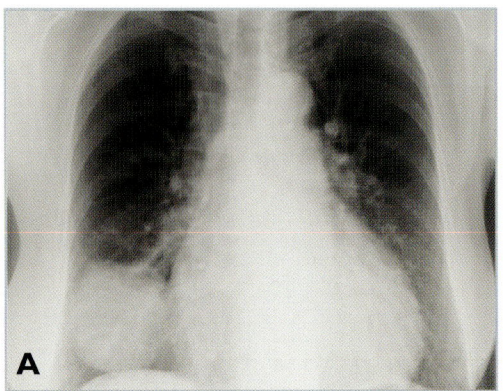 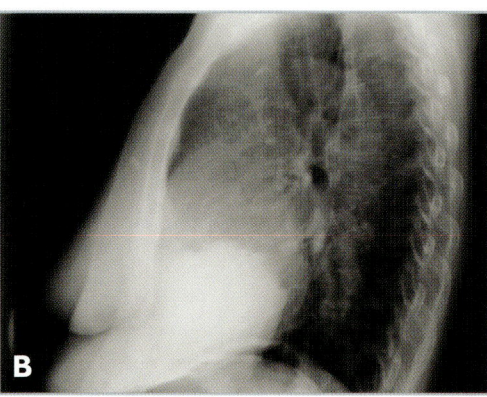

Figure 25-20. Solitary fibrous tumor of the pleura. **A,** Posteroanterior chest radiograph of a 56-year-old nonsmoker with new-onset hypertrophic pulmonary osteoarthropathy, revealing a large homogenous mass in the right lower lung field. **B,** Lateral chest radiograph showing the mass in the right lower lung zone. At surgery, the tumor was confined to the right major fissure. Solitary fibrous tumors of the pleura are neoplasms derived from mesenchymal cells located in the submesothelial lining of the pleura and represent 10% of pleural neoplasms. Unlike malignant mesothelioma, this tumor is unrelated to asbestos exposure. Approximately 50% of patients are asymptomatic at the time of diagnosis. Two paraneoplastic syndromes that occur frequently with solitary fibrous tumor of the pleura are hypertrophic pulmonary osteoarthropathy and hypoglycemia. Symptomatic hypoglycemia is seen in 4% of patients and is secondary to the production of insulin-like growth factor II. Most patients are cured with surgical resection, but the tumor recurs in 10% of cases [43–46].

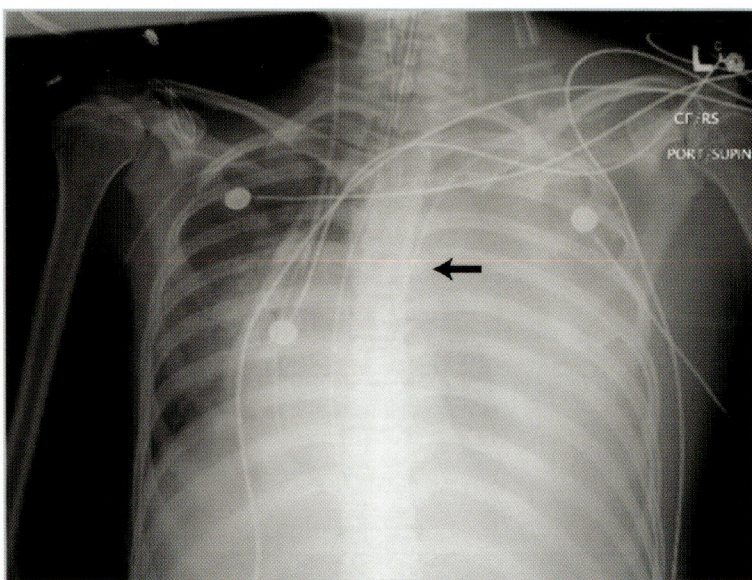

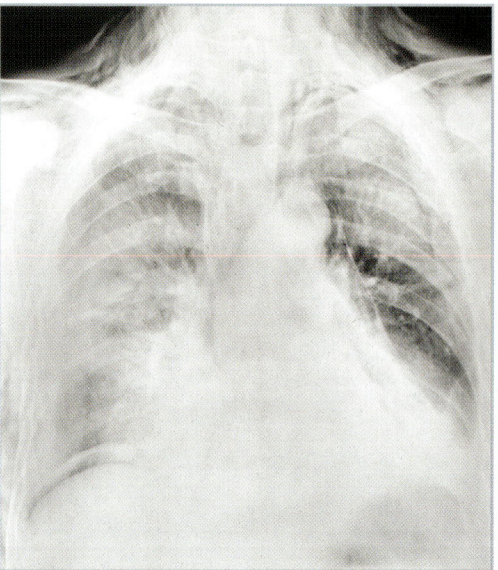

Figure 25-21. A 19-year-old HIV-positive patient developed the acute onset of hypotension and oxygen desaturation after surgery and the placement of a left subclavian catheter. A supine chest radiograph showed a massive tension hydrothorax resulting from extravascular migration of the left subclavian catheter, with infusion of total parenteral nutrition with lipid into the mediastinum and the left pleural space. Note the abnormal position of the left subclavian catheter (*arrow*) and evidence of tension with a marked contralateral mediastinal shift to the right. Thoracentesis revealed a whitish fluid, confirming the diagnosis.

Figure 25-22. Boerhaave's syndrome is caused by rupture of the esophagus—usually from violent retching. As a consequence, air and stomach contents leak into the surrounding tissue and into the left pleural space. This chest radiograph shows a small left pleural effusion and mediastinal and subcutaneous emphysema. Free peritoneal air is evident between the liver and the right hemidiaphragm.

Classification and Causes of Pneumothorax

Classification	Causes	Classification	Causes
Spontaneous		Iatrogenic	Barotrauma
Primary	No clinical lung disease		Mechanical ventilation
Secondary	Clinical presence of lung disease		Procedure-related
	Airway diseases		Central venous catheter placement
	Chronic obstructive pulmonary disease		Thoracentesis
	Status asthmaticus		Endotracheal intubation
	Cystic fibrosis		Tracheostomy
	Interstitial lung diseases		Cardiopulmonary resuscitation
	Lymphangioleiomyomatosis		Bronchoscopy
	Langerhans' cell histiocytosis		Nasogastric tube placement
	Stage IV sarcoidosis	Trauma	Blunt chest trauma
	Pulmonary infections		Penetrating chest trauma
	Pneumocystis carinii		Rib fracture
	Necrotizing pneumonia		Esophageal rupture
	Tuberculosis		Tracheobronchial injury

Figure 25-23. Classification and causes of pneumothorax.

Radiographic Signs of Pleural Effusion and Pneumothorax in the Supine Patient

Diagnosis	Radiographic Signs	Diagnosis	Radiographic Signs
Pleural effusion		Pneumothorax	Hyperlucency in anteromedial and subpulmonic recesses
Small effusion	Veil-like opacity		Deep sulcus sign
Moderate-to-large effusion	Silhouetting of diaphragm		Apical capping
	Evidence of fluid between chest wall and lung		Air interposed between visceral pleura and medistinal structures
Massive effusion	Complete opacification of hemithorax	Tension pneumothorax	Depression of hemidiaphragm
	Contralateral mediastinal shift		Increased volume of hemithorax
			Widening of intercostal spaces
			Contralateral tracheal deviation
			Contralateral mediastinal shift

Figure 25-24. Radiographic signs of pleural effusion and pneumothorax in the supine patient.

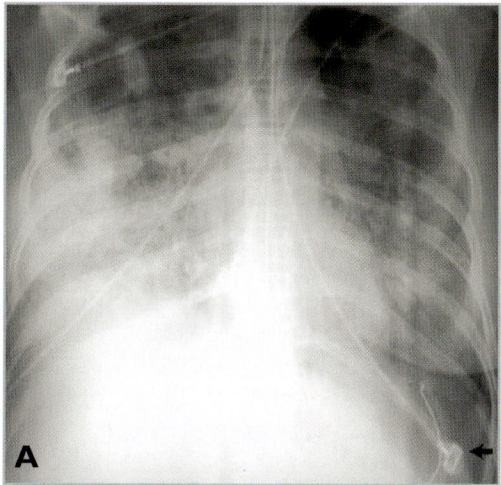 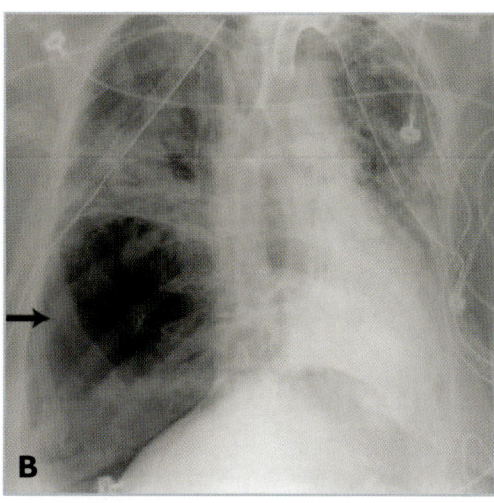

Figure 25-25. A, Chest radiograph of a critically ill patient with a deep sulcus sign on the left (*arrow*), consistent with the diagnosis of a pneumothorax. **B,** Chest radiograph of a critically ill patient on mechanical ventilation with the presence of a right loculated tension pneumothorax (*arrow*). Note the increase in volume of the right hemithorax, the depression of the right hemidiaphragm, and the contralateral mediastinal shift.

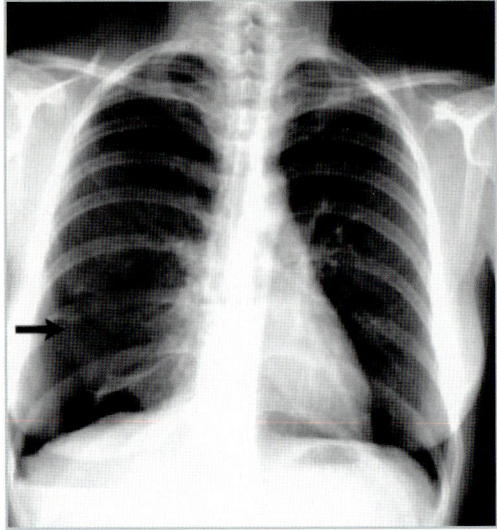

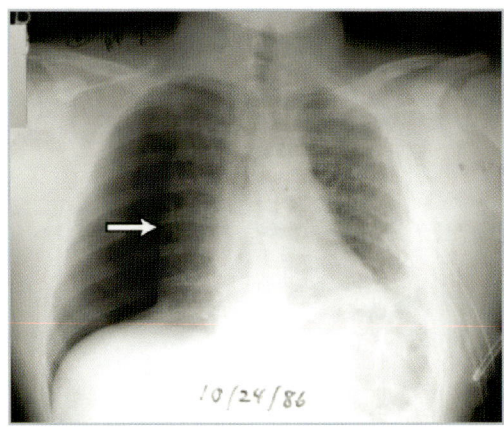

Figure 25-26. Catamenial pneumothorax. Chest radiograph of a 31-year-old nonsmoking woman with multiple spontaneous right-sided pneumothoraces who presented with acute onset of pleuritic chest pain and dyspnea. There is a large right-sided pneumothorax; the arrow signifies the 1 mm visceral pleural line. Excluding smoking, which is a contributor to spontaneous pneumothorax, the development of spontaneous pneumothorax has a limited differential in premenopausal women; this differential includes thoracic endometriosis, lymphangioleiomyomatosis, and Marfan and Ehlers-Danlos syndromes. Catamenial pneumothorax is the most common manifestation of thoracic endometriosis. Other manifestations of thoracic endometriosis include catamenial hemothorax, catamenial hemoptysis, and lung nodules. Patients typically present 24 to 48 hours after the onset of menstruation. Catamenial pneumothorax occurs exclusively on the right. In most patients, pelvic endometriosis has been diagnosed several years earlier. Suppression of ovulation prevents recurrence in less than 50% of patients, and pleurodesis is usually required [47–49].

Figure 25-27. Spontaneous pneumothorax in the setting of pulmonary Langerhans' cell histiocytosis. The posteroanterior chest radiograph demonstrates a large right-sided pneumothorax under tension (arrow) in the setting of fine reticulonodular infiltrates and thin-walled cysts throughout the left lung parenchyma. Two large-bore chest tubes are seen in the left pleural space because of the development of spontaneous pneumothorax. Langerhans' cell histiocytosis is a rare lung disease usually seen in smokers, who may present with pneumothorax [50,51]. Chest radiographs usually demonstrate diffuse reticular, reticulonodular, or cystic lesions with a predilection for the mid- to upper lung fields. The costophrenic angles are usually spared. Both nodular and cystic components are present concomitantly [52]. Spontaneous pneumothorax occurs in 6% to 25% of patients, with a recurrence rate approaching 50%.

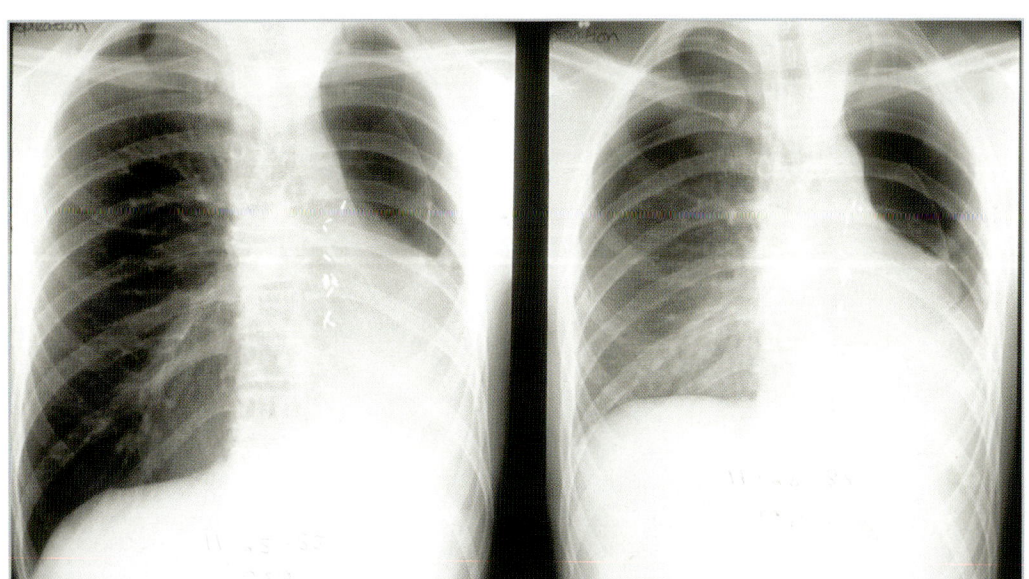

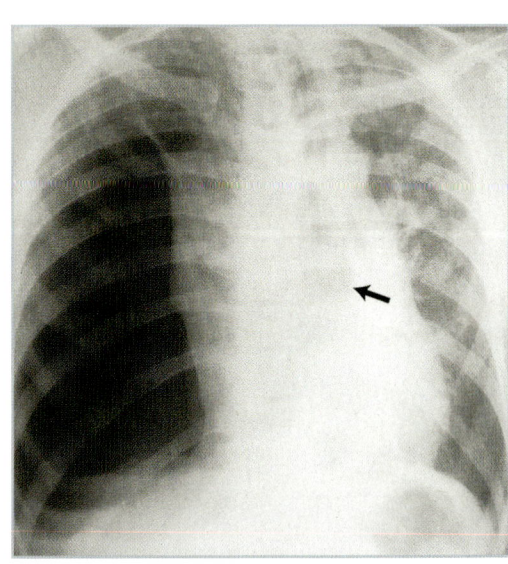

Figure 25-28. This patient developed a right sided pneumothorax and previously has had a left pneumonectomy. The *left* chest radiograph shows a large right pneumothorax with contralateral mediastinal shift and herniation of the right lung into the left pneumonectomy space. The radiograph on the *right* shows partial resolution of the right pneumothorax and decreased contralateral mediastinal shift. Herniation of the right lung into the left pneumonectomy space is still present.

Figure 25-29. Chest radiograph showing a right-sided tension pneumothorax (arrow). The right hemithorax is hyperinflated, and the lung is completely collapsed. Tethering of the right upper lobe to the apical chest wall is visible. The mediastinum is shifted to the left. A tension pneumothorax is an emergency; drainage must be performed immediately.

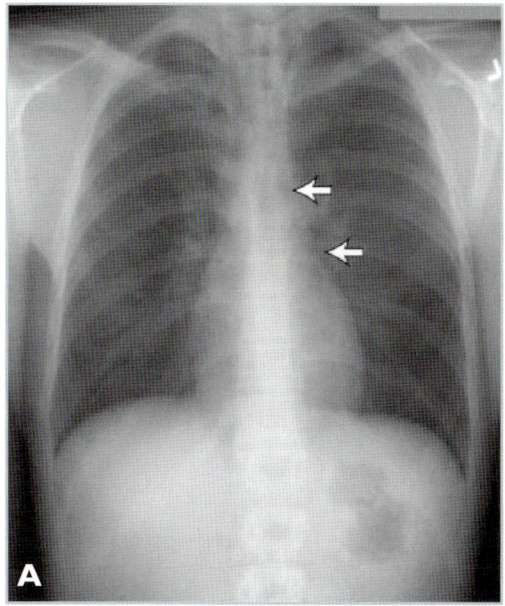 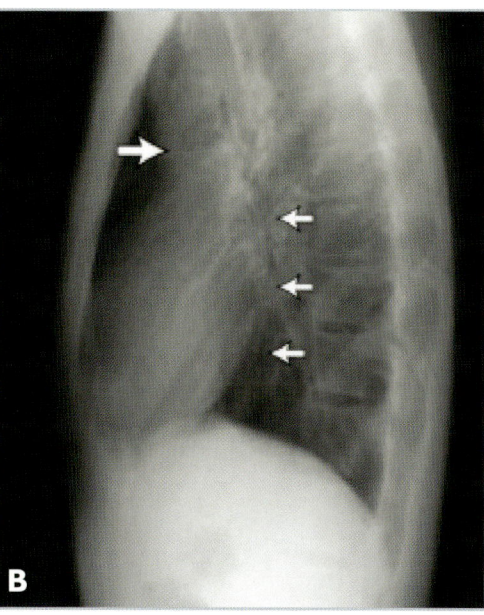

Figure 25-30. Pneumomediastinum. Pneumomediastinum following crack cocaine use in a 35-year-old man. **A,** Posteroanterior chest radiograph showing air along the left heart border, with air tracking up into the upper mediastinum (*arrows*). **B,** The presence of the pneumomediastinum (*arrows*) is also demonstrated on the lateral chest radiograph. Pneumomediastinum is defined as extra-alveolar air confined to the mediastinum without an accompanying infection or inflammatory disorder. The pathophysiology of pneumomediastinum following crack cocaine use involves alveolar wall rupture from an intense Valsalva maneuver. Air then moves proximally along the bronchovascular bundle into the mediastinum.

REFERENCES

1. Sahn A: Pleural diseases. In *American College of Chest Physicians Pulmonary Board Review*. Northbrook, IL: American College of Chest Physicians; 2003:131–152.

2. Rockey DC, Cello JP: Pancreaticopleural fistula: a report of 7 patients and review of the literature. *Medicine* 1990, 69:332–344.

3. Maringhini A, Ciambra M, Patti R, *et al.*: Ascites, pleural, and pericardial effusions in acute pancreatitis: a prospective study of the incidence, natural history, and prognostic role. *Dig Dis Sci* 1996, 41:848–852.

4. Kaye MD: Pleuropulmonary complications of pancreatitis. *Thorax* 1968, 23:297–305.

5. Berger HW, Rammohan G, Neff MS, *et al.*: Uremic pleural effusion: a study in 14 patients on chronic dialysis. *Ann Intern Med* 1975, 82:362–364.

6. Jarratt MJ, Sahn SA: Pleural effusions in hospitalized patients receiving long-term hemodialysis. *Chest* 1995, 108:470–474.

7. Galen MA, Steinberg SM, Lowrie EG, *et al.*: Hemorrhagic pleural effusions in patients undergoing chronic hemodialysis. *Ann Intern Med* 1975, 82:359–361.

8. Rodelas R, Rakowski TA, Argy WP, *et al.*: Fibrosing uremic pleuritis during hemodialysis. *JAMA* 1980, 243:2424–2425.

9. Gilbert L, Ribot S, Frankel H, *et al.*: Fibrinous uremic pleuritis: a surgical entity. *Chest* 1975, 67:53–56.

10. Sahn SA: The pleura: state of the art. *Am Rev Respir Dis* 1988, 138:184–234.

11. Allanson JE, Hall JG, Hughes HE, *et al.*: Noonan syndrome: the changing phenotype. *Am J Med Genet* 1985, 21:507–514.

12. Mendez HMN, Opitz JM: Noonan syndrome: a review. *Am J Med Genet* 1985, 21:493–506.

13. Lanning P, Simila S, Suramo I, *et al.*: Lymphatic abnormalities in Noonan's syndrome. *Pediatr Radiol* 1978, 7:106–109.

14. Prasad R, Singh K, Singh R: Bilateral congenital chylothorax with Noonan syndrome. *Indian Pediatr* 2002, 39:975–976.

15. Goens MB, Campbell D, Wiggins JW: Spontaneous chylothorax in Noonan syndrome. Treatment with prednisone. *Am J Dis Child* 1992, 146:1453–1456.

16. Sahn SA, Iseman MD: Tuberculous empyema. *Semin Respir Infect* 1999, 14:82–87.

17. Hulnick DH, Naidich DP, McCauley DI: Pleural tuberculosis evaluated by computed tomography. *Radiology* 1983, 149:759–765.

18. Tatsumura T, Koyama S, Yamamoto K, *et al.*: A new technique for one-stage eradication of long-standing chronic thoracic empyema. *J Thorac Cardiovasc Surg* 1990, 99:410–415.

19. Yim APC: The role of video-assisted thoracoscopic surgery in the management of pulmonary tuberculosis. *Chest* 1996, 110:829–832.

20. Shepherd MP: Plombage in the 1980s. *Thorax* 1985, 40:328–340.

21. Harrison LH Jr: Current aspects of the surgical management of tuberculosis. *Surg Clin North Am* 1980, 60:883–895.

22. Rosenow EC III, DeRemee RA, Dines DE: Chronic nitrofurantoin pulmonary reactions: report of five cases. *N Engl J Med* 1968, 279:1258–1262.

23. Holmberg L, Boman G: Pulmonary reactions to nitrofurantoin: 447 cases reported to the Swedish adverse drug reaction committee. *Eur J Respir Dis* 1981, 62:180–189.

24. Geller M, Flaherty DK, Dickee HA, *et al.*: Lymphopenia in acute nitrofurantoin pleuropulmonary disease. *J Allergy Clin Immunol* 1977, 49:445–448.

25. Israel HL, Diamond P: Recurrent pulmonary infiltration and pleural effusion due to nitrofurantoin sensitivity. *N Engl J Med* 1962, 266:1024–1026.

26. Haus BM, Stark P, Shofer SC, *et al.*: Massive pulmonary pseudotumor. *Chest* 2003, 124:758–760.

27. O'Brien RF, Cohn DL: Serosanguineous pleural effusions in AIDS-associated Kaposi's sarcoma. *Chest* 1989, 96:460–466.

28. Ognibene FP, Steis RG, Macher AM, *et al.*: Kaposi's sarcoma causing pulmonary infiltrates and respiratory failure in the acquired immunodeficiency syndrome. *Ann Intern Med* 1985, 102:471–475.

29. Knowles DM, Cesarman E: The Kaposi's sarcoma–associated herpesvirus (human herpesvirus-8) in Kaposi's sarcoma, malignant lymphoma, and other diseases. *Ann Oncol* 1997, 8:123–129.

30. Bragg GD, Chor PJ, Murray KA, *et al.*: Lymphoproliferative disorders of the lung: histopathology, clinical manifestations, and imaging features. *Am J Roentgenol* 1994, 163:273–281.

31. Sider L, Weiss AJ, Smith MD, *et al.*: Varied appearance of AIDS-related lymphoma in the chest. *Radiology* 1989, 171:629–632.

32. Eisner MD, Kaplan LD, Herndier B, *et al.*: The pulmonary manifestations of AIDS-related non-Hodgkin's lymphoma. *Chest* 1996, 110:729–736.

33. Hillerdal G: Rounded atelectasis: clinical experience with 74 patients. *Chest* 1989, 95:836–841.

34. Lynch DA, Gamsu G, Ray CS, *et al.*: Asbestos-related focal lung masses: manifestations on conventional and high-resolution CT scans. *Radiology* 1988, 169:603–607.

35. Wagner JC, Sleggs CA, Marchand P: Diffuse pleural mesothelioma and asbestos exposure in northwestern Cape Province. *Br J Ind Med* 1960, 17:260.

36. Pisani RJ, Colby TV, William DE: Malignant mesothelioma of the pleura. *Mayo Clin Proc* 1988, 63:1234–1244.

37. Antman KH: Natural history and epidemiology of malignant mesothelioma. *Chest* 1993, 103:373–376.

38. Sheibani K, Esteban J, Bailey A, *et al.*: Immunopathologic and molecular studies as an aid to the diagnosis of malignant mesothelioma. *Hum Pathol* 1992, 23:107–116.

39. Sugarbaker DJ, Heher EC, Lee TH, *et al.*: Extrapleural pneumonectomy, chemotherapy, and radiotherapy in the treatment of diffuse malignant pleural mesothelioma. *J Thorac Cardiovasc Surg* 1991, 101:10–15.

40. Ball DL, Cruickshank DG: The treatment of malignant mesothelioma of the pleura: review of five-year experience, with special reference to radiotherapy. *Am J Clin Oncol* 1990, 13:4–9.

41. Allen KB, Faber LP, Warren WH: Malignant pleural mesothelioma: extrapleural pneumonectomy and pleurectomy. *Chest Surg Clin North Am* 1994, 4:113–126.

42. Alberts AS, Falkson F, Goedhals L, *et al.*: Malignant pleural mesothelioma: a disease unaffected by current therapeutic maneuvers. *J Clin Oncol* 1988, 6:527–535.

43. Mitchell JD: Solitary fibrous tumor of the pleura. *Semin Thorac Cardiovasc Surg* 2003, 15:305–309.

44. Mezzetti M: Surgical experience of 15 solitary benign fibrous tumor of the pleura. *Crit Rev Oncol Hematol* 2003, 47:29–33.

45. Briselli M, Mack EJ, Dickerson GR: Solitary fibrous tumor of the pleura: eight new cases and review of 360 cases in the literature. *Cancer* 1981, 47:2678–2689.

46. Axelrod L, Ron D: Insulin-like growth factor II and the riddle of tumor-induced hypoglycemia. *N Engl J Med* 1988, 319:1477–1478.

47. Joseph J, Sahn SA: Thoracic endometriosis syndrome: new observations from an analysis of 110 cases. *Am J Med* 1996, 100:164–170.

48. Olive DL, Schwartz IB: Endometriosis. *N Engl J Med* 1993, 328:1759–1769.

49. Hibbard LT, Schumann WR, Goldstein GE: Thoracic endometriosis: a review and report of two cases. *Am J Obstet Gynecol* 1981, 140:227–232.

50. Vassallo R, Ryu JH, Colby TV, *et al.*: Pulmonary Langerhans'-cell histiocytosis. *N Engl J Med* 2000, 342:1969–1978.

51. Tazi A, Soler P, Hance AJ: Adult pulmonary Langerhans' cell histiocytosis. *Thorax* 2000, 55:405–416.

52. Moore AD, Godwin JD, Muller NL, *et al.*: Pulmonary histiocytosis X: comparison of radiographic and CT findings. *Radiology* 1989, 172:249–254.

INDEX

A

Acinetobacter pneumonia, 123
Acquired immunodeficiency syndrome.
　See HIV/AIDS
Acute exacerbations of chronic bronchitis, 99–115
　antibiotics in, 106–112
　bronchodilators in, 115
　causes of, 103–105
　clinical presentation of, 102
　corticosteroids in, 113
　costs of, 108
　disease severity and, 105
　epidemiology of, 99–102
　factors in poor treatment outcomes of, 106
　noninvasive positive pressure ventilation in, 114
　sputum in, 102
　treatment algorithm and strategies for, 112, 115
Adenocarcinoma of the lung, 253
Adenoid cystic carcinoma, 273
Airway clearance therapy, 56
Airways
　anatomy of, 70–71
　in asthma, 3–8, 20–23
　in chronic obstructive pulmonary disease, 31–32
　in cystic fibrosis, 50–51, 53
　in lung cancer, 264
Allergy
　in asthma, 3, 5
American Thoracic Society asthma severity criteria, 15–16
Amyloid
　pleural, 296
Aneurysm
　aortic, 308
Ankylosing spondylitis, 203–204
Antibiotics, 57–59, 106–112
Anticholinergics, 28, 40
Anticoagulation, 228, 231–233, 236
Anti-IgE therapy, 23
Anti-inflammatory agents, 59–60
Antiretroviral agents, 135
Antituberculous agents, 130–132
Aortic abnormalities, 308–309
Apnea
　sleep, 88–92
Aspergillosis, 144–145, 150–151
Asthma, 1–13
　assessment of control in, 10–11
　bronchiolitis in, 74
　chronic obstructive pulmonary disease overlap with, 30
　chronic obstructive pulmonary disease *versus*, 35
　diagnosis of, 6–8
　economic impact of, 3
　epidemiology of, 1–2
　mortality risk factors in, 13
　overview of, 1
　pathophysiology of, 3–6
　severe, 15–24.
　　See also Severe asthma
　severity assessment and classification in, 9, 12–13
　treatment of, 12–13
Asthma Control Test, 11
Atelectasis, 325

B

Bacterial infections
　in acute exacerbations of chronic bronchitis, 103–112
　in cystic fibrosis, 50–52, 58–59
　in HIV/AIDS, 137, 139
Biofilm formation, 119
Blastomycosis, 152–157
Boerhaave's syndrome, 326
Bone marrow transplantation, 75, 79–80
Breast cancer metastases, 314
Breathing
　sleep disordered, 85–97.
　　See also Sleep disordered breathing
Bronchial metastases, 315–315, 317
Bronchioalveolar cell carcinoma, 253
Bronchiolar disorders, 69–82.
　See also specific disorders
　cellular/exudative reaction predominant, 71–72
　clinical syndromes in, 77–82
　history of, 70
　mesenchymal reaction predominant, 73–76
　overview of, 69, 71
Bronchiolitis
　classification and history of, 69–71, 76
　constrictive, 69, 74–75, 78–82
　follicular, 81
　as interstitial lung disease, 183
　mycobacterial, 72
　viral, 71–72
Bronchiolitis obliterans, 69–71, 75, 78–81
Bronchiolitis obliterans organizing pneumonia, 69–71, 73, 76, 78
Bronchitis
　acute exacerbations of chronic, 99–115.
　　See also Acute exacerbations of chronic bronchitis
Bronchoalveolar lavage
　for hypersensitivity pneumonitis, 219
　for solitary pulmonary nodule, 285
　for ventilator-associated pneumonia, 122
Bronchodilators, 28, 40, 115
Bronchogenic cyst, 308
Bronchoscopy, 258, 284, 285
Bronchus sign, 285

C

Calcium channel blockers, 244–245
Cancer
　See also Lung cancer; specific cancer types
　lung, 249–266
　metastatic to lungs, 311–318
　thymic, 305

Candidiasis, 147–149
Carcinoid tumors, 269–272
Cardiac catheterization, 236
Catamenial pneumothorax, 328
Central sleep apnea, 90–91
Chest wall tumors, 292, 294, 296–299.
  See also specific tumors
Children
  asthma exacerbation risk in, 11
  cystic fibrosis in, 45–63
  tuberculosis in, 129
Cholangiocarcinoma, 146
Chondrosarcoma
  chest wall, 295, 297
Choriocarcinoma, 306, 315–316
Chronic bronchitis
  acute exacerbations of, 99–115
Chronic eosinophilic pneumonia, 186–187
Chronic obstructive pulmonary disease, 27–43
  acute exacerbations of, 41–42, 99, 101–115
  asthma overlap with, 30
  asthma versus, 35
  diagnosis of, 36–37
  disorders included in, 27
  epidemiology of, 27–29, 99
  genetics of, 31
  mortality and survival data on, 100–100
  natural history of, 30, 101
  overview of, 27–29, 99
  pathophysiology of, 28, 31–35
  risk factors in, 31
  severity assessment in, 37–38
  smoking and, 28–31, 39, 99
  surgical intervention in, 28, 42
  symptoms and systemic features of, 28, 35, 38
  treatment of, 38–43, 106–115
Churg-Strauss syndrome, 208–209, 212–213
Chylothorax, 322
Coccidioidomycosis, 141
Colorimetric diagnostic tumor sensing, 276
Connective tissue disease, 193–205
  ankylosing spondylitis as, 203–204
  autoantibodies in, 205
  drug toxicity in, 195, 204
  overview of, 193–194
  polymyositis and dermatomyositis as, 201–202
  progressive systemic sclerosis as, 200–201
  pulmonary manifestations of, 195
  rheumatoid arthritis as, 198–199
  systemic lupus erythematosus as, 196–197
Constrictive bronchiolitis, 69, 74–75, 78–82
Corticosteroids
  in acute exacerbations of chronic bronchitis, 113
  in asthma, 12, 23, 38
  in chronic obstructive pulmonary disease, 28, 41
  in cystic fibrosis, 60
  pulmonary effects of, 144
  in sarcoidosis, 162, 175
Cryptococcosis, 157
Cryptogenic organizing pneumonia, 73
Cyclic alternating patterns
  in sleep disordered breathing, 88–97
Cystic fibrosis, 45–64
  adults with, 63–64
  airway clearance therapy in, 56
  clinical manifestations of, 53–54
  diagnosis of, 55
  epidemiology of, 46, 63–64
  gene therapy in, 61
  genetics of, 46–49, 55
  lung transplantation in, 60–61
  overview of, 45
  pathophysiology of, 49–52
  pharmacotherapy in, 57–60
  prognosis in, 63
  surveillance in, 56
  treatment overview of, 62
Cystic fibrosis transmembrane regulator gene, 45–48, 55
Cysts
  mediastinal bronchogenic, 308
Cytokines
  in acute exacerbations of chronic bronchitis, 103
  in asthma, 4, 21
  in chronic obstructive pulmonary disease, 43
Cytomegalovirus pneumonia, 145

D

Deep vein thrombosis, 223.
  See also Venous thromboembolism
Dermatomyositis and polymyositis, 201–202
Desmoid chest wall tumor, 297
Desquamative interstitial pneumonia, 182–183
Diffuse idiopathic neuroendocrine cell hyperplasia, 81
Diffuse panbronchiolitis, 77

E

Economic impact of lung disease, 3, 108
Emphysema
  See Chronic obstructive pulmonary disease
Empyema
  tuberculous, 323
Endocarditis, 119
Endothelin antagonists, 236
Environmental factors
  in asthma, 3, 16
  in hypersensitivity pneumonitis, 185, 215
  in lung cancer, 251
  in toxic fume bronchiolitis obliterans, 78–79
Eosinophilia, 19, 21, 320
Epoprostenol, 236, 244–246
Escherichia coli pneumonia, 144
Ewing's sarcoma
  chest wall, 295
Exercise
  in cystic fibrosis, 56
  in idiopathic pulmonary hypertension, 236

F

Factor Xa inhibitors, 228–229
Fibrosing uremic pleuritis, 322
Follicular bronchiolitis, 81

Fondaparinux, 228–229
Fungal infections, 147–158. *See also* specific disorders
   classification of, 158
   in immunocompromise, 141, 144–145
   overview of, 147

G

Ganglioneuroma
   mediastinal, 309
Gene therapy
   in cystic fibrosis, 61
Genetics
   of chronic obstructive pulmonary disease, 31
   of cystic fibrosis, 46–49, 55
   of idiopathic pulmonary hypertension, 238
   of severe asthma, 16
Genotyping in tuberculosis, 126–127
Germ cell tumors
   mediastinal, 305
Goblet cell hyperplasia, 22
Graft *versus* host disease, 75, 79–80
Granulomas
   in sarcoidosis, 161, 163–164, 166, 169–170, 172

H

Hamartoma, 272, 282
Heparin, 228
Histiocytoma
   malignant fibrous, 296
Histiocytosis
   pulmonary Langerhans' cell, 188–189, 328
Histoplasmosis, 141, 147, 151–152
HIV/AIDS
   chest imaging in, 139–143
   epidemiology of, 138–139
   opportunistic infections in, 137, 139–144, 147, 152
   overview of, 137
   tuberculosis in, 129, 135
Hodgkin's lymphoma, 308
Horner's syndrome, 255
Hospital-acquired pneumonia, 117–124
Human immunodeficiency virus.
 See HIV/AIDS
Hydrothorax, 326
Hypersensitivity pneumonitis, 185–186, 215–221
   causes of, 185, 216–217
   diagnosis of, 217, 220
   features of, 185–186, 215, 218–220
   overview of, 215
   treatment and prognosis of, 221
Hypertension
   idiopathic pulmonary arterial, 235–246
Hypertrophic pulmonary osteoarthropathy, 256
Hypopnea and hypoventilation during sleep, 93, 97

I

Ibuprofen, 59–60
Idiopathic bronchiolitis, 73–74, 82
Idiopathic pulmonary alveolar proteinosis, 187
Idiopathic pulmonary arterial hypertension, 235–246
   classification of, 237
   diagnosis of, 235–236, 240–242
   epidemiology of, 240
   features of, 235, 240, 242
   genetics of, 238
   overview of, 235–237
   pathogenesis of, 239–240
   prognosis of, 237, 244–246
   risk factors in, 238
   treatment of, 236, 243–244
Idiopathic pulmonary fibrosis, 181
Immune reconstitution syndrome, 129, 143
Immunocompromise
   HIV-related, 137–144.
    See also HIV/AIDS
   non-HIV-related, 144–146
Infections.
 See also Lower respiratory tract infections; specific disorders and pathogens
   in cystic fibrosis, 50–52, 58–59
   fungal, 141, 144–145, 147–158
   in immunocompromise, 137, 139–146
   nosocomial, 117–124
   opportunistic, 137, 139–151
   parasitic, 146
   viral, 145
Infective endocarditis, 119
Infertility in cystic fibrosis, 64
Inflammation
   in asthma, 3–5, 19–23
   in bronchiolitis, 71
   in chronic obstructive pulmonary disease, 33–35, 41
   in cystic fibrosis, 49, 51
   in sarcoidosis, 161, 164, 169–170
Inflammatory bowel disease, 82
Interstitial lung disease, 179–190.
 See also Interstitial pneumonia; other disorders
   Bronchiolitis-associated, 183
   diagnosis of, 180
   etiology of, 180
   idiopathic pulmonary alveolar proteinosis as, 187
   idiopathic pulmonary fibrosis as, 181
   Langerhans' cell histiocytosis as, 188–189
   lymphangioleiomyomatosis as, 189–190
   overview of, 179
   pneumonia as, 181–187
Interstitial pneumonia
   chronic eosinophilic, 186–187
   desquamative, 182–183
   hypersensitivity, 185–186
   lymphocytic, 184
   nonspecific, 183–184
   usual, 181–182

J

Juvenile papillomatosis, 274–275

K

Kaposi's sarcoma, 142, 324

L

Langerhans' cell histiocytosis, 188–189, 328
Large cell lung carcinoma, 253
Legionellosis, 144
Leukotriene modifiers, 23
Liposarcoma
   chest wall, 298
Lobectomy, 263
Low molecular weight heparin, 228
Lower respiratory tract infections.
  See also Infections; specific infections
    acute exacerbation of chronic bronchitis as, 99–115
    fungal, 147, 150–154, 157–158
    in HIV/AIDS and immunocompromise, 137–146
    mycobacterial, 125–136
    nosocomial, 117–124
Lung cancer, 249–266
   acquired risk factors for, 251–252
   classification of, 253–254, 256
   clinical features of, 254–256
   diagnosis of, 256–261
   epidemiology of, 249–250
   metastatic, 263
   overview of, 249
   paraneoplastic syndromes in, 255
   pathogenesis of, 252
   prognosis of, 265–266, 281
   screening for, 266
   solitary pulmonary nodule in, 280–281, 283
   staging of, 256, 261–262, 281
   treatment of, 256, 263–264
   tumor markers in, 253
Lung transplantation
   bronchiolitis after, 80
   in cystic fibrosis, 60–61
   cytomegalovirus pneumonia after, 145
   in sarcoidosis, 162
Lupus pernio, 170
Lymph node enlargement
   mediastinal, 307
Lymphangioleiomyomatosis, 189–190
Lymphangitic carcinomatosis, 314, 325
Lymphocytic interstitial pneumonitis, 142–143, 184
Lymphoma, 142, 299, 308, 325

M

Malignant fibrous histiocytoma, 296
Malignant pleural mesothelioma, 291–293, 296–298, 325–326
Matrix metalloproteinase, 20
Mediastinal anatomy, 301–302
Mediastinal masses, 301–309
   anterior, 304–306
   diagnosis of, 302–304
   frequency and distribution of, 304
   middle, 304, 307–309
   overview of, 301
   posterior, 304, 309
Mediastinoscopy, 260, 303
Mesenchymal lung tumors, 275

Mesothelioma
   malignant pleural, 291–293, 296–298, 325–326
Metastatic disease, 311–318
   treatment and prognosis in, 317–318
Microscopic polyangiitis, 208–212
Moxifloxacin, 110
Mucocele, 54
Mucoepidermoid carcinoma, 273–274
Mucolytic therapy, 57
Mucous gland tumors, 273–274
Mucus hypersecretion, 22, 32
Mucus plaques, 50–51
Mycobacterial infections, 125–136
   bronchiolitis in, 72
   in cystic fibrosis, 58
   nontuberculous, 125, 135–136
   overview of, 125
   tuberculous, 125–135.
    See also Tuberculosis

N

Nasal polyps, 54
National Emphysema Treatment trial, 42
Needle aspiration
   for lung cancer, 259–260
   for mediastinal masses, 304
   for solitary pulmonary nodule, 285–286
Neoplasms.
  See also Lung cancer; specific tumors
    malignant pulmonary, 249–266
    mediastinal, 301–309
    pleural and chest wall, 291–299
    pulmonary other than lung cancer, 269–276
Neurogenic mediastinal tumors, 309
Nitrofurantoin toxicity, 324
Nocardiosis, 145
Nodule
   solitary pulmonary, 279–287
Non-Hodgkin's lymphoma, 142, 299, 325
Noninvasive positive pressure ventilation, 114
Noonan's syndrome, 322
Nosocomial infections, 117–124.
  See also specific disorders and pathogens
    classification of, 117
    diagnosis of, 121–122
    histology of, 117, 123–124
    overview of, 117
    pathogenesis of, 118–119
    prevention of, 120
    radiography of, 117, 119
    treatment of, 123–124

O

Obesity in asthma, 6
Obstructive sleep apnea, 89, 91–92
Ofloxacin, 109
Oleothorax, 323
Opportunistic infections, 137, 139–151.
  See also specific pathogens
Osteoarthropathy, 256

Osteosarcoma
    chest wall, 295
Oxygen therapy, 41

P

Panbronchiolitis
    diffuse, 77
Pancreatic pleural fistula, 321
Papilloma, 274–275
Paraganglioma
    mediastinal, 309
Paraneoplastic syndromes in lung cancer, 255
Parasitic infections, 146
Penicillium marneffei, 158
Percutaneous needle aspiration, 259, 285–286
Peribronchiolar metaplasia, 75
Plasmacytoma
    chest wall, 295, 297–298
Pleural disease, 319–329
    Boerhaave's syndrome, 326
    chylothorax as, 322
    effusions as, 321–322, 327
    fluid formation in, 320
    hydrothorax as, 326
    lymphangitic carcinomatosis as, 325
    neoplastic, 291–297, 324–326
    oleothorax as, 323
    overview of, 319
    pleurisy as, 322
    pleuritis as, 322
    pneumomediastinum as, 329
    pneumothorax as, 327–328
    pseudotumor as, 324
Pleural fluid analysis, 320–321
Pneumocystis pneumonia, 137, 140–141, 143
Pneumomediastinum, 329
Pneumonectomy, 263, 293
Pneumonia
    bronchiolitis obliterans organizing, 69–71, 73, 76, 78
    in HIV/AIDS, 137, 139
    interstitial, 181–187
    nosocomial, 117–124
Pneumonitis
    hypersensitivity, 185–186, 215–221
Pneumothorax, 327–328
Polyangiitis
    microscopic, 208–212
Polymyositis and dermatomyositis, 201–202
Positive pressure ventilation, 114
Positron emission tomography, 258, 284, 303
Postural drainage and percussion, 56
Pregnancy
    asthma management in, 13
    in cystic fibrosis, 64
    idiopathic pulmonary hypertension in, 236–237
Progressive systemic sclerosis, 200–201
Pseudomonas infection, 117, 123
Pseudotumor, 324
Pulmonary alveolar proteinosis, 187
Pulmonary arterial hypertension
    idiopathic, 235–246
Pulmonary embolism, 223.
    See also Venous thromboembolism
Pulmonary fibrosis, 181
Pulmonary function testing
    in asthma, 7, 18
    in chronic obstructive pulmonary disease, 30, 36–38, 101
    in cystic fibrosis, 46
    in hypersensitivity pneumonitis, 218
Pulmonary metastases, 311–318
Pulmonary nodules
    metastatic, 312–313
    solitary, 279–287
Pulmonary vasculitis, 207–213

R

Radon
    in lung cancer, 251
Respiratory syncytial virus infection, 71–72
Respiratory tract infections
    lower.
        See Lower respiratory tract infections; specific disorders
Rheumatoid arthritis, 81, 198–199, 322
Rivaroxaban, 229
Rounded atelectasis, 325

S

Sarcoidosis, 161–176
    ACCESS criteria for organ involvement in, 173
    cardiac, 171
    central nervous system, 172
    clinical features of, 169–173
    cutaneous, 170
    diagnosis of, 162, 165–169
    epidemiology of, 163
    immunopathogenesis of, 161, 163–164
    overview of, 161–162
    pulmonary, 161–162, 164–169, 173–175
    treatment of, 162, 174–176
Seminoma
    mediastinal, 306
Severe asthma, 15–24
  See also Asthma
    defined, 15
    different phenotype in, 20
    differential diagnosis of, 17
    epidemiology of, 16
    overview of, 15
    pathology of, 18–23
    physiology of, 17–18
    risk of life-threatening, 17
    treatment of, 23–24
Sleep apnea, 88–92
Sleep disordered breathing, 85–97
    central apnea as, 90
    flow limitation as, 94–95
    hypopnea as, 93, 97
    hypoventilation as, 94
    mixed obstructive and central apnea as, 91
    nomenclature of, 87

obstructive sleep apnea as, 89, 92
overview of, 85
pattern definition and scoring in, 88, 97
persistent respiratory effort as, 96
predisposing factors in, 86
signs and symptoms of, 86
Small cell lung carcinoma, 253, 262–263, 266
Smoking
chronic obstructive pulmonary disease and, 28–31, 39
in lung cancer, 251–252
Soft tissue sarcoma
chest wall, 295, 298
Solitary fibrous tumor of the pleura, 292, 296, 298, 326
Solitary pulmonary nodule, 279–287
diagnosis of, 280–286
management of, 286–287
overview of, 279
patterns of, 282–283, 285
prevalence of malignancy in, 280–281, 283
radiographic definition of, 279
Spirometry in asthma, 7, 11
Sporotrichosis, 157
Sputum cytology, 102, 258
Squamous cell lung cancer, 253
Stains
in tuberculosis, 127
Staphylococcal nosocomial infection, 120, 123–124
Streptococcal pneumonia, 139
Streptococcus pneumoniae
penicillin-resistant, 103
Superior vena cava syndrome, 255
Surgery
for chronic obstructive pulmonary disease, 28, 42
for lung cancer, 261, 263
for malignant mesothelioma, 293–294
for pulmonary metastases, 317
for venous thromboembolism, 232–233
Sweat testing in cystic fibrosis, 45, 55
Systemic lupus erythematosus, 196–197

T

Tension pneumothorax, 328
Teratoma
mediastinal, 306
Thoracentesis, 260
Thoracoscopy, 259, 286
Thoracotomy, 261, 285–286
Thromboembolism
venous, 223–233.
See also Venous thromboembolism
Thrombolysis, 230
Thrombus
autopsy specimen of, 227–228
Thymic tumors, 305
Thyroid cancer metastasis, 313
Toxic fume bronchiolitis obliterans, 78–79
Tracheobronchial metastases, 315–317

Transbronchial needle aspiration, 259–260
Tuberculin skin test, 128
Tuberculosis
clinical presentation of, 129–130
conditions associated with, 128
diagnosis of, 127–128
empyema in, 323
epidemiology of, 126
genotyping of, 126–127
in HIV/AIDS, 134–135, 140
latent, 133
multidrug-resistant, 134
overview of, 125
transmission prevention of, 135
treatment of, 130–135
Tumor emboli, 316
Tumors
See also Lung cancer; specific tumors
malignant pulmonary, 249–266
mediastinal, 301–309
pleural and chest wall, 291–299, 325
pulmonary other than lung cancer, 269–276
solitary pulmonary nodule as, 279–287

U

Ultrasound-guided transbronchial needle aspiration, 260
Usual interstitial pneumonia, 1810182

V

Vasculitis, 207–213
Churg-Strauss syndrome as, 208–209, 212–213
features of, 209–210
management of, 208, 213
microscopic polyangiitis as, 208–212
overview of, 207
Wegener's granulomatosis as, 207, 209–211
Vasodilators, 244
Venous thromboembolism, 223–233
diagnosis of, 225–228
epidemiology of, 224
overview of, 223
prevention of, 233
treatment of, 228–233
Ventilator-associated pneumonia
diagnosis of, 121–122
pathogenesis of, 118–119
prevention of, 120
treatment of, 123–124
Video-assisted thoracoscopy, 286
Viral infections
in acute exacerbations of chronic bronchitis, 104
post-transplant, 145
respiratory syncytial, 71–72

W

Wegener's granulomatosis, 207, 209–211, 307